Hematopoietic Stem Cell Transplantation

Guest Editors

MAX J. COPPES, MD, PhD, MBA,
TERRY J. FRY, MD, AND
CRYSTAL L. MACKALL, MD

PEDIATRIC CLINICS
OF NORTH AMERICA

www.pediatric.theclinics.com

February 2010 • Volume 57 • Number 1

SAUNDERS an imprint of ELSEVIER, Inc.

W.B. SAUNDERS COMPANY
A Division of Elsevier Inc.

1600 John F. Kennedy Boulevard • Suite 1800 • Philadelphia, Pennsylvania 19103-2899

http://www.theclinics.com

THE PEDIATRIC CLINICS OF NORTH AMERICA Volume 57, Number 1
February 2010 ISSN 0031-3955, ISBN-13: 978-1-4377-1852-2

Editor: Carla Holloway
Developmental Editor: Theresa Collier

Photocopying
Single photocopies of single articles may be made for personal use as allowed by national copyright laws. Permission of the Publisher and payment of a fee is required for all other photocopying, including multiple or systematic copying, copying for advertising or promotional purposes, resale, and all forms of document delivery. Special rates are available for educational institutions that wish to make photocopies for non-profit educational classroom use. For information on how to seek permission visit www.elsevier.com/permissions or call: (+44) 1865 843830 (UK)/(+1) 215 239 3804 (USA).

Derivative Works
Subscribers may reproduce tables of contents or prepare lists of articles including abstracts for internal circulation within their institutions. Permission of the Publisher is required for resale or distribution outside the institution. Permission of the Publisher is required for all other derivative works, including compilations and translations (please consult www.elsevier.com/permissions).

Electronic Storage or Usage
Permission of the Publisher is required to store or use electronically any material contained in this journal, including any article or part of an article (please consult www.elsevier.com/permissions). Except as outlined above, no part of this publication may be reproduced, stored in a retrieval system or transmitted in any form or by any means, electronic, mechanical, photocopying, recording or otherwise, without prior written permission of the Publisher.

Notice
No responsibility is assumed by the Publisher for any injury and/or damage to persons or property as a matter of products liability, negligence or otherwise, or from any use or operation of any methods, products, instructions or ideas contained in the material herein. Because of rapid advances in the medical sciences, in particular, independent verification of diagnoses and drug dosages should be made.

Although all advertising material is expected to conform to ethical (medical) standards, inclusion in this publication does not constitute a guarantee or endorsement of the quality or value of such product or of the claims made of it by its manufacturer.

The Pediatric Clinics of North America (ISSN 0031-3955) is published bimonthly by Elsevier Inc., 360 Park Avenue South, New York, NY 10010-1710. Months of issue are February, April, June, August, October, and December. Periodicals postage paid at New York, NY and additional mailing offices. Subscription prices are $167.00 per year (US individuals), $378.00 per year (US institutions), $227.00 per year (Canadian individuals), $503.00 per year (Canadian institutions), $270.00 per year (international individuals), $503.00 per year (international institutions), $83.00 per year (US students and residents), and $142.00 per year (international and Canadian residents and students). To receive students/resident rare, orders must be accompanied by name of affiliated institution, date of term, and the signature of program/residency coordinator on institution letterhead. Orders will be billed at individual rate until proof of status is received. Foreign air speed delivery is included in all *Clinics* subscription prices. All prices are subject to change without notice. **POSTMASTER:** Send address changes to *The Pediatric Clinics of North America*, Elsevier Health Sciences Division, Subscription Customer Service, 3251 Riverport Lane, Maryland Heights, MO 63043. **Customer Service: 1-800-654-2452 (US and Canada). From outside of the US and Canada: 1-314-447-8871. Fax: 1-314-447-8029. For print support, E-mail: JournalsCustomerService-usa@elsevier.com. For online support, E-mail: JournalsOnlineSupport-usa@elsevier.com.**

Reprints. For copies of 100 or more, of articles in this publication, please contact the Commercial Reprints Department, Elsevier Inc., 360 Park Avenue South, New York, NY 10010-1710. Tel.: 212-633-3812; Fax: 212-462-1935; E-mail: reprints@elsevier.com.

The Pediatric Clinics of North America is also published in Spanish by McGraw-Hill Inter-americana Editores S.A., Mexico City, Mexico; in Portuguese by Riechmann and Affonso Editores, Rua Comandante Coelho 1085, CEP 21250, Rio de Janeiro, Brazil; and in Greek by Althayia SA, Athens, Greece.

The Pediatric Clinics of North America is covered in *MEDLINE/PubMed (Index Medicus), Excerpta Medica, Current Contents, Current Contents/Clinical Medicine, Science Citation Index, ASCA, ISI/BIOMED,* and *BIOSIS*.

Printed in the United States of America.

GOAL STATEMENT

The goal of the *Pediatric Clinics of North America* is to keep practicing physicians and residents up to date with current clinical practice in pediatrics by providing timely articles reviewing the state-of-the-art in patient care.

ACCREDITATION

The *Pediatric Clinics of North America* is planned and implemented in accordance with the Essential Areas and Policies of the Accreditation Council for Continuing Medical Education (ACCME) through the joint sponsorship of the University Of Virginia School Of Medicine and Elsevier. The University Of Virginia School of Medicine is accredited by the ACCME to provide continuing medical education for physicians.

The University of Virginia School of Medicine designates this educational activity for a maximum of 15 *AMA PRA Category 1 Credits*™ for each issue, 90 credits per year. Physicians should only claim credit commensurate with the extent of their participation in the activity.

The American Medical Association has determined that physicians not licensed in the US who participate in this CME activity are eligible for a maximum of 15 *AMA PRA Category 1 Credits*™ for each issue, 90 credits per year.

Credit can be earned by reading the text material, taking the CME examination online at http://www.theclinics.com/home/cme, and completing the evaluation. After taking the test, you will be required to review any and all incorrect answers. Following completion of the test and evaluation, your credit will be awarded and you may print your certificate.

FACULTY DISCLOSURE/CONFLICT OF INTEREST

The University of Virginia School of Medicine, as an ACCME accredited provider, endorses and strives to comply with the Accreditation Council for Continuing Medical Education (ACCME) Standards of Commercial Support, Commonwealth of Virginia statutes, University of Virginia policies and procedures, and associated federal and private regulations and guidelines on the need for disclosure and monitoring of proprietary and financial interests that may affect the scientific integrity and balance of content delivered in continuing medical education activities under our auspices.

The University of Virginia School of Medicine requires that all CME activities accredited through this institution be developed independently and be scientifically rigorous, balanced and objective in the presentation/discussion of its content, theories and practices.

All authors/editors participating in an accredited CME activity are expected to disclose to the readers relevant financial relationships with commercial entities occurring within the past 12 months (such as grants or research support, employee, consultant, stock holder, member of speakers bureau, etc.). The University of Virginia School of Medicine will employ appropriate mechanisms to resolve potential conflicts of interest to maintain the standards of fair and balanced education to the reader. Questions about specific strategies can be directed to the Office of Continuing Medical Education, University of Virginia School of Medicine, Charlottesville, Virginia.

The faculty and staff of the University of Virginia Office of Continuing Medical Education have no financial affiliations to disclose.

The authors/editors listed below have identified no financial or professional relationships for themselves or their spouse/partner:
Mario Abinun, MD, PhD, FRCPCH, FRCP; Nabil M. Ahmed, MD, MPH; Peter Bader, MD; Kristin Baird, MD; K. Scott Baker, MD, MS; Lynne M. Ball, MD, PhD; David Barrett, MD, PhD; Jaap J. Boelens, MD, PhD; Dorine Bresters, MD, PhD; Richard K. Burt, MD; Marina Cavazzana-Calvo, MD, PhD; Jacqueline M. Cornish, MD; Alain Fischer, MD, PhD; Jonathan D. Fish, MD; Terry J. Fry, MD (Guest Editor); Stephan A. Grupp, MD, PhD; Rupert Handgretinger, MD, PhD; Helen E. Heslop, MD; Carla Holloway (Acquisitions Editor); Lakshmanan Krishnamurti, MD; Joanne Kurtzberg, MD; Peter Lang, MD, PhD; Arjan C. Lankester, PhD; Franco Locatelli, MD; Guido Lucarelli, MD; Crystal L. Mackall, MD (Guest Editor); Margaret L. MacMillan, MD; Parinda Metha, MD; Francesca Milanetti, MD; Suhag H Parikh, MD; Charles Peters, MD; Christina Peters, MD; Vinod K. Prasad, MD, MRCP; Karen Rheuban, MD (Test Author); Jane E. Sande, MD; Kirk R. Schultz, MD; Frans J. Smiers, MD, PhD; Franklin O. Smith, MD; Jan Stary, MD; Colin G. Steward, MD, PhD; Paul Szabolcs, MD; Paul Veys, MBBS, FRCP, FRCPath, FRCPCH; Júlio C. Voltarelli, MD, PhD; Alan S. Wayne, MD; Andre Willasch, MD; and Robert F. Wynn, MD, MRCP, FRCPath.

The authors/editors listed below identified the following professional or financial affiliations for themselves or their spouse/partner:
Paul A. Carpenter, MBBS is an industry funded research/investigator for Quintiles, Inc. and Novartis Pharmaceutical Corporation.
Kenneth Cooke, MD is on the Speakers Bureau for Enzon Pharmaceuticals, and is an industry funded research/investigator for Amgen Inc.
Max J Coppes, MD, PhD, MBA (Guest Editor) is on the Advisory Committee/Board of Astellas Pharma and Kiadis.
R. Maarten Egeler, MD, PhD has CMO 20% employment with Kiadis Pharma.
Jakub Tolar, MD, PhD is on the Speakers' Bureau for Genzyme.

Disclosure of Discussion of Non-FDA Approved Uses for Pharmaceutical Products and/or Medical Devices
The University of Virginia School of Medicine, as an ACCME provider, requires that all faculty presenters identify and disclose any off-label uses for pharmaceutical and medical device products. The University of Virginia School of Medicine recommends that each physician fully review all the available data on new products or procedures prior to clinical use.

TO ENROLL

To enroll in the Pediatric Clinics of North America Continuing Medical Education program, call customer service at 1-800-654-2452 or visit us online at www.theclinics.com/home/cme. The CME program is available to subscribers for an additional fee of $195.00

Contributors

GUEST EDITORS

MAX J. COPPES, MD, PhD, MBA
Senior Vice President, Center for Cancer and Blood Disorders, Children's National Medical Center; Professor of Medicine, Pediatrics, and Oncology, Georgetown University, Washington, DC

TERRY J. FRY, MD
Chief, Division of Blood and Marrow Transplantation/Immunology, Center for Cancer and Blood Disorders, Children's National Medical Center, Washington, DC

CRYSTAL L. MACKALL, MD
Chief, Pediatric Oncology Branch, Center for Cancer Research, National Cancer Institute, National Institutes of Health, Bethesda, Maryland

AUTHORS

MARIO ABINUN, MD, PhD, FRCPCH, FRCP
Consultant in Paediatric Immunology, Children's BMT Unit, Department of Paediatrics, Newcastle upon Tyne Hospitals NHS Foundation Trust; Honorary Clinical Senior Lecturer, Institute for Cellular Medicine, Newcastle University, Newcastle General Hospital, Newcastle upon Tyne, United Kingdom

NABIL AHMED, MD, MPH
Assistant Professor, Department of Pediatrics, Center for Cell and Gene Therapy, Baylor College of Medicine, Houston, Texas

PETER BADER, MD, PhD
Division for Stem Cell Transplantation, Hospital for Children and Adolescents III, Goethe University, Frankfurt am Main, Germany

KRISTIN BAIRD, MD
Staff Clinician, Pediatric Oncology Branch, Center for Cancer Research, National Cancer Institute, National Institutes of Health, Bethesda, Maryland

K. SCOTT BAKER, MD, MS
Professor of Pediatrics, Director, Survivorship Program, Member, Fred Hutchinson Cancer Research Center, University of Washington, Seattle, Washington

LYNNE M. BALL, MD, PhD
Leiden University Medical Centre, Department of Pediatrics, Leiden, The Netherlands

DAVID BARRETT, MD, PhD
Instructor in Pediatrics, Division of Oncology, Children's Hospital of Philadelphia, Philadelphia, Pennsylvania

JAAP J. BOELENS, MD, PhD
Department of Pediatrics, Blood and Marrow Transplantation Program, UMC Utrecht, Wilhelmina Children's Hospital, Utrecht, The Netherlands

DORINE BRESTERS, MD, PhD
Department of Pediatric Immunology, Hemato-Oncology, and Bone Marrow Transplantation, Leiden University Medical Center, Leiden, The Netherlands

RICHARD K. BURT, MD
Director, Division of Immunotherapy, Department of Medicine, Northwestern University Feinberg School of Medicine, Chicago, Illinois

PAUL A. CARPENTER, MBBS
Associate Member, Clinical Research Division, Fred Hutchinson Cancer Research Center; Associate Professor of Pediatrics, Department of Pediatrics, University of Washington, Seattle, Washington

MARINA CAVAZZANA-CALVO, MD, PhD
Department of Biotherapy, Hôpital Necker Enfants-Malades, Assistance Publique – Hôpitaux de Paris, Université Paris Descartes; Clinical Investigation Center in Biotherapy, Groupe Hospitalier Ouest, Assistance Publique – Hôpitaux de Paris and INSERM, Paris, France

KENNETH COOKE, MD
Ohio Eminent Scholar and Leonard C Hanna Professor in Stem Cell and Regenerative Medicine; Director, Pediatric Blood and Marrow Transplantation Program; Director, Multidisciplinary Initiative in Graft-vs-Host Disease, Case Western Reserve University School of Medicine; Rainbow Babies and Children's Hospital, Cleveland, Ohio

JACQUELINE M. CORNISH, MD
Director, Paediatric Stem Cell Transplantation, Head of Division, Women's and Children's Services, Bristol Royal Hospital for Children, Bristol, United Kingdom

R. MAARTEN EGELER, MD, PhD
Professor, Department of Pediatric Immunology, Hematology, and Oncology, Bone Marrow Transplantation and Auto-immune Diseases, Leiden University Medical Center, Leiden, The Netherlands

ALAIN FISCHER, MD, PhD
Department of Pediatrics, Immunology & Hematology Unit, Hôpital Necker Enfants-Malades, Assistance Publique – Hôpitaux de Paris, Université Paris Descartes, Paris, France

JONATHAN D. FISH, MD
Assistant Professor of Pediatrics, Division of Pediatric Hematology/Oncology and Stem Cell Transplantation, Schneider Children's Hospital, New Hyde Park, New York

TERRY J. FRY, MD
Chief, Division of Blood and Marrow Transplantation/Immunology, Center for Cancer and Blood Disorders, Children's National Medical Center, Washington, DC

STEPHAN A. GRUPP, MD, PhD
Assistant Professor of Pediatrics, CCCR Director of Translational Research, Division of Oncology, Children's Hospital of Philadelphia; Department of Pediatrics, University of Pennsylvania School of Medicine; Department of Pathology and Laboratory Medicine, Children's Hospital of Philadelphia, Philadelphia, Pennsylvania

RUPERT HANDGRETINGER, MD, PhD
Children's University Hospital, Tuebingen, Germany

HELEN E. HESLOP, MD
Professor, Department of Pediatrics and Medicine, Center for Cell and Gene Therapy, Baylor College of Medicine and The Methodist Hospital, Houston, Texas

LAKSHMANAN KRISHNAMURTI, MD
Division of Hematology/Oncology/Bone Marrow Transplantation, Children's Hospital of Pittsburgh of UPMC, Pittsburgh, Pennsylvania

JOANNE KURTZBERG, MD
Professor of Pediatrics and Pathology, Division of Pediatric Blood and Marrow Transplantation, Duke University Medical Center, Durham, North Carolina

PETER LANG, MD, PhD
Children's University Hospital, Tuebingen, Germany

ARJAN C. LANKESTER, MD, PhD
Leiden University Medical Centre, Department of Pediatrics, Leiden, The Netherlands

FRANCO LOCATELLI, MD
Professor, University of Pavia, Ospedale Pediatrico Bambino Gesu, Roma; Director, Pediatric Haematology/Oncology Fondazione, IRCCS Policlinico San Matteo, Pavia, Italy

GUIDO LUCARELLI, MD
Director, International Centre for Transplantation in Thalassemia and Sickle Cell Anemia, Mediterranean Institute of Hematology, Rome, Italy

CRYSTAL L. MACKALL, MD
Chief, Pediatric Oncology Branch, Center for Cancer Research, National Cancer Institute, National Institutes of Health, Bethesda, Maryland

MARGARET L. MACMILLAN, MD
Associate Professor of Pediatrics, Blood and Marrow Transplant Program, Department of Pediatrics, University of Minnesota Medical School, Minneapolis, Minnesota

PARINDA MEHTA, MD
Cincinnati Children's Hospital Medical Center and the University of Cincinnati College of Medicine, Cincinnati, Ohio

FRANCESCA MILANETTI, MD
Visiting Scholar, Division of Immunotherapy, Department of Medicine, Northwestern University Feinberg School of Medicine, Chicago, Illinois; Medico Specializzando, Division of Rheumatology and Clinical Immunology, Department of Medicine, Sapienza Università di Roma, II Facoltà di Medicina e Chirurgia, A.O.S. Andrea, Rome, Italy

SUHAG H. PARIKH, MD
Assistant Professor of Pediatrics, Division of Pediatric Blood and Marrow Transplantation, Duke University Medical Center, Durham, North Carolina

CHARLES PETERS, MD
Director, Pediatric Hematology-Oncology, Sanford Children's Hospital; Professor of Pediatrics, Sanford School of Medicine, The University of South Dakota, Sioux Falls, South Dakota

CHRISTINA PETERS, MD
Professor of Pediatrics, Stem Cell Transplantation Unit, St Anna Children's Hospital, Kinderspitalgasse, Vienna, Austria

VINOD K. PRASAD, MD, MRCP
Assistant Professor, Department of Pediatrics, Blood and Marrow Transplant Program, Duke University Medical Center, Duke University School of Medicine, Durham, North Carolina

JANE E. SANDE, MD
Associate Professor of Pediatrics, Medical Director, Blood and Marrow Transplant Program, Division of BMT and Immunology, Center for Cancer and Blood Disorders, Children's National Medical Center, The George Washington University, Washington, DC

KIRK R. SCHULTZ, MD
Director, Childhood Cancer Research Program of BC Children's Hospital and the Child and Family Research Institute; Professor of Pediatrics, BC Children's Hospital, Vancouver, British Columbia, Canada

FRANS J. SMIERS, MD, PhD
Leiden University Medical Center, Department of Pediatrics, Hematology Oncology and BMT Unit, Leiden, The Netherlands

FRANKLIN O. SMITH, MD
Cincinnati Children's Hospital Medical Center and the University of Cincinnati College of Medicine, Cincinnati, Ohio

JAN STARY, MD
Department of Pediatric Hematology and Oncology, University Hospital Motol and Charles University, Prague, Czech Republic

COLIN G. STEWARD, MD, PhD
Reader in Stem Cell Transplantation, Department of Cellular & Molecular Medicine, School of Medical Sciences, University of Bristol; Consultant in BMT for Genetic Diseases, BMT Unit, Royal Hospital for Children, Bristol, United Kingdom

PAUL SZABOLCS, MD
Department of Pediatrics, Pediatric Blood and Marrow Transplant Program, Duke University Medical Center; Department of Immunology, Duke University, Durham, North Carolina

JAKUB TOLAR, MD, PhD
Assistant Professor, Department of Pediatrics, Division of Pediatric Blood and Marrow Transplantation, University of Minnesota School of Medicine, Minneapolis, Minnesota

PAUL VEYS, MBBS, FRCP, FRCPath, FRCPCH
Department of BMT, Great Ormond Street Hospital for Children NHS Trust, London, United Kingdom

JULIO C. VOLTARELLI, MD, PhD
Director, Bone Marrow Transplantation Unit, Department of Clinical Medicine, School of Medicine of Ribeirão Preto, University of São Paulo, Hemocentro-RP, Campus USP, Ribeirão Preto, Brazil

ALAN S. WAYNE, MD
Clinical Director, Senior Clinician Head, Hematologic Diseases Section, Pediatric Oncology Branch, Center for Cancer Research, National Cancer Institute, National Institutes of Health, Bethesda, Maryland

ANDRE WILLASCH, MD
Division for Stem Cell Transplantation, Hospital for Children and Adolescents III, Goethe University, Frankfurt am Main, Germany

ROBERT F. WYNN, MD, MRCP, FRCPath
Director, Blood and Marrow Transplant Programme; Consultant Paediatric Haematologist, Department of Paediatric Haematology and Oncology, Royal Manchester Children's Hospital, Manchester, United Kingdom

Contents

Preface   xvii

Max J. Coppes, Terry J. Fry, and Crystal L. Mackall

Hematopoietic Stem Cell Transplantation for Leukemia   1

Alan S. Wayne, Kristin Baird, and Maarten Egeler

> Leukemia represents the most common pediatric malignancy, accounting
> for approximately 30% of all cancers in children less than 20 years of age.
> Most children diagnosed with leukemia are cured without hematopoietic
> stem cell transplantation (HSCT), but for some high-risk subgroups, allo-
> geneic HSCT plays an important role in their therapeutic approach. The
> characteristics of these high-risk subgroups and the role of HSCT in child-
> hood leukemias are discussed.

**Stem Cell Source and Outcome After Hematopoietic Stem Cell Transplantation
(HSCT) in Children and Adolescents with Acute Leukemia**   27

Christina Peters, Jacqueline M. Cornish, Suhag H. Parikh,
and Joanne Kurtzberg

> Allogeneic hematopoietic stem cell transplantation from siblings, unrelated
> donors or HLA mismatched family members has become an important
> procedure to offer a chance of cure to children and adolescents with acute
> leukemia at high risk of relapse and those with certain genetic diseases.
> Bone marrow (BM) was the only stem cell source for many years. During
> the past 15 years, peripheral blood stem cells from granulocyte colony-
> stimulating factor (G-CSF) mobilized healthy donors, or umbilical cord
> blood from related or unrelated donors, have become available. Each
> stem cell source has different risks/benefits for patients and donors, the
> choice depending not only on availability, but also on HLA compatibility
> and urgency of the HSCT. This review will analyze the advantages and lim-
> itations of each of these options, and the main criteria which can be ap-
> plied when choosing the appropriate stem cell source for pediatric
> transplant recipients with acute leukemia.

Autologous and Allogeneic Cellular Therapies for High-risk Pediatric Solid Tumors   47

David Barrett, Jonathan D. Fish, and Stephan A. Grupp

> Since the 1950s, the overall survival of children with cancer has gone from
> almost zero to approaching 80%. Although there have been notable suc-
> cesses in treating solid tumors such as Wilms tumor, some childhood solid
> tumors have continued to elude effective therapy. With the use of mega-
> therapy techniques such as tandem transplantation, dose escalation has
> been pushed to the edge of dose-limiting toxicities, and any further im-
> provements in event-free survival will have to be achieved through novel
> therapeutic approaches. This article reviews the status of autologous
> and allogeneic hematopoietic stem cell transplantation (HSCT) for many
> pediatric solid tumor types. Most of the clinical experience in transplant
> for pediatric solid tumors is in the autologous setting, so some general

principles of autologous HSCT are reviewed. The article then examines HSCT for diseases such as Hodgkin disease, Ewing sarcoma, and neuroblastoma, and the future of cell-based therapies by considering some experimental approaches to cell therapies.

The Graft-Versus-Tumor Effect in Pediatric Malignancy   67

Terry J. Fry, Andre Willasch, and Peter Bader

Because severe forms of the graft-versus-host reaction directed against normal tissues (also termed graft-versus-host disease [GVHD]) also contribute to morbidity and mortality following allogeneic hematopoietic stem cell transplantation, major efforts have focused on strategies to separate GVHD from the potentially beneficial immune reactivity against tumor (also called the graft-versus-tumor [GVT] effect). This article focuses on the data supporting the contribution of the GVT effect to cure of malignancy, what is known about the biology of the GVT reaction, and, finally, strategies to manipulate the GVT effect to increase the potency of HSCT.

T-cell-based Therapies for Malignancy and Infection in Childhood   83

Nabil Ahmed, Helen E. Heslop, and Crystal L. Mackall

One major advance in T-cell-based immunotherapy in the last 20 years has been the molecular definition of numerous viral and tumor antigens. Adoptive T-cell transfer has shown definite clinical benefit in the prophylaxis and treatment of viral infections that develop in pediatric patients after allogeneic transplant and in posttransplant lymphoproliferative disease associated with Epstein-Barr virus. Developing adoptive T-cell therapies for other malignancies presents additional challenges. This article describes the recent advances in T-cell-based therapies for malignancy and infection in childhood and strategies to enhance the effector functions of T cells and optimize the cellular product, including gene modification and modulation of the host environment.

Immunotherapy in the Context of Hematopoietic Stem Cell Transplantation: The Emerging Role of Natural Killer Cells and Mesenchymal Stromal Cells   97

Arjan C. Lankester, Lynne M. Ball, Peter Lang, and Rupert Handgretinger

Immunotherapy in the context of hematopoietic stem cell transplantation has been dominated for many years by T-cell- and dendritic-cell-based treatment modalities. During the last decade, insight into the biology of natural killer (NK) cells and mesenchymal stromal cells (MSC) has rapidly increased and resulted in NK- and MSC-based therapeutic strategies in clinical practice. This article reviews current knowledge of the biology and clinical aspects of NK cells and MSC.

Current International Perspectives on Hematopoietic Stem Cell Transplantation for Inherited Metabolic Disorders   123

Jaap J. Boelens, Vinod K. Prasad, Jakub Tolar, Robert F. Wynn, and Charles Peters

Inherited metabolic disorders (IMD) or inborn errors of metabolism are a diverse group of diseases arising from genetic defects in lysosomal enzymes or peroxisomal function. These diseases are characterized by devastating systemic processes affecting neurologic and cognitive function, growth and development, and cardiopulmonary status. Onset in infancy or early childhood is typically accompanied by rapid deterioration. Early death is a common outcome. Timely diagnosis and immediate referral to an IMD specialist are essential steps in management of these disorders. Treatment recommendations are based on the disorder, its phenotype including age at onset and rate of progression, severity of clinical signs and symptoms, family values and expectations, and the risks and benefits associated with available therapies such as allogeneic hematopoietic stem cell transplantation (HSCT). This review discusses indications for HSCT and outcomes of HSCT for selected IMD. An international perspective on progress, limitations, and future directions in the field is provided.

Bone Marrow Transplantation for Inherited Bone Marrow Failure Syndromes   **147**

Parinda Mehta, Franco Locatelli, Jan Stary, and Franklin O. Smith

The inherited bone marrow failure (BMF) syndromes are characterized by impaired hematopoiesis and cancer predisposition. Most inherited BMF syndromes are also associated with a range of congenital anomalies. Progress in improving the outcomes for children with inherited BMF syndromes has been limited by the rarity of these disorders, as well as disease-specific genetic, molecular, cellular, and clinical characteristics that increase the risks of complications associated with hematopoietic stem cell transplantation (HSCT). As a result, the ability to develop innovative transplant approaches to circumvent these problems has been limited. Recent progress has been made, as best evidenced in studies adding fludarabine to the preparative regimen for children undergoing unrelated donor HSCT for Fanconi anemia. The rarity of these diseases coupled with the far more likely incremental improvements that will result from ongoing research will require prospective international clinical trials to improve the outcome for these children.

Hematopoietic Stem Cell Transplantation for Osteopetrosis   **171**

Colin G. Steward

Osteopetrosis is the generic name for a group of diseases caused by deficient formation or function of osteoclasts, inherited in either autosomal recessive or dominant fashion. Osteopetrosis varies in severity from a disease that may kill infants to an incidental radiological finding in adults. It is increasingly clear that prognosis is governed by which gene is affected, making detailed elucidation of the cause of the disease a critical component of optimal care, including the decision on whether hematopoietic stem cell transplantation is appropriate. This article reviews the characteristics and management of osteopetrosis.

Hematopoietic Stem Cell Transplantation for Hemoglobinopathies: Current Practice and Emerging Trends   **181**

Frans J. Smiers, Lakshmanan Krishnamurti, and Guido Lucarelli

Despite improvements in the management of thalassemia major and sickle cell disease, treatment complications are frequent and life expectancy remains diminished for these patients. Hematopoietic stem cell transplantation (HSCT) is the only curative option currently available. Existing results for HSCT in patients with hemoglobinopathy are excellent and still improving. New conditioning regimens are being used to reduce treatment-related toxicity and new donor pools accessed to increase the number of patients who can undergo HSCT.

Bone Marrow Transplantation for Primary Immunodeficiency Diseases　　**207**

Paul Szabolcs, Marina Cavazzana-Calvo, Alain Fischer, and Paul Veys

Advances in immunology have led to a breathtaking expansion of recognized primary immunodeficiency diseases (PID) with over 120 disease-related genes identified. In North America alone more than 1000 children have received allogeneic blood or marrow transplant over the past 30 years, with the majority surviving long term. This review presents results and highlights challenges and notable advances, including novel less toxic conditioning regimens, to transplant the more common and severe forms of PID. HLA-matched sibling donors remain the ideal option, however, advances in living donor unrelated HSCT and banked umbilical cord blood grafts provide hope for all children with severe PID.

Autologous Hematopoietic Stem Cell Transplantation for Childhood Autoimmune Disease　　**239**

Francesca Milanetti, Mario Abinun, Julio C. Voltarelli, and Richard K. Burt

Autologous and allogeneic hematopoietic stem cell transplantation (HSCT) can be used in the management of patients with autoimmune disorders. Experience gained in adults has helped to better define the conditioning regimens required and appropriate selection of patients who are most likely to benefit from autologous HSCT. The field has been shifting toward the use of safer and less intense nonmyeloablative regimens used earlier in the disease course before patients accumulate extensive irreversible organ damage. This article reviews the experience of using autologous HSCT in treating the most common childhood autoimmune and rheumatic diseases, primarily juvenile idiopathic arthritis, systemic lupus erythematosus, and diabetes mellitus.

Management of Acute Graft-Versus-Host Disease in Children　　**273**

Paul A. Carpenter and Margaret L. MacMillan

Acute graft-versus-host disease (aGVHD) remains a major cause of morbidity and mortality after allogeneic hematopoietic stem cell transplantation (HSCT) in children. Although 30% to 50% of children respond to corticosteroids as initial therapy, the optimal initial or second-line therapies have not yet been determined. Newer approaches with combination therapy, novel agents, monoclonal antibodies, and/or cellular therapies show some promise but require prospective well-designed trials that include children to establish their efficacy. This article reviews the clinical presentation, treatment, and practical management guidelines for children with aGVHD.

Chronic Graft-Versus-Host Disease (GVHD) in Children   **297**

Kristin Baird, Kenneth Cooke, and Kirk R. Schultz

Five-year survival rates for childhood cancer now exceed 80% and with the significant progress made by the transplant community in developing less toxic conditioning regimens and in the treatment of posttransplant complications, allo-hematopoietic stem cell transplantation (HSCT) contributes significantly to that population of long-term survivors. In this context, the acute and long-term toxicities of chronic graft-versus-host disease (cGVHD) have an ever-increasing effect on organ function, quality of life, and survival; patients and families who initially felt great relief to be cured from the primary disease, now face the challenge of a chronic debilitating illness for which preventative and treatment strategies are suboptimal. Hence, the development of novel strategies that reduce and/or control cGVHD, preserve graft-versus-tumor effects, facilitate engraftment and immune reconstitution, and enhance survival after allo-HSCT represents one of the most significant challenges facing physician-scientists and patients.

The Burden of Cure: Long-term Side Effects Following Hematopoietic Stem Cell Transplantation (HSCT) in Children   **323**

K. Scott Baker, Dorine Bresters, and Jane E. Sande

Children who survive hematopoietic stem cell transplantation (HSCT) are at risk for an inordinate number of long-term side effects. Late effects can be secondary to the underlying diagnosis for which the transplant is performed, prior treatment of the disease, the transplant preparative regimen, treatment of the complications of transplant, and immunologic interactions between the graft and the host. This article describes the risks and manifestations of the most commonly reported late effects in survivors of pediatric HSCT.

Index   **343**

FORTHCOMING ISSUES

April 2010
Solid Organ Transplantation
Vicky Lee Ng, MD, FRCPC, and
Sandy Feng, MD, PhD,
Guest Editors

June 2010
Pediatric Sports Medicine
Dilip R. Patel, MD, and
Donald E. Greydanus, MD,
Guest Editors

August 2010
Birthmarks of Medical Significance
Beth A. Drolet, MD, and
Maria C. Garzon, MD, *Guest Editors*

RECENT ISSUES

December 2009
**Health Issues in Indigenous Children: An
Evidence-Based Approach for the General
Pediatrician**
Anne B. Chang, MBBS, MPHTM, PhD,
FRACP, and Rosalyn Singleton, MD MPH,
Guest Editors

October 2009
Nutritional Deficiencies
Praveen S. Goday, MD, CNSP, and
Timothy S. Sentongo, MD,
Guest Editors

August 2009
Pediatric Quality
Leonard G. Feld, MD, PhD, MMM, FAAP,
and Shabnam Jain, MD, FAAP,
Guest Editors

RELATED INTEREST

Immunology and Allergy Clinics Volume 30, Issue 1 (February 2010), Volume 30,
Issue 2 (May 2010)
Hematopoietic Stem Cell Transplantation for Immunodeficiency: Parts I and II
Chaim M. Roifman, MD, FRCPC, FCACB, *Guest Editor*
www.immunology.theclinics.com

THE CLINICS ARE NOW AVAILABLE ONLINE!

Access your subscription at:
www.theclinics.com

Preface

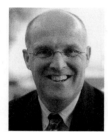 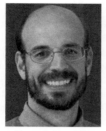 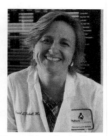

Max J. Coppes, MD, PhD, MBA   Terry J. Fry, MD   Crystal L. Mackall, MD

Guest Editors

After 2 decades of studies in animals and failed attempts in humans,[1] which provided critical ground work for the field of hematopoietic stem cell transplantation (HSCT)[2], the first successful bone marrow transplant was performed in 1968 by Dr Robert Good and colleagues[3] in a child with severe combined immune deficiency. Thus, the field of HSCT (a term now used to include blood stem cell transplants using bone marrow, peripheral blood, or umbilical cord blood) had its beginnings in pediatrics. This was rapidly followed by success in aplastic anemia and leukemia.[4,5] At present, more than 15,000 allogeneic HSCTs are performed annually worldwide, with more than a quarter of them in children. In the 4 decades since the first successful HSCT, the fundamental principal of the procedure has not changed—the infusion of hematopoietic stem cells into a conditioned recipient to treat cancer, to correct a poorly functioning bone marrow or immune system, or to treat other genetic or metabolic diseases (almost exclusively in children). However, the details of HSCT have undergone dramatic changes resulting in significant improvements in outcome. The purpose of this issue of *Pediatric Clinics of North America* is to review current challenges facing pediatric HSCT in a single volume. Each section summarizes the state of the art and provides a discussion of how specific areas of HSCT have evolved. There are articles focused on specific indications for bone marrow transplant, including leukemia ("Hematopoietic Stem Cell Transplantation for Leukemia" and "The Graft-Versus-Tumor Effect in Pediatric Malignancy"), solid tumors ("Autologous and Allogeneic Cellular Therapies for High-Risk Pediatric Solid Tumors"), hemoglobinopathies ("Hematopoietic Stem Cell Transplantation for Hemoglobinopathies: Current Practice and Emerging Trends"), immune deficiencies ("Bone Marrow Transplantation for Primary Immunodeficiency Diseases"), metabolic disorders ("Current International Perspectives on Hematopoietic Stem Cell Transplantation for Inherited Metabolic Disorders"), bone marrow failure ("Bone Marrow Transplantation for Inherited Bone Marrow Failure Syndromes"), and other nonmalignant conditions such as osteopetrosis ("Hematopoietic Stem Cell Transplantation for Osteopetrosis"). Also included are discussions of stem cell source ("Stem Cell Source and Outcome After Hematopoietic

Pediatr Clin N Am 57 (2010) xvii–xix
doi:10.1016/j.pcl.2010.01.021
0031-3955/10/$ – see front matter © 2010 Elsevier Inc. All rights reserved.

Stem Cell Transplantation in Children and Adolescents with Acute Leukemia") and graft-versus-host disease ("Management of Acute Graft-Versus-Host Disease in Children" and "Chronic Graft-Versus-Host Disease in Children"). Given the current emphasis in the field on using the donor immune system to target residual cancer cells or to treat infections, there are also articles focused on cancer vaccines, cell therapies, and other immune-based therapies ("T-cell-based Therapies for Malignancy and Infection in Childhood" and "Immunotherapy in the Context of Hematopoietic Stem Cell Transplantation: The Emerging Role of Natural Killer Cells and Mesenchymal Stromal Cells"). Finally, one article ("The Burden of Cure: Long Term Side Effects Following Hematopoietic Stem Cell Transplantation in Children") addresses the important issue of long-term side effects in the increasing number of survivors of pediatric HSCT. Although the highly specialized nature of HSCT might suggest that this issue is primarily a resource for transplant physicians, the diversity of diseases that are treated and protean effects (both acute and late) on pediatric recipients illustrate that HSCT is, in fact, of broad interest to the pediatric community. We hope that this issue will provide a comprehensive review of important topics in this continuously evolving field for all pediatric practitioners.

Max J. Coppes, MD, PhD, MBA
Center for Cancer and Blood Disorders
Children's National Medical Center
4 West Wing
111 Michigan Avenue, NW
Washington, DC 20010, USA

Medicine, Pediatrics, and Oncology
Georgetown University
Washington, DC, USA

Terry J. Fry, MD
Division of Blood and Marrow Transplantation/Immunology
Center for Cancer and Blood Disorders
Children's National Medical Center
1 West Wing
111 Michigan Avenue, NW
Washington, DC 20010, USA

Crystal L. Mackall, MD
Center for Cancer Research
National Cancer Institute, NIH
10-CRC, 1W-3750
10 Center Drive MSC 1104
Bethesda, MD 20892-1104, USA

E-mail addresses:
MCoppes@cnmc.org (M.J. Coppes)
tfry@cnmc.org (T.J. Fry)
cm35c@nih.gov (C.L. Mackall)

REFERENCES

1. Bortin MM. A compendium of reported human bone marrow transplants. Transplantation 1970;9:571–87.

2. Appelbaum FR, Forman SJ, Negrin RS, et al, editors. Thomas' hematopoietic cell transplantation. 4th edition. West Sussex (UK): Wiley-Blackwell; 2007. p. 3–7.
3. Gatti RA, Meuwissen HJ, Allen HD, et al. Immunological reconstitution of sex-linked lymphopenic immunological deficiency. Lancet 1968;2:1366–9.
4. Thomas ED, Storb R, Clift RA, et al. Bone-marrow transplantation (second of two parts). N Engl J Med 1975;292:895–902.
5. Thomas E, Storb R, Clift RA, et al. Bone-marrow transplantation (first of two parts). N Engl J Med 1975;292:832–43.

Hematopoietic Stem Cell Transplantation for Leukemia

Alan S. Wayne, MD[a,*], Kristin Baird, MD[a],
R. Maarten Egeler, MD, PhD[b]

KEYWORDS

- Leukemia • Hematopoietic stem cell transplantation
- HSCT • Pediatric

Leukemia represents the most common pediatric malignancy, accounting for approximately 30% of all cancers in children less than 20 years of age. Acute lymphoblastic leukemia (ALL) is the most frequent, accounting for approximately 23% of childhood cancers. Acute myeloid leukemia (AML) accounts for approximately 4% of pediatric cancer diagnoses and 20% of childhood leukemia. Chronic myelogenous leukemia (CML) is rare and accounts for approximately 1% of all pediatric cancer, although it accounts for 10% of leukemias in older adolescents. Juvenile myelomonocytic leukemia (JMML) is infrequent, accounting for about 2% of leukemias and 25% of myelodysplastic syndrome in childhood.[1] Most children diagnosed with leukemia are cured without hematopoietic stem cell transplantation (HSCT), but for some high-risk subgroups, allogeneic HSCT plays an important role in their therapeutic approach.

ALL

Prognostic Variables and Risk Stratification at Diagnosis

Clinical and biologic features are used to subtype, risk stratify, and assign therapy at diagnosis. Initial risk group assignment is made based on age, peripheral white blood cell count (WBC), central nervous system (CNS) involvement, and phenotype.[2] Phenotypic classification is determined by flow cytometry of lineage-associated cell surface markers. Most cases of ALL are of precursor B cell (pre-B) phenotype (CD10, CD19, HLA-DR, TDT+), 10% to 20% are T cell (CD2, CD3, CD5, and/or CD7+), and <5% are mature B cell or Burkitt type (CD20, surface-IgM+).

[a] Pediatric Oncology Branch, Center for Cancer Research, National Cancer Institute, National Institutes of Health, Building 10, Room 1-3750, 9000 Rockville Pike, MSC 1104, Bethesda, MD 20892-1104, USA
[b] Department of Pediatric Immunology, Hematology, Oncology, Bone Marrow Transplantation and Auto-immune Diseases, Leiden University Medical Center, PO Box 9600, 2300 RC Leiden, The Netherlands
* Corresponding author.
E-mail address: waynea@mail.nih.gov

Pediatr Clin N Am 57 (2010) 1–25
doi:10.1016/j.pcl.2009.11.005
0031-3955/10/$ – see front matter

Cytogenetic studies are subsequently used to further define the risk of relapse. The t(12;21) translocation, the most frequent recurrent chromosomal translocation associated with childhood ALL, is identified in approximately 25% of cases and this is associated with a favorable prognosis.[3–6] Gene rearrangements of the mixed-lineage leukemia (MLL) gene located at 11q23 is the most common cytogenetic finding in infants with ALL, and has an extremely poor prognosis.[7–10] The so-called Philadelphia chromosome (Ph+), which results from a translocation between chromosomes 9 and 22, t(9;22), also confers adverse risk.[11] The t(1;19) translocation is also associated with an increased risk of relapse, but this can be offset by therapy intensification.[12,13] Hyperdiploidy, which most often includes trisomies of chromosomes 4, 7, and/or 10, carries a favorable prognosis.[14–18] Hypodiploid cases are at higher risk of relapse.[19–22] Recently, gene expression analysis has been shown to allow further discrimination in risk classification and prediction of treatment response.[23]

The initial response to therapy has important prognostic usefulness. A rapid early response (RER), defined as a marrow blast count less than 5% within 7 to 14 days, or clearance of peripheral blasts within 7 to 10 days, has a better outcome than when the response is slower (SER).[24–30] Response to therapy can be further quantified by flow cytometric or molecular analysis of minimal residual disease (MRD), which has been shown to correlate with outcome.[31,32]

Nontransplant Therapy

Approximately 80% of children with ALL are cured with chemotherapy, the intensity of which is determined by risk group assignment and treatment stratification. Most patients fall into the standard risk category characterized by age between 1 and 9 years, WBC <50,000/μL, B-precursor phenotype, and absence of high-risk chromosomal abnormalities. Therapy for B-precursor and T cell ALL consists of induction, consolidation/intensification/re-induction, CNS sterilization, and maintenance for 2 to 3 years.[33–40] Individuals with mature B cell phenotype are treated using Burkitt lymphoma regimens, which most commonly include dose- and sequence-intensive, short-course combination chemotherapy.[41–43]

The prognosis after relapse of ALL depends on the duration of the first remission (CR1) and the site of relapse.[44–47] Outcome after short CR1 duration (<12–18 months) is very poor, as is the prognosis for individuals who are unable to achieve a second remission. Those with isolated extramedullary relapse fair better than those with marrow relapse.[48,49]

Transplantation

There have been no large, prospective, controlled clinical trials to evaluate the relative efficacy of allogeneic HSCT in comparison with chemotherapy for childhood ALL. However, multiple comparative studies suggest that relapse rates are lower after HSCT.[50] Some of the benefits of relapse-free survival are offset by transplant-associated morbidity and mortality.[51] Consequently, HSCT is usually reserved for the management of relapse and it is rarely used for children in CR1 except for those with extremely high-risk features (**Fig. 1; Table 1**). Results of recent trials of HSCT for children and adolescents with ALL in second remission (CR2) are presented in **Table 2**. For those with HLA-matched sibling donors, allogeneic HSCT in second remission is considered standard. Unrelated donor HSCT is usually reserved for those at high risk of relapse with chemotherapy (**Figs. 1** and **2**). The approach in individual cases varies based on risk/benefit analysis, donor options, and access to transplantation. The American Society for Blood and Marrow Transplantation (ASBMT) has

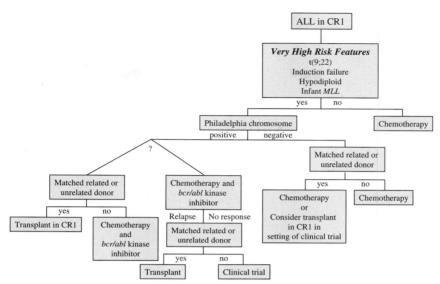

Fig. 1. ALL: algorithm for transplantation in first remission.

published consensus guidelines for the use of HSCT in childhood ALL (**Table 3**).[50] Suggested algorithms for HSCT in pediatric ALL are presented in **Figs. 1** and **2**.

A retrospective matched cohort analysis performed by the Children's Oncology Group (COG) and International Bone Marrow Transplant Registry (IBMTR) compared matched related HSCT with chemotherapy for children with ALL in CR2. Leukemia-free survival and relapse rates were better after HSCT in all patient groups regardless of the CR1 duration.[51] In a more recent study from the COG and IBMTR, overall survival, leukemia-free survival, and treatment-related mortality were superior for patients with a short CR1 duration (<36 months) who underwent HSCT with total body irradiation (TBI)-based conditioning regimens (vs chemotherapy and non-TBI transplant regimens). For those with a late relapse (≥36 months CR1 duration), outcomes were equivalent in the chemotherapy and TBI transplant groups. Those treated with HSCT without TBI had higher risk of relapse and inferior disease-free survival (DFS) rates regardless of CR1 duration.[64]

Despite the lower relapse rates after HSCT, this approach carries the risk of transplant-associated mortality and morbidity (eg, graft-versus-host disease [GVHD]). Further, chemotherapy alone can be effective. Approximately 30% to 40% of children who sustain a late relapse (≥36 months CR1 duration) may achieve long-term DFS with aggressive chemotherapy alone.[45–47,51,66,67]

Decisions about the role for and timing of HSCT for children with relapsed ALL are commonly individualized based on biologic, clinical, treatment, and donor factors (see **Fig. 2**). Transplant is usually recommended for children with relapse who have HLA-matched sibling donors irrespective of other prognostic factors. An alternative approach for those with a long CR1 duration is to reserve HSCT in the event of another relapse. For individuals who sustain bone marrow relapse during front-line therapy or within 6 months of completion of therapy the prognosis is poor with chemotherapy alone, and HSCT with an alternative (ie, unrelated or HLA-mismatched related) donor should be considered. HSCT is also often considered for T-cell ALL with marrow relapse. Additional factors that place an individual at high risk of subsequent relapse

Table 1
Results of HSCT for pediatric patients with ALL in first remission

Study Group	Dates of Study	High Risk Indicator	Patients (n)	Outcome (Years)	References
Toronto	1985–2001	t(9;22)	11 MRD, MUD 10 chemo	53% EFS (4)	Sharathkumar, 2004[52]
UKALL-X UKALL-XI	1985–1990 1990–1997	WBC >100,000/μL ± t(9;22), near-haploid, induction failure	76 MRD, 25 MUD 351 chemo	45% EFS (10) 39% EFS (10)	Wheeler, 2000[53]
AIEOP/GITMO	1986–1994	WBC >100,000/μL, BFM risk index >1.7, t(9;22), t(8;11), steroid resistance, T-cell disease, induction failure	30 MRD 130 chemo	58% DFS (4) 48% DFS (4)	Uderzo, 1997[54]
NOPHO	1981–1991	WBC >100,000/μL	22 MRD 44 chemo[a] 405 chemo[b]	73% DFS (10) 50% DFS (10) 59% DFS (10)	Saarinen, 1996[55]
IBMTR	1978–1990	t(9;22)	33 MRD	38% DFS (2)	Barrett, 1992[56]
Groupe d'Etude de la Greffe de Moelle Osseuse	1980–1987	t(9;22) WBC >100,000/μL, induction failure	32 MRD	84% DFS (2.5)	Bordigoni, 1989[57]

Abbreviations: chemo, chemotherapy; DFS, disease-free survival; EFS, event-free survival; MRD, matched related donor; MUD, matched unrelated donor.
[a] Matched control patients.
[b] Unmatched patients.

Table 2
Results of HSCT for pediatric patients with ALL in second remission

Study Group	Dates of Study	Patients (n)	Outcome (Years)	References
BFM	1985–1991	51 MRD	52% EFS (5)	Dopfer, 1991[58]
IBMTR/POG	1983–1991	255 MRD	40% DFS (5)	Barrett, 1994[51]
		255 chemo	17% DFS (5)	
Leiden	1982–1991	25 MRD	44% DFS (4)	Hoogerbrugge,
		97 chemo	24% DFS (4)	1995[59]
AIEOP/GITMO	1980–1990	57 MRD	41% DFS (5)	Uderzo, 1995[60]
		230 chemo	21% DFS (5)	
Paris	1983–1993	42 MRD	53% (4)	Moussalem, 1995[61]
UKALL-X	1985–1990	83 MRD, 27 MUD	40% EFS (5)	Wheeler, 1998[62]
		61 ABMT	34% EFS (5)	
		261 chemo	26% EFS (5)	
UKALL-R1	1991–1995	63 MRD	46% EFS (5)	Harrison, 2000[63]
		41 MUD	54% EFS (5)	
		15 ABMT, 89 chemo	43% EFS (5)	
IBMTR/COG	1991–1997	CR1 <36 months		Eapen, 2006[64]
		92 MRD + TBI	32% OS (8)	
		19 MRD no TBI	44% OS (8)	
		110 chemo	18% OS (8)	
		CR1 ≥36 months		
		61 MRD + TBI	66% OS (8)	
		14 MRD no TBI	63% OS (8)	
		78 chemo	32% OS (8)	
COG	1995–1998	32 MRD	42% DFS (3)	Gaynon, 2006[45]
		19 MUD	29% DFS (3)	
		23 chemo	30% DFS (3)	

Abbreviations: ABMT, autologous bone marrow transplant; chemo, chemotherapy; DFS, disease-free survival; EFS, event-free survival; MRD, matched related donor; MUD, matched unrelated donor; OS, overall survival; TBI, total body irradiation.

or that limit the ability to administer chemotherapy (eg, allergy, organ toxicity) also warrant consideration of HSCT.

HSCT in first remission has no proven benefits for patients defined as high risk by WBC count, gender, and age. However, transplantation is commonly considered for those at very high risk of relapse with standard therapy (eg, hypodiploidy, induction

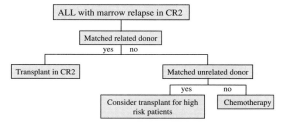

Fig. 2. ALL: algorithm for transplantation in second remission.

Table 3
HSCT for pediatric ALL: 2005 ASBMT Expert Panel Consensus[50]

Recommendation	Indication	References
HSCT in CR1	Benefit demonstrated for matched related donor HSCT for Philadelphia chromosome+ only	Wheeler, 2000[53]
		Chessells, 1992[65]
		Arico, 2000[11]
	Not recommended for other high-risk patients, except in the setting of a clinical trial	Uderzo, 1997[54]
HSCT in CR2 with prior bone marrow relapse	Recommended for those with matched related donors	Barrett, 1994[51]
		Wheeler, 1998[62]
	Evidence insufficient to recommend unrelated donor HSCT	Uderzo, 1995[60]
		Harrison, 2000[63]

failure) (see **Fig. 1**, **Table 1**). Although historically HSCT has been considered for children with Ph+ ALL,[11,68] the addition of imatinib mesylate, a tyrosine kinase inhibitor, to chemotherapy seems to have improved nontransplant outcome,[69] diminishing the role of HSCT as upfront therapy. The role of HSCT for other very high-risk groups should be considered in the setting of a clinical trial.[50] HSCT in infants <18 months old, especially those with *MLL* rearrangements remains controversial because of the high risk of adverse effects of transplant conditioning in such young patients.[70] Some series report outcomes following HSCT in CR1 that may be superior to chemotherapy.[38,71–73] However, others show no definitive benefit compared with intensive chemotherapy.[74–76] A IBMTR database review report 3-year probabilities of DFS of approximately 50% after HLA-matched sibling and unrelated donor transplantation in CR1 for infants with ALL.[64]

Conditioning Regimens

Multiple studies indicate that TBI-based transplant conditioning regimens are associated with lower risk of relapse compared with chemotherapy-only regimens for children with ALL.[50,64,77,78] Second HSCT using TBI has been successful for children who have relapsed after a busulfan-based preparative regimen.[79]

Disease Status

Individuals with ALL should be transplanted in complete remission (CR) and there is little to no role for HSCT in patients with ALL who are not in CR.[80] Recent data indicate that the MRD level at the time of HSCT correlates with outcome. Children with no detectable MRD (<1 leukemia cell in 10,000 bone marrow cells) have excellent post-transplant outcomes.[81] In addition, many series report that patients transplanted in earlier remissions fare better than those with a history of multiple relapses, although such studies are subject to significant selection bias.

Donor Selection

Outcomes of alternative donor transplantation have improved in recent years and several groups report equivalent outcomes to HLA-identical sibling donors using matched unrelated, partially matched related, partially mismatched unrelated cord blood, and haploidentical donors.[82–89] Donor T cell depletion and improvements in supportive care of infection and GVHD have improved the outcomes of such alternative donor transplants. However, T cell depletion is associated with increased risk of graft rejection, mixed chimerism, delayed immune reconstitution, and infectious complications. Treatment-associated mortality remains high, exceeding 20% in published series of alternative donor transplants for ALL, due in part to the high-risk nature of patients treated with that approach. Rates of extensive chronic GVHD also remain high after alternative donor transplants.[85–87]

Second Transplants

For patients who relapse following allogeneic HSCT for ALL, a second transplant may be possible, although the outlook is very poor.[90] This approach carries a high risk of mortality as a result of progressive disease and/or treatment-associated toxicity. Although remission can be obtained in as many as 50% to 70% of patients, the duration is typically short and only 10% to 30% achieve long-term event-free survival. The prognosis is better for those with longer remission duration after the first HSCT.[84,91,92] Donor leukocyte infusion (DLI) has a limited role in the setting of ALL and posttransplant relapse, although successful remission induction with withdrawal of immunosuppression and/or DLI has been reported in a small percentage of cases (discussed elsewhere in this issue).[93–97]

AML
Prognostic Variables and Risk Stratification at Diagnosis

The French-American-British (FAB) classification system categorizes AML into 7 distinct subtypes based on morphology and phenotype. AML subtype and other clinical and biologic features that influence outcome have recently been used to stratify treatment.[98]

Nontransplant Therapy

In most cases AML treatment consists of intensive induction, consolidation, and CNS-directed chemotherapy. Approximately 75% to 90% of children with AML achieve a CR and increasing the treatment intensity of induction improves DFS rates.[99–101] Postremission consolidation chemotherapy is essential and can be delivered in standard doses or as high-dose therapy with autologous stem cell rescue with similar DFS rates.[102–110] Despite treatment intensification the outcome is guarded for most children with AML, and only about 50% are cured with chemotherapy alone.[111] Individuals with acute promyelocytic leukemia (FAB M3) have a better prognosis, with 80% DFS rates observed when all-*trans*-retinoic acid is added during induction and a maintenance phase.[112–115] Young children with trisomy 21 who develop AML also have excellent outcomes and require less intensive therapy.[116–118]

Transplantation

Given the relatively poor outcome for pediatric patients with AML, allogeneic HSCT has commonly been used as consolidation in CR1. There have been multiple genetic randomization studies of matched related allogeneic HSCT in which individuals who have matched sibling donors are assigned to transplantation. Allogeneic HSCT confers a lower risk of relapse and improves DFS compared with chemotherapy with or without autologous rescue (**Table 4**).[99–101,104,106–109,119–122] However, clinical benefits can be offset by transplant-related morbidity and mortality, which may eliminate any overall survival advantage in low-risk groups.[100,123–126] Consequently, there is some debate as to whether allogeneic HSCT should be used in CR1 or CR2 for AML in childhood.[126–128] The ASBMT has published consensus guidelines for the use of HSCT in pediatric AML (**Table 5**)[104] and a suggested approach is presented in **Fig. 3**.

Table 4
Results of HSCT as postremission therapy for childhood AML in first remission

Study Group	DFS			Median Follow-up (Years)	References
	Matched Related Donor HSCT (%)	Chemotherapy (%)	Autologous HSCT (%)		
AML-80	43	31	–	6	Dahl, 1990[119]
AIEOP LAM-87	51[a]	27	21	5	Amadori, 1993[107]
CCG-213	54[a]	37	–	5	Wells, 1994[120]
CCG-251	45[a]	32	–	8	Nesbit, 1994[121]
POG-8821	52[a]	36	38	3	Ravindranath, 1996[106]
MRC AML-10	61[a]	46	68[b]	7	Stevens, 1998[100]
AML BFM-93	64	61	–	5	Creutzig, 2001[99]
CCG-2891	55[a]	47	42	8	Woods, 2001[108]
LAME-89/91	72[a]	48	–	6	Perel, 2002[101] Aladjidi, 2003[122]

[a] $P \leq .05$ allogeneic versus others.
[b] $P \leq .05$ autologous versus chemotherapy.

In the United States, matched related sibling donor HSCT is the most common consolidation therapy used for children with AML in CR1 outside specific low-risk groups.[104] This approach is based largely on clinical trials conducted by the Pediatric Oncology Group (POG) and the Children's Cancer Group (CCG).[132,133] Both groups reported superior outcomes for high- and intermediate-risk patients treated with HSCT in CR1. The 5-year overall survival rate for patients transplanted with a matched sibling donor in CR1 ranges from 52% to 72% (see **Table 4**).[99–101,104,108,122,132,133]

Long-term DFS can be achieved in approximately 30% of children with AML who are transplanted in CR2 with either matched unrelated or mismatched related

Table 5
HSCT for pediatric AML: 2007 ASBMT Expert Panel Consensus[104]

Recommendation	Indication	References
HSCT in CR1	Benefit demonstrated for matched related donor HSCT	Alonzo, 2005[129] Woods, 2001[108] Ravindranath, 1996[106] Wells, 1994[120] Nesbit, 1994[121] Amadori, 1993[107]
HSCT in CR2	Recommended for those with matched related donors Evidence insufficient to recommend unrelated donor HSCT, except in the setting of a clinical trial	Aladjidi, 2003[122] Pession, 2000[130] Gorin, 1996[131]

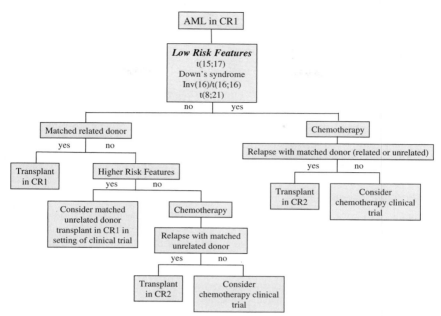

Fig. 3. AML: algorithm for transplantation.

donors.[122] Consequently, HSCT is sometimes reserved for management of patients who relapse after chemotherapy, especially for low-risk groups[128] or those without sibling donors. ASBMT consensus guidelines recommend HSCT in CR2 only for patients with matched related donors, as evidence supporting unrelated donor HSCT is lacking.[104]

Conditioning Regimens

Comparative clinical trials in adults reveal similar results with busulfan/cyclophospha-mide compared with TBI/cyclophosphamide.[134] Pediatric studies are limited, although no obvious differences are apparent.[135] In general, busulfan/cyclophospha-mide is the most commonly used pretransplant preparative regimen for pediatric AML.

Disease Status

In most of the published series of HSCT for pediatric AML, transplantation is per-formed for patients in remission.[104] Although some individuals with AML who undergo HSCT in relapse can achieve long-term DFS,[80] small pediatric studies suggest that the percentage of pretransplant blasts correlates with posttransplant relapse and that outcomes are improved when HSCT is performed in remission.[136,137]

Donor Selection

Donors mismatched for natural killer cell (NK) killer immunoglobulin-like receptor may improve posttransplant outcome in AML as a result of allogeneic NK-cell mediated antileukemic effects,[138] an approach that is currently under study in pediatric AML (see the article by Lankester and colleagues elsewhere in this issue).

Second Transplants

As in ALL, the outcome of second transplants for children with AML varies based on the interval since prior transplantation.[139]

CML
Prognostic Variables and Risk Stratification at Diagnosis

CML is characterized by the presence of the Philadelphia chromosome and the associated translocation product *bcr/abl*. CML has 3 defined clinical phases: chronic, accelerated, and blast crisis; most patients present with chronic phase. Response to treatment and survival correlate with phase of disease. Blast crisis is clinically indistinguishable from acute leukemia and treatment responses are short-lived.

Nontransplant Therapy

The kinase activity of the *bcr/abl* fusion protein is inhibited by imatinib mesylate (Gleevec) and related kinase inhibitors, and these agents have transformed the approach to treatment with CML.[140] Imatinib induces CR in most patients with chronic phase CML, although continuous treatment seems to be required and resistance may develop.[141,142] Thus, there is as yet no evidence that this new class of kinase inhibitors will be curative and they cannot be recommended as a replacement for allogeneic HSCT in children who have an HLA-matched donor.[143] Several criteria have been proposed for deciding when to proceed from kinase inhibitor therapy to HSCT, including loss of therapeutic response or failure to achieve a complete hematologic response by 3 months or a substantial cytogenetic response by 3 to 6 months of treatment.[144]

Transplantation

Allogeneic HSCT is the only proven cure for CML and donor availability should be considered soon after diagnosis for all children with this disorder. Posttransplant DFS rates are inversely related to age and exceed 80% for young children with matched sibling donors in first chronic phase.

Conditioning Regimens

Busulfan/cyclophosphamide is the most common preparative regimen used for pediatric patients with CML undergoing HSCT.

Disease Status

Results are best when HSCT is performed in first chronic phase and with a shorter diagnosis-to-transplant interval. Success is substantially diminished for the accelerated phase or blast crisis and attempts should be made to induce a second chronic phase before transplant.[145,146]

Donor Selection

In general, pediatric patients have relatively low risk of transplant-related mortality and results are similar with matched unrelated and related donors. Thus, unrelated donor HSCT is usually recommended for those who lack sibling donors.[140,143,146–149]

Second Transplants

DLIs have been well shown in adult studies and in a small pediatric series to be effective in the management of posttransplant relapse of chronic phase CML.[95] When DLI is unsuccessful, second transplants should be considered, especially in cases in which there was no prior development of GVHD.[97]

JMML AND MYELODYSPLASTIC SYNDROMES
Prognostic Variables and Risk Stratification at Diagnosis

The myelodysplastic syndromes (MDS) represent a heterogeneous group of disorders characterized by ineffective hematopoiesis, impaired maturation of myeloid progenitors, cytopenias, dysplastic changes, and a propensity for the development of AML.[150,151] The major diagnostic groups within MDS encountered in pediatric patients include JMML, myeloid leukemia of Down syndrome, and MDS occurring de novo and secondary to previous therapy or preexisting disorders.[152–154] Pediatric MDS carries a poor prognosis and clinical variables have little practical usefulness in guiding therapy.[155–158]

Nontransplant Therapy

Therapeutic options are limited in MDS and in general, outcome is guarded. Some patients with MDS initially have an indolent course without therapy.[157] AML-type chemotherapy is associated with low response and high relapse rates.[151,158] JMML is resistant to therapy. Although chemotherapy may reduce disease burden, responses are usually short-lived and the disease rapidly progresses with a median survival of approximately 1 year.[159] The European Working Group of MDS (EWOG-MDS) in Childhood reported a retrospective analysis of 110 cases of JMML. The probability of survival at 10 years was 6% for the nontransplant group versus 39% after transplantation.[156]

Transplantation

HSCT is considered the only curative treatment of childhood MDS and JMML. Given the low response rates to nontransplant therapies, and because failure rates after HSCT seem lower when HSCT is performed soon after diagnosis, strong consideration should be given to early transplantation, especially when a matched sibling donor is available. DFS rates of 50% to 64% are reported with HSCT. Results of the largest published transplant series for children with MDS and JMML are summarized in **Table 6**.[160–166] Individuals with JMML who develop GVHD have a lower incidence of relapse.[150,167]

Conditioning Regimens

Busulfan- and TBI-based pretransplant preparative regimens have both been used for pediatric MDS and JMML, and neither has been shown to be superior. Results with second transplants suggest that radiation may be advantageous (see later discussion). Given the risks of radiation in young children, however, busulfan-based regimens are most commonly used for children with JMML.

Disease Status

Outcome may be improved for individuals transplanted with lower blast percentage and induction chemotherapy is commonly used for patients with elevated bone marrow blasts to induce a CR before HSCT.[158,168] However, definitive recommendations cannot be made given the paucity of data.

Donor Selection

Given the poor prognosis without transplant and the favorable results of matched unrelated donor HSCT in pediatrics, transplantation is usually recommended for

Table 6
Results of HSCT for pediatric patients with MDS and JMML

Patients (n)	Survival (Years)					References
	RA/RARS	RAEB	RAEB/T	MDS/AML	JMML	
48 MRD 52 MUD					55% EFS (5) 49% EFS (5)	Locatelli, 2005[160]
30 MRD, 27 MMRD, 30 MUD, 7 MMUD	59% EFS (3) 74% OS (3)	58% EFS (3) 68% OS (3)	18% EFS (3) 18% OS (3)		27% EFS (3) 33% OS (3)	Yusuf, 2004[161]
46 MUD					24% DFS (2)	Smith, 2002[162]
9 MUD, 3 MMRD					64% EFS (3)	Bunin, 1999[163]
131 MRD	52% DFS (5) 57% OS (5)	34% DFS (5) 42% OS (5)	19% DFS (5) 24% OS (5)	26% DFS (5) 28% OS (5)		Runde, 1998[164]
60 MRD 19 MUD					36% OS (4) 31% OS (4)	Arico,[a] 1997[165]
14 MRD, 1 MMRD, 7 MUD, 2 MMUD (second HSCT)					32% DFS (5)	Yoshimi, 2007[166]

Abbreviations: MRD, matched related donor; MMRD, mismatched related donor; MUD, matched unrelated donor; MMUD, mismatched unrelated donor.
[a] Review article.

children with JMML and MDS without regard to the donor type (see **Table 6**).[151,160,162,163,165]

Second Transplants

Initial management of posttransplant relapse should include withdrawal of immuno-suppression and/or DLI, although this is frequently ineffective. In contrast with other types of leukemia, children with JMML have outcomes after second HSCT that are comparable with the results of first transplant.[166] The EWOG-MDS observed several important factors for second transplants for JMML. Most patients received transplants from the same donor, but with reduced GVHD prophylaxis and using TBI-based regimens (vs busulfan-based conditioning) compared with the first transplant. Chronic GVHD was significantly associated with improved DFS after second HSCT. There was no apparent effect of the interval between transplants.[160]

GENERAL CONSIDERATIONS IN THE USE OF HSCT FOR CHILDHOOD LEUKEMIA
GVHD and the Graft-Versus-Leukemia Effect

As noted earlier, an allogeneic graft-versus-leukemia (GVL) effect is an important component of the curative potential of HSCT for certain leukemias. Thus, interventions designed to decrease the incidence and severity of GVHD must be balanced against the risk of leukemic relapse.

Late Effects

Leukemia remains the leading indication for HSCT in pediatrics and with improvements in posttransplant DFS rates, acute and long-term toxicities have an increasing effect on organ function, quality of life, and overall survival. The risks of conditioning regimens on the developing child should be closely considered during pretransplant planning.

Reduced Intensity Conditioning Regimens

Reduced intensity pretransplant regimens have been developed to decrease the toxicity associated with myeloablative conditioning. Based on positive results in adults with hematologic malignancies, pilot studies of reduced intensity conditioning regimens have been conducted in pediatric populations.[169] Because of the potency of the GVL effect in CML, this approach is particularly appealing for that disorder. However, safety and efficacy in the more common acute leukemias of childhood have yet to be demonstrated.

THE FUTURE OF HSCT FOR PEDIATRIC LEUKEMIAS

Allogeneic HSCT will likely continue to play a part in the curative treatment of childhood leukemias well into the future. Scientific discovery and technological advances in transplant immunology, cancer biology, and supportive care will continue to transform the approach to HSCT. As discussed elsewhere in this issue, novel approaches to donor selection, graft source and manipulation, immunotherapy, and tumor-directed targeted treatment with applications in hematologic malignancies are being developed and advanced in the pediatric setting. Alternative donors have assumed an increasing role in HSCT for pediatric leukemias, especially umbilical cord blood in the United States and haploidentical donors in Europe. It is hoped that such strategies will lead to continued decreases in transplant-associated toxicities and improvements in relapse-free and overall survival for children with leukemia.

REFERENCES

1. Edited by National Cancer Institute SP. In: Gloeckler Ries LAPC, Bunin GR, Reis LAG SM, et al, editors. Cancer incidence and survival among children and adolescents: United States SEER Program 1975–1995, vol. 99. NIH Publication; 1999. p. 1–16.
2. Smith M, Arthur D, Camitta B, et al. Uniform approach to risk classification and treatment assignment for children with acute lymphoblastic leukemia. J Clin Oncol 1996;14:18–24.
3. McLean TW, Ringold S, Neuberg D, et al. TEL/AML-1 dimerizes and is associated with a favorable outcome in childhood acute lymphoblastic leukemia. Blood 1996;88:4252–8.
4. Borkhardt A, Cazzaniga G, Viehmann S, et al. Incidence and clinical relevance of TEL/AML1 fusion genes in children with acute lymphoblastic leukemia enrolled in the German and Italian multicenter therapy trials. Associazione Italiana Ematologia Oncologia Pediatrica and the Berlin-Frankfurt-Munster Study Group. Blood 1997;90:571–7.
5. Uckun FM, Pallisgaard N, Hokland P, et al. Expression of TEL-AML1 fusion transcripts and response to induction therapy in standard risk acute lymphoblastic leukemia. Leuk Lymphoma 2001;42:41–56.
6. Kanerva J, Saarinen-Pihkala UM, Niini T, et al. Favorable outcome in 20-year follow-up of children with very-low-risk ALL and minimal standard therapy, with special reference to TEL-AML1 fusion. Pediatr Blood Cancer 2004;42: 30–5.
7. Johansson B, Moorman AV, Haas OA, et al. Hematologic malignancies with t(4;11)(q21;q23) – a cytogenetic, morphologic, immunophenotypic and clinical study of 183 cases. European 11q23 Workshop participants. Leukemia 1998;12: 779–87.
8. Pui CH, Frankel LS, Carroll AJ, et al. Clinical characteristics and treatment outcome of childhood acute lymphoblastic leukemia with the t(4;11)(q21;q23): a collaborative study of 40 cases. Blood 1991;77:440–7.
9. Crist W, Boyett J, Pullen J, et al. Clinical and biologic features predict poor prognosis in acute lymphoid leukemias in children and adolescents: a Pediatric Oncology Group review. Med Pediatr Oncol 1986;14:135–9.
10. Reaman G, Zeltzer P, Bleyer WA, et al. Acute lymphoblastic leukemia in infants less than one year of age: a cumulative experience of the Children's Cancer Study Group. J Clin Oncol 1985;3:1513–21.
11. Arico M, Valsecchi MG, Camitta B, et al. Outcome of treatment in children with Philadelphia chromosome-positive acute lymphoblastic leukemia. N Engl J Med 2000;342:998–1006.
12. Crist WM, Carroll AJ, Shuster JJ, et al. Poor prognosis of children with pre-B acute lymphoblastic leukemia is associated with the t(1;19)(q23;p13): a Pediatric Oncology Group study. Blood 1990;76:117–22.
13. Uckun FM, Sensel MG, Sather HN, et al. Clinical significance of translocation t(1;19) in childhood acute lymphoblastic leukemia in the context of contemporary therapies: a report from the Children's Cancer Group. J Clin Oncol 1998; 16:527–35.
14. Harris MB, Shuster JJ, Carroll A, et al. Trisomy of leukemic cell chromosomes 4 and 10 identifies children with B-progenitor cell acute lymphoblastic leukemia with a very low risk of treatment failure: a Pediatric Oncology Group study. Blood 1992;79:3316–24.

15. Moorman AV, Richards SM, Martineau M, et al. Outcome heterogeneity in childhood high-hyperdiploid acute lymphoblastic leukemia. Blood 2003;102: 2756–62.
16. Charrin C, Thomas X, Ffrench M, et al. A report from the LALA-94 and LALA-SA groups on hypodiploidy with 30 to 39 chromosomes and near-triploidy: 2 possible expressions of a sole entity conferring poor prognosis in adult acute lymphoblastic leukemia (ALL). Blood 2004;104:2444–51.
17. Heerema NA, Sather HN, Sensel MG, et al. Prognostic impact of trisomies of chromosomes 10, 17, and 5 among children with acute lymphoblastic leukemia and high hyperdiploidy (>50 chromosomes). J Clin Oncol 2000;18:1876–87.
18. Sutcliffe MJ, Shuster JJ, Sather HN, et al. High concordance from independent studies by the Children's Cancer Group (CCG) and Pediatric Oncology Group (POG) associating favorable prognosis with combined trisomies 4, 10, and 17 in children with NCI Standard-Risk B-precursor Acute Lymphoblastic Leukemia: a Children's Oncology Group (COG) initiative. Leukemia 2005;19:734–40.
19. Harrison CJ, Moorman AV, Broadfield ZJ, et al. Three distinct subgroups of hypodiploidy in acute lymphoblastic leukaemia. Br J Haematol 2004;125:552–9.
20. Heerema NA, Nachman JB, Sather HN, et al. Hypodiploidy with less than 45 chromosomes confers adverse risk in childhood acute lymphoblastic leukemia: a report from the children's cancer group. Blood 1999;94:4036–45.
21. Raimondi SC, Zhou Y, Mathew S, et al. Reassessment of the prognostic significance of hypodiploidy in pediatric patients with acute lymphoblastic leukemia. Cancer 2003;98:2715–22.
22. Pui CH, Carroll AJ, Raimondi SC, et al. Clinical presentation, karyotypic characterization, and treatment outcome of childhood acute lymphoblastic leukemia with a near-haploid or hypodiploid less than 45 line. Blood 1990;75:1170–7.
23. Mullighan CG, Downing JR. Genome-wide profiling of genetic alterations in acute lymphoblastic leukemia: recent insights and future directions. Leukemia 2009;23:1209–18.
24. Gaynon PS, Desai AA, Bostrom BC, et al. Early response to therapy and outcome in childhood acute lymphoblastic leukemia: a review. Cancer 1997; 80:1717–26.
25. Steinherz PG, Gaynon PS, Breneman JC, et al. Cytoreduction and prognosis in acute lymphoblastic leukemia–the importance of early marrow response: report from the Childrens Cancer Group. J Clin Oncol 1996;14:389–98.
26. Arico M, Basso G, Mandelli F, et al. Good steroid response in vivo predicts a favorable outcome in children with T-cell acute lymphoblastic leukemia. The Associazione Italiana Ematologia Oncologia Pediatrica (AIEOP). Cancer 1995; 75:1684–93.
27. Gajjar A, Ribeiro R, Hancock ML, et al. Persistence of circulating blasts after 1 week of multiagent chemotherapy confers a poor prognosis in childhood acute lymphoblastic leukemia. Blood 1995;86:1292–5.
28. Rautonen J, Hovi L, Siimes MA. Slow disappearance of peripheral blast cells: an independent risk factor indicating poor prognosis in children with acute lymphoblastic leukemia. Blood 1988;71:989–91.
29. Griffin TC, Shuster JJ, Buchanan GR, et al. Slow disappearance of peripheral blood blasts is an adverse prognostic factor in childhood T cell acute lymphoblastic leukemia: a Pediatric Oncology Group study. Leukemia 2000;14:792–5.
30. Panzer-Grumayer ER, Schneider M, Panzer S, et al. Rapid molecular response during early induction chemotherapy predicts a good outcome in childhood acute lymphoblastic leukemia. Blood 2000;95:790–4.

31. van Dongen JJ, Seriu T, Panzer-Grumayer ER, et al. Prognostic value of minimal residual disease in acute lymphoblastic leukaemia in childhood. Lancet 1998; 352:1731–8.
32. Coustan-Smith E, Sancho J, Hancock ML, et al. Clinical importance of minimal residual disease in childhood acute lymphoblastic leukemia. Blood 2000;96: 2691–6.
33. Nachman JB, Sather HN, Sensel MG, et al. Augmented post-induction therapy for children with high-risk acute lymphoblastic leukemia and a slow response to initial therapy. N Engl J Med 1998;338:1663–71.
34. Schrappe M, Reiter A, Ludwig WD, et al. Improved outcome in childhood acute lymphoblastic leukemia despite reduced use of anthracyclines and cranial radiotherapy: results of trial ALL-BFM 90. German-Austrian-Swiss ALL-BFM Study Group. Blood 2000;95:3310–22.
35. Richards S, Burrett J, Hann I, et al. Improved survival with early intensification: combined results from the Medical Research Council childhood ALL randomised trials, UKALL X and UKALL XI. Medical Research Council Working Party on Childhood Leukaemia. Leukemia 1998;12:1031–6.
36. Silverman LB, Gelber RD, Dalton VK, et al. Improved outcome for children with acute lymphoblastic leukemia: results of Dana-Farber Consortium Protocol 91–01. Blood 2001;97:1211–8.
37. Amylon MD, Shuster J, Pullen J, et al. Intensive high-dose asparaginase consolidation improves survival for pediatric patients with T cell acute lymphoblastic leukemia and advanced stage lymphoblastic lymphoma: a Pediatric Oncology Group study. Leukemia 1999;13:335–42.
38. Pui CH, Sandlund JT, Pei D, et al. Improved outcome for children with acute lymphoblastic leukemia: results of Total Therapy Study XIIIB at St Jude Children's Research Hospital. Blood 2004;104:2690–6.
39. Goldberg JM, Silverman LB, Levy DE, et al. Childhood T-cell acute lymphoblastic leukemia: the Dana-Farber Cancer Institute acute lymphoblastic leukemia consortium experience. J Clin Oncol 2003;21:3616–22.
40. Reiter A, Schrappe M, Ludwig WD, et al. Intensive ALL-type therapy without local radiotherapy provides a 90% event-free survival for children with T-cell lymphoblastic lymphoma: a BFM group report. Blood 2000;95:416–21.
41. Magrath I, Adde M, Shad A, et al. Adults and children with small non-cleaved-cell lymphoma have a similar excellent outcome when treated with the same chemotherapy regimen. J Clin Oncol 1996;14:925–34.
42. Atra A, Imeson JD, Hobson R, et al. Improved outcome in children with advanced stage B-cell non-Hodgkin's lymphoma (B-NHL): results of the United Kingdom Children Cancer Study Group (UKCCSG) 9002 protocol. Br J Cancer 2000;82:1396–402.
43. Bowman WP, Shuster JJ, Cook B, et al. Improved survival for children with B-cell acute lymphoblastic leukemia and stage IV small noncleaved-cell lymphoma: a Pediatric Oncology Group study. J Clin Oncol 1996;14:1252–61.
44. Chessells JM. Relapsed lymphoblastic leukaemia in children: a continuing challenge. Br J Haematol 1998;102:423–38.
45. Gaynon PS, Harris RE, Altman AJ, et al. Bone marrow transplantation versus prolonged intensive chemotherapy for children with acute lymphoblastic leukemia and an initial bone marrow relapse within 12 months of the completion of primary therapy: Children's Oncology Group study CCG-1941. J Clin Oncol 2006;24:3150–6.

46. Raetz EA, Borowitz MJ, Devidas M, et al. Reinduction platform for children with first marrow relapse of acute lymphoblastic leukemia: a Children's Oncology Group study [corrected]. J Clin Oncol 2008;26:3971–8.
47. Nguyen K, Devidas M, Cheng SC, et al. Factors influencing survival after relapse from acute lymphoblastic leukemia: a Children's Oncology Group study. Leukemia 2008;22:2142–50.
48. Ritchey AK, Pollock BH, Lauer SJ, et al. Improved survival of children with isolated CNS relapse of acute lymphoblastic leukemia: a Pediatric Oncology Group study. J Clin Oncol 1999;17:3745–52.
49. Buchanan GR, Boyett JM, Pollock BH, et al. Improved treatment results in boys with overt testicular relapse during or shortly after initial therapy for acute lymphoblastic leukemia. A Pediatric Oncology Group study. Cancer 1991;68:48–55.
50. Hahn T, Wall D, Camitta B, et al. The role of cytotoxic therapy with hematopoietic stem cell transplantation in the therapy of acute lymphoblastic leukemia in children: an evidence-based review. Biol Blood Marrow Transplant 2005;11:823–61.
51. Barrett AJ, Horowitz MM, Pollock BH, et al. Bone marrow transplants from HLA-identical siblings as compared with chemotherapy for children with acute lymphoblastic leukemia in a second remission. N Engl J Med 1994;331:1253–8.
52. Sharathkumar A, Saunders EF, Dror Y, et al. Allogeneic bone marrow transplantation vs chemotherapy for children with Philadelphia chromosome-positive acute lymphoblastic leukemia. Bone Marrow Transplant 2004;33:39–45.
53. Wheeler KA, Richards SM, Bailey CC, et al. Bone marrow transplantation versus chemotherapy in the treatment of very high-risk childhood acute lymphoblastic leukemia in first remission: results from Medical Research Council UKALL X and XI. Blood 2000;96:2412–8.
54. Uderzo C, Valsecchi MG, Balduzzi A, et al. Allogeneic bone marrow transplantation versus chemotherapy in high-risk childhood acute lymphoblastic leukaemia in first remission. Associazione Italiana di Ematologia ed Oncologia Pediatrica (AIEOP) and the Gruppo Italiano Trapianto di Midollo Osseo (GITMO). Br J Haematol 1997;96:387–94.
55. Saarinen UM, Mellander L, Nysom K, et al. Allogeneic bone marrow transplantation in first remission for children with very high-risk acute lymphoblastic leukemia: a retrospective case-control study in the Nordic countries. Nordic Society for Pediatric Hematology and Oncology (NOPHO). Bone Marrow Transplant 1996;17:357–63.
56. Barrett AJ, Horowitz MM, Ash RC, et al. Bone marrow transplantation for Philadelphia chromosome-positive acute lymphoblastic leukemia. Blood 1992;79:3067–70.
57. Bordigoni P, Vernant JP, Souillet G, et al. Allogeneic bone marrow transplantation for children with acute lymphoblastic leukemia in first remission: a cooperative study of the Groupe d'Etude de la Greffe de Moelle Osseuse. J Clin Oncol 1989;7:747–53.
58. Dopfer R, Henze G, Bender-Gotze C, et al. Allogeneic bone marrow transplantation for childhood acute lymphoblastic leukemia in second remission after intensive primary and relapse therapy according to the BFM- and CoALL-protocols: results of the German Cooperative Study. Blood 1991;78:2780–4.
59. Hoogerbrugge PM, Gerritsen EJ, Does-van den Berg AV, et al. Case-control analysis of allogeneic bone marrow transplantation versus maintenance chemotherapy for relapsed ALL in children. Bone Marrow Transplant 1995;15:255–9.

60. Uderzo C, Valsecchi MG, Bacigalupo A, et al. Treatment of childhood acute lymphoblastic leukemia in second remission with allogeneic bone marrow transplantation and chemotherapy: ten-year experience of the Italian Bone Marrow Transplantation Group and the Italian Pediatric Hematology Oncology Association. J Clin Oncol 1995;13:352–8.
61. Moussalem M, Esperou Bourdeau H, Devergie A, et al. Allogeneic bone marrow transplantation for childhood acute lymphoblastic leukemia in second remission: factors predictive of survival, relapse and graft-versus-host disease. Bone Marrow Transplant 1995;15:943–7.
62. Wheeler K, Richards S, Bailey C, et al. Comparison of bone marrow transplant and chemotherapy for relapsed childhood acute lymphoblastic leukaemia: the MRC UKALL X experience. Medical Research Council Working Party on Childhood Leukaemia. Br J Haematol 1998;101:94–103.
63. Harrison G, Richards S, Lawson S, et al. Comparison of allogeneic transplant versus chemotherapy for relapsed childhood acute lymphoblastic leukaemia in the MRC UKALL R1 trial. MRC Childhood Leukaemia Working Party. Ann Oncol 2000;11:999–1006.
64. Eapen M, Raetz E, Zhang MJ, et al. Outcomes after HLA-matched sibling transplantation or chemotherapy in children with B-precursor acute lymphoblastic leukemia in a second remission: a collaborative study of the Children's Oncology Group and the Center for International Blood and Marrow Transplant Research. Blood 2006;107:4961–7.
65. Chessells JM, Bailey C, Wheeler K, et al. Bone marrow transplantation for high-risk childhood lymphoblastic leukaemia in first remission: experience in MRC UKALL X. Lancet 1992;340:565–8.
66. Buchanan GR, Rivera GK, Pollock BH, et al. Alternating drug pairs with or without periodic reinduction in children with acute lymphoblastic leukemia in second bone marrow remission: a Pediatric Oncology Group study. Cancer 2000;88:1166–74.
67. Sadowitz PD, Smith SD, Shuster J, et al. Treatment of late bone marrow relapse in children with acute lymphoblastic leukemia: a Pediatric Oncology Group study. Blood 1993;81:602–9.
68. Balduzzi A, Valsecchi MG, Uderzo C, et al. Chemotherapy versus allogeneic transplantation for very-high-risk childhood acute lymphoblastic leukaemia in first complete remission: comparison by genetic randomisation in an international prospective study. Lancet 2005;366:635–42.
69. Schultz KRBW, Slayton W, Aledo A, et al. Improved early event free survival in children with Philadelphia chromosome-positive acute lymphoblastic leukemia with intensive imatinib in combination with high dose chemotherapy: Children's Oncology Group (COG) study AALL0031 [abstract]. Blood 2007; 110:4a.
70. Eapen M, Rubinstein P, Zhang MJ, et al. Comparable long-term survival after unrelated and HLA-matched sibling donor hematopoietic stem cell transplantations for acute leukemia in children younger than 18 months. J Clin Oncol 2006; 24:145–51.
71. Jacobsohn DA, Hewlett B, Morgan E, et al. Favorable outcome for infant acute lymphoblastic leukemia after hematopoietic stem cell transplantation. Biol Blood Marrow Transplant 2005;11:999–1005.
72. Kosaka Y, Koh K, Kinukawa N, et al. Infant acute lymphoblastic leukemia with MLL gene rearrangements: outcome following intensive chemotherapy and hematopoietic stem cell transplantation. Blood 2004;104:3527–34.

73. Silverman LB, Weinstein HJ. Treatment of childhood leukemia. Curr Opin Oncol 1997;9:26–33.
74. Pui CH, Chessells JM, Camitta B, et al. Clinical heterogeneity in childhood acute lymphoblastic leukemia with 11q23 rearrangements. Leukemia 2003;17:700–6.
75. Luciani M, Rana I, Pansini V, et al. Infant leukaemia: clinical, biological and therapeutic advances. Acta Paediatr Suppl 2006;95:47–51.
76. Nagayama J, Tomizawa D, Koh K, et al. Infants with acute lymphoblastic leukemia and a germline MLL gene are highly curable with use of chemotherapy alone: results from the Japan Infant Leukemia Study Group. Blood 2006;107:4663–5.
77. Davies SM, Ramsay NK, Klein JP, et al. Comparison of preparative regimens in transplants for children with acute lymphoblastic leukemia. J Clin Oncol 2000; 18:340–7.
78. Bunin N, Aplenc R, Kamani N, et al. Randomized trial of busulfan vs total body irradiation containing conditioning regimens for children with acute lymphoblastic leukemia: a Pediatric Blood and Marrow Transplant Consortium study. Bone Marrow Transplant 2003;32:543–8.
79. Shah AJ, Lenarsky C, Kapoor N, et al. Busulfan and cyclophosphamide as a conditioning regimen for pediatric acute lymphoblastic leukemia patients undergoing bone marrow transplantation. J Pediatr Hematol Oncol 2004;26:91–7.
80. Sullivan KM, Weiden PL, Storb R, et al. Influence of acute and chronic graft-versus-host disease on relapse and survival after bone marrow transplantation from HLA-identical siblings as treatment of acute and chronic leukemia. Blood 1989;73:1720–8.
81. Bader P, Kreyenberg H, Henze GH, et al. Prognostic value of minimal residual disease quantification before allogeneic stem-cell transplantation in relapsed childhood acute lymphoblastic leukemia: the ALL-REZ BFM Study Group. J Clin Oncol 2009;27:377–84.
82. Dini G, Valsecchi MG, Micalizzi C, et al. Impact of marrow unrelated donor search duration on outcome of children with acute lymphoblastic leukemia in second remission. Bone Marrow Transplant 2003;32:325–31.
83. Bunin N, Carston M, Wall D, et al. Unrelated marrow transplantation for children with acute lymphoblastic leukemia in second remission. Blood 2002; 99:3151–7.
84. Saarinen-Pihkala UM, Gustafsson G, Ringden O, et al. No disadvantage in outcome of using matched unrelated donors as compared with matched sibling donors for bone marrow transplantation in children with acute lymphoblastic leukemia in second remission. J Clin Oncol 2001;19:3406–14.
85. Green A, Clarke E, Hunt L, et al. Children with acute lymphoblastic leukemia who receive T-cell-depleted HLA mismatched marrow allografts from unrelated donors have an increased incidence of primary graft failure but a similar overall transplant outcome. Blood 1999;94:2236–46.
86. Oakhill A, Pamphilon DH, Potter MN, et al. Unrelated donor bone marrow transplantation for children with relapsed acute lymphoblastic leukaemia in second complete remission. Br J Haematol 1996;94:574–8.
87. Fleming DR, Henslee-Downey PJ, Romond EH, et al. Allogeneic bone marrow transplantation with T cell-depleted partially matched related donors for advanced acute lymphoblastic leukemia in children and adults: a comparative matched cohort study. Bone Marrow Transplant 1996;17:917–22.
88. Ball LM, Lankester AC, Bredius RG, et al. Graft dysfunction and delayed immune reconstitution following haploidentical peripheral blood hematopoietic stem cell transplantation. Bone Marrow Transplant 2005;35(Suppl 1):S35–8.

89. Lang P, Greil J, Bader P, et al. Long-term outcome after haploidentical stem cell transplantation in children. Blood Cells Mol Dis 2004;33:281–7.

90. Bosi A, Laszlo D, Labopin M, et al. Second allogeneic bone marrow transplantation in acute leukemia: results of a survey by the European Cooperative Group for Blood and Marrow Transplantation. J Clin Oncol 2001;19:3675–84.

91. Schroeder H, Gustafsson G, Saarinen-Pihkala UM, et al. Allogeneic bone marrow transplantation in second remission of childhood acute lymphoblastic leukemia: a population-based case control study from the Nordic countries. Bone Marrow Transplant 1999;23:555–60.

92. Sanders JE, Thomas ED, Buckner CD, et al. Marrow transplantation for children with acute lymphoblastic leukemia in second remission. Blood 1987; 70:324–6.

93. Lawson SE, Darbyshire PJ. Use of donor lymphocytes in extramedullary relapse of childhood acute lymphoblastic leukaemia following bone marrow transplantation. Bone Marrow Transplant 1998;22:829–30.

94. Atra A, Millar B, Shepherd V, et al. Donor lymphocyte infusion for childhood acute lymphoblastic leukaemia relapsing after bone marrow transplantation. Br J Haematol 1997;97:165–8.

95. Collins RH Jr, Shpilberg O, Drobyski WR, et al. Donor leukocyte infusions in 140 patients with relapsed malignancy after allogeneic bone marrow transplantation. J Clin Oncol 1997;15:433–44.

96. Helg C, Starobinski M, Jeannet M, et al. Donor lymphocyte infusion for the treatment of relapse after allogeneic hematopoietic stem cell transplantation. Leuk Lymphoma 1998;29:301–13.

97. Porter DL, Collins RH Jr, Hardy C, et al. Treatment of relapsed leukemia after unrelated donor marrow transplantation with unrelated donor leukocyte infusions. Blood 2000;95:1214–21.

98. Absalon MJ, Smith FO. Treatment strategies for pediatric acute myeloid leukemia. Expert Opin Pharmacother 2009;10:57–79.

99. Creutzig U, Ritter J, Zimmermann M, et al. Improved treatment results in high-risk pediatric acute myeloid leukemia patients after intensification with high-dose cytarabine and mitoxantrone: results of Study Acute Myeloid Leukemia-Berlin-Frankfurt-Munster 93. J Clin Oncol 2001;19:2705–13.

100. Stevens RF, Hann IM, Wheatley K, et al. Marked improvements in outcome with chemotherapy alone in paediatric acute myeloid leukemia: results of the United Kingdom Medical Research Council's 10th AML trial. MRC Childhood Leukaemia Working Party. Br J Haematol 1998;101:130–40.

101. Perel Y, Auvrignon A, Leblanc T, et al. Impact of addition of maintenance therapy to intensive induction and consolidation chemotherapy for childhood acute myeloblastic leukemia: results of a prospective randomized trial, LAME 89/91. J Clin Oncol 2002;20:2774–82.

102. Capizzi RL, Poole M, Cooper MR, et al. Treatment of poor risk acute leukemia with sequential high-dose ARA-C and asparaginase. Blood 1984; 63:694–700.

103. Woods WG, Ruymann FB, Lampkin BC, et al. The role of timing of high-dose cytosine arabinoside intensification and of maintenance therapy in the treatment of children with acute nonlymphocytic leukemia. Cancer 1990;66:1106–13.

104. Oliansky DM, Rizzo JD, Aplan PD, et al. The role of cytotoxic therapy with hematopoietic stem cell transplantation in the therapy of acute myeloid leukemia in children: an evidence-based review. Biol Blood Marrow Transplant 2007;13: 1–25.

105. Bleakley M, Lau L, Shaw PJ, et al. Bone marrow transplantation for paediatric AML in first remission: a systematic review and meta-analysis. Bone Marrow Transplant 2002;29:843–52.

106. Ravindranath Y, Yeager AM, Chang MN, et al. Autologous bone marrow transplantation versus intensive consolidation chemotherapy for acute myeloid leukemia in childhood. Pediatric Oncology Group. N Engl J Med 1996;334: 1428–34.

107. Amadori S, Testi AM, Arico M, et al. Prospective comparative study of bone marrow transplantation and postremission chemotherapy for childhood acute myelogenous leukemia. The Associazione Italiana Ematologia ed Oncologia Pediatrica Cooperative Group. J Clin Oncol 1993;11:1046–54.

108. Woods WG, Neudorf S, Gold S, et al. A comparison of allogeneic bone marrow transplantation, autologous bone marrow transplantation, and aggressive chemotherapy in children with acute myeloid leukemia in remission. Blood 2001;97:56–62.

109. Feig SA, Lampkin B, Nesbit ME, et al. Outcome of BMT during first complete remission of AML: a comparison of two sequential studies by the Children's Cancer Group. Bone Marrow Transplant 1993;12:65–71.

110. Burnett AK, Goldstone AH, Stevens RM, et al. Randomised comparison of addition of autologous bone-marrow transplantation to intensive chemotherapy for acute myeloid leukaemia in first remission: results of MRC AML 10 trial. UK Medical Research Council Adult and Children's Leukaemia Working Parties. Lancet 1998;351:700–8.

111. Razzouk BI, Estey E, Pounds S, et al. Impact of age on outcome of pediatric acute myeloid leukemia: a report from 2 institutions. Cancer 2006;106:2495–502.

112. Ortega JJ, Madero L, Martin G, et al. Treatment with all-trans retinoic acid and anthracycline monochemotherapy for children with acute promyelocytic leukemia: a multicenter study by the PETHEMA Group. J Clin Oncol 2005;23: 7632–40.

113. Testi AM, Biondi A, Lo Coco F, et al. GIMEMA-AIEOPAIDA protocol for the treatment of newly diagnosed acute promyelocytic leukemia (APL) in children. Blood 2005;106:447–53.

114. De Botton S, Chevret S, Sanz M, et al. Additional chromosomal abnormalities in patients with acute promyelocytic leukaemia (APL) do not confer poor prognosis: results of APL 93 trial. Br J Haematol 2000;111:801–6.

115. Fenaux P, Chevret S, Guerci A, et al. Long-term follow-up confirms the benefit of all-trans retinoic acid in acute promyelocytic leukemia. European APL group. Leukemia 2000;14:1371–7.

116. Ravindranath Y, Abella E, Krischer JP, et al. Acute myeloid leukemia (AML) in Down's syndrome is highly responsive to chemotherapy: experience on Pediatric Oncology Group AML Study 8498. Blood 1992;80:2210–4.

117. Gamis AS, Woods WG, Alonzo TA, et al. Increased age at diagnosis has a significantly negative effect on outcome in children with Down syndrome and acute myeloid leukemia: a report from the Children's Cancer Group Study 2891. J Clin Oncol 2003;21:3415–22.

118. Massey GV. Transient leukemia in newborns with Down syndrome. Pediatr Blood Cancer 2005;44:29–32.

119. Dahl GV, Kalwinsky DK, Mirro J Jr, et al. Allogeneic bone marrow transplantation in a program of intensive sequential chemotherapy for children and young adults with acute nonlymphocytic leukemia in first remission. J Clin Oncol 1990;8:295–303.

120. Wells RJ, Woods WG, Buckley JD, et al. Treatment of newly diagnosed children and adolescents with acute myeloid leukemia: a Childrens Cancer Group study. J Clin Oncol 1994;12:2367–77.
121. Nesbit ME Jr, Buckley JD, Feig SA, et al. Chemotherapy for induction of remission of childhood acute myeloid leukemia followed by marrow transplantation or multiagent chemotherapy: a report from the Childrens Cancer Group. J Clin Oncol 1994;12:127–35.
122. Aladjidi N, Auvrignon A, Leblanc T, et al. Outcome in children with relapsed acute myeloid leukemia after initial treatment with the French Leucemie Aique Myeloide Enfant (LAME) 89/91 protocol of the French Society of Pediatric Hematology and Immunology. J Clin Oncol 2003;21:4377–85.
123. Watson M, Buck G, Wheatley K, et al. Adverse impact of bone marrow transplantation on quality of life in acute myeloid leukaemia patients; analysis of the UK Medical Research Council AML 10 Trial. Eur J Cancer 2004;40:971–8.
124. Cassileth PA, Harrington DP, Appelbaum FR, et al. Chemotherapy compared with autologous or allogeneic bone marrow transplantation in the management of acute myeloid leukemia in first remission. N Engl J Med 1998;339:1649–56.
125. Zittoun RA, Mandelli F, Willemze R, et al. Autologous or allogeneic bone marrow transplantation compared with intensive chemotherapy in acute myelogenous leukemia. European Organization for Research and Treatment of Cancer (EORTC) and the Gruppo Italiano Malattie Ematologiche Maligne dell'Adulto (GIMEMA) Leukemia Cooperative Groups. N Engl J Med 1995;332:217–23.
126. Burnett AK, Wheatley K, Goldstone AH, et al. The value of allogeneic bone marrow transplant in patients with acute myeloid leukaemia at differing risk of relapse: results of the UK MRC AML 10 trial. Br J Haematol 2002;118:385–400.
127. Chen AR, Alonzo TA, Woods WG, et al. Current controversies: which patients with acute myeloid leukaemia should receive a bone marrow transplantation?–an American view. Br J Haematol 2002;118:378–84.
128. Creutzig U, Reinhardt D. Current controversies: which patients with acute myeloid leukaemia should receive a bone marrow transplantation?–a European view. Br J Haematol 2002;118:365–77.
129. Alonzo TA, Wells RJ, Woods WG, et al. Postremission therapy for children with acute myeloid leukemia: the children's cancer group experience in the transplant era. Leukemia 2005;19:965–70.
130. Pession A, Rondelli R, Paolucci P, et al. Hematopoietic stem cell transplantation in childhood: report from the bone marrow transplantation group of the Associazione Italiana Ematologia Oncologia Pediatrica (AIEOP). Haematologica 2000;85:638–46.
131. Gorin NC, Labopin M, Fouillard L, et al. Retrospective evaluation of autologous bone marrow transplantation vs allogeneic bone marrow transplantation from an HLA identical related donor in acute myelocytic leukemia. A study of the European Cooperative Group for Blood and Marrow Transplantation (EBMT). Bone Marrow Transplant 1996;18:111–7.
132. Ravindranath Y, Chang M, Steuber CP, et al. Pediatric Oncology Group (POG) studies of acute myeloid leukemia (AML): a review of four consecutive childhood AML trials conducted between 1981 and 2000. Leukemia 2005;19:2101–16.
133. Smith FO, Alonzo TA, Gerbing RB, et al. Long-term results of children with acute myeloid leukemia: a report of three consecutive Phase III trials by the Children's Cancer Group: CCG 251, CCG 213 and CCG 2891. Leukemia 2005;19:2054–62.

134. Ferry C, Socie G. Busulfan-cyclophosphamide versus total body irradiation-cyclophosphamide as preparative regimen before allogeneic hematopoietic stem cell transplantation for acute myeloid leukemia: what have we learned? Exp Hematol 2003;31:1182–6.

135. Michel G, Gluckman E, Esperou-Bourdeau H, et al. Allogeneic bone marrow transplantation for children with acute myeloblastic leukemia in first complete remission: impact of conditioning regimen without total-body irradiation–a report from the Societe Francaise de Greffe de Moelle. J Clin Oncol 1994;12:1217–22.

136. Woodard P, Barfield R, Hale G, et al. Outcome of hematopoietic stem cell transplantation for pediatric patients with therapy-related acute myeloid leukemia or myelodysplastic syndrome. Pediatr Blood Cancer 2006;47:931–5.

137. Woolfrey AE, Gooley TA, Sievers EL, et al. Bone marrow transplantation for children less than 2 years of age with acute myelogenous leukemia or myelodysplastic syndrome. Blood 1998;92:3546–56.

138. Hsu KC, Keever-Taylor CA, Wilton A, et al. Improved outcome in HLA-identical sibling hematopoietic stem-cell transplantation for acute myelogenous leukemia predicted by KIR and HLA genotypes. Blood 2005;105:4878–84.

139. Meshinchi S, Leisenring WM, Carpenter PA, et al. Survival after second hematopoietic stem cell transplantation for recurrent pediatric acute myeloid leukemia. Biol Blood Marrow Transplant 2003;9:706–13.

140. Pulsipher MA. Treatment of CML in pediatric patients: should imatinib mesylate (STI-571, Gleevec) or allogeneic hematopoietic cell transplant be front-line therapy? Pediatr Blood Cancer 2004;43:523–33.

141. Druker BJ, Guilhot F, O'Brien SG, et al. Five-year follow-up of patients receiving imatinib for chronic myeloid leukemia. N Engl J Med 2006;355:2408–17.

142. Shah NP. Loss of response to imatinib: mechanisms and management. Hematology Am Soc Hematol Educ Program 2005;183–7.

143. Kolb EA, Pan Q, Ladanyi M, et al. Imatinib mesylate in Philadelphia chromosome-positive leukemia of childhood. Cancer 2003;98:2643–50.

144. Goldman JM, Marin D. Management decisions in chronic myeloid leukemia. Semin Hematol 2003;40:97–103.

145. Wassmann B, Pfeifer H, Scheuring U, et al. Therapy with imatinib mesylate (Glivec) preceding allogeneic stem cell transplantation (SCT) in relapsed or refractory Philadelphia-positive acute lymphoblastic leukemia (Ph+ALL). Leukemia 2002;16:2358–65.

146. Weisdorf DJ, Anasetti C, Antin JH, et al. Allogeneic bone marrow transplantation for chronic myelogenous leukemia: comparative analysis of unrelated versus matched sibling donor transplantation. Blood 2002;99:1971–7.

147. Goldman JM, Druker BJ. Chronic myeloid leukemia: current treatment options. Blood 2001;98:2039–42.

148. Gratwohl A, Hermans J, Goldman JM, et al. Risk assessment for patients with chronic myeloid leukaemia before allogeneic blood or marrow transplantation. Chronic Leukemia Working Party of the European Group for Blood and Marrow Transplantation. Lancet 1998;352:1087–92.

149. Silver RT, Woolf SH, Hehlmann R, et al. An evidence-based analysis of the effect of busulfan, hydroxyurea, interferon, and allogeneic bone marrow transplantation in treating the chronic phase of chronic myeloid leukemia: developed for the American Society of Hematology. Blood 1999;94:1517–36.

150. Stary J, Locatelli F, Niemeyer CM. Stem cell transplantation for aplastic anemia and myelodysplastic syndrome. Bone Marrow Transplant 2005;35(Suppl 1): S13–6.

151. Niemeyer CM, Kratz CP, Hasle H. Pediatric myelodysplastic syndromes. Curr Treat Options Oncol 2005;6:209–14.
152. Hasle H, Niemeyer CM, Chessells JM, et al. A pediatric approach to the WHO classification of myelodysplastic and myeloproliferative diseases. Leukemia 2003;17:277–82.
153. Mandel K, Dror Y, Poon A, et al. A practical, comprehensive classification for pediatric myelodysplastic syndromes: the CCC system. J Pediatr Hematol Oncol 2002;24:596–605.
154. Occhipinti E, Correa H, Yu L, et al. Comparison of two new classifications for pediatric myelodysplastic and myeloproliferative disorders. Pediatr Blood Cancer 2005;44:240–4.
155. Hasle H, Baumann I, Bergstrasser E, et al. The International Prognostic Scoring System (IPSS) for childhood myelodysplastic syndrome (MDS) and juvenile myelomonocytic leukemia (JMML). Leukemia 2004;18:2008–14.
156. Niemeyer CM, Arico M, Basso G, et al. Chronic myelomonocytic leukemia in childhood: a retrospective analysis of 110 cases. European Working Group on Myelodysplastic Syndromes in Childhood (EWOG-MDS). Blood 1997;89: 3534–43.
157. Hasle H, Arico M, Basso G, et al. Myelodysplastic syndrome, juvenile myelomonocytic leukemia, and acute myeloid leukemia associated with complete or partial monosomy 7. European Working Group on MDS in Childhood (EWOG-MDS). Leukemia 1999;13:376–85.
158. Woods WG, Barnard DR, Alonzo TA, et al. Prospective study of 90 children requiring treatment for juvenile myelomonocytic leukemia or myelodysplastic syndrome: a report from the Children's Cancer Group. J Clin Oncol 2002;20: 434–40.
159. Freedman MH, Estrov Z, Chan HS. Juvenile chronic myelogenous leukemia. Am J Pediatr Hematol Oncol 1988;10:261–7.
160. Locatelli F, Nollke P, Zecca M, et al. Hematopoietic stem cell transplantation (HSCT) in children with juvenile myelomonocytic leukemia (JMML): results of the EWOG-MDS/EBMT trial. Blood 2005;105:410–9.
161. Yusuf U, Frangoul HA, Gooley TA, et al. Allogeneic bone marrow transplantation in children with myelodysplastic syndrome or juvenile myelomonocytic leukemia: the Seattle experience. Bone Marrow Transplant 2004;33:805–14.
162. Smith FO, King R, Nelson G, et al. Unrelated donor bone marrow transplantation for children with juvenile myelomonocytic leukaemia. Br J Haematol 2002;116: 716–24.
163. Bunin N, Saunders F, Leahey A, et al. Alternative donor bone marrow transplantation for children with juvenile myelomonocytic leukemia. J Pediatr Hematol Oncol 1999;21:479–85.
164. Runde V, de Witte T, Arnold R, et al. Bone marrow transplantation from HLA-identical siblings as first-line treatment in patients with myelodysplastic syndromes: early transplantation is associated with improved outcome. Chronic Leukemia Working Party of the European Group for Blood and Marrow Transplantation. Bone Marrow Transplant 1998;21:255–61.
165. Arico M, Biondi A, Pui CH. Juvenile myelomonocytic leukemia. Blood 1997;90: 479–88.
166. Yoshimi A, Mohamed M, Bierings M, et al. Second allogeneic hematopoietic stem cell transplantation (HSCT) results in outcome similar to that of first HSCT for patients with juvenile myelomonocytic leukemia. Leukemia 2007;21: 556–60.

167. Yoshimi A, Bader P, Matthes-Martin S, et al. Donor leukocyte infusion after hematopoietic stem cell transplantation in patients with juvenile myelomonocytic leukemia. Leukemia 2005;19:971–7.
168. Creutzig U, Bender-Gotze C, Ritter J, et al. The role of intensive AML-specific therapy in treatment of children with RAEB and RAEB-t. Leukemia 1998;12: 652–9.
169. Kletzel M, Jacobsohn D, Tse W, et al. Reduced intensity transplants (RIT) in pediatrics: a review. Pediatr Transplant 2005;9(Suppl 7):63–70.

Stem Cell Source and Outcome After Hematopoietic Stem Cell Transplantation (HSCT) in Children and Adolescents with Acute Leukemia

Christina Peters, MD[a],*, Jacqueline M. Cornish, MD[b],
Suhag H. Parikh, MD[c], Joanne Kurtzberg, MD[c]

KEYWORDS

- Bone marrow • Peripheral blood stem cells
- Umbilical Cord blood • Allogeneic stem cell transplantation
- Children • Adolescents • Acute Leukemia

The scientific basis of clinical Hematopoietic Stem Cell Transplantation (HSCT) was established with the seminal animal experiments of Jacobson and Lorenz performed in 1949 and 1950, demonstrating a protective effect of infusion of splenic or BM cells on lethally irradiated mice.[1,2] While the impetus for these initial "irradiation protection" experiments was generated by concerns for radiation induced marrow damage resulting from nuclear explosions during WWII, its therapeutic potential to cure inherited and naturally acquired diseases of the hematopoietic and immune systems was soon recognized. Early attempts at allogeneic BM transplantation were unsuccessful because of graft rejection or leukemic relapse. With the discovery and understanding of the role of the human leukocyte antigen (HLA) system in tolerance and rejection of transplanted donor cells in 1958, the knowledge of which has rapidly evolved since, the field has advanced rapidly.[3,4] The first successful allogeneic HSCTs were

[a] Stem Cell Transplantation Unit, St Anna Children's Hospital, Kinderspitalgasse 6, A-1090 Vienna, Austria
[b] Paediatric Stem Cell Transplantation, Women's and Children's Services, Bristol Royal Hospital for Children, Bristol, BS2 8BJ, UK
[c] Division of Pediatric Blood and Marrow Transplantation, Duke University Medical Center, Box 3350, Durham, NC 27705, USA
* Corresponding author.
E-mail address: christina.peters@stanna.at

Pediatr Clin N Am 57 (2010) 27–46
doi:10.1016/j.pcl.2010.01.004
0031-3955/10/$ – see front matter © 2010 Elsevier Inc. All rights reserved.

pediatric.theclinics.com

performed for children with severe combined immune deficiency (SCID) in 1968 by Drs Robert Good and Jon van Rood using BM from HLA matched sibling donors.[5,6] This was followed by increasing number of HSCTs in the subsequent years. In 1977, the Seattle team, led by E. Donnall Thomas, reported outcomes of 100 patients with refractory acute leukemia undergoing HLA *matched related donor bone marrow* transplantation with total body irradiation (TBI) based regimen, of which 13 patients survived long-term, a remarkable achievement for a disease that was regarded as incurable at that time.[7] Many patients in need of a transplant lacked a matched related donor limiting wider applicability of HSCT at this time. The first successful *matched unrelated donor bone marrow* transplant was performed in Seattle in 1979 in a patient with refractory leukemia, who successfully engrafted and did not have graft-versus-host-disease (GVHD).[8,9] Even though the patient died of recurrent leukemia 2 years post-transplant, this experience demonstrated feasibility of matched unrelated donor HSCT and was instrumental in the eventual establishment of the National Marrow Donor Program (NMDP) in 1986,[9] 12 years after the Anthony Nolan Donor Register had been established in London. Similar registries have since been established in several other countries. Currently there is tremendous international collaboration among these registries and very effective exchange of donor marrow for patients in need.

It was shown for the first time in 1962 that hematopoietic progenitor cells from the peripheral blood (*peripheral blood progenitor cells, PBPC*) were capable of restoring radiation induced aplasia in mice.[10] However, the very low concentration of PBPCs in unmanipulated peripheral blood was a major barrier to their use in clinical transplantation. With the discovery of G-CSF and its ability to mobilize CD34+ hematopoietic progenitors into peripheral blood and improvements in pheresis technology, this approach became feasible and, since 1995, has resulted in a significant increase in use of PBPCs, with 60%–70% of current allogeneic transplants for adult recipients worldwide using PBPC as the graft source in place of BM.[11] While most of these transplants are from HLA-matched related and unrelated adult donors, graft manipulation (T-cell depletion and megadose CD34+ transplantation) has opened up the possibility of transplantation across broader HLA barriers, such as in mismatched family member donor (haploidentical) transplants. Martelli and co-workers showed that CD34+ selected PBSC from full-haplotype mismatched donors could overcome graft rejection and graft versus host disease (GVHD) in patients with acute leukemia.[12]

Over the past two decades, *umbilical cord blood (UCB)* has emerged as a viable graft source for HSCT. In the mid-1980s, Dr Ted Boyse, an immunologist at Memorial Sloan Kettering Cancer Center, demonstrated restoration of marrow function in lethally irradiated mice with placental blood from near term mouse donors. In the same period, Dr Hal Broxmeyer demonstrated that human UCB was a rich source of hematopoietic progenitor cells, that cord blood progenitors had higher proliferative capacity as compared with BM cells and also that they could be readily cryopreserved.[13] The first use of UCB as a source of hematopoietic stem cells for transplantation was reported in 1988 following an international, multi-institutional collaboration, when a 6-yr-old boy with Fanconi anemia from the USA underwent a successful transplant in Paris.[14] The source of the donor cells was umbilical cord blood from his unaffected, HLA-matched sibling. Currently, more than 20 years post-transplant, he is durably engrafted, immunologically competent, with normal hematopoietic function and overall good health. This proved that UCB harvested from a single donor contained sufficient dose of stem cells for successful reconstitution of a pediatric patient. An increasing number of HLA matched related UCB transplants were performed in the subsequent 5 years, demonstrating acceptable rates of engraftment and a lower incidence of GVHD as compared with BM.[15]

In 1992, the first public unrelated UCB bank was established at the New York Blood Center by Dr Pablo Rubinstein to explore the use of banked umbilical cord blood from unrelated donors for HSCT.[16] In 1993, the first unrelated UCB transplant was performed in a young child with acute leukemia at Duke University Medical Center using an unrelated cord blood donor from the New York Blood Center. The outcomes of 25 successive transplants with unrelated umbilical cord blood banked at the New York Blood Center, and transplanted at Duke University, were reported in 1996.[17] Important observations in these patients and subsequent reports from other centers and registries including the University of Minnesota, New York Blood Center, the Center for International Blood and Marrow Transplant Research (CIBMTR) and the European Cord Blood Registry, (Eurocord)[18–21] demonstrated that (i) unrelated cord blood could engraft in children undergoing myeloablative therapy for treatment of leukemia, hemoglobinopathies, inherited immunodeficiency syndromes and other genetic diseases, (ii) reasonable outcomes could be achieved using partially HLA mismatched grafts, (iii) the incidence and severity of acute and chronic GVHD was lower and milder than that seen with matched unrelated BM transplants, (iv) graft versus leukemia effect (GVL) was preserved, (v) cell dose strongly correlated with clinical outcomes including time to engraftment and probability of overall engraftment and survival and (vi) engraftment times were observed to be slower than that of BM or mobilized PBSC.

A prospective study (COBLT) and several retrospective analyses have further established cord blood's place in allogeneic transplantation.[21–24] Underscoring the growing need to increase cord blood inventories and to create a centralized donor database (Single Point of Access, SPA, registry) and coordinating centers for unrelated cord blood and adult donors, the Stem Cell Therapeutics and Research Act was enacted in the USA in 2005. An international inventory of most of the adult unrelated donors as well as cord blood donor units is maintained by Bone Marrow Donors Worldwide (www.bmdw.org). As of late 2009, it is estimated to have HLA data from 63 registries and 128 cord blood banks accounting for more than 13 million adult donors and nearly 400,000 cord blood units.

Autologous BM or *peripheral blood* is not recommended in the treatment of acute leukemia due to an increased incidence of relapse. Autologous cord blood is also not recommended for treatment of malignant conditions because of concerns of presence of disease.[25] Autologous transplant does have a role in the treatment of solid tumors such as neuroblastoma and brain tumors, mainly by enabling the delivery of high dose chemotherapy.

In summary, the various hematopoietic stem cell sources in use today are: BM, PBPC, and UCB. These stem cell sources are commonly derived from HLA matched related donors (MRD) or from alternative donors, eg, HLA-matched adult unrelated donors (MUD), HLA mismatched family donors or cryopreserved umbilical cord blood from HLA-matched or partially mismatched related or unrelated donors. This review will address the advantages and limitations of the different stem cell sources from the range of potential donors.

PROCUREMENT OF GRAFT AND DONOR SAFETY
General Concepts

All HSCT donors must undergo donor screening using testing and screening questionnaires that are in compliance with the applicable laws of their country. Generally donors are screened, within 30 days of their donation, for infectious diseases that can be transmitted through the blood, eg, Human Immunodeficiency Virus (HIV) 1 and 2, Human T-lymphotropic virus (HTLV) 1 and 2, Cytomegalovirus (CMV), Hepatitis

B and C, West Nile virus, Syphilis and Chagas disease. Many transplant centers also screen donors for herpes simplex virus (HSV), varicella zoster virus (VZV), Toxoplasmosis and Epstein Barr virus (EBV). Medical history questionnaires target risk factors for transmission of genetic or infectious diseases. All donors must have a screening physical examination and must give written informed consent for donation. In the case of children, their parents or legal guardians provide consent. In the case of cord blood donors, the mother of the baby provides consent.

Bone marrow

Bone marrow harvest from minors BM harvest from sibling donors is the most common method of obtaining hematopoietic progenitor and stem cells. In a survey among European pediatric HSCT centers almost all performed this procedure under general anesthesia of the donor. Only a small minority offer BM collection under local/spinal anesthesia, or use both anesthetic options.[26] BM harvest is commonly achieved by repeated insertion of large bore needles into the posterior iliac crests (generally 50–200 times on both sides). This technique of multiple site needle aspiration is not appropriate for young children as the extent of tissue damage due to the smaller size of their bones, post procedure inflammation, chronic scarring and postoperative discomfort is generally unacceptable. Multiple aspirations from one puncture site by repositioning the harvest needle within the bone, are an alternative and preferable practice to limit the number of bone entry sites.

Special attention has to be given to the circulating blood volume of a pediatric donor, and transfusion of irradiated, ABO-compatible red cells might be indicated during or after the BM collection.[27] A directed donor unit might be procured in advance of the procedure, or, in larger donors, an autologous unit of blood might be donated a few weeks before the procedure. All donors should be placed on iron supplementation a minimum of a few weeks before and 2–3 months after a BM harvest, unless blood is transfused during or shortly after the procedure.

An alternative method is described by Kletzel and colleagues using a semi-automated processing technique to salvage red blood cells from pediatric BM donors to minimize the risk of severe anemia following BM harvest and ABO incompatibility in the recipient. Sixty healthy, HLA-matched, pediatric BM donors with a median age 8.0 years (2–19) were studied. The viability before and after cell processing was 99%, with reduced risk of post-bone marrow harvest anemia, decreased volume infused into the donor, and enriching the mononuclear and CD34+ cell population, without affecting hematopoietic reconstitution.[28]

Another option is the administration of recombinant human erythropoietin (rh-Epo) to normal pediatric BM donors. Martinez and colleagues have evaluated the efficacy of administering rh-Epo to 11 healthy BM donors weighing less than 30 kg. For three weeks before harvesting, the donors received 100 units/kg/day rh-Epo subcutaneously and oral iron supplementation (2.5 mg/kg twice daily). Six children with hematocrit values below the normal ranges for their ages after BM harvesting, received 150 units/kg rh-Epo three times a week for 2 additional weeks and oral iron supplementation at the same dose. No rh-Epo side-effects were observed. Hematocrit values before harvesting increased to between 5.7 and 18.5% (mean 10.6 ± 1.2) above the baseline values ($P = .0001$). Hematocrit after harvesting decreased to between 4 and 19.5% (mean, 11.1) below the day 0 pre-harvest values. On day +15 all but one patient had a hematocrit value greater than or equal to baseline value. No patient required transfusion during or after BM harvest.[29] However, as this product is not licensed for this indication and the fact that there is no long term safety data with this approach, we strongly discourage incorporation of this practice in routine marrow harvest from healthy pediatric donors.

Pediatric marrow donor safety data is limited to publications from small single-institution studies. Buckner described the Seattle experience with 128 children less than age 10, and an additional 343 donors between the ages of 10 and 19. As with adults, life threatening complications in donors under the age of 20 undergoing BM harvest were rare (2/507, 0.39%).[27] Sanders described harvests from 23 donors under the age of 2 years. None of these donors experienced major difficulties following the harvest. Three donors had significant medical problems diagnosed during the pre-donation evaluation. All harvests were performed from the posterior iliac crests under general anesthesia. Irradiated blood transfusions were given to 85% of these younger donors during the procedure, due to the large volume of marrow required for older, larger recipients. The volume of marrow obtained ranged from 11.5 to 19.3 mL/kg donor weight and contained from 2.5 to 10.4 × 10(8) nucleated cells/kg donor weight.[30] No fatal complications were reported in a recent analysis of Halter and colleagues in donors below 20 years of age. Three pediatric donors with severe adverse events were reported, two BM (cardiac arrest, pulmonary edema) and one PBPC donor (transfusion related acute lung injury).[31] However, the potential risk of blood transfusion associated side effects (eg, infections, tranfusion related acute lung injury, hemolytic transfusion reactions) have to be considered.[32,33]

The most frequent side effects of marrow harvest are mild and self-limiting such as fatigue, transient anemia and local pain at the harvest site(s). Risks of general anesthesia are no greater than for any other surgical procedure. The procedure rarely results in long term morbidities or life-threatening complications. However, it is important that the team responsible for information, pre-harvest physical examination, donor clearance, general anesthesia and BM collection is experienced in all of the necessary procedures.

Despite the growing numbers of pediatric sibling stem cell donors, little information is available on the potential for adverse psychological responses in the pediatric donor population. Wiener and colleagues investigated eight published reports assessing the pediatric sibling donor experience. Studies were generally small (n<44) and cross-sectional. Results suggested a range of psychological distress responses, with greater distress in the pediatric donor than non-donor siblings. They strongly suggest that for these youngsters, psychological distress exists before, during, or after stem cell donation and transplantation, due to disease impact on the family, irrespective of outcome. Recommendations include future longitudinal research on sibling donor psychological status, identification of sibling donors at high risk of disturbed responses, and development of educational and specific interventions for this generally overlooked but invaluable pediatric population.[34] In general, in the case of a pediatric donor, it has been suggested that there may be a benefit to the donor as well as the patient.[35,36]

Bone marrow harvest from adults BM harvest from adults is technically the same as with pediatric donors. Minor adverse events, such as transient syncope, headache, and minor local infections occur in 6%–20% of marrow harvests. However, severe adverse events related to harvest are rare (0.1–0.3%) and risk of death is estimated to be ~1 in 10,000 (0.0001%). Thus, careful donor selection and follow up are required to ensure donor safety.[37]

Peripheral blood progenitor cells (PBPC)
PBPC collection from G-CSF stimulated pediatric sibling donors Peripheral blood apheresis is performed following G-CSF administration, and usually takes about 4–6

hours per day. The number of collections depends on the number of stem cells collected with each procedure. Though the PBPC donation procedures in adult and pediatric donors are technically similar, there are medical risks and complications of PBSC collection that are more likely in pediatric donors. These include difficulty with vascular access with possible need for central venous catheter placement, need for anesthesia or sedation, low platelet count, anemia, need for red blood cell or volume priming before apheresis, vasovagal complications, shifts in blood volume with resultant cardiovascular changes, hypocalcemia due to citrate anticoagulant (or iatrogenic hypercalcemia due to supplementation), hypotension, nausea, and vomiting. In the event that enough stem cells cannot be collected by apheresis, a BM harvest may need to be performed in addition to supplement the graft.[38–41] Another concern is the risk of developing a hematological malignancy in previously healthy individuals who have received hematopoietic growth factors. It is known that siblings of patients with cancer have an increased risk of leukemia and other cancers. It is difficult therefore to assess an additive risk of developing leukemia after short term exposure to G-CSF.[42–45] However, recent publications do report small numbers of different types of leukemia, predominantly acute myeloid leukemia, after G-CSF administration before PBPC donation.[46–48]

In spite of limited safety data in pediatric donors, G-CSF-mobilized stem cell or G-CSF primed BM harvest is an accepted practice in many pediatric transplant centers. Data between 1996 and 2003 from more than 50 centers reporting to the Pediatric Blood and Marrow Consortium (PBMTC) has shown an average of 23% of all matched sibling transplants (30–60/y) have used PBPC collection.[49–51] Results from 3 separate studies in children using PBSCs as a stem-cell source in matched-related donor transplantations have shown a chronic GVHD disease rate of 63% to 75%,[52–54] That was twice of what is expected in pediatric patients receiving unstimulated BM.[55]

Nine major U.S. centers reported the administration of G-CSF to pediatric donors before a marrow harvest, as part of a PBMTC pilot study on the use of G-CSF primed marrow as a stem cell source in pediatric patients. This trial demonstrated that priming with a dose of G-CSF (5 µg/kg) results in nucleated and CD34$^+$ cell yields that were comparable with PBSC collections and greater than that achieved in BM collections, while avoiding the high CD3$^+$ cell collections typical for PBSCs.[56]

As no clear benefit over conventional BM transplantation for a pediatric donor could be demonstrated, and as G-CSF is not licensed for pediatric donors, PBPC-collection and G-CSF stimulation might appropriately be reserved for exceptional use in siblings following multidisciplinary team discussion and ethical committee approval or as part of an ongoing research study.

PBPC collection from G-CSF stimulated adult donors In a prospective study of 2,408 unrelated adult PBPC donors who donated between 1999–2004 with a median follow up of 49 months, the overall incidence of serious adverse events was 0.6%. The most common side effects were bone pain, headache, fatigue, hypocalcemia and thrombocytopenia. Complete recovery was universal and no long term effects were noted that could be attributed to PBPC harvest. Women and obese donors were at increased risk of adverse events. While no increase in the incidence of malignancies was noted in this cohort, continued long-term follow up of donors is important.[49]

Umbilical cord blood
Procurement, processing, cryopreservation and banking Cord blood, known to be rich in hematopoietic stem cells and typically discarded with the placenta at birth, can be collected without physical risk to the mother or baby. It can be collected from the

delivered placenta (*ex utero*) or during the third stage of labor (*in utero*). Many public cord blood banks employ dedicated staff to perform *ex utero* collections away from the delivery room so that the privacy of the family is preserved and obstetricians are not distracted from their usual practices. Alternatively, obstetricians or midwives perform in utero collections while waiting for the placenta to deliver. In either case, after sterile preparation, the umbilical vein is punctured with a 17-gauge needle attached to a sterile, closed system collection bag containing citrate phosphate dextrose anticoagulant, which is positioned lower than the placenta. Blood flows from the placenta through the cord, by gravity into the bag over approximately 9–10 minutes. Experienced collectors harvest an average of 110 mL from a single placenta. The cord blood unit is labeled and subsequently sent to the bank for processing, testing, cryopreservation, and storage.

There are two types of cord blood banks, public and private. Public cord blood banks store cord blood units donated voluntarily by women after delivering normal term babies. The mother and family give written consent for donation, agree to donor screening and give up all rights to the cord blood which, if qualified, is listed on an unrelated donor registry. Unrelated transplant programs use cord blood units from public banks for transplantation of patients lacking other suitable donors. The costs of the donation, procurement, testing, storage and distribution are borne by the public cord blood bank.

Private banks, which are for-profit entities, store "directed donations" collected by obstetricians from babies born into families who save the cord blood for the use of that family. They may intend to use the cord blood for the baby itself for future use in treating degenerative diseases (autologous donation), although indications for this are unproven, or for another family member in need of future transplantation (eg, genetic or malignant diseases of the blood, immune system or inborn errors of metabolism). Families have to pay private banks for this service. Despite aggressive marketing by some private banks, evidence that such future use will be efficacious in currently lacking. Another misleading pitch by some banks to parents is that autologous cord blood could be used if the child developed leukemia in the future. However, childhood leukemia is very uncommon and most such children can be cured with conventional chemotherapy alone and in those who fail this approach, allogeneic transplantation is the treatment of choice. The fact that leukemic cells can be seen in autologous cord blood of children presenting with leukemia from 1–11 years of age is another reason to advise against the use of autologous cord blood to treat pediatric patients with malignancies.[57-60]

CLINICAL OUTCOMES AFTER ALLOGENEIC HSCT IN PEDIATRIC ACUTE LEUKEMIAS BY STEM CELL SOURCE

Today, HSCT is established as a curative therapy for a variety of malignant and nonmalignant diseases in adults and children. Relapsed or refractory acute leukemia is the most common childhood malignancy and also the most common indication for allogeneic HSCT.

Matched Related Donors

Bone marrow transplantation from HLA identical siblings
Acute lymphoid leukemia (ALL) More than 70% of pediatric patients with ALL are cured with chemotherapy alone. Certain characteristics predict a very poor response to chemotherapy, such as the presence of Philadelphia chromosome (Ph+), hypodiploidy, infant leukemia with MLL gene rearrangement and slow response to chemotherapy (>28 days to achieve CR1). Transplant is indicated in such patients in first complete remission (CR1) to decrease the risk of relapse and improve leukemia free

survival (LFS). Arico and colleagues pooled data on 326 patients with Ph+ ALL from multiple institutions and concluded that matched sibling BMT was superior to chemotherapy and other types of transplantation with 5-yr LFS of 65% with transplant versus. 25% with chemotherapy ($P<.001$) and a decreased risk of relapse with transplant (RR 0.3, $P<.001$).[61] Only few studies have directly compared outcomes of transplant versus chemotherapy in CR1, reflecting the challenges of conducting clinical trials in this population. Balduzzi and colleagues[62] showed in a prospective multicenter trial that allogeneic HSCT from HLA matched sibling donors was superior to chemotherapy alone in children with very high risk ALL in CR1. Furthermore, the BFM-Study group showed a superiority of allogeneic HSCT compared with chemotherapy alone in high-risk childhood T-cell ALL.[63] A minority of studies have failed to show a survival benefit from transplant in CR1.[64]

For patients with ALL who relapse and achieve a second or subsequent remission (CR2 or beyond), LFS after matched sibling transplant ranges from 35%–65% for ALL in CR2 and 20%–30% for patients in CR3 or beyond. For children with relapsed ALL it has been shown that MRD HSCT improves survival compared with chemotherapy alone.[65] The length of first remission is prognostic in patients with relapsed ALL. The most comprehensive data comes from retrospective registry analysis by Eapen and colleagues, who compared 188 pediatric patients receiving chemotherapy on POG studies with 186 patients undergoing matched sibling BMT. Patients with short CR1 (<36 months after diagnosis) had a significant decrease in relapse risk (RR 0.49, $P<.001$) with TBI containing regimens as compared with chemotherapy alone. Also noted was the fact that transplant did not provide benefit over chemotherapy for patients with a longer CR1 ($\geq$36 months).[66] In contrast, Gaynon and colleagues[67] found no benefit for MRD transplant in ALL patients with early relapse. In general, patients with isolated extramedullary relapse respond well to chemotherapy alone, and transplant is not indicated, the notable exception being CNS relapse very close (<18 months) to diagnosis.

Acute myeloid leukemia (AML) In AML patients, outcomes after chemotherapy were very poor in the 1970s. As such, patients with available matched sibling donor have traditionally received allogeneic transplant – so called 'biologic randomization'. The outcomes of several of these studies indicate benefit of allogeneic transplant over chemotherapy in pediatric patients with AML in CR1.[68–70] Horan and colleagues[70] found that MRD BMT is an effective treatment for pediatric patients with intermediate risk AML in first CR. Woods and colleagues[68] found superiority for BMT from MRD in children and adolescents. In a systematic review and meta-analysis, 6 trials with donor versus. no donor comparisons were analyzed (total number of patients was 1486). The overall result of this meta-analysis showed an advantage for matched sibling transplantation.[69] With increasing intensity of upfront chemotherapy, the gap between outcomes of chemotherapy and HSCT may be narrowing. However, at present, the American Society of Blood and Marrow Transplantation recommends transplant in CR1 for AML patients, if a matched sibling donor is available. In Europe, there is a trend to refrain from HSCT in first remission, reserving this option in case of relapse hoping to avoid early and late sequelae associated with HSCT.[71]

Patients with AML who relapse after chemotherapy can achieve remission after treatment with agents such as mitoxantrone and ARA-C about 70%–75% of the time as reported by the French group. The 5-year overall survival (OS) of these patients after allogeneic HSCT in CR2 was approximately 40%–50%. Thus one-third of relapsed patients could be salvaged with transplant. Early relapse (<12 months after CR1) was predictive of poor outcome.[72]

Peripheral blood progenitor cell transplantation from HLA identical siblings In recent years there have been PBPC transplantations from MRD in children with acute leukemias. Early outcomes data on the use of PBPC transplantation in pediatric patients suggest rapid engraftment, with comparable relapse risk, but increased incidence of chronic GVHD.[52–54]

The first comparison between BM and PBPC in children was a single center observation in 16 pediatric patients, where a faster engraftment and a higher incidence of acute GVHD was noted but no difference in OS.[73] The only available multicenter, retrospective analysis comparing PBPC versus BM transplant in patients (age: 8–20 years) with ALL or AML came from the IBMTR and showed a higher mortality after PBPCT. Outcomes of PBPCTs in 143 patients were compared with 630 BM transplants. The patient cohort was not completely comparable as PBPC recipients were older and more likely to have advanced leukemia, more likely to receive growth factors, and higher cell doses, and have undergone HSCT more recently. The PBPC donors tended to be older than BM donors. Donor age was highly correlated with recipient age in both groups: median 18 years (4–36) for PBPC donors and median 14 years (2–37) for BM donors. Hematopoietic recovery was faster after PBPC transplantation. Risks of grade II - IV acute GVHD were similar, but chronic GVHD risk was higher after PBPC transplantation. While the risk of leukemic relapse was similar between the two groups, overall mortality was higher resulting in a 10% decrease in OS in the group receiving PBPCs.[55]

Umbilical cord blood (UCB) transplantation from HLA identical siblings UCB transplantation (UCBT) from matched related siblings has been performed since 1988, demonstrating acceptable outcomes when sufficient cell dose is infused.[14,15] Wagner and colleagues reported 44 patients undergoing sibling donor UCBT. Indication for transplant was acute leukemia in 18 of these patients. The majority of patients received a UCB unit that was fully matched or had 1 antigen mismatch. The probability of event-free survival was 46%.[15] Smythe and colleagues[74] reported three transplantations in children with ALL from cryopreserved sibling UCB. Two patients died from relapse, and one was alive 4 years after the procedure. Outcome data comparing HSCT using UCB versus. BM from HLA identical siblings is scant. Rocha and colleagues studied the records of 113 children who received an UCB from a HLA-identical sibling transplanted between 1990 and 1997, and compared them with the records of 2052 children who were transplanted using BM from HLA-identical siblings during the same period. The recipients of UCB were younger than the recipients of BM (median age, 5 years vs 8 years; $P<.001$), weighed less and were less likely to have received methotrexate for GVHD prophylaxis. Multivariate analysis demonstrated a lower risk of acute GVHD (relative risk, 0.41; $P = .001$) and chronic GVHD (relative risk, 0.35; $P = .02$) among recipients of UCB transplants. When compared with recovery after BM transplantation, the likelihood of recovery of the neutrophil count and the platelet count was significantly lower in the first month after UCB transplantation, although overall engraftment rates were similar. Mortality was similar in both groups. Deaths related to infection from any cause and hemorrhage were more common in the UCB group, whereas deaths related to GVHD, interstitial pneumonitis, and organ failure were more common in the BM group The number of relapse related deaths was similar in the two groups. OS was not statistically different between the two groups.[75]

Matched Unrelated Donors

Since only 20%–25% of children with an indication for allogeneic HSCT have a MRD, the availability of volunteer HLA matched unrelated donors (MUD) has widened the donor pool over the past decade. The chance of finding a suitable donor mainly depends on ethnic group (ranging from 60%–70% for Caucasians to <10% for patients belonging to ethnic minorities) and the frequency of the HLA phenotype of the patient.[76] High-resolution DNA matching of HLA class I and II of unrelated donors and recipients have impacted outcome with reduced morbidity and mortality over the last decade.[77–81] Consequently, the use of unrelated donors is now acceptable in children lacking an HLA identical sibling.

Retrospective studies over the past years have shown reduced early toxicity, especially acute and chronic GVHD, lower TRM, and similar relapse rates compared with the early reported MUD-BMT experience.[77,82–87] It is likely that improved outcomes have resulted not only from better HLA matching, but also from the use of intensified GVHD prophylaxis by in vivo or in vitro T cell depletion. Many HSCT units, in Europe in particular, have pioneered the use of monoclonal and polyclonal antibodies (eg, different types of anti-thymocyte globulins, alemtuzumab, OKT3) to effectively deplete T cells in vivo. Finally, supportive care has improved over time, in particular faster and more accurate diagnosis of infections, and more effective antimicrobial, antiviral and antifungal therapies.

A limitation to evaluating current HSCT data is the usually heterogeneous nature of the patient population, with different diseases, disease stage and leukemic burden.[88] Therefore, the BFM and IBFM-study groups are prospectively comparing the outcome of MUD with MRD HSCT, at a well defined disease stage of ALL. The interim analysis shows that allogeneic HSCTs from a MUD, typed with high resolution techniques, and the use of in vivo T-cell depletion with ATG, have identical outcome to MRD HSCTs, with low TRM (~5%) in both cases.[89] Another consideration for children and adolescents when searching for a MUD is donor age, and it has been demonstrated that age was the only donor characteristic significantly associated with overall and disease-free survival, younger donor age being associated with the most favorable outcomes.[90]

No specific pediatric study has investigated the effect of MUD-PBPCT in children, however, a retrospective analysis of the NMDP for pediatric patients showed that the improvement of survival over time after BMT from a MUD was not similarly observed in unmodified PBPC recipients due to GVHD-associated mortality, suggesting unmodified PBPC may not be the optimal stem cell source for children.[91] In contrast, a single center evaluation showed no difference with respect to TRM, relapse and survival in a small cohort of pediatric patients.[92]

Unrelated Umbilical Cord Blood Transplantation (UUCBT)

UCBT has some advantages over other graft sources, the most important ones being the feasibility of performing mismatched transplants and easy, quick access (**Table 1**). The main limitation is the cell dose delivered by a single cord blood unit.[18] Since the first UUCBT in 1993, it is estimated that over 15,000 UUCBTs have been performed worldwide. Results from Eurocord in 95 childhood AML-patients, the majority of whom had high risk disease, and 1 or 2 antigen mismatched donors, showed a 2-year LFS of 42% in CR1, 50% in CR2, and 21% for children not in CR. Cumulative incidence of neutrophil recovery was 78%, acute GVHD was 35%, and 100-day TRM was 20%.[93] Another retrospective analysis from Eurocord compared the outcomes of UUCBTs with BM transplants in 541 children with acute leukemia. Patients underwent UUCBT (n = 99), T-cell–depleted unrelated BMTs (n = 180), or un-manipulated unrelated BMT (n = 262). Compared with unmanipulated unrelated BMT recipients, UCB recipients had delayed hematopoietic recovery, increased 100 day TRM and decreased acute GVHD. T-cell–depleted unrelated BMT recipients had decreased

Table 1
Comparison of stem cell sources

| | MRD | Alternative Donors | | |
		MUD	Unrelated UCB	Haploidentical PBSC with TCD
Availability	+	++	+++	++++
Donor risk	+	++	0	++
Time to procurement	+	+++	+	+
Cost	+	+++	+++	+++
Time to engraftment	+	+	+++	+
GVHD risk	+	+++	++	+
GVL effect	++	++	++	+
Infections	+	++	+++	+++
Relapse	+	+	+	+++

Abbreviations: MRD, matched related donor; MUD, matched unrelated donor; UCB, umbilical cord blood.

acute GVHD and increased risk of relapse, which was not statistically significant. After day 100 post transplant, the 3 groups achieved similar results in terms of relapse. Chronic GVHD was decreased after T-cell–depleted unrelated BMTs and UUCBTs, and overall mortality was higher in the T-cell–depleted unrelated BMTs recipients, also not significant.[20]

Reporting on data from the CIBMTR, Eapen and colleagues compared outcomes of 503 children (<16 years) with acute leukemia undergoing UUCBT with outcomes of 282 BMT recipients. Five-year LFS was similar in allele matched BMTs to that after transplantation from UUCB, mismatched for either one or two antigens and possibly higher after transplants of HLA-matched UUCB. TRM rates were higher after transplants of two-antigen HLA-mismatched UUCB, and possibly after one-antigen HLA-mismatched low-cell-dose UUCB transplants. Relapse rates were lower after two-antigen HLA-mismatched UUCB transplants. In this report, cell dose and HLA match affected the risk of TRM; recipients of two-antigen and one-antigen mismatched UUCB with low cell dose had worse outcomes.[94] A retrospective analysis showed similar survival between MUD BMTs and UUCB-recipients with up to 2 HLA mismatches.[95]

Comparing UUCBT with haploidentical T-cell depleted PBSCT in children with ALL showed that failure of engraftment was significantly higher following UUCBT than after haplo-HSCT (23 vs 11%, $P = .007$). Acute II-IV GVHD was higher in the UUCBT-group. Relapse incidence was higher in haploidentical HSCT recipients compared with UUCBT. TRM and LFS were, however, not significantly different.[96]

Taken together, these studies show that UUCB transplant outcomes are comparable with those of MUD transplants, but decreased incidence of engraftment or delayed engraftment is one of the relative drawbacks. Newer strategies to enhance engraftment, such as combining two cord blood units,[97] supplementing cord blood with haploidentical donor cells,[98] third party mesenchymal cells,[99] ex vivo expansion[100] and better HLA matching may mitigate these issues, and decrease the incidence of graft failure and GVHD incidence for children with acute leukemias.[101]

Mismatched Family Donors

If pediatric patients with very high risk features of acute leukemia lack a suitable HLA compatible related or unrelated donor, another option available is allogeneic PBPCT from a T-cell depleted haploidentical parental donor. Like UCB, almost immediate access to an allogeneic stem cell product is assured in almost all patients. To date, no general recommendation for these alternative donors (UCB and mismatched family donors) can be given as no randomized or prospective studies have investigated the outcomes in comparable pediatric and adolescent groups. **Table 1** provides a guide to comparison of outcomes of different graft sources.

The outcomes of adult patients who underwent PBPC transplant from G-CSF mobilized haploidentical donors is widely published.[12,102] As described in adults, with the modern techniques of either 'positive' CD34+ selection using immunomagnetic columns or more recently, with 'negative' CD34+ selection by CD3/CD19 depletion approach, a megadose of CD34+ cells can be obtained that can overcome the increased tendency to graft rejection and enough CD3+ T-cell depletion can be achieved, decreasing the risk of GVHD substantially.[103] As discussed elsewhere in this book, there is also evidence of role of NK alloreactivity in mediating graft-versus-leukemia (GVL) effect in this mismatched haploidentical setting, particularly in patients with AML.[102] While T-cell depletion has been necessary to decrease GVHD, the consequent delay in immune reconstitution is responsible for the two major challenges (i) the very high risk of post-transplant infections, and (ii) increased relapse rates.

Only limited data are available on the results of haploidentical transplantation in pediatric patients with acute leukemias.[104–107] Children and adolescents with acute leukemias which have not responded adequately to chemotherapy are, by definition, a high risk population with co-morbidities which increase the risk of infectious and toxic complications after transplant. In contrast to adult patients, children with AML are likely to have poor outcomes after haploidentical HSCT, particularly if not in CR at the time of transplantation, suggesting different disease biology in this age group.[108] In a recent analysis of the EBMT Acute Leukemia and Pediatric Diseases Working Parties, 118 children with high-risk ALL who received haploidentical HSCT after a myeloablative regimen had a 3-year LFS of 32% for patients in CR1, 28% for patients in CR2 or CR3, and 0% for children who were not in remission. This information shows the importance of remission status before the transplant procedure. Furthermore, relapse incidence and TRM tended to be different, though not statistically different, between centers that performed greater than 10 haploidentical transplants in the observation period compared with centers with less than 10 transplants. In the more experienced centers TRM was 27% and relapse incidence 24%, compared with 41% TRM and 41% relapse incidence in the less experienced centers ($P = .10$).[109] Such transplants, may therefore require considerable expertise, and should perhaps be undertaken in highly experienced centers.[110]

To overcome the period of profound immune deficiency, several strategies have been developed, and include the adoptive transfer of pathogen-specific antigens and disease-directed cell therapies.[111–117] As parents are in most cases available for additional cell support in the post-transplant period, these approaches are likely to improve the outcomes after haploidentical HSCT.

SUMMARY

- Children with acute leukemias who have an indication for an allogeneic HSCT, as defined by national chemotherapy groups and protocols, should have HLA typing performed as soon as the potential need for transplant is realized, to identify the best available donor and the most appropriate stem cell source.
- If an HLA genoidentical sibling or related donor is available, HSCT with BM as the source is still the first choice, followed by a matched related donor cord blood

unit with a sufficient cell dose (generally $>3 \times 10^7$/kg). If lower UCB cell doses are present, the UCB unit can be supplemented with a smaller amount of BM from the sibling ($\geq 2 \times 10^7$/kg). PBPC from G-CSF stimulated minor sibling donors should only be undertaken in exceptional situations (eg, second stem cell donation, contraindication for general anesthesia, no informed consent for BM harvest) as G-CSF is not licensed for healthy children. Furthermore, the literature so far has not shown an advantage for children receiving unmanipulated PBPC from siblings or unrelated donors.

- If no HLA-genoidentical sibling or related donor is available, a search for an unrelated donor is indicated. Generally, donor selection can be prioritized as follows:

MRD, 10/10 or 9/10 MUD, 6/6 or 5/6 UCB with a cell dose $>3 \times 10^7$/kg, 4/6 UCB with a cell dose of $>5 \times 10^7$/kg, less than 9/10 MUD or haploidentical family donor. If an unrelated donor is needed urgently, UUCB with sufficient stem cell dose or a graft from a haplo-identical family-member may be an acceptable option.

- In all of these situations, the enrolment of patients into prospective clinical trials will best help to identify the appropriate treatment strategy within a comparable disease cohort and result in better outcome for children overall.

REFERENCES

1. Jacobson L, Marks E, Robson M, et al. Effect of spleen protection on mortality following X-irradiation. J Lab Clin Med 1949;34:1538–43.
2. Lorenz E, Uphoff D, Reid T, et al. Modification of irradiation injury in mice and guinea pigs by bone marrow injections. J Natl Cancer Inst 1951;12:197–201.
3. Dausset J. Iso-leuco-anticorps. Acta Haematologica 1958;20:156–66.
4. Van Rood J, Eernisse J, Van Leeuwen A. Leucocyte antibodies in sera from pregnant women. Nature 1958;181:1735–6.
5. De Koning J, Van Bekkum DW, Dicke KA, et al. Transplantation of bone-marrow cells and fetal thymus in an infant with lymphopenic immunological deficiency. Lancet 1969;1(7608):1223–7.
6. Gatti RA, Meuwissen HJ, Allen HD, et al. Immunological reconstitution of sex-linked lymphopenic immunological deficiency. Lancet 1968;2(7583):1366–9.
7. Thomas ED, Buckner CD, Banaji M, et al. One hundred patients with acute leukemia treated by chemotherapy, total body irradiation, and allogeneic marrow transplantation. Blood 1977;49(4):511–33.
8. Hansen J, Clift R, Thomas E, et al. Transplantation of marrow from an unrelated donor to a patient with acute leukemia. N Engl J Med 1979;303(10):565–7.
9. McCullough J, Perkins HA, Hansen J. The national marrow donor program with emphasis on the early years. Transfusion 2006;46(7):1248–55.
10. Goodman JW, Hodgson GS. Evidence for stem cells in the peripheral blood of mice. Blood 1962;19(6):702–14.
11. Gratwohl A, Baldomero H, Schwendener A, et al. The EBMT activity survey 2007 with focus on allogeneic HSCT for AML and novel cellular therapies. Bone Marrow Transplant 2009;43(4):275–91.
12. Aversa F, Tabilio A, Velardi A, et al. Treatment of high-risk acute leukemia with T-cell-depleted stem cells from related donors with one fully mismatched HLA haplotype. N Engl J Med 1998;339(17):1186–93.
13. Broxmeyer HE, Douglas GW, Hangoc G, et al. Human umbilical cord blood as a potential source of transplantable hematopoietic stem/progenitor cells. Proc Natl Acad Sci U S A 1989;86(10):3828–32.

14. Gluckman E, Broxmeyer H, Auerbach A, et al. Hematopoietic reconstitution in a patient with Fanconi's Anemia by means of umbilical-cord blood from an HLA-identical sibling. N Engl J Med 1989;321(17):1174–8.

15. Wagner J, Kernan N, Steinbuch M, et al. Allogeneic sibling umbilical-cord-blood transplantation in children with malignant and non-malignant disease. Lancet 1995;346(8969):214–9.

16. Rubinstein P, Dobrila L, Rosenfield RE, et al. Processing and cryopreservation of placental/umbilical cord blood for unrelated bone marrow reconstitution. Proc Natl Acad Sci U S A 1995;92(22):10119–22.

17. Kurtzberg J, Laughlin M, Graham ML, et al. Placental blood as a source of hematopoietic stem cells for transplantation into unrelated recipients. N Engl J Med 1996;335(3):157–66.

18. Rubinstein P, Carrier C, Scaradavou A, et al. Outcomes among 562 recipients of placental-blood transplants from unrelated donors. N Engl J Med 1998;339(22):1565–77.

19. Gluckman E, Rocha V, Boyer-Chammard A, et al. Outcome of cord-blood transplantation from related and unrelated donors. N Engl J Med 1997;337(6):373–81.

20. Rocha V, Cornish J, Sievers EL, et al. Comparison of outcomes of unrelated bone marrow and umbilical cord blood transplants in children with acute leukemia. Blood 2001;97(10):2962–71.

21. Barker JN, Davies SM, DeFor T, et al. Survival after transplantation of unrelated donor umbilical cord blood is comparable to that of human leukocyte antigen-matched unrelated donor bone marrow: results of a matched-pair analysis. Blood 2001;97(10):2957–61.

22. Fraser J, Cairo M, Wagner E, et al. Cord Blood Transplantation Study (COBLT): cord blood bank standard operating procedures. J Hematother 1998;7(6):521–61.

23. Kurtzberg J, Wall DA, Wagner JE, et al. Results of the Cord Blood Transplantation Study (COBLT): clinical outcomes of 193 unrelated donor umbilical cord blood transplantations in pediatric patients with malignant conditions. Biol Blood Marrow Transplant 2005;11(2):2 [abstract: 6].

24. Kurtzberg J, Prasad VK, Carter SL, et al. Results of the Cord Blood Transplantation Study (COBLT): clinical outcomes of unrelated donor umbilical cord blood transplantation in pediatric patients with hematologic malignancies. Blood 2008;112(10):4318–27.

25. Rowley J. Backtracking leukemia to birth. Nat Med 1998;4(2):150–1.

26. Peters C, Ladenstein R, Ochsenreiter W, et al. Survey of supportive care standards for paediatric allogeneic stem cell transplantation patients in Europe: a first report from the EBMT Paediatric Diseases Working Party. Bone Marrow Transplant 1996;18(Suppl 2):17–24.

27. Buckner CD, Clift RA, Sanders JE, et al. Marrow harvesting from normal donors. Blood 1984;64(3):630–4.

28. Kletzel M, Olszewski M, Danner-Koptik K, et al. Red cell salvage and reinfusion in pediatric bone marrow donors. Bone Marrow Transplant 1999;24(4):385–8.

29. Martinez AM, Sastre A, Munoz A, et al. Recombinant human erythropoietin (rh-Epo) administration to normal child bone marrow donors. Bone Marrow Transplant 1998;22(2):137–8.

30. Sanders J, Buckner CD, Bensinger WI, et al. Experience with marrow harvesting from donors less than two years of age. Bone Marrow Transplant 1987;2(1):45–50.

31. Halter J, Kodera Y, Ispizua AU, et al. Severe events in donors after allogeneic hematopoietic stem cell donation. Haematologica 2009;94(1):94–101.
32. Vamvakas EC, Blajchman MA. Transfusion-related mortality: the ongoing risks of allogeneic blood transfusion and the available strategies for their prevention. Blood 2009;113(15):3406–17.
33. Traineau R, Elghouzzi MH, Bierling P. [Update on infectious risks associated with blood products]. Rev Prat 2009;59(1):86–9 [in French].
34. Wiener LS, Steffen-Smith E, Fry T, et al. Hematopoietic stem cell donation in children: a review of the sibling donor experience. J Psychosoc Oncol 2007;25(1):45–66.
35. Delany L, Month S, Savulescu J, et al. Altruism by proxy: volunteering children for bone marrow donation. Br Med J 1996;312(7025):240–3.
36. Pentz RD, Haight AE, Noll RB, et al. The ethical justification for minor sibling bone marrow donation: a Case Study. Oncologist 2008;13(2):148–51.
37. Horowitz MM, Confer DL. Evaluation of hematopoietic stem cell donors. Hematology Am Soc Hematol Educ Program 2005;469–75.
38. Grupp SA, Cohn SL, Wall D, et al. Collection, storage, and infusion of stem cells in children with high-risk neuroblastoma: saving for a rainy day. Pediatr Blood Cancer 2006;46(7):719–22.
39. Lipton JM. Peripheral blood as a stem cell source for hematopoietic cell transplantation in children: is the effort in vein? Pediatr Transplant 2003;7(Suppl 3):65–70.
40. Pulsipher MA, Chitphakdithai P, Logan BR, et al. Donor, recipient, and transplant characteristics as risk factors after unrelated donor PBSC transplantation: beneficial effects of higher CD34+ cell dose. Blood 2009;114(13):2606–16.
41. Sevilla J, Gonzalez-Vicent M, Madero L, et al. Large volume leukapheresis in small children: safety profile and variables affecting peripheral blood progenitor cell collection. Bone Marrow Transplant 2003;31(4):263–7.
42. Bortin MM, D'Amaro J, Bach FH, et al. HLA associations with leukemia. Blood 1987;70(1):227–32.
43. Calin GA, Trapasso F, Shimizu M, et al. Familial cancer associated with a polymorphism in ARLTS1. N Engl J Med 2005;352(16):1667–76.
44. Goldin LR, Pfeiffer RM, Li X, et al. Familial risk of lymphoproliferative tumors in families of patients with chronic lymphocytic leukemia: results from the Swedish Family-Cancer Database. Blood 2004;104(6):1850–4.
45. Ripert M, Menegaux F, Perel Y, et al. Familial history of cancer and childhood acute leukemia: a French population-based case-control study. Eur J Cancer Prev 2007;16(5):466–70.
46. Bennett CL, Evens AM, Andritsos LA, et al. Haematological malignancies developing in previously healthy individuals who received haematopoietic growth factors: report from the Research on Adverse Drug Events and Reports (RADAR) project. Br J Haematol 2006;135(5):642–50.
47. Hsia CC, Linenberger M, Howson-Jan K, et al. Acute myeloid leukemia in a healthy hematopoietic stem cell donor following past exposure to a short course of G-CSF. Bone Marrow Transplant 2008;42(6):431–2.
48. Makita K, Ohta K, Mugitani A, et al. Acute myelogenous leukemia in a donor after granulocyte colony-stimulating factor-primed peripheral blood stem cell harvest. Bone Marrow Transplant 2004;33(6):661–5.
49. Pulsipher MA, Chitphakdithai P, Miller JP, et al. Adverse events among 2408 unrelated donors of peripheral blood stem cells: results of a prospective trial from the National Marrow Donor Program. Blood 2009;113(15):3604–11.

50. Pulsipher MA, Levine JE, Hayashi RJ, et al. Safety and efficacy of allogeneic PBSC collection in normal pediatric donors: the Pediatric Blood and Marrow Transplant Consortium Experience (PBMTC) 1996–2003. Bone Marrow Transplant 2004;35(4):361–7.

51. Pulsipher MA, Nagler A, Iannone R, et al. Weighing the risks of G-CSF administration, leukopheresis, and standard marrow harvest: ethical and safety considerations for normal pediatric hematopoietic cell donors. Pediatr Blood Cancer 2006;46(4):422–33.

52. Diaz MA, Vicent MG, Gonzalez ME, et al. Risk assessment and outcome of chronic graft-versus-host disease after allogeneic peripheral blood progenitor cell transplantation in pediatric patients. Bone Marrow Transplant 2004;34(5):433–8.

53. Levine JE, Wiley J, Kletzel M, et al. Cytokine-mobilized allogeneic peripheral blood stem cell transplants in children result in rapid engraftment and a high incidence of chronic GVHD. Bone Marrow Transplant 2000;25(1):13–8.

54. Watanabe T, Takaue Y, Kawano Y, et al. HLA-identical sibling peripheral blood stem cell transplantation in children and adolescents. Biol Blood Marrow Transplant 2002;8(1):26–31.

55. Eapen M, Horowitz MM, Klein JP, et al. Higher mortality after allogeneic peripheral-blood transplantation compared with bone marrow in children and adolescents: the histocompatibility and alternate stem cell source working committee of the international bone marrow transplant registry. J Clin Oncol 2004;22(24):4872–80.

56. Frangoul H, Nemecek ER, Billheimer D, et al. A prospective study of G-CSF primed bone marrow as a stem-cell source for allogeneic bone marrow transplantation in children: a Pediatric Blood and Marrow Transplant Consortium (PBMTC) study. Blood 2007;110(13):4584–7.

57. Committee on Obstetric Practice, Committee on Genetics. ACOG committee opinion number 399, February 2008: umbilical cord blood banking. Obstet Gynecol 2008;111(2 Pt 1):475–7.

58. Ballen KK, Barker JN, Stewart SK, et al. Collection and preservation of cord blood for personal use. Biol Blood Marrow Transplant 2008;14(3):356–63.

59. Kurtzberg J, Lyerly AD, Sugarman J. Untying the Gordian knot: policies, practices, and ethical issues related to banking of umbilical cord blood. J Clin Invest 2005;115(10):2592–7.

60. Lubin BH, Shearer WT. Cord blood banking for potential future transplantation. Pediatrics 2007;119(1):165–70.

61. Arico M, Valsecchi MG, Camitta B, et al. Outcome of treatment in children with Philadelphia chromosome-positive acute lymphoblastic leukemia. N Engl J Med 2000;342(14):998–1006.

62. Balduzzi A, Valsecchi MG, Uderzo C, et al. Chemotherapy versus allogeneic transplantation for very-high-risk childhood acute lymphoblastic leukaemia in first complete remission: comparison by genetic randomisation in an international prospective study. Lancet 2005;366(9486):635–42.

63. Schrauder A, Reiter A, Gadner H, et al. Superiority of allogeneic hematopoietic stem-cell transplantation compared with chemotherapy alone in high-risk childhood T-cell acute lymphoblastic leukemia: results from ALL-BFM 90 and 95. J Clin Oncol 2006;24(36):5742–9.

64. Wheeler KA, Richards SM, Bailey CC, et al. Bone marrow transplantation versus chemotherapy in the treatment of very high-risk childhood acute lymphoblastic leukemia in first remission: results from Medical Research Council UKALL X and XI. Blood 2000;96(7):2412–8.

65. Wheeler K, Richards S, Bailey C, et al. Comparison of bone marrow transplant and chemotherapy for relapsed childhood acute lymphoblastic leukaemia: the MRC UKALL X experience. Medical research council working party on childhood leukaemia. Br J Haematol 1998;101(1):94–103.

66. Eapen M, Raetz E, Zhang M-J, et al. Outcomes after HLA-matched sibling transplantation or chemotherapy in children with B-precursor acute lymphoblastic leukemia in a second remission: a collaborative study of the Children's Oncology Group and the center for international blood and marrow transplant research. Blood 2006;107(12):4961–7.

67. Gaynon PS, Harris RE, Altman AJ, et al. Bone marrow transplantation versus prolonged intensive chemotherapy for children with acute lymphoblastic leukemia and an initial bone marrow relapse within 12 months of the completion of primary therapy: children's Oncology Group Study CCG-1941. J Clin Oncol 2006;24(19):3150–6.

68. Woods WG, Neudorf S, Gold S, et al. A comparison of allogeneic bone marrow transplantation, autologous bone marrow transplantation, and aggressive chemotherapy in children with acute myeloid leukemia in remission: a report from the Children's Cancer Group. Blood 2001;97(1):56–62.

69. Bleakley M, Lau L, Shaw PJ, et al. Bone marrow transplantation for paediatric AML in first remission: a systematic review and meta-analysis. Bone Marrow Transplant 2002;29(10):843–52.

70. Horan JT, Alonzo TA, Lyman GH, et al. Impact of disease risk on efficacy of matched related bone marrow transplantation for pediatric acute myeloid leukemia: the Children's Oncology Group. J Clin Oncol 2008;26(35): 5797–801.

71. Messerer D, Engel J, Hasford J, et al. Impact of different post-remission strategies on quality of life in patients with acute myeloid leukemia. Haematologica 2008;93(6):826–33.

72. Aladjidi N, Auvrignon A, Leblanc T, et al. Outcome in children with relapsed acute myeloid leukemia after initial treatment with the French leucemie aique myeloide enfant (LAME) 89/91 protocol of the French Society of Pediatric Hematology and Immunology. J Clin Oncol 2003;21(23):4377–85.

73. Meisel R, Enczmann J, Balzer S, et al. Similar survival following HLA-identical sibling transplantation for standard indication in children with haematologic malignancies: a single center comparison of mobilized peripheral blood stem cell with bone marrow transplantation. Klin Padiatr 2005; 217(3):135–41.

74. Smythe J, Armitage S, McDonald D, et al. Directed sibling cord blood banking for transplantation: the 10-year experience in the national blood service in England. Stem Cells 2007;25(8):2087–93.

75. Rocha V, Wagner JE, Sobocinski KA, et al. Graft-versus-host disease in children who have received a cord-blood or bone marrow transplant from an HLA-identical sibling. N Engl J Med 2000;342(25):1846–54.

76. Rocha V, Locatelli F. Searching for alternative hematopoietic stem cell donors for pediatric patients. Bone Marrow Transplant 2008;41(2):207–14.

77. Cornish J. Unrelated donor transplant for acute leukaemia in children–the UK experience. Pathol Biol (Paris) 2005;53(3):167–70.

78. Green A, Clarke E, Hunt L, et al. Children with acute lymphoblastic leukemia who receive T-cell-depleted HLA mismatched marrow allografts from unrelated donors have an increased incidence of primary graft failure but a similar overall transplant outcome. Blood 1999;94(7):2236–46.

79. Marks DI, Bird JM, Vettenranta K, et al. T cell-depleted unrelated donor bone marrow transplantation for acute myeloid leukemia. Biol Blood Marrow Transplant 2000;6(6):646–53.
80. Oakhill A, Pamphilon DH, Potter MN, et al. Unrelated donor bone marrow transplantation for children with relapsed acute lymphoblastic leukaemia in second complete remission. Br J Haematol 1996;94(3):574–8.
81. Vettenranta K, Saarinen-Pihkala UM, Cornish J, et al. Pediatric marrow transplantation for acute leukemia using unrelated donors and T-replete or -depleted grafts: a case-matched analysis. Bone Marrow Transplant 2000; 25(4):395–9.
82. Dini G, Cancedda R, Locatelli F, et al. Unrelated donor marrow transplantation: an update of the experience of the Italian Bone Marrow Group (GITMO). Haematologica 2001;86(5):451–6.
83. Dini G, Valsecchi MG, Micalizzi C, et al. Impact of marrow unrelated donor search duration on outcome of children with acute lymphoblastic leukemia in second remission. Bone Marrow Transplant 2003;32(3):325–31.
84. Eapen M, Rubinstein P, Zhang MJ, et al. Comparable long-term survival after unrelated and HLA-matched sibling donor hematopoietic stem cell transplantations for acute leukemia in children younger than 18 months. J Clin Oncol 2006; 24(1):145–51.
85. Garderet L, Labopin M, Gorin NC, et al. Patients with acute lymphoblastic leukaemia allografted with a matched unrelated donor may have a lower survival with a peripheral blood stem cell graft compared to bone marrow. Bone Marrow Transplant 2003;31(1):23–9.
86. Cornish JM, Pamphilon DH, Potter MN, et al. Unrelated donor bone marrow transplant in childhood ALL. The role of T-cell depletion. Bone Marrow Transplant 1996;18(Suppl 2):31–5.
87. Oakhill A, Pamphilon DH, Potter MN, et al. Unrelated donor bone marrow transplantation for children with relapsed acute lymphoblastic leukaemia in second complete remission. Br J Haematol 1996;93(3):674–6.
88. Locatelli F, Zecca M, Messina C, et al. Improvement over time in outcome for children with acute lymphoblastic leukemia in second remission given hematopoietic stem cell transplantation from unrelated donors. Leukemia 2002;16(11): 2228–37.
89. Schrauder A, Stackelberg A, Bader P, et al. Reduction of treatment related mortality after stem cell transplantation in children and adolescents with ALL undergoing allogeneic stem cell transplantation. Biol Blood Marrow Transplant 2009;15(2):80.
90. Kollman C, Howe CW, Anasetti C, et al. Donor characteristics as risk factors in recipients after transplantation of bone marrow from unrelated donors: the effect of donor age. Blood 2001;98(7):2043–51.
91. MacMillan ML, Davies SM, Nelson GO, et al. Twenty years of unrelated donor bone marrow transplantation for pediatric acute leukemia facilitated by the National Marrow Donor Program. Biol Blood Marrow Transplant 2008;14(Suppl 9):16–22.
92. Meisel R, Laws HJ, Balzer S, et al. Comparable long-term survival after bone marrow versus peripheral blood progenitor cell transplantation from matched unrelated donors in children with hematologic malignancies. Biol Blood Marrow Transplant 2007;13(11):1338–45.
93. Michel G, Rocha V, Chevret S, et al. Unrelated cord blood transplantation for childhood acute myeloid leukemia: a Eurocord Group analysis. Blood 2003; 102(13):4290–7.

94. Eapen M, Rubinstein P, Zhang MJ, et al. Outcomes of transplantation of unrelated donor umbilical cord blood and bone marrow in children with acute leukaemia: a comparison study. Lancet 2007;369(9577):1947–54.
95. Dalle JH, Duval M, Moghrabi A, et al. Results of an unrelated transplant search strategy using partially HLA-mismatched cord blood as an immediate alternative to HLA-matched bone marrow. Bone Marrow Transplant 2004; 33(6):605–11.
96. Hough RLM, Michel G, Locatelli F, et al. Outcomes of fully haplo-identical haematopoietic stem cell transplantation compared to unrelated cord blood transplantation in children with acute lymphoblastic leukaemia. A retrospective analysis on behalf of Eurocord, PDWP and ALWP of EBMT. Bone Marrow Transplant 2007;39:S1–3.
97. Barker JN, Weisdorf DJ, DeFor TE, et al. Transplantation of 2 partially HLA-matched umbilical cord blood units to enhance engraftment in adults with hematologic malignancy. Blood 2005;105(3):1343–7.
98. Fernández MN, Regidor C, Cabrera R, et al. Unrelated umbilical cord blood transplants in adults: early recovery of neutrophils by supportive co-transplantation of a low number of highlypurified peripheral blood CD34+ cells from an HLA-haploidentical donor. Exp Hematol 2003;31(6):535–44.
99. Gonzalo-Daganzo R, Regidor C, Martin-Donaire T, et al. Results of a pilot study on the use of third-party donor mesenchymal stromal cells in cord blood transplantation in adults. Cytotherapy 2009;11(3):278–88.
100. Kelly SS, Sola CBS, de Lima M, et al. Ex vivo expansion of cord blood. Bone Marrow Transplant 2009;44(10):673–81.
101. Hwang WY, Samuel M, Tan D, et al. A meta-analysis of unrelated donor umbilical cord blood transplantation versus unrelated donor bone marrow transplantation in adult and pediatric patients. Biol Blood Marrow Transplant 2007;13(4):444–53.
102. Ruggeri L, Capanni M, Urbani E, et al. Effectiveness of donor natural killer cell alloreactivity in mismatched hematopoietic transplants. Science 2002; 295(5562):2097–100.
103. Handgretinger R, Lang P. The history and future prospective of haplo-identical stem cell transplantation. Cytotherapy 2008;10(5):443–51.
104. Lang P, Schumm M, Greil J, et al. A comparison between three graft manipulation methods for haploidentical stem cell transplantation in pediatric patients: preliminary results of a pilot study. Klin Padiatr 2005;217(6):334–8.
105. Marks DI, Khattry N, Cummins M, et al. Haploidentical stem cell transplantation for children with acute leukaemia. Br J Haematol 2006;134(2):196–201.
106. Peters C. Another step forward towards improved outcome after HLA-haploidentical stem cell transplantation. Leukemia 2004;18(11):1769–71.
107. Klingebiel T, Handgretinger R, Lang P, et al. Haploidentical transplantation for acute lymphoblastic leukemia in childhood. Blood Rev 2004;18(3):181–92.
108. Lang P, Greil J, Bader P, et al. Long-term outcome after haploidentical stem cell transplantation in children. Blood Cells Mol Dis 2004;33(3):281–7.
109. Klingebiel T, Cornish J, Labopin M, et al. Results and factors influencing outcome after fully haploidentical hematopoietic stem cell transplant in children with very-high risk acute lymphoblastic leukemia - impact of center size: an analysis on behalf of the Acute Leukemia and Pediatric Disease Working Parties of the European Blood and Marrow Transplant group. Blood 2009. DOI:10.1182/blood-2009-03-207001. [Epub ahead of Print].

110. Ball LM, Lankester AC, Bredius RG, et al. Graft dysfunction and delayed immune reconstitution following haploidentical peripheral blood hematopoietic stem cell transplantation. Bone Marrow Transplant 2005;35(Suppl 1):S35–8.
111. Perruccio K, Tosti A, Burchielli E, et al. Transferring functional immune responses to pathogens after haploidentical hematopoietic transplantation. Blood 2005;106(13):4397–406.
112. Velardi A, Ruggeri L, Capanni M, et al. Immunotherapy with alloreactive natural killer cells in haploidentical haematopoietic transplantation. Hematol J 2004; 5(Suppl 3):S87–90.
113. Feuchtinger T, Richard C, Pfeiffer M, et al. Adenoviral infections after transplantation of positive selected stem cells from haploidentical donors in children: an update. Klin Padiatr 2005;217(6):339–44.
114. Handgretinger R, Chen X, Pfeiffer M, et al. Cellular immune reconstitution after haploidentical transplantation in children. Biol Blood Marrow Transplant 2008; 14(1 Suppl 1):59–65.
115. Montagna D, Maccario R, Locatelli F. Expansion of antileukaemia CTL lines and clones for adoptive cell therapy in paediatric patients given allogeneic haematopoietic stem cell transplantation. Int J Immunogenet 2008;35(4–5):389–93.
116. Locatelli F, Comoli P, Montagna D, et al. Innovative approaches of adoptive immune cell therapy in paediatric recipients of haematopoietic stem cell transplantation. Best Pract Res Clin Haematol 2004;17(3):479–92.
117. Comoli P, Maccario R, Locatelli F, et al. Adoptive transfer of herpesvirusspecific cytotoxic T lymphocytes in transplant recipients. Herpes 2000;7(1):9–12.

Autologous and Allogeneic Cellular Therapies for High-risk Pediatric Solid Tumors

David Barrett, MD, PhD[a], Jonathan D. Fish, MD[d],
Stephan A. Grupp, MD, PhD[a,b,c],*

KEYWORDS
- Hematopoietic stem cell transplantation
- Pediatric solid tumors • Cell-based therapies

Since the 1950s, the overall survival (OS) of children with cancer has gone from almost zero to approaching 80%. Although there have been notable successes in treating solid tumors such as Wilms tumor, some childhood solid tumors, exemplified by diseases like high-risk neuroblastoma and metastatic sarcomas, have continued to elude effective therapy.[1] With the use of megatherapy techniques such as tandem transplantation, dose escalation has been pushed to the edge of dose-limiting toxicities, and any further improvements in event-free survival (EFS) will have to be achieved through novel therapeutic approaches.

This article reviews the status of autologous and allogeneic hematopoietic stem cell transplantation (HSCT) for many pediatric solid tumor types. Most of the clinical experience in transplant for pediatric solid tumors is in the autologous setting, so some general principles of autologous HSCT are reviewed, followed by an examination of HSCT for diseases such as Hodgkin disease, Ewing sarcoma, and neuroblastoma.

[a] Division of Oncology, Children's Hospital of Philadelphia, 3006 Colket Translational Research Building, 3501 Civic Center Boulevard, Philadelphia, PA 19104, USA
[b] Department of Pediatrics, University of Pennsylvania School of Medicine, 34th and Civic Center Boulevard, Philadelphia, PA, USA
[c] Department of Pathology and Laboratory Medicine, Children's Hospital of Philadelphia, 34th and Civic Center Boulevard, Philadelphia, PA 19104, USA
[d] Division of Pediatric Hematology/Oncology and Stem Cell Transplantation, Schneider Children's Hospital, 26901 76th Avenue, New Hyde Park, NY 11040, USA
* Corresponding author. Division of Oncology, Children's Hospital of Philadelphia, 3006 Colket Translational Research Building, 3501 Civic Center Boulevard, Philadelphia, PA 19104.
E-mail address: grupp@email.chop.edu

Pediatr Clin N Am 57 (2010) 47–66
doi:10.1016/j.pcl.2010.01.001
0031-3955/10/$ – see front matter © 2010 Elsevier Inc. All rights reserved.

pediatric.theclinics.com

The article then looks to the future of cell-based therapies by considering some experimental approaches to effector cell therapies.

PRINCIPLES OF AUTOLOGOUS HSCT

Before the introduction of high-dose chemotherapy (HDC) with autologous stem cell rescue (also called autologous HSCT), marrow tolerance was the limiting factor in the escalation of chemotherapy for the treatment of malignancies. With the ability to safely harvest, store, and reinfuse a patient's own hematopoietic stem cells, doses of cytotoxic therapies for cancer could safely proceed beyond marrow tolerance, thereby allowing more intense treatment of certain malignancies. Two approaches to the use of HDC with stem cell rescue are (1) myeloablative regimens, meaning that no hematopoietic recovery can occur without the stored HSCs, and (2) submyeloablative HDC regimens in which stem cell rescue is used to speed recovery, decrease toxicity, and decrease the interval between courses of chemotherapy, although it is not absolutely required for engraftment.[2,3] Although the increased treatment intensity may improve disease-free survival for patients with some malignancies, this must be balanced with the increased treatment-related mortality associated with the higher doses of cytotoxic agents, and the potential late effects of more intense cytotoxic treatments and radiotherapeutic regimens in young children. Criteria that may help define circumstances in which HDC with stem cell rescue would be most beneficial include (1) a tumor with good response to induction chemotherapy, but a poor 3- or 5-year EFS, and (2) an HDC regimen that can use multiple agents active against the disease, especially if the agents differ from those used during induction therapy. Although the use of HDC with stem cell rescue is controversial in most diseases, diseases such as Hodgkin disease and high-risk neuroblastoma (discussed later) meet the design criteria listed earlier and have shown improved outcomes in clinical trials.

HODGKIN DISEASE

Although most pediatric patients with Hodgkin disease achieve excellent long-term survival with standard chemotherapy and low-dose radiation therapy, with EFS and OS of 80% and 90%, respectively, many patients have refractory disease or experience relapse.[4–6] Poor prognosis in these relapsed patients is associated with chemotherapy-resistant disease, short time to relapse (<1 year), extranodal disease at relapse, and poor performance status in adult patients.[7,8]

Adult studies comparing conventional salvage therapy with HDC with autologous stem cell rescue show the benefit of the HSCT approach in relapsed disease.[9–11] Following up on a pilot study in 1991 that suggested HSCT might be a better frontline therapy for high-risk patients, a randomized trial was conducted comparing conventional therapy with HSCT.[12,13] Using a foundation of 4 cycles of ABVD (adriamycin, bleomycin, vinblastine, dacarbazine), patients with high-risk features (high lactate dehydrogenase level, mediastinal mass, >1 extranodal site, anemia, or inguinal disease) were assigned to either 4 more cycles of ABVD or HSCT. There was no difference in EFS or OS, discouraging HSCT as frontline therapy for high-risk patients. Linch and colleagues[14] compared a standard intensified HDC regimen (bis-chloroethyl-nitrosourea [BCNU], etoposide, cytarabine and melphalan [BEAM]) and autologous stem cell rescue with mini-BEAM in a randomized trial for relapsed and refractory adult patients, finding improved EFS and lower relapse rate in the intensified arm but similar OS. A large randomized study of patients aged 16 to 60 years with relapsed Hodgkin disease compared 4 cycles of nonmyeloablative Dexa-BEAM with 2 cycles of

Dexa-BEAM plus a high-dose BEAM with HSCT. EFS was 55% at 3 years for the HSCT group and only 34% for conventional therapy (P = .019).[15] In both trials, the lack of difference in OS may be in part because patients who relapsed after conventional therapy went on to receive HSCT and were salvaged by that regimen.

As the incidence of Hodgkin disease places it in an age group of mostly adolescents and young adults, many studies have pooled pediatric patients (<18 years) with older patients for study. A case-control series examining HSCT in children less than 16 years old at diagnosis compared with a population older than 16 years found progression-free survival was similar (39% vs 48%), as were most of the secondary measures and subgroup analysis between these older and younger patients.[16] This study also confirmed chemotherapy-resistant disease is a poor prognostic factor in children and adults. A retrospective analysis of 51 children receiving autologous HSCT compared with 78 children receiving conventional salvage therapy did not find an advantage to HSCT, but may have been biased because the group proceeding to transplant had more adverse disease characteristics,[17] a common issue with such retrospective analyses. Baker and colleagues[18] reported on patients less than 21 years old at time of transplant for relapsed or refractory Hodgkin disease: 5-year OS was 43% and EFS 31%, and no difference was observed in 3 age brackets (<13 years, 13–18 years, and 19–21 years). As HSCT became more common, smaller case series were published in children from Spain, Germany, and Austria that again identified the presence of bulky or extranodal disease at time of HSCT as an independent poor prognostic factor in children.[19,20]

The role of allogeneic HSCT has also been investigated for relapsed Hodgkin disease. Although early use of myeloablative regimens and allogeneic HSCT resulted in high transplant-related mortality (TRM) without much indication of benefit, some groups have reported disease regression with donor lymphocyte infusions (DLIs), suggesting a graft-versus-lymphoma effect is possible.[21,22] There have been no randomized comparisons of allogeneic and autologous transplant for relapsed Hodgkin disease. A single-center study from the Fred Hutchinson Cancer Research Center comparing 53 patients receiving allogeneic HSCT with controls receiving autologous HSCT found a significantly lower relapse rate in the allogeneic recipients (45% vs 76%).[23] EFS was not significantly different, and in the allogeneic transplant group the competing risk of TRM was high (53%). The role of reduced intensity conditioning (RIC) regimens in the allogeneic transplant setting is being investigated to reduce TRM and potentially expand the graft-versus-lymphoma effect. A recent report from Europe compared 89 patients receiving an RIC allogeneic HSCT with 79 patients receiving a traditional myeloablative regimen.[24] About half of these patients had received a prior HSCT, and all were heavily pretreated. OS was superior in the RIC group (28% vs 22%) despite a higher relapse rate (57% vs 30%). This finding was likely a result of the significant reduction in TRM in the RIC group (23% vs 46%). A recurring theme in these patients is the poor prognostic indicators of chemotherapy-resistant disease and presence of bulky disease at time of transplant. This study continues a trend of earlier single-center reviews, and suggests that RIC allogeneic HSCT, either alone or coupled to an autologous HSCT, may have a role in the treatment of multiply relapsed patients with Hodgkin disease.[21,25,26]

Although autologous HSCT is the treatment of choice for relapsed or refractory Hodgkin disease, the addition of newer agents such as monoclonal antibodies and tyrosine kinase inhibitors to conventional regimens has not been studied in a randomized fashion against HSCT. In addition, patients with chemotherapy-resistant disease or bulky disease at time of HSCT still do poorly. RIC allogeneic HSCT should be considered for patients who relapse following autologous HSCT, and more study is needed to further identify ways to reduce TRM and increase the potential of graft versus lymphoma.

NON-HODGKIN LYMPHOMA

Pediatric non-Hodgkin lymphoma (NHL) consists mainly of Burkitt, lymphoblastic, diffuse large B cell, and anaplastic large cell lymphoma. Conventional chemotherapy remains the frontline treatment of choice, with long-term survival in the 60% to 90% range depending on histology.[27–29] Relapsed disease carries a more dismal prognosis, and autologous HSCT has been investigated for these high-risk patients. A Children's Cancer Group (CCG) study for relapsed lymphoma did not find a benefit for autologous HSCT for these patients, as EFS was not significantly changed compared with other salvage regimens.[30] A comprehensive review by Gross and colleagues[31] found that some patients with relapsed NHL can be salvaged by autologous or allogeneic HSCT. As with Hodgkin disease, chemotherapy-resistant disease and disease status at time of transplant significantly affect survival. As most single-center experiences include multiple types of NHL to acquire enough cases for review, separating effects within each subtype is difficult. A trend toward improved salvage with allogeneic HSCT in lymphoblastic lymphoma is seen, although this is biased by the greater number of patients who underwent this procedure compared with autologous HSCT. As the numbers of pediatric patients with relapsed or refractory NHL remain small, studying the role of autologous and allogeneic HSCT against conventional therapy is difficult.

EWING SARCOMA

Ewing sarcoma is the second most common bone tumor in children after osteosarcoma, and carries a 70% long-term survival for localized disease. The backbone of this therapy includes surgical resection, anthracycline and alkylator chemotherapy (typically doxorubicin and ifosfamide), and in some cases radiation therapy. Patients with metastases, however, have a worse outcome (4-year OS 39%) and survival after relapse is also dismal (10-year OS 10%).[32–35] Escalation of therapy in patients with metastatic Ewing sarcoma with the core treatment agents ifosfamide, doxorubicin, and cyclophosphamide or addition of ifosfamide/etoposide to a standard regimen seemed only to increase short-term toxicity and secondary myelodysplasia.[35]

In higher-risk patients with Ewing sarcoma, autologous HSCT has been investigated for poor prognostic groups such as patients with large, unresectable tumors, patients with metastatic disease, or that subset of stage-4 patients with metastases outside the lung (the highest risk group). A CCG study of 36 patients with Ewing sarcoma metastatic to the bone marrow at diagnosis investigated the efficacy of melphalan, etoposide, and total body irradiation (TBI) followed by autologous HSCT. This treatment led to no improvement in 2-year survival (20%) compared with conventional therapy.[36] These disappointing results were replicated in 3 other studies, using allogeneic and autologous stem cell sources, with high rates of TRM raising further concerns.[37–39] The ongoing EuroEWING-99 trial has a study question comparing autologous HSCT with intensified standard therapy for patients with a poor local response or with lung metastases. Patients are randomized after a standardized vincristine, ifosfamide, doxorubicin, and etoposide (VIDE) induction phase. The data collection is ongoing.

For those patients who have relapsed Ewing sarcoma, the outlook is grim, with a 10% 5-year OS.[40] In 2 single-center studies, 32 patients with relapsed Ewing sarcoma underwent megatherapy (26 with autologous HSCT, 6 with allogeneic HSCT).

Fifteen of 32 patients were reported as long-term survivors, although they represent a rare subgroup that was able to achieve a second remission in this disease,[38,41] and it is unclear if HSCT provides an advantage to intensified standard chemotherapy in these small highly selected groups. A common observation is that the outcome of megatherapy or autologous HSCT in the presence of gross residual disease is exceptionally poor (5-year OS 19%).[42] Nevertheless, there are enough data to support design of studies comparing autologous HSCT with standard intensified therapy for high-risk and relapsed patients, and we look forward to the results of the EuroEWING-99 trial.

RHABDOMYOSARCOMA

Rhabdomyosarcoma is the most common sarcoma of childhood, and children with low- or intermediate-risk disease have excellent long-term survival rates with standard chemotherapy approaches. As with neuroblastoma, high-risk patients continue to do poorly despite intensification of nonmyeloablative chemotherapy as in the IRS-III and IRS-IV trials (5-year OS 30% for metastatic disease, group IV).[43,44] In vitro and in vivo studies of relapsed rhabdomyosarcoma samples suggest sensitivity to melphalan, and based on this finding HSCT approaches to relapsed or high-risk rhabdomyosarcoma were designed.[45,46] Of 98 HSCTs for relapsed or progressive rhabdomyosarcoma in children performed up to 1994 in Europe, the OS was not different from historical controls at 20%.[47] Single-institution studies with various criteria to define high-risk rhabdomyosarcoma have replicated these data, with children in remission status receiving megatherapy achieving some degree of long-term OS, although it is unclear if this is superior to intensified conventional therapy.[48] Although a randomized trial of autologous HSCT as a consolidation for high-risk patients without gross residual disease could be contemplated, there is little support for this approach in the current literature.

NEUROBLASTOMA

Neuroblastoma is the most common extracranial solid malignancy of childhood, and has a broad spectrum of clinical presentations and behavior. Although low- and intermediate-risk neuroblastoma are mostly curable,[49,50] high-risk neuroblastoma has proven refractory to conventional treatment modalities.[1,51,52] Despite the unsatisfactory responses to conventional therapies, some improvements in outcome have been achieved through the escalation of therapeutic intensity.[53] Although even the most intense conventional therapy results in long-term EFS of less than 40%, improvements can be achieved through the addition of consolidation therapy with high-dose therapies that exceed marrow tolerance. This improvement was originally achieved through the harvest, storage, and reinfusion of autologous bone marrow capable of reestablishing trilinear hematopoiesis,[52] and later replicated using peripheral blood stem cells (PBSC).[54] Even with this intensified consolidation therapy, outcomes still remained poor. However, the ability to collect adequate PBSC in small children, along with the decreased TRM associated with their use, has allowed for even more intense consolidation therapy by enabling tandem autologous HSCT. Early studies suggest that this is a feasible approach that may improve outcomes.[51,55]

Early, Non-Randomized Studies

Having acquired the ability to safely harvest, store, and reinfuse HSC, investigators in the late 1980s and early 1990s began exploring the hypothesis that increased treatment intensity beyond marrow tolerance would improve survival in patients with high-risk neuroblastoma. Multiple early single-arm or retrospective studies suggested that autologous HSCT might improve the EFS of these patients, although none of the studies were randomized and may have been influenced by selection bias.[56–61] The largest retrospective analysis was performed through the European Group for Bone Marrow Transplantation in 1997; 1070 transplants for high-risk patients with neuroblastoma were analyzed, and the 2-year survival among the group of patients who had reached an SCT procedure was 49%. Most relapses occurred within the first 18 months following transplant, and there were no survivors amongst the group of 48 patients who relapsed and underwent a second HSCT. Late relapses were found as long as 7 years from transplant.[62]

Randomized Trials

The promise suggested by these early studies propelled prospective evaluation of autologous HSCT for high-risk neuroblastoma. The largest of the randomized, prospective studies was a phase III trial performed by the CCG. In CCG-3891, patients were randomized to a consolidation regimen consisting of autologous bone marrow transplant versus continuation chemotherapy. Following consolidation, patients were then randomized to biologic therapy with 13-*cis*-retinoic acid (a maturational agent) versus no further therapy.[52] The study found that those treated with autologous HSCT had a significantly better EFS than those treated with chemotherapy alone. It was also noted that treatment with 13-*cis*-retinoic acid further improved outcome among patients without progressive disease. With an estimated 38% EFS 3.7 years from diagnosis in the best group, this study helped establish autologous HSCT followed by 6 months of oral *cis*-retinoic acid therapy as the new standard of care for these patients, and represented an important step forward in the treatment of high-risk neuroblastoma. Despite its important results, this study was subject to the challenges of a complex treatment plan and the 2 × 2 factorial design. Of 579 eligible patients, 379 underwent the first randomization, and 258 patients underwent the second, thereby reducing the population of patients being studied to approximately 50 patients in each of the 4 treatment groups. Other studies of autologous HSCT in high-risk neuroblastoma have since built on the results of CCG-3891.[2,51,63] Conditioning regimens used in subsequent studies have varied widely, with the greatest difference being that some studies have used TBI in the conditioning regimen whereas others did not. There have been no randomized trials of the use of TBI during conditioning, and although it may improve outcomes, it also results in significant late effects in those who survive treatment. Thus, although the use of radiotherapy to the tumor bed is standard care in neuroblastoma, the use of TBI remains controversial. Overall, these studies have led to the current core standard for neuroblastoma treatment: 5 or 6 cycles of induction chemotherapy, surgery, radiotherapy (at a minimum to the tumor bed), and autologous HSCT followed by oral cis-retinoic acid. To this treatment, GD2-targeted immunotherapy may now be added based on recent data from the Children's Oncology Group (COG) ANBL0032 study presented at the American Society of Clinical Oncology meeting in 2009, which showed a superior outcome in patients who received this immunotherapy in addition to cis-retinoic acid.

Tandem Transplantation

Given the evidence that dose intensity correlates with outcome, and that HDC with autologous stem cell rescue renders a statistically significant improvement in survival, it was logical to examine sequential courses of HDC with stem cell rescue, otherwise known as tandem transplant. Tandem transplantation allows for even greater dose intensity in consolidation, with the potential to introduce different active agents at each transplant. An early attempt to use this technique was complicated by unacceptable TRM, primarily related to extended periods of neutropenia following the transplants.[64] Although initially discouraging, this study, like CCG-3891, was conducted using bone marrow as the stem cell source. Other stem cell sources, specifically PBSC, can provide more rapid engraftment and faster recovery times than bone marrow. The more rapid engraftment of PBSC results in decreased days with severe neutropenia and a shorter duration of mucositis, thereby resulting in a lower rate of infectious complications. With the high TRM found using bone marrow as the stem cell source for tandem transplantation, PBSC became an attractive alternative. Despite the challenges inherent in collecting PBSC from patients with high-risk neuroblastoma (young age at diagnosis, small size, and blood volume), clinicians can now safely, effectively, and routinely perform this procedure.[65] Following the switch from bone marrow to PBSC, several groups have retested the tandem transplant approach, with more promising results.[2,51,63] The largest of these studies was conducted for 6 years at 4 cooperating institutions. The study was designed using early collection of PBSC, CD34 selection as a purging method (discussed later) and 2 myeloablative regimens containing distinct agents: (1) carboplatin, etoposide, and cyclophosphamide, followed by (2) melphalan and TBI. TRM in this study was 6%, and included 2 patients who died of Epstein-Barr virus lymphoproliferative disease (EBV-LPD). Post-HSCT immunosuppression is discussed later. Longer follow-up of this treatment approach in a large phase II cohort has shown a 3-year EFS from diagnosis of consecutively enrolled patients of 55% (most recent update shown in **Fig. 1**). A second multiple-cycle autologous HSCT study, performed using 3 sequential HSCT procedures, found comparable results in 3-year EFS (57%), although there appeared to be instability of the curve out to 4 to 5 years.[2] In that study, 19 of the 25 patients completed the second autologous HSCT and 17 went on to the third. Only 1 late TRM was observed. Based on these promising results, the current open phase III COG trial, ANBL0532, is testing single versus tandem transplant as consolidation therapy for high-risk neuroblastoma.

Processing of Stem Cells

In addition to increasing dose intensity, graft manipulation has been used to attempt to improve survival following autologous HSCT in neuroblastoma. Engineering of the HSC graft is possible to remove or expand desired cell populations. The most researched manipulation in the context of neuroblastoma has been purging of malignant cells before the infusion of the HSC product. Research in the 1990s suggested that clonogenic tumor cells can be infused with an HSC graft, and that these cells can result in relapse of the malignancy.[66] This finding led to trials in neuroblastoma addressing the question of whether purging stem cell products of tumor cells could further improve posttransplant overall and disease-free survival. There are 2 methods to purge an HSCT product of tumor cells: either positive selection of HSC, leading to the exclusion of tumor cells, or negative selection designed specifically to remove malignant cells. Positive selection of CD34 expressing cells is the primary technique available to most stem cell laboratories. CD34 is an antigen expressed on HSC and progenitors of all hematopoietic lineages, and positive selection of CD34 would result in the exclusion of neuroblastoma from the graft, assuming that the neuroblastoma cells themselves do not express CD34. Concerns have indeed been raised that some neuroblastoma cells may express either CD34, or surface epitopes cross-reactive with the anti-CD34 monoclonal antibodies necessary for the selection process.[67,68] Our data have not confirmed this hypothesis,[69] and we, along with others, have used CD34 selection as a purging technique for PBSC products in the clinical setting.[70]

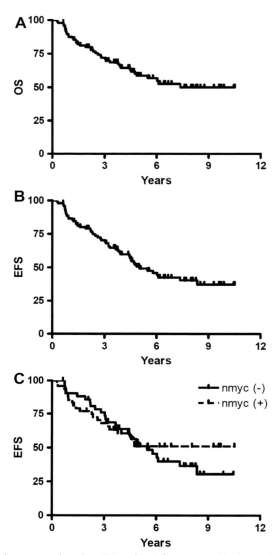

Fig. 1. Kaplan-Meier curves showing OS and EFS for consecutively treated patients under-going tandem autologous HSCT for high-risk neuroblastoma. The patients were conditioned with carboplatin/etoposide/cyclophosphamide for the first autologous HSCT procedure, fol-lowed by melphalan/TBI for the second. (*A*) OS from diagnosis, (*B*) EFS from diagnosis, and (*C*) EFS from diagnosis stratified by MYCN (nMYC) amplification. (*Modified from* Fish JD, Grupp SA. Stem cell transplantation for neuroblastoma. Bone Marrow Transplant 2008;41:162; with permission.)

Automated processes are available that are capable of selecting the CD34+ cell population away from the 99% of peripheral blood mononuclear cells that are irrele-vant for engraftment, including T cells and any tumor cells that do not express CD34. Of these automated technologies, the Isolex 300i device (Baxter, Deerfield, IL, USA) is approved by the US Food and Drug Administration, and the Miltenyi

CliniMACS device is approved in Europe and may become available in the United States. In negative selection, the most widely used technique in neuroblastoma has been antitumor monoclonal antibodies followed by a magnetic depletion step.[71,72] Although the evidence suggests that purging of bone marrow may be important, PBSC are less likely to contain tumor cells than bone marrow, and no study to date has shown that purging itself improves outcome. The COG has assessed whether graft manipulation through negative selection improves survival. COG A3973 is a recently completed, phase III, randomized comparison of purged versus unpurged PBSC given in the context of autologous HSCT for high-risk neuroblastoma. Data from this trial have yet to be published, but preliminary analyses have shown no advantage for patients receiving a purged PBSC product (S Kreissman and W London, unpublished data, 2008). The 2-year EFS was 51% in the unpurged group and 47% in the purged group ($P = .47$). The overall estimated 3-year EFS was 40%.

In 2010, the standard treatment of a patient with newly diagnosed high-risk neuroblastoma is based on the premise that maximal tolerable intensity of therapy yields maximal positive outcomes. The clinical trials outlined earlier have resulted in a therapeutic backbone of multicycle induction, PBSC collection early in induction, testing of the PBSC product for neuroblastoma contamination, as complete surgical resection as possible without organ sacrifice, autologous HSCT, and local radiotherapy, followed by biologic therapy and immunotherapy. It is an imposing package, and in the quest to improve outcomes further, the current phase III COG ANBL0532 trial is testing single versus tandem transplant as consolidation therapy. Although maximum tolerable intensity of cytotoxic therapy has been achieved, the outcomes for patients with high-risk neuroblastoma remain poor, with a 5-year OS less than 50%. Having reached an effective limit in chemotherapeutic intensity with tandem transplant, future trials need to focus on targeted therapies or immunotherapy in the hope of improving outcomes for children afflicted with this disease.

High-Dose mIBG with Stem Cell Rescue

The neuroendocrine nature of neuroblastoma makes it amenable to therapy with radiopharmaceutical agents also. Arising from the adrenal medulla, 90% to 95% of neuroblastomas show characteristic uptake of catecholamines and their derivatives, making them attractive radiopharmaceutical agents. Metaiodobenzylguanidine (mIBG) is an aralkylguanidine analog of catecholamine precursors, first reported in 1979, that can be labeled with ^{123}I or ^{131}I and imaged with a γ-camera.[73] The first report using mIBG for diagnosis and localization of neuroblastoma was in 1985.[74] Since that time, diagnostic imaging with [^{123}I-m]IBG has become the standard of care.

[^{131}I-m]IBG is a higher-energy releasing isotope that has been used for therapy for neuroblastoma since the mid-1980s. A review of the literature in 1999 showed an objective response rate to [^{131}I-m]IBG of 35% across multiple small studies, and a phase I study of its efficacy showed a response rate of 37% in children with relapsed neuroblastoma.[75,76] The dose-limiting toxicity of the [^{131}I-m]IBG is hematologic, although the marrow failure associated with high-dose [^{131}I-m]IBG can be overcome using stem cell rescue.[77,78] Building on these findings, several groups began to incorporate high-dose [^{131}I-m]IBG into the conditioning regimen for autologous HSCT. Initial, small-scale pilot studies showed the tolerability of high-dose [^{131}I-m]IBG combined with standard myeloablative chemotherapy.[79–81] This finding led to a larger, phase I study that again reported good tolerability of this combination in patients with refractory neuroblastoma but also reported an OS of 58%.[82] A phase II study combining high-dose [^{131}I-m]IBG and intensive chemotherapy as consolidation is under way for patients with high-risk neuroblastoma. Novel modalities for using this unique radiopharmaceutical in the treatment of neuroblastoma promise further improvements in outcomes for patients with high-risk disease.

ALLOGENEIC HSCT

Allogeneic transplant for solid tumors of childhood has been studied in a limited fashion and is rarely pursued, which may partly be a result of the neuroblastoma experience, in which allogeneic marrow sources were not superior to purged autologous sources (see later discussion).[83,84] No convincing evidence of any graft-versus-solid-tumor effect has been shown in pediatric patients, although case reports continue to be suggestive. In contrast, some of the earliest reports of allogeneic graft-versus-solid-tumor reports were in adult metastatic renal cell carcinoma,[85] in which 4 of 50 patients receiving myeloablative therapy and allogeneic stem cells were long-term survivors. A few other reports of allogeneic activity against adult tumors exist, including colon carcinoma, ovarian carcinoma, and prostate carcinoma.[86–88] In a review of these adult case reports and other small series, Ringden and colleagues[89] comment that the allogeneic effect may be a blunt application of immunotherapy that could be much more specifically applied with monoclonal antibodies without TRM.

The potential benefit of immunotherapy or cellular therapy for solid tumors should not be discounted; however, pure myeloablation and allogeneic reconstitution does not seem to provide any specific benefit for pediatric solid tumors in the face of the considerable risk of graft-versus-host disease (GVHD) and TRM. A recent report from Japan using a model of a murine bladder tumor, RIC, and allogeneic reconstitution followed by DLI showed some antitumor effect.[90] A recent case report from France observed that an adult patient undergoing RIC and allogeneic transplant for acute myelogenous leukemia had concomitant regression of a malignant renal tumor.[91]

Similarly, the potential to harness an immunotherapeutic effect has led some groups to study allogeneic HSCT for high-risk or relapsed neuroblastoma. A case report in 2003 described a patient in whom residual disease noted following a haploidentical HSCT fully resolved 3 years later, hinting at a potential graft-versus-neuroblastoma effect.[92] However, although the promise of a graft-versus-malignancy effect has been well described in allogeneic transplant for liquid tumors, it has yet to be convincingly shown in the setting of solid tumors.[93] Two studies published in 1994 compared allogeneic with autologous HSCT for high-risk neuroblastoma. The first compared the outcomes of 20 patients who underwent a single, human leukocyte antigen (HLA)-matched sibling donor transplant with 36 patients who underwent autologous transplants following identical TBI-containing conditioning regimens. Four of 20 allogeneic patients experienced TRM, compared with 3 of 36 autologous patients $(P = .21)$. The relapse rate among allogeneic HSCT patients was 69%, compared with 46% for autologous HSCT patients $(P = .14)$, and the estimated progression-free survival rates 4 years after HSCT were 25% for allogeneic HSCT patients and 49% for autologous HSCT patients $(P = .051)$.[84] A second case-controlled study compared 17 allogeneic and 34 autologous cases. It found no difference in progression-free survival (35% and 41% at 2 years, respectively).[94] Although these initial results do not show any clear benefit of allogeneic versus autologous HSCT for high-risk neuroblastoma, the advent of RIC regimens has provided the possibility that reduction of TRM allows for the detection of a therapeutic benefit. The limited data available to date indicate that there is no current role for allogeneic transplant for solid tumors in pediatric patients outside the context of well-designed clinical trials.

CELLULAR IMMUNOTHERAPY

Having reached an effective limit in chemotherapeutic intensity with tandem transplant, any further improvement of survival in children with high-risk neuroblastoma will have to come from novel therapeutic approaches. The most immediate hope for an effective different treatment modality lies in immunotherapy. Although several groups have published on the potential benefit of antineuroblastoma monoclonal antibodies,[95,96] this section focuses on potential cellular immunotherapies.

T-Cell Augmentation for Neuroblastoma

There were 3 cases of EBV-LPD among patients treated on the CHOP/DFCI tandem transplant study for neuroblastoma.[97] EBV-LPD is associated with significant immunosuppression and is usually uncommon following autologous HSCT. The Mackall group[98,99] has suggested that T-cell depletion that is produced by CD34 selection (as used in that study) may not increase immunosuppression. However, the CHOP/DFCI experience suggests that the combination of the use of a CD34-selected PBSC product and tandem transplant including TBI may be significantly more immunosuppressive than conventional autologous HSCT using unmanipulated PBSC.[70,97]

Regardless of the regimen used, the issue of immunosuppression induced by autologous HSCT is extremely important when considering alternative approaches to treating high-risk neuroblastoma. Although there is some suggestion that tandem HSCT may improve outcome in these patients (see earlier discussion), it is indisputable that the limit of dose escalation has been reached. An alternative approach is required. T-cell-based therapies, possibly paired with a cancer vaccine, represent a major area to explore novel treatments.[100,101] However, the limitations are clear: T cells, which may have antitumor efficacy, are not suited to treating bulk disease and are almost certainly best used at the point of minimal residual disease. This is the point reached after chemotherapy, surgery, radiation, and HSCT. Immunotherapy or tumor vaccines should be used as quickly as possible after completion of conventional therapy, but this is also a point where numbers of T cells and effector function are minimal to absent. One solution to this problem is to provide T cells to the patient in an attempt to speed immunologic recovery. This solution also has the potential to harness a profoundly lymphopenic environment supportive of homeostatic expansion. The passenger T cells provided with a PBSC product, although large in number, do not provide this solution, as recovery of cellular immunity after standard autologous HSCT takes many months.

The authors have recently tested an alternative approach in studies at the University of Pennsylvania and Children's Hospital of Philadelphia. The cell product used in all of these studies is ex vivo activated and expanded autologous T cells, using an artificial antigen-presenting cell of anti-CD3 and anti-CD28 activating antibodies coupled to beads.[102] The glucose monophosphate cell-manufacturing process produces a highly activated polyclonal T-cell population, with a T-cell repertoire representative of the full repertoire of the input of the cells into the culture.[103,104] We have referred to the infusion of these activated T cells into lymphodepleted patients as T-cell augmentation (TCA). We have completed a phase I trial of TCA in adult and pediatric patients with high-risk lymphoma following autologous CD34-selected PBSCT,[105] showing promising normalization of lymphocyte counts. In many cases, an absolute lymphocytosis was observed following TCA, suggesting that homeostatic T-cell proliferation was induced.

Ongoing studies have tested TCA in patients with high-risk neuroblastoma (S Grupp, unpublished data, 2009). In a series of studies, we are assessing the effect of TCA on immune reconstitution in these profoundly immunodeficient patients. These patients are an interesting group for studying TCA, as the need for HSCT is known at diagnosis and T cells may thus be collected before exposure to any immunosuppressive chemotherapy. Some of our preliminary results are presented in **Fig. 2**. Patients receiving a CD34-selected PBSC product have slow recovery of CD4+ T cells, which is significantly and strikingly improved after TCA given on day 12 after PBSC infusion. CD4 recovery is even more rapid when the infusion time is moved to day 2, with supranormal lymphocyte and T-cell counts apparent as soon as 10 days after TCA. Among patients receiving TCA on day 2, we have observed lymphocyte counts on day 12 post-HSCT as high at 10,000/μL. Four of these patients experienced an engraftment syndrome clinically indistinguishable from autologous GVHD, with fever, a rash characteristic of GVHD and, in the 2 cases in which skin biopsies were performed, biopsies were consistent with the appearance of GVHD as well. In the current study, we are assessing the effect of TCA on response to 2 vaccines (Prevnar conjugate vaccine and influenza vaccine). Preliminary analysis of the patients receiving Prevnar on day 12 post-SCT shows protective antipneuomococcal antibody titers to multiple serotypes as early as day 30 (S Grupp, unpublished data, 2009), which supports the hypothesis that TCA could be used to support an anticancer immunization strategy early after HSCT and achievement of minimal residual disease. Similar results in patients with myeloma receiving TCA and Prevnar vaccination have recently been published by June and coworkers.[106]

A possible target for a therapeutic cancer vaccine could be the cancer antigen survivin. Survivin is expressed in neuroblastoma, with expression correlating with adverse outcome.[107,108] In our studies, we have observed high expression of survivin in all tested tumor biopsies from high-risk patients with neuroblastoma.[109] We have found that most patients who are HLA-A2+, and are thus assessable for T cells recognizing survivin by tetramer staining, have such T cells. These T cells can be expanded and will kill allogeneic and autologous neuroblastoma in the appropriate HLA context. When whole neuroblastoma RNA is transfected into antigen-presenting cells and these cells are used to expand T cells with neuroblastoma specificity, the immunodominant epitope in the effector T-cell response is survivin.[109]

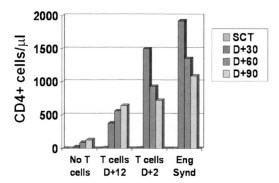

Fig. 2. Effect of TCA on peripheral blood CD4 cell recovery after immunoablative and myeloablative tandem HSCT for neuroblastoma. Patients were given autologous, costimulated, activated T-cell infusions on the indicated day after the second HSCT. In 4 patients, an engraftment syndrome (Eng Synd) was observed, consisting of a pruritic rash with or without fever. This correlated with higher CD4 counts after TCA. Similar results were seen in the CD8 count (data not shown).

Chimeric Immunoreceptors

Although antineuroblastoma monoclonal antibodies have had promising results, antibody-mediated antitumor activity may be dependent on functional adaptive immunity. Patients with neuroblastoma have been heavily treated with cytotoxic chemotherapy and radiation, with resulting immunosuppression, lymphopenia, and dysfunctional T cells. Although these challenges may be partly overcome by the TCA strategy described earlier, direct tumor targeting of neuroblastoma by T cells is additionally hampered by a paucity of tumor-specific antigens, and by the requirement for antigen processing and MHC-restricted antigen presentation. These immune-evasion strategies may be confronted through the generation of a chimeric immunoreceptor (CIR). The CIR is an engineered T-cell receptor (TCR) comprised of an antibody-like extracellular domain fused to an intracellular, functional TCR domain. The CIR was first described by Eshhar in 1993,[110] and has been developed and extended over the last 15 years. The first report of CIR-modified T cells specific for neuroblastoma was published in 2001,[111] and research since that time has led to an early-phase clinical trial published in 2007.[112] To redirect T cells safely against a tumor, the CIR must target a tumor-specific antigen that is minimally expressed on normal tissues.

In the Park trial, the investigators targeted the L1 cell-adhesion molecule (L1-CAM). L1-CAM is expressed on neuroblastoma cells and to a lesser extent on normal adrenal medulla and sympathetic ganglia. The trial was designed to test the feasibility harvesting, genetic modification, expansion, and reinfusion of autologous T cells, and safety. The feasibility was successfully tested, and there were no neural toxicities associated with the infusions. Although outcome was not a primary measure of the trial, there was at least 1 patient with a complete response. An important study in 2008 from the Brenner group used the CIR approach, engineering Epstein-Barr virus-specific cytotoxic T lymphocytes (EBV-CTLs) to express a CIR recognizing GD2 and using these cells in a clinical trial of 11 patients. The use of EBV-CTLs was chosen to address the issue of persistence in the recipient, as conventionally activated T cells used in clinical trials have often shown poor persistence and expansion. The study showed better persistence of the EBV-CTLs compared with activated T cells. Four patients had responses.[113] These trials, and others examining the use of CIR-modified T cells in other malignancies, have shown the feasibility of using genetic modification to redirect autologous T cells against malignancies. As technologies improve, and the experience with CIRs increases, harnessing a patient's own immune system in the treatment for high-risk pediatric cancers will likely become a promising new therapeutic frontier.

SUMMARY

In designing future therapies, consideration will have to include the long-term consequences of those therapies. As an example, although almost 1 in 2 patients with high-risk neuroblastoma may become long-term survivors with intensive multimodal therapy, their quality of life must also be considered. A recent case series examining 23 survivors of high-risk neuroblastoma treated with autologous HSCT showed that these patients can experience long-term complications including growth failure (100%), pubertal failure (83%), hearing impairment (73%), orthopedic complications (63%), renal impairment (47%), and thyroid abnormalities (36%).[114] These complications serve as a reminder that although the imperative to cure children with this terrible disease is strong, those designing therapeutic interventions must recall the motto "cure is not enough".

REFERENCES

1. Maris JM, Hogarty MD, Bagatell R, et al. Neuroblastoma. Lancet 2007; 369(9579):2106–20.
2. Kletzel M, Katzenstein HM, Haut PR, et al. Treatment of high-risk neuroblastoma with triple-tandem high-dose therapy and stem-cell rescue: results of the Chicago Pilot II Study. J Clin Oncol 2002;20(9):2284–92.
3. Kreissman SG, Rackoff W, Lee M, et al. High dose cyclophosphamide with carboplatin: a tolerable regimen suitable for dose intensification in children with solid tumors. J Pediatr Hematol Oncol 1997;19(4):309–12.
4. Aisenberg AC. Problems in Hodgkin's disease management. Blood 1999;93(3): 761–79.
5. Dorffel W, Luders H, Ruhl U, et al. Preliminary results of the multicenter trial GPOH-HD 95 for the treatment of Hodgkin's disease in children and adolescents: analysis and outlook. Klin Padiatr 2003;215(3):139–45.
6. Schellong G, Potter R, Bramswig J, et al. High cure rates and reduced long-term toxicity in pediatric Hodgkin's disease: the German-Austrian multicenter trial DAL-HD-90. The German-Austrian Pediatric Hodgkin's Disease Study Group. J Clin Oncol 1999;17(12):3736–44.
7. Balwierz W, Armata J, Moryl-Bujakowska A, et al. Chemotherapy combined with involved-field radiotherapy for 177 children with Hodgkin's disease treated in 1983–1987. Acta Paediatr Jpn 1991;33(6):703–8.
8. Schellong G, Bramswig JH, Hornig-Franz I, et al. Hodgkin's disease in children: combined modality treatment for stages IA, IB, and IIA. Results in 356 patients of the German/Austrian Pediatric Study Group. Ann Oncol 1994;5(Suppl 2):113–5.
9. Anselmo AP, Meloni G, Cavalieri E, et al. Conventional salvage chemotherapy vs. high-dose therapy with autografting for recurrent or refractory Hodgkin's disease patients. Ann Hematol 2000;79(2):79–82.
10. Ferme C, Mounier N, Divine M, et al. Intensive salvage therapy with high-dose chemotherapy for patients with advanced Hodgkin's disease in relapse or failure after initial chemotherapy: results of the Groupe d'Etudes des Lymphomes de l'Adulte H89 Trial. J Clin Oncol 2002;20(2):467–75.
11. Yuen AR, Horning SJ. Recent advances in the treatment of Hodgkin's disease. Curr Opin Hematol 1997;4(4):286–90.
12. Carella AM, Carlier P, Congiu A, et al. Autologous bone marrow transplantation as adjuvant treatment for high-risk Hodgkin's disease in first complete remission after MOPP/ABVD protocol. Bone Marrow Transplant 1991;8(2):99–103.
13. Federico M, Bellei M, Brice P, et al. High-dose therapy and autologous stem-cell transplantation versus conventional therapy for patients with advanced Hodgkin's lymphoma responding to front-line therapy. J Clin Oncol 2003;21(12):2320–5.
14. Linch DC, Winfield D, Goldstone AH, et al. Dose intensification with autologous bone-marrow transplantation in relapsed and resistant Hodgkin's disease: results of a BNLI randomised trial. Lancet 1993;341(8852):1051–4.
15. Schmitz N, Pfistner B, Sextro M, et al. Aggressive conventional chemotherapy compared with high-dose chemotherapy with autologous haemopoietic stem-cell transplantation for relapsed chemosensitive Hodgkin's disease: a randomised trial. Lancet 2002;359(9323):2065–71.
16. Williams CD, Goldstone AH, Pearce R, et al. Autologous bone marrow transplantation for pediatric Hodgkin's disease: a case-matched comparison with adult patients by the European Bone Marrow Transplant Group Lymphoma Registry. J Clin Oncol 1993;11(11):2243–9.

17. Stoneham S, Ashley S, Pinkerton CR, et al. Outcome after autologous hemopoietic stem cell transplantation in relapsed or refractory childhood Hodgkin disease. J Pediatr Hematol Oncol 2004;26(11):740–5.
18. Baker KS, Gordon BG, Gross TG, et al. Autologous hematopoietic stem-cell transplantation for relapsed or refractory Hodgkin's disease in children and adolescents. J Clin Oncol 1999;17(3):825–31.
19. Claviez A, Tiemann M, Luders H, et al. Impact of latent Epstein-Barr virus infection on outcome in children and adolescents with Hodgkin's lymphoma. J Clin Oncol 2005;23(18):4048–56.
20. Verdeguer A, Pardo N, Madero L, et al. Autologous stem cell transplantation for advanced Hodgkin's disease in children. Spanish group for BMT in children (GETMON), Spain. Bone Marrow Transplant 2000;25(1):31–4.
21. Anderlini P, Swanston N, Rashid A, et al. Evidence of a graft-versus-Hodgkin lymphoma effect in the setting of extensive bone marrow involvement. Biol Blood Marrow Transplant 2008;14(4):478–80.
22. Thomson KJ, Peggs KS, Smith P, et al. Superiority of reduced-intensity allogeneic transplantation over conventional treatment for relapse of Hodgkin's lymphoma following autologous stem cell transplantation. Bone Marrow Transplant 2008;41(9):765–70.
23. Anderson JE, Litzow MR, Appelbaum FR, et al. Allogeneic, syngeneic, and autologous marrow transplantation for Hodgkin's disease: the 21-year Seattle experience. J Clin Oncol 1993;11(12):2342–50.
24. Sureda A, Robinson S, Canals C, et al. Reduced-intensity conditioning compared with conventional allogeneic stem-cell transplantation in relapsed or refractory Hodgkin's lymphoma: an analysis from the Lymphoma Working Party of the European Group for Blood and Marrow Transplantation. J Clin Oncol 2008;26(3):455–62.
25. Alvarez I, Sureda A, Caballero MD, et al. Nonmyeloablative stem cell transplantation is an effective therapy for refractory or relapsed Hodgkin lymphoma: results of a Spanish prospective cooperative protocol. Biol Blood Marrow Transplant 2006; 12(2):172–83.
26. Peggs KS, Hunter A, Chopra R, et al. Clinical evidence of a graft-versus-Hodgkin's-lymphoma effect after reduced-intensity allogeneic transplantation. Lancet 2005;365(9475):1934–41.
27. Cairo MS, Gerrard M, Sposto R, et al. Results of a randomized international study of high-risk central nervous system B non-Hodgkin lymphoma and B acute lymphoblastic leukemia in children and adolescents. Blood 2007; 109(7):2736–43.
28. Link MP, Shuster JJ, Donaldson SS, et al. Treatment of children and young adults with early-stage non-Hodgkin's lymphoma. N Engl J Med 1997;337(18): 1259–66.
29. Seidemann K, Tiemann M, Schrappe M, et al. Short-pulse B-non-Hodgkin lymphoma-type chemotherapy is efficacious treatment for pediatric anaplastic large cell lymphoma: a report of the Berlin-Frankfurt-Munster Group Trial NHL-BFM 90. Blood 2001;97(12):3699–706.
30. Kobrinsky NL, Sposto R, Shah NR, et al. Outcomes of treatment of children and adolescents with recurrent non-Hodgkin's lymphoma and Hodgkin's disease with dexamethasone, etoposide, cisplatin, cytarabine, and l-asparaginase, maintenance chemotherapy, and transplantation: Children's Cancer Group Study CCG-5912. J Clin Oncol 2001;19(9):2390–6.

31. Gross TG, Hale GA, He W, et al. Hematopoietic stem cell transplantation for refractory or recurrent non-Hodgkin lymphoma in children and adolescents. Biol Blood Marrow Transplant 2009. [Epub ahead of print].
32. Chen AR. High-dose therapy with stem cell rescue for pediatric solid tumors: rationale and results. Pediatr Transplant 1999;3(Suppl 1):78–86.
33. Leavey PJ, Collier AB. Ewing sarcoma: prognostic criteria, outcomes and future treatment. Expert Rev Anticancer Ther 2008;8(4):617–24.
34. Leavey PJ, Mascarenhas L, Marina N, et al. Prognostic factors for patients with Ewing sarcoma (EWS) at first recurrence following multi-modality therapy: a report from the Children's Oncology Group. Pediatr Blood Cancer 2008; 51(3):334–8.
35. Miser JS, Goldsby RE, Chen Z, et al. Treatment of metastatic Ewing sarcoma/ primitive neuroectodermal tumor of bone: evaluation of increasing the dose intensity of chemotherapy–a report from the Children's Oncology Group. Pediatr Blood Cancer 2007;49(7):894–900.
36. Meyers PA, Krailo MD, Ladanyi M, et al. High-dose melphalan, etoposide, total-body irradiation, and autologous stem-cell reconstitution as consolidation therapy for high-risk Ewing's sarcoma does not improve prognosis. J Clin Oncol 2001;19(11):2812–20.
37. Burdach S, Meyer-Bahlburg A, Laws HJ, et al. High-dose therapy for patients with primary multifocal and early relapsed Ewing's tumors: results of two consecutive regimens assessing the role of total-body irradiation. J Clin Oncol 2003;21(16):3072–8.
38. Burdach S, van Kaick B, Laws HJ, et al. Allogeneic and autologous stem-cell transplantation in advanced Ewing tumors. An update after long-term follow-up from two centers of the European Intergroup Study EICESS. Stem-Cell Transplant Programs at Dusseldorf University Medical Center, Germany and St. Anna Kinderspital, Vienna, Austria. Ann Oncol 2000;11(11):1451–62.
39. Oberlin O, Rey A, Desfachelles AS, et al. Impact of high-dose busulfan plus melphalan as consolidation in metastatic Ewing tumors: a study by the Société Française des Cancers de l'Enfant. J Clin Oncol 2006;24(24):3997–4002.
40. Bacci G, Ferrari S, Longhi A, et al. Therapy and survival after recurrence of Ewing's tumors: the Rizzoli experience in 195 patients treated with adjuvant and neoadjuvant chemotherapy from 1979 to 1997. Ann Oncol 2003;14(11):1654–9.
41. Barker LM, Pendergrass TW, Sanders JE, et al. Survival after recurrence of Ewing's sarcoma family of tumors. J Clin Oncol 2005;23(19):4354–62.
42. Ladenstein R, Philip T, Gardner H. Autologous stem cell transplantation for solid tumors in children. Curr Opin Pediatr 1997;9(1):55–69.
43. Crist W, Gehan EA, Ragab AH, et al. The Third Intergroup Rhabdomyosarcoma Study. J Clin Oncol 1995;13(3):610–30.
44. Lager JJ, Lyden ER, Anderson JR, et al. Pooled analysis of phase II window studies in children with contemporary high-risk metastatic rhabdomyosarcoma: a report from the Soft Tissue Sarcoma Committee of the Children's Oncology Group. J Clin Oncol 2006;24(21):3415–22.
45. Houghton JA, Cook RL, Lutz PJ, et al. Melphalan: a potential new agent in the treatment of childhood rhabdomyosarcoma. Cancer Treat Rep 1985;69(1):91–6.
46. Lazarus HM, Herzig RH, Graham-Pole J, et al. Intensive melphalan chemotherapy and cryopreserved autologous bone marrow transplantation for the treatment of refractory cancer. J Clin Oncol 1983;1(6):359–67.
47. Koscielniak E, Klingebiel TH, Peters C, et al. Do patients with metastatic and recurrent rhabdomyosarcoma benefit from high-dose therapy with

hematopoietic rescue? Report of the German/Austrian Pediatric Bone Marrow Transplantation Group. Bone Marrow Transplant 1997;19(3):227–31.

48. Pinkerton CR, Groot-Loonen J, Barrett A, et al. Rapid VAC high dose melphalan regimen, a novel chemotherapy approach in childhood soft tissue sarcomas. Br J Cancer 1991;64(2):381–5.

49. Bagatell R, Rumcheva P, London WB, et al. Outcomes of children with intermediate-risk neuroblastoma after treatment stratified by MYCN status and tumor cell ploidy. J Clin Oncol 2005;23(34):8819–27.

50. Simon T, Spitz R, Faldum A, et al. New definition of low-risk neuroblastoma using stage, age, and 1p and MYCN status. J Pediatr Hematol Oncol 2004;26(12): 791–6.

51. Grupp SA, Stern JW, Bunin N, et al. Tandem high-dose therapy in rapid sequence for children with high-risk neuroblastoma. J Clin Oncol 2000;18(13): 2567–75.

52. Matthay KK, Villablanca JG, Seeger RC, et al. Treatment of high-risk neuroblastoma with intensive chemotherapy, radiotherapy, autologous bone marrow transplantation, and 13-cis-retinoic acid. Children's Cancer Group. N Engl J Med 1999;341(16):1165–73.

53. Cheung NV, Heller G. Chemotherapy dose intensity correlates strongly with response, median survival, and median progression-free survival in metastatic neuroblastoma. J Clin Oncol 1991;9(6):1050–8.

54. Berthold F, Boos J, Burdach S, et al. Myeloablative megatherapy with autologous stem-cell rescue versus oral maintenance chemotherapy as consolidation treatment in patients with high-risk neuroblastoma: a randomised controlled trial. Lancet Oncol 2005;6(9):649–58.

55. George RE, Li S, Medeiros-Nancarrow C, et al. High-risk neuroblastoma treated with tandem autologous peripheral-blood stem cell-supported transplantation: long-term survival update. J Clin Oncol 2006;24(18):2891–6.

56. Dini G, Lanino E, Garaventa A, et al. Myeloablative therapy and unpurged autologous bone marrow transplantation for poor-prognosis neuroblastoma: report of 34 cases. J Clin Oncol 1991;9(6):962–9.

57. Dini G, Philip T, Hartmann O, et al. Bone marrow transplantation for neuroblastoma: a review of 509 cases. EBMT Group. Bone Marrow Transplant 1989; 4(Suppl 4):42–6.

58. Kushner BH, O'Reilly RJ, Mandell LR, et al. Myeloablative combination chemotherapy without total body irradiation for neuroblastoma. J Clin Oncol 1991;9(2): 274–9.

59. Matthay KK. Impact of myeloablative therapy with bone marrow transplantation in advanced neuroblastoma. Bone Marrow Transplant 1996;18(Suppl 3):S21–4.

60. Matthay KK, O'Leary MC, Ramsay NK, et al. Role of myeloablative therapy in improved outcome for high risk neuroblastoma: review of recent Children's Cancer Group results. Eur J Cancer 1995;31(4):572–5.

61. Pole JG, Casper J, Elfenbein G, et al. High-dose chemoradiotherapy supported by marrow infusions for advanced neuroblastoma: a Pediatric Oncology Group study. J Clin Oncol 1991;9(1):152–8.

62. Philip T, Ladenstein R, Lasset C, et al. 1070 myeloablative megatherapy procedures followed by stem cell rescue for neuroblastoma: 17 years of European experience and conclusions. European Group for Blood and Marrow Transplant Registry Solid Tumour Working Party. Eur J Cancer 1997;33(12):2130–5.

63. Grupp SA, Stern JW, Bunin N, et al. Rapid-sequence tandem transplant for children with high-risk neuroblastoma. Med Pediatr Oncol 2000;35(6):696–700.

64. Philip T, Ladenstein R, Zucker JM, et al. Double megatherapy and autologous bone marrow transplantation for advanced neuroblastoma: the LMCE2 study. Br J Cancer 1993;67(1):119–27.

65. Grupp SA, Cohn SL, Wall D, et al. Collection, storage, and infusion of stem cells in children with high-risk neuroblastoma: saving for a rainy day. Pediatr Blood Cancer 2006;46(7):719–22.

66. Rill DR, Santana VM, Roberts WM, et al. Direct demonstration that autologous bone marrow transplantation for solid tumors can return a multiplicity of tumorigenic cells. Blood 1994;84(2):380–3.

67. Hafer R, Voigt A, Gruhn B, et al. Neuroblastoma cells can express the hemato-poietic progenitor cell antigen CD34 as detected at surface protein and mRNA level. J Neuroimmunol 1999;96(2):201–6.

68. Voigt A, Hafer R, Gruhn B, et al. Expression of CD34 and other haematopoietic anti-gens on neuroblastoma cells: consequences for autologous bone marrow and peripheral blood stem cell transplantation. J Neuroimmunol 1997;78(1–2):117–26.

69. Donovan J, Temel J, Zuckerman A, et al. CD34 selection as a stem cell purging strategy for neuroblastoma: preclinical and clinical studies. Med Pediatr Oncol 2000;35(6):677–82.

70. Kanold J, Yakouben K, Tchirkov A, et al. Long-term results of CD34(+) cell trans-plantation in children with neuroblastoma. Med Pediatr Oncol 2000;35(1):1–7.

71. Reynolds CP, Seeger RC, Vo DD, et al. Model system for removing neuroblas-toma cells from bone marrow using monoclonal antibodies and magnetic immu-nobeads. Cancer Res 1986;46(11):5882–6.

72. Seeger RC, Vo DD, Ugelstad J, et al. Removal of neuroblastoma cells from bone marrow with monoclonal antibodies and magnetic immunobeads. Prog Clin Biol Res 1986;211:285–93.

73. Wieland DM, Swanson DP, Brown LE, et al. Imaging the adrenal medulla with an I-131-labeled antiadrenergic agent. J Nucl Med 1979;20(2):155–8.

74. Geatti O, Shapiro B, Sisson JC, et al. Iodine-131 metaiodobenzylguanidine scin-tigraphy for the location of neuroblastoma: preliminary experience in ten cases. J Nucl Med 1985;26(7):736–42.

75. Tepmongkol S, Heyman S. 131I MIBG therapy in neuroblastoma: mechanisms, rationale, and current status. Med Pediatr Oncol 1999;32(6):427–31 [discussion: 432].

76. Matthay KK, DeSantes K, Hasegawa B, et al. Phase I dose escalation of 131I-metaiodobenzylguanidine with autologous bone marrow support in refractory neuroblastoma. J Clin Oncol 1998;16(1):229–36.

77. DuBois SG, Messina J, Maris JM, et al. Hematologic toxicity of high-dose iodine-131-metaiodobenzylguanidine therapy for advanced neuroblastoma. J Clin Oncol 2004;22(12):2452–60.

78. Goldberg SS, DeSantes K, Huberty JP, et al. Engraftment after myeloablative doses of 131I-metaiodobenzylguanidine followed by autologous bone marrow transplantation for treatment of refractory neuroblastoma. Med Pediatr Oncol 1998;30(6):339–46.

79. Corbett R, Pinkerton R, Tait D, et al. [131I]metaiodobenzylguanidine and high-dose chemotherapy with bone marrow rescue in advanced neuroblastoma. J Nucl Biol Med 1991;35(4):228–31.

80. Gaze MN, Wheldon TE, O'Donoghue JA, et al. Multi-modality megatherapy with [131I]meta-iodobenzylguanidine, high dose melphalan and total body irradia-tion with bone marrow rescue: feasibility study of a new strategy for advanced neuroblastoma. Eur J Cancer 1995;31(2):252–6.

81. Klingebiel T, Bader P, Bares R, et al. Treatment of neuroblastoma stage 4 with 131I-meta-iodo-benzylguanidine, high-dose chemotherapy and immunotherapy. A pilot study. Eur J Cancer 1998;34(9):1398–402.

82. Matthay KK, Tan JC, Villablanca JG, et al. Phase I dose escalation of iodine-131-metaiodobenzylguanidine with myeloablative chemotherapy and autologous stem-cell transplantation in refractory neuroblastoma: a New Approaches to Neuroblastoma Therapy Consortium Study. J Clin Oncol 2006;24(3):500–6.

83. Graham-Pole J. The role of marrow autografting in neuroblastoma. Bone Marrow Transplant 1989;4(1):3.

84. Matthay KK, Seeger RC, Reynolds CP, et al. Allogeneic versus autologous purged bone marrow transplantation for neuroblastoma: a report from the Children's Cancer Group. J Clin Oncol 1994;12(11):2382–9.

85. Childs RW, Clave E, Tisdale J, et al. Successful treatment of metastatic renal cell carcinoma with a nonmyeloablative allogeneic peripheral-blood progenitor-cell transplant: evidence for a graft-versus-tumor effect. J Clin Oncol 1999;17(7):2044–9.

86. Bay JO, Fleury J, Choufi B, et al. Allogeneic hematopoietic stem cell transplantation in ovarian carcinoma: results of five patients. Bone Marrow Transplant 2002;30(2):95–102.

87. Uhlin M, Okas M, Karlsson H, et al. Increased frequency and responsiveness of PSA-specific T cells after allogeneic hematopoetic stem-cell transplantation. Transplantation 2009;87(4):467–72.

88. Zetterquist H, Hentschke P, Thorne A, et al. A graft-versus-colonic cancer effect of allogeneic stem cell transplantation. Bone Marrow Transplant 2001;28(12):1161–6.

89. Ringden O, Karlsson H, Olsson R, et al. The allogeneic graft-versus-cancer effect. Br J Haematol 2009;147(5):614–33.

90. Kamiryo Y, Eto M, Yamada H, et al. Donor CD4 T cells are critical in allogeneic stem cell transplantation against murine solid tumor. Cancer Res 2009;69(12):5151–8.

91. Gac AC, Chantepie S, Leporrier M, et al. Full response of a localized renal tumour after reduced-intensity conditioned hematopoietic stem cell transplantation. Case Report Med 2009;2009:879765.

92. Inoue M, Nakano T, Yoneda A, et al. Graft-versus-tumor effect in a patient with advanced neuroblastoma who received HLA haplo-identical bone marrow transplantation. Bone Marrow Transplant 2003;32(1):103–6.

93. Srinivasan R, Barrett J, Childs R. Allogeneic stem cell transplantation as immunotherapy for nonhematological cancers. Semin Oncol 2004;31(1):47–55.

94. Ladenstein R, Lasset C, Hartmann O, et al. Comparison of auto versus allografting as consolidation of primary treatments in advanced neuroblastoma over one year of age at diagnosis: report from the European Group for Bone Marrow Transplantation. Bone Marrow Transplant 1994;14(1):37–46.

95. Cheung NK, Kushner BH, Kramer K. Monoclonal antibody-based therapy of neuroblastoma. Hematol Oncol Clin North Am 2001;15(5):853–66.

96. Simon T, Hero B, Faldum A, et al. Consolidation treatment with chimeric anti-GD2-antibody ch14.18 in children older than 1 year with metastatic neuroblastoma. J Clin Oncol 2004;22(17):3549–57.

97. Powell JL, Bunin NJ, Callahan C, et al. An unexpectedly high incidence of Epstein-Barr virus lymphoproliferative disease after CD34+ selected autologous peripheral blood stem cell transplant in neuroblastoma. Bone Marrow Transplant 2004;33(6):651–7.

98. Mackall CL, Fleisher TA, Brown MR, et al. Lymphocyte depletion during treatment with intensive chemotherapy for cancer. Blood 1994;84:2221–8.

99. Mackall CL, Stein D, Fleisher TA, et al. Prolonged CD4 depletion after sequential autologous peripheral blood progenitor cell infusions in children and young adults. Blood 2000;96:754–62.

100. June CH. Adoptive T cell therapy for cancer in the clinic. J Clin Invest 2007; 117(6):1466–76.

101. June CH. Principles of adoptive T cell cancer therapy. J Clin Invest 2007;117(5): 1204–12.

102. Levine BL, Ueda Y, Craighead N, et al. CD28 ligands CD80 (B7-1) and CD86 (B&-2) induce long-term autocrine growth of CD4+ T cells and induce similar patterns of cytokine secretion in vitro. Int Immunol 1995;7:891–904.

103. Levine BL, Bernstein W, Craighead N, et al. Ex vivo replicative potential of adult human peripheral blood CD4+ T cells. Transplant Proc 1997;29:2028.

104. Levine BL, Cotte J, Small CC, et al. Large-scale production of CD4+ T cells from HIV-1-infected donors after CD3/CD28 costimulation. J Hematother 1998;7: 437–48.

105. Laport GG, Levine BL, Stadtmauer EA, et al. Adoptive transfer of costimulated T cells induces lymphocytosis in patients with relapsed/refractory non-Hodgkin lymphoma following CD34+-selected hematopoietic cell transplantation. Blood 2003;102:2004–13.

106. Rapoport AP, Stadtmauer EA, Aqui N, et al. Restoration of immunity in lymphopenic individuals with cancer by vaccination and adoptive T-cell transfer. Nat Med 2005;11(11):1230–7.

107. Islam A, Kageyama H, Takada N, et al. High expression of Survivin, mapped to 17q25, is significantly associated with poor prognostic factors and promotes cell survival in human neuroblastoma. Oncogene 2000;19(5):617–23.

108. Azuhata T, Scott D, Takamizawa S, et al. The inhibitor of apoptosis protein survivin is associated with high-risk behavior of neuroblastoma. J Pediatr Surg 2001;36(12):1785–91.

109. Coughlin CM, Fleming MD, Carroll RG, et al. Immunosurveillance and survivin-specific T-cell immunity in children with high-risk neuroblastoma. J Clin Oncol 2006;24(36):5725–34.

110. Eshhar Z, Waks T, Gross G, et al. Specific activation and targeting of cytotoxic lymphocytes through chimeric single chains consisting of antibody-binding domains and the gamma or zeta subunits of the immunoglobulin and T-cell receptors. Proc Natl Acad Sci U S A 1993;90(2):720–4.

111. Rossig C, Bollard CM, Nuchtern JG, et al. Targeting of G(D2)-positive tumor cells by human T lymphocytes engineered to express chimeric T-cell receptor genes. Int J Cancer 2001;94(2):228–36.

112. Park JR, Digiusto DL, Slovak M, et al. Adoptive transfer of chimeric antigen receptor re-directed cytolytic T lymphocyte clones in patients with neuroblastoma. Mol Ther 2007;15(4):825–33.

113. Pule MA, Savoldo B, Myers GD, et al. Virus-specific T cells engineered to coexpress tumor-specific receptors: persistence and antitumor activity in individuals with neuroblastoma. Nat Med 2008;14(11):1264–70.

114. Trahair TN, Vowels MR, Johnston K, et al. Long-term outcomes in children with high-risk neuroblastoma treated with autologous stem cell transplantation. Bone Marrow Transplant 2007;40(8):741–6.

The Graft-Versus-Tumor Effect in Pediatric Malignancy

Terry J. Fry, MD[a],*, Andre Willasch, MD[b], Peter Bader, MD, PhD[b]

KEYWORDS

- Graft-versus-host disease
- Allogeneic hematopoietic stem cell transplantation
- Graft-versus-tumor effect • Graft-versus-host reaction
- Graft-versus-leukemia

Transplantation of hematopoietic stem cells from either bone marrow, peripheral blood, or umbilical cord blood from one individual to another following the administration of high doses of cytotoxic chemotherapy or radiation therapy (allogeneic hematopoietic stem cell transplantation [allo HSCT]) can cure malignancy. Indeed, this approach is the standard of care for children with acute leukemias at high risk of recurrence following chemotherapy. When allo HSCT was initially developed as a treatment for cancer, the concept was largely based on the opportunity to administer lethally myeloablative doses of cytoxic therapy to eradicate leukemia within the normal bone marrow with rescue provided by the donor hematopoietic stem cells. However, as experience with this procedure progressed, it became apparent the immune reactivity of the donor immune system against the recipient, termed *graft-versus-host reaction*, was associated with diminished risk of relapse, indicating that the curative potential of allo HSCT for cancer is multifactorial. Because severe forms of the graft-versus-host reaction directed against normal tissues (also termed *graft-versus-host disease* [GVHD]) also contribute to morbidity and mortality following allo HSCT, major efforts have focused on strategies to separate GVHD from the potentially beneficial immune reactivity against tumor (also called the *graft-versus-tumor* [GVT] effect). This article focuses on the data supporting the contribution of the GVT effect

[a] Division of Blood and Marrow Transplantation/Immunology, Center for Cancer and Blood Disorders, Children's National Medical Center, 1 West Wing, 111 Michigan Avenue, NW, Washington, DC 20010, USA
[b] Division for Stem Cell Transplantation, Hospital for Children and Adolescents III, Goethe University, Theodor-Stern Kai 7, 60590 Frankfurt am Main, Germany
* Corresponding author.
E-mail address: tfry@cnmc.org

Pediatr Clin N Am 57 (2010) 67–81
doi:10.1016/j.pcl.2009.12.002
0031-3955/10/$ – see front matter © 2010 Elsevier Inc. All rights reserved.

to cure of malignancy, what is known about the biology of the GVT reaction, and, finally, strategies to manipulate the GVT effect to increase the potency. Discussions about the biology and treatment of GVHD, and about the closely related topic of tumor-directed immunotherapeutic strategies to treat pediatric cancer, are contained in other articles in this issue.

EVIDENCE FOR GRAFT-VERSUS-TUMOR REACTIVITY

Although HSCT was originally conceived as an approach to replace defective or cancer-containing bone marrow and to rescue the patient from lethal doses of chemo-radiotherapy, it was eventually recognized that the transplant offered additional advantages in terms of preventing cancer relapse. In fact, the first evidence for an allogeneic antileukemic effect came earlier from murine models where it was observed that radiation alone was not curative in all cases of leukemia, but that the addition of immunologically disparate allogeneic bone marrow could improve the likelihood of leukemia eradication.[1] The earliest publications of large series of allogeneic transplants undertaken for leukemia in the late 1970s noted that the development of acute or chronic GVHD was associated with decreased risk of relapse.[2,3] The role of T cells in the GVT reaction was demonstrated first in preclinical models and subsequently in humans where increased relapse counterbalanced the beneficial effect of T cell depletion for GVHD in patients with leukemia.[4,5] The dramatic effect of GVHD on relapse emerged from a retrospective review of a large series of transplants for leukemia performed at multiple centers.[6] In this study, the risk of relapse was shown to be significantly affected by type of transplant or the development of GVHD with the highest relapse risk in patients undergoing transplants from genetically identical twins (also reported in other studies).[7] The next highest risk of relapse was seen in recipients of transplants using T cell–depleted grafts and in recipients of transplants from T cell–containing grafts not developing GVHD. The lowest risk of relapse occurred in patients with acute or chronic GVHD. There appears to be a graft-versus-leukemia (GVL) effect (measured by decreased risk of relapse) even in the absence of clinically evident GVHD, suggesting that these two immunologic aspects of transplant can be separated. Additional evidence for the GVL effect comes from data demonstrating that the level of immune suppression given to prevent GVHD can also affect the risk of relapse.[8] Finally, as will be discussed in more detail, manipulation of the immunologic milieu in the recipient with recurrent leukemia posttransplant through rapid withdrawal of immune suppression or the infusion of donor-derived lymphocytes (donor lymphocyte infusion [DLI]) can induce responses (and even remission in some cases), providing direct evidence for the GVL effect.[9] Indeed, for recurrent chronic myelogenous leukemia (CML) detected posttransplant while still in chronic phase, the likelihood of inducing remission with DLI may be as a high as 70% to 80%, thus representing the most potent form of cancer immunotherapy.[10,11] A number of recent publications have comprehensively reviewed the GVL effect.[12–14]

THE POTENCY OF GRAFT-VERSUS-TUMOR VARIES BY MALIGNANCY

Multiple studies assessing response to DLI have indicated that the potency of the GVT reaction differs depending on the type of malignancy for which the transplant was performed.[10,11,15–18] As indicated above, success is greatest when the GVT effect is used to treat recurrent disease posttransplant in patients with CML detected at low levels. However, as the disease burden increases and patients with CML are treated in more advanced stages, the response rate declines dramatically with only 10% to 30% of patients treated in blast crisis achieving remission. The response rate to DLI in acute myelogenous leukemia (AML) approximates that observed in CML treated in blast crisis, suggesting that a major factor determining the effectiveness of the GVT reaction is the pace of the disease.

Although disease burden and pace clearly contribute to the effectiveness of the GVT reaction, other factors certainly contribute as well, as indicated by the lower response for the GVT effect in acute lymphoblastic leukemia (ALL), the most common form of pediatric leukemia. There is definite evidence for the existence of a GVT effect in ALL, particularly in children.[19,20] However, the potency of this effect is certainly lower than that for CML and, probably, AML, although in the latter case studies have been conflicting. Because of this apparent low potency, clinicians have shown little enthusiasm for treating recurrent ALL posttransplant with discontinuation of immune suppression or DLI, although reports of remission being achieved using these maneuvers have been reported.[21,22] Regardless, the poor response rate indicates a clear need for strategies to enhance the GVT reaction in ALL.

In terms of solid tumors, the best evidence for the GVT effect comes from studies in lymphoma in adults (reviewed by Grigg and Ritchie).[23] As with leukemia, there are likely to be differences in potency, depending on the type of lymphoma. Non-Hodgkin lymphoma histology is less diverse in pediatrics, with the vast majority of lymphomas being high grade. Given the small numbers of pediatric lymphomas treated with allo HSCT, it is not possible to draw firm conclusions. However, recent retrospective analyses suggest the presence of a graft-versus-lymphoma effect in B and T lymphoblastic lymphoma.[24] Hodgkin disease may also be targeted by an allogeneic GVT effect. Finally, in terms of nonhematologic malignancies, there have been multiple reports of a GVT effect in adult renal cell carcinoma and some reports of a GVT effect in other solid tumors.[25-27] However, although there are case reports and small series of allo HSCT in pediatric solid tumors,[28-32] definitive data are lacking. Allo HSCT in pediatric solid tumors is the focus of several ongoing studies.

BIOLOGY OF GRAFT-VERSUS-TUMOR

Multiple lines of evidence support the notion that the immune system can prevent the development of cancer, can contribute to controlling the growth of cancer, and can be harnessed to treat established cancer. A detailed discussion of these topics is beyond the scope of this article but has been extensively reviewed elsewhere,[33,34] as well as in other articles of this issue. Thus, the concept that the donor immune system that recovers following allogeneic bone marrow transplant can target the recipient's tumor is consistent with a large body of data on the ability for the autologous immune system to recognize cancer. However, it has also been recognized that the growing tumor often acquires features that enable it to escape the patient's own immune system, a development termed *immunologic tolerance*.[35] Thus, the most simplistic explanation for the GVT effect is the replacement of an immune system that has been rendered tolerant by the tumor by an immune system that has not been made tolerant. While this is certainly a major contributor to the potency of the GVT reaction, there are many other layers of complexity. Perhaps the most obvious is the presence of multiple genetic differences between donor and recipient giving rise to new antigenic targets for the donor immune system to recognize. Indeed, it has long been recognized that genetic mismatch at the major histocompatibility loci (also termed *tissue rejection antigens*) can result in rapid rejection of solid organs due in part to a high precursor frequency of lymphocytes (particularly T cells) recognizing proteins derived from nonself versions of these highly polymorphic genes. However, even when a donor fully matched at these genes can be identified (as in the case of a matched sibling), multiple minor antigenic differences (eg, proteins derived from the Y chromosome in sex-mismatched transplants) remain and can serve as targets for GVHD or the GVT effect.[36] Because even minor antigenic differences are still recognized as nonself, they can induce more potent immune reactivity than can autologous immune responses recognizing self antigens on tumors. Thus, genetic disparity between donor and recipient likely serves as a major contributor to the potency of the GVT effect. Indeed, it has recently been demonstrated that when allo HSCT is performed from a major histocompatibility complex–mismatched donor (termed *haploidentical* as in a parental donor for a child), leukemic relapse can be associated with loss of expression of the disparate major histocompatibility complex haplotype under immunologic pressure from the donor.[37] In addition, the recent report of the association of GVT responses with specific HLA antigen disparities in a large series of patients has further contributed to our developing understanding of the mechanism of the GVT effect.[38]

For many disparate antigens between donor and recipient, broader expression on multiple normal tissues can make it challenging to separate GVHD from the GVT effect. Indeed, multiple clinical studies have shown that the severity of GVHD is linked to the risk of relapse.[6,39] However, recent retrospective data have demonstrated that the GVT effect from matched unrelated donors (predicted to have greater genetic disparity at minor histocompatibility antigens than siblings) was not more potent than in related donor transplants.[40] Furthermore, there is evidence for the GVT effect even in the absence of clinical GVHD.[6,41,42] Restricted expression of minor histocompatibility antigens on the cancer (or at least in the compartment in which the cancer resides, such as bone marrow in the case of leukemia) provides the potential for some selectivity of the GVT reaction.[36,43] Finally, since the donor immune system will not have been exposed to the malignancy, tolerance to tumor-restricted antigens that can serve as targets of an autologous antitumor immune response may not have occurred. Indeed, donor-derived responses to the leukemia-associated antigens derived from the Wilms tumor 1 (*WT1*) and proteinase 3 (*PR3*) genes have been identified in allo HSCT recipients[44] and responses to these antigens are associated with reduced risk of relapse.[45] Several potential targets of an allogeneic GVT response are summarized in **Fig. 1**. Ultimately, the potency of the GVT effect is likely to be derived from the composite immune reactivity against histocompatibility antigens

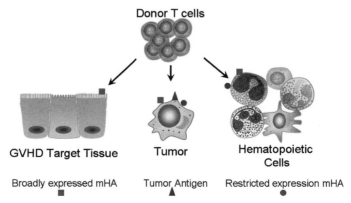

Fig. 1. Potential targets of a graft-versus-malignancy reaction following allogeneic blood or marrow transplantation. mHA, minor histocompatibility antigen.

(minor or major, depending on the degree of donor-recipient matching) and tumor antigen-directed immunity. Thus, manipulating the relative contribution of tumor-directed reactivity and responses to more broadly expressed antigens may be a potential strategy to increase the selectivity of the GVT effect (as discussed elsewhere in this issue).

While T cells mediate immunity, other immune cells also contribute to the GVT reaction. Recent data have demonstrated that, as with T cell responses, clinical responses to the GVT effect are associated with the development of antibody responses to tumor-specific antigens derived from immunoglobulin gene rearrangements in lymphoid malignancies[46–50] or from more broadly expressed minor histocompatibility antigens, such as HY.[51]

Adaptive immune responses (T cell or B cell) clearly play a major role in the GVT effect as depletion of donor T cells from the infused allograft and poor lymphocyte reconstitution following allo HSCT can result in increased risk of relapse, including pediatric ALL. However, activation of the nonspecific innate immune system can modulate the potency of an adaptive immune response (reviewed by Zitvogel and colleagues).[52] Following allo HSCT, heightened innate immune activation is induced by inflammation from the preparative regimen and is a central feature of the pathophysiology of GVHD.[53] Thus, it is likely that the potency of antigen-specific adaptive GVL responses may be modulated by increased innate immunity present in the post–allo HSCT environment and the impact can likely be both beneficial or detrimental, depending upon the setting.[54,55]

Natural killer (NK) cells are also capable of mediating a potent GVT effect, particularly early after HSCT.[56] Unlike T and B lymphocytes that generate an antigen receptor that recognizes a specific target, NK cells mediate cell killing. This characteristic is based in part on lack of self (discussed elsewhere in this issue). Thus, depending on degree and type of matching, donor NK cells can have varying degrees of reactivity. Indeed, multiple retrospective studies have shown that, for AML, NK reactivity is associated with a markedly decreased risk of relapse.[57] Interestingly, although NK cell–mediated GVT effect was originally associated with AML and believed to have a minimal effect in ALL, recent data have suggested that pediatric ALL may be more susceptible to NK cells than adult ALL.[58] However, the NK cell effect, while potent, is transient and limited to early post–allo HSCT before T cell recovery.[59] Thus, the optimization of the GVT effect to prevent relapse long term may require the memory associated with adaptive immune responses.

STRATEGIES TO ENHANCE GRAFT-VERSUS-TUMOR

The clinical GVT effect plays an important role in curing children with acute leukemia treated with allo HSCT. In recent years, different approaches aimed at augmenting or inducing an immune GVL effect have been used to treat relapsed leukemia after allogeneic bone marrow transplant.[9,11,60–66] Such approaches include abrupt cessation[67] or rapid tapering of immune suppression[68]; administration of cytokines, such as interleukin 2[61,66,69]; and DLI with or without cytokines.[70,71] As discussed above, although the benefit of immunotherapy for CML is well documented,[9,11,18,72–74] there are fewer reports of success in patients with acute leukemia.[61–63,70,75] Furthermore, clinical response to immunotherapy has usually been associated with measurable GVHD, possibly caused by high doses of donor cells given to patients in frank hematological relapse. However, there is evidence that low doses of donor T cells may also induce an effective GVT effect and produce long-term remission in patients whose leukemia burden is small.[40,70,76,77]

Guimond and colleagues[78] demonstrated that mixed hematopoietic chimerism (mixed donor and recipient cells) in T and NK cell subpopulations can frequently distinguish pediatric patients with leukemia relapse from children in remission, but such mixed hematopoietic chimerism is not useful for making the similar distinctions among adult patients. These findings support the hypothesis that a state of mixed hematopoietic chimerism may reduce the clinical GVT effect of alloreactive donor-derived effector cells in patients with acute leukemia and may facilitate the proliferation of residual malignant cells that may have survived the preparative regimen. Barrios and colleagues[79] could show in 133 patients with acute leukemia that patients with increasing mixed hematopoietic chimerism had a significantly elevated risk of relapse. Based on these studies, several consecutive trials were initiated evaluating the hypothesis that relapse of acute leukemia could be prevented by preemptive immunotherapy on the basis of chimerism analysis.[80–82] A large, prospective multicenter trial including patients with ALL demonstrated that (1) serial analysis of chimerism reliably identifies patients with highest risk of relapse and (2) that overt hematological relapse of ALL can primarily be prevented by withdrawal of immune suppression (cyclosporine A [CSA]) or administration of low-dose DLI based on chimerism analyses.[83] As indicated earlier, the presence of a GVT reaction in patients with ALL has been suggested by the higher incidence of relapse in the absence of GVHD[2,6,84] or with the use of T cell–depleted allografts.[5] These results are consistent with the finding that the highest incidence of increasing mixed hematopoietic chimerism was detected in those patients who received T cell–depleted stem cells. This supports a model wherein that T cell depletion substantially reduces the alloreactive potential of the graft, facilitates the recurrence of autologous hematopoiesis, and allows the reexpansion of underlying disease.[85–87] Molecular evidence of persisting or reappearing recipient cells may be a reflection of either survival of leukemic cells, or of survival of normal host hematopoietic cells, or of a combination of both. Surviving host normal hematopoietic cells may, in turn, facilitate the reemergence of a malignant cell clone by inhibiting immune competent donor effector cells. **Fig. 2** illustrates the posttransplant course of a patient suffering from pre–B cell ALL transplanted in second remission from a matched unrelated donor. The patient developed decreasing donor

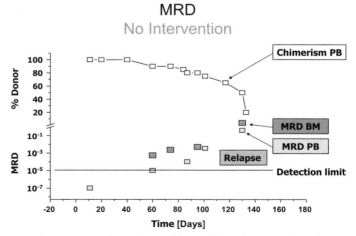

Fig. 2. Posttransplant course of a patient with B cell ALL (UPN1776): no intervention. BM, bone marrow; MRD, minimal residual disease; PB, peripheral blood.

chimerism posttransplant without the detection of leukemic cells or minimal residual disease (MRD). Consequently the patient became MRD positive and finally, demonstrated definitive relapse. This outcome is in concordance with patients treated for CML where it has been clearly demonstrated that reappearance of host hematopoietic cells in the mononuclear cell fraction precedes hematological relapse.[88] Based on these findings, the development of mixed hematopoietic chimerism has been considered to reduce the potency of the GVT effect.[88,89]

As mentioned above, support for the GVL effect in patients with ALL was documented in a study from Locatelli and colleagues,[90] who reported that lower-dose CSA reduced the risk of relapse in children with acute leukemia receiving allo HSCT transplants from human leukocyte antigen–identical siblings. Slavin and colleagues[70] reported the first successful implementation of DLI in a patient with ALL relapsed after allo HSCT. Since that time, experience with immunotherapy had shown that DLI initiated during frank hematological relapse induced complete remission in fewer than 10% of patients with ALL and in fewer than 25% of patients with AML.[10,67,91,92] If tumor burden was reduced by chemotherapy before DLI, the rate of complete response significantly improved (to 33% in ALL and 37% in AML).[93,94] These results suggested that immunotherapy offered the greatest benefit to patients with acute leukemia if administered before hematological relapse occurs.[70,76,77] **Fig. 3** illustrates the posttransplant course of a patient suffering from common-ALL transplanted in second remission from a matched unrelated donor. An MRD level of 1E-03 (1 in 1000 bone marrow cells) was detected before transplant. Posttransplant, the patient was 95% donor chimera. CSA was withdrawn, and a DLI administered to augment the GVT effect, which was associated with return to full donor chimerism. On day 60, after an MRD level of greater than 1E-04 (1 in 10,000 bone marrow cells) was detected, a second DLI was given and the patient developed GVHD grade 1. This was associated with eradication of MRD followed by long-term remission.

Therefore, it is desirable to identify early those patients who have the greatest risk of relapse and to deliver preemptive immunotherapy to them. Immunotherapy after allo HSCT can strengthen the alloreactive potential of the graft and augment the GVL

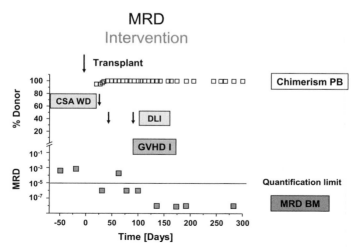

Fig. 3. Posttransplant course of a patient with c-ALL (UPN3710): intervention. BM, bone marrow; c-ALL, common ALL; PB, peripheral blood; WD, withdrawal.

effect (discussed elsewhere in this issue). Additionally, the implementation of treatment in an early phase of impending relapse offers a greater potential for therapeutic benefit with taper of immunosuppressive agents (eg, CSA, mycophenolate mofetil) or with low-dose DLI, approaches less likely to cause severe acute GVHD.[95] We hypothesize that the increase of donor chimerism after withdrawal of immunosuppressive drug clears residual disease by reinducing or augmenting the GVL effect. This GVL response is considered to be a complex, multistep process that involves activation of donor T cells by antigens, clonal expansion of activated T cells, and differentiation of these cells into helper or cytotoxic effectors. However, clonal expansion of transfused T cells is not likely to occur before 3 to 4 weeks after infusion. This delay could allow rapidly evolving leukemia cells to proliferate and progress to overt relapse before the donor graft has a chance to augment the GVL effect. In the majority of patients who do not respond to DLI, leukemia progresses to frank hematological relapse. In such cases, the diagnosis of imminent relapse was likely too late or the administered cell doses may have been too small to treat disease recurrence by induction of a GVL effect.

LIMITATIONS OF GRAFT-VERSUS-LEUKEMIA ENHANCING STRATEGIES

Chimerism analysis provides information about the alloreactivity or tolerance induction of the graft and thereby may serve as a "prognostic factor" more than as an indirect marker for minimal residual disease (MRD). However, it is important to stress that, due to the low sensitivity, chimerism analysis (approximately 1%) is not a reliable procedure for the detection of MRD. As a consequence of this, immunotherapy might be started too late if solely based on chimerism testing.

After transplantation, MRD monitoring in addition to chimerism analysis enables the detection of impending relapse in a substantial percentage of children undergoing transplantation for ALL. Consequently, these analyses have served as the basis for treatment intervention to avoid graft rejection, maintain engraftment, and treat imminent relapse. We retrospectively investigated the MRD load of patients who received DLI on the basis of increasing mixed hematopoietic chimerism. MRD was assessed when immunotherapy was initiated. It could be shown that patients who had an MRD load of greater than 1E-03 did not benefit from intervention. In contrast, patients whose MRD load was less than 1E-03 when immunotherapy was started had a fair chance to clear their disease (**Fig. 4**). These findings highlight the potentially important role for concomitant MRD analysis in addition to chimerism posttransplant.[96]

Few prospective data are available to evaluate the significance of MRD monitoring posttransplant. The first study was published by Knechtli and colleagues[97] in 1998. In this study, MRD was assessed using a polymerase chain reaction–based analysis of immunglobulin- and T cell receptor–gene rearrangements, followed by a resolution using a semiquantitative dot blot hybridization approach. The investigators demonstrated that persistent MRD positivity was an unfavorable predictor for event-free survival.[97] These results were later confirmed by smaller series of patients either using immunophenotyping of leukemia-associated antigens[98] or molecular-based quantitative polymerase chain reaction approaches,[99–101] all indicating that MRD is a predictor for unfavorable outcome.

Recently, the ALL-REZ BFM Study Group (Acute Lymphoblastic Leukemia Relapse Study of the Berlin-Frankfurt-Münster Group) monitored MRD in 92 pediatric ALL patients after allo HSCT to identify patients with the highest risk for relapse for whom preemptive treatment may be offered. The probability of event-free survival and relapse-free survival for MRD-negative patients was 0.55 and 0.77 respectively

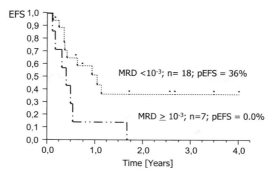

Fig. 4. The level of MRD at the time of further immunotherapy determines the success rate to avoid hematological relapse in children with ALL after allogeneic bone marrow transplant. Retrospective assessment of quantitative characterization of MRD levels are shown in children with ALL who received preemptive DLI on the basis of increasing mixed hematopoietic chimerism. EFS, event-free survival; pEFS, probability of event-free survival. (*From* Pulsipher MA, Bader P, Klingebiel T, et al. Allogeneic transplantation for pediatric acute lymphoblastic leukemia: the emerging role of peritransplantation minimal residual disease/chimerism monitoring and novel chemotherapeutic, molecular, and immune approaches aimed at preventing relapse. Biol Blood Marrow Transplant 2008;15(Suppl 1):62–71; with permission.)

compared with 0.48 and 0.62 respectively in MRD-positive patients less than 1E-04 and compared with 0.09 and 0.11 respectively in MRD-positive patients equal to or greater than 1E-04 (event-free survival: $P<.005$; relapse-free survival: $P<.001$). Patients who remained persistent MRD negative showed a probability of relapse-free survival of 0.78 compared with 0.5 in patients with a decrease of MRD and compared with only 0.1 in patients who developed an increase of MRD equal or above 1E-04 and of 0.0 in patients with MRD levels remaining permanently above 1E-04 ($P<.001$). Consequently, MRD monitoring after transplantation enables identification of individual patients with highest risk for relapse who may benefit from intervention.[102]

SUMMARY

An immunologic GVT effect contributes substantially to the curative potential of allo HSCT. The basis for the GVT effect is multifactorial and involves complex immunobiology that is only recently becoming understood. The potency of this reaction is dependent, in part, on the underlying malignancy being treated and is linked to the severity of GVHD. However, the GVT effect is observed in the absence of GVHD and ongoing studies are addressing how best to separate the beneficial aspect of the GVT effect from the morbidity and mortality associated with GVHD. One approach involves careful monitoring for recipient chimerism with early intervention by withdrawal of immunosupression or the infusion of donor lymphocytes. Given that therapeutic response to this approach is more likely with early detection of relapse, high-sensitivity methodology to detect relapse may increase the success of the GVT effect. Finally, emerging immune-based therapies (discussed elsewhere in this issue) offer the potential for further success using the GVT reaction. If, through these approaches, we can come to rely less on the conditioning regimen, then we will be able to perform allo HSCT with less long-term toxicity, which would be especially beneficial for treating children.

REFERENCES

1. Barnes DW, Corp MJ, Loutit JF, et al. Treatment of murine leukaemia with X rays and homologous bone marrow; preliminary communication. Br Med J 1956;2: 626–7.
2. Weiden PL, Flournoy N, Thomas ED, et al. Antileukemic effect of graft-versus-host disease in human recipients of allogeneic-marrow grafts. N Engl J Med 1979;300:1068–73.
3. Weiden PL, Flournoy N, Sanders JE, et al. Antileukemic effect of graft-versus-host disease contributes to improved survival after allogeneic marrow transplantation. Transplant Proc 1981;13:248–51.
4. Goldman JM, Gale RP, Horowitz MM, et al. Bone marrow transplantation for chronic myelogenous leukemia in chronic phase. Increased risk for relapse associated with T-cell depletion. Ann Intern Med 1988;108:806–14.
5. Marmont AM, Horowitz MM, Gale RP, et al. T-cell depletion of HLA-identical transplants in leukemia. Blood 1991;78:2120–30.
6. Horowitz MM, Gale RP, Sondel PM, et al. Graft-versus-leukemia reactions after bone marrow transplantation. Blood 1990;75:555–62.
7. Ringden O, Zwaan F, Hermans J, et al. European experience of bone marrow transplantation for leukemia. Transplant Proc 1987;19:2600–4.
8. Bacigalupo A, Van Lint MT, Occhini D, et al. Increased risk of leukemia relapse with high-dose cyclosporine A after allogeneic marrow transplantation for acute leukemia. Blood 1991;77:1423–8.
9. Kolb HJ, Mittermuller J, Clemm C, et al. Donor leukocyte transfusions for treatment of recurrent chronic myelogenous leukemia in marrow transplant patients. Blood 1990;76:2462–5.
10. Collins RH Jr, Shpilberg O, Drobyski WR, et al. Donor leukocyte infusions in 140 patients with relapsed malignancy after allogeneic bone marrow transplantation. J Clin Oncol 1997;15:433–44.
11. Kolb HJ, Schattenberg A, Goldman JM, et al. Graft-versus-leukemia effect of donor lymphocyte transfusions in marrow grafted patients. Blood 1995;86:2041–50.
12. Kolb HJ. Graft-versus-leukemia effects of transplantation and donor lymphocytes. Blood 2008;112:4371–83.
13. Ringden O, Karlsson H, Olsson R, et al. The allogeneic graft-versus-cancer effect. Br J Haematol 2009;147(5):614–33.
14. Barrett AJ. Understanding and harnessing the graft-versus-leukaemia effect. Br J Haematol 2008;142:877–88.
15. Collins RH Jr, Goldstein S, Giralt S, et al. Donor leukocyte infusions in acute lymphocytic leukemia. Bone Marrow Transplant 2000;26:511–6.
16. Porter DL, Collins RH Jr, Hardy C, et al. Treatment of relapsed leukemia after unrelated donor marrow transplantation with unrelated donor leukocyte infusions. Blood 2000;95:1214–21.
17. Shiobara S, Nakao S, Ueda M, et al. Donor leukocyte infusion for Japanese patients with relapsed leukemia after allogeneic bone marrow transplantation: indications and dose escalation. Ther Apher 2001;5:40–5.
18. Mackinnon S, Papadopoulos EB, Carabasi MH, et al. Adoptive immunotherapy evaluating escalating doses of donor leukocytes for relapse of chronic myeloid leukemia after bone marrow transplantation: separation of graft-versus-leukemia responses from graft-versus-host disease. Blood 1995;86:1261–8.
19. Appelbaum FR. Graft versus leukemia (GVL) in the therapy of acute lymphoblastic leukemia (ALL). Leukemia 1997;11(Suppl 4):S15–7.

20. Atra A, Millar B, Shepherd V, et al. Donor lymphocyte infusion for childhood acute lymphoblastic leukaemia relapsing after bone marrow transplantation. Br J Haematol 1997;97:165–8.
21. Kanamori H, Sasaki S, Yamazaki E, et al. Eradication of minimal residual disease during graft-versus-host reaction induced by abrupt discontinuation of immuno-suppression following bone marrow transplantation in a patient with Ph1-ALL. Transpl Int 1997;10:328–30.
22. Rymes NL, Murray JA, Holmes JA. Abrupt cessation of immunosuppression in a patient with persistent acute lymphoblastic leukaemia following allogeneic transplantation. Clin Lab Haematol 1996;18:45–6.
23. Grigg A, Ritchie D. Graft-versus-lymphoma effects: clinical review, policy proposals, and immunobiology. Biol Blood Marrow Transplant 2004;10:579–90.
24. Gross TG, Hale GA, He W, et al. Hematopoietic stem cell transplantation for refractory or recurrent non-Hodgkin lymphoma in children and adolescents. Biol Blood Marrow Transplant 2009. [Epub ahead of print].
25. Childs R, Chernoff A, Contentin N, et al. Regression of metastatic renal-cell carcinoma after nonmyeloablative allogeneic peripheral-blood stem-cell trans-plantation. N Engl J Med 2000;343:750–8.
26. Demirer T, Barkholt L, Blaise D, et al. Transplantation of allogeneic hematopoi-etic stem cells: an emerging treatment modality for solid tumors. Nat Clin Pract Oncol 2008;5:256–67.
27. Srinivasan R, Barrett J, Childs R. Allogeneic stem cell transplantation as immu-notherapy for nonhematological cancers. Semin Oncol 2004;31:47–55.
28. Capitini CM, Derdak J, Hughes MS, et al. Unusual sites of extraskeletal metas-tases of Ewing sarcoma after allogeneic hematopoietic stem cell transplanta-tion. J Pediatr Hematol Oncol 2009;31:142–4.
29. Hosono A, Makimoto A, Kawai A, et al. Segregated graft-versus-tumor effect between CNS and non-CNS lesions of Ewing's sarcoma family of tumors. Bone Marrow Transplant 2008;41:1067–8.
30. Lucas KG, Schwartz C, Kaplan J. Allogeneic stem cell transplantation in a patient with relapsed Ewing sarcoma. Pediatr Blood Cancer 2008;51:142–4.
31. Lang P, Pfeiffer M, Muller I, et al. Haploidentical stem cell transplantation in patients with pediatric solid tumors: preliminary results of a pilot study and anal-ysis of graft versus tumor effects. Klin Padiatr 2006;218:321–6.
32. Inaba H, Handgretinger R, Furman W, et al. Allogeneic graft-versus-hepatoblas-toma effect. Pediatr Blood Cancer 2006;46:501–5.
33. Dunn GP, Koebel CM, Schreiber RD. Interferons, immunity and cancer immu-noediting. Nat Rev Immunol 2006;6:836–48.
34. Gattinoni L, Powell DJ Jr, Rosenberg SA, et al. Adoptive immunotherapy for cancer: building on success. Nat Rev Immunol 2006;6:383–93.
35. Dunn GP, Old LJ, Schreiber RD. The immunobiology of cancer immunosurveil-lance and immunoediting. Immunity 2004;21:137–48.
36. Goulmy E. Minor histocompatibility antigens: from transplantation problems to therapy of cancer. Hum Immunol 2006;67:433–8.
37. Vago L, Perna SK, Zanussi M, et al. Loss of mismatched HLA in leukemia after stem-cell transplantation. N Engl J Med 2009;361:478–88.
38. Kawase T, Matsuo K, Kashiwase K, et al. HLA mismatch combinations associ-ated with decreased risk of relapse: implications for the molecular mechanism. Blood 2009;113:2851–8.
39. Gratwohl A, Hermans J, Apperley J, et al. Acute graft-versus-host disease: grade and outcome in patients with chronic myelogenous leukemia. Working

Party Chronic Leukemia of the European Group for Blood and Marrow Transplantation. Blood 1995;86:813–8.

40. Or R, Ackerstein A, Nagler A, et al. Allogeneic cell-mediated and cytokine-activated immunotherapy for malignant lymphoma at the stage of minimal residual disease after autologous stem cell transplantation. J Immunother 1998;21:447–53.

41. Ringden O, Labopin M, Gluckman E, et al. Graft-versus-leukemia effect in allogeneic marrow transplant recipients with acute leukemia is maintained using cyclosporin A combined with methotrexate as prophylaxis. Acute Leukemia Working Party of the European Group for Blood and Marrow Transplantation. Bone Marrow Transplant 1996;18:921–9.

42. Ringden O, Labopin M, Gorin NC, et al. Is there a graft-versus-leukaemia effect in the absence of graft-versus-host disease in patients undergoing bone marrow transplantation for acute leukaemia? Br J Haematol 2000;111:1130–7.

43. Mutis T. Targeting alloreactive donor T-cells to hematopoietic system-restricted minor histocompatibility antigens to dissect graft-versus-leukemia effects from graft-versus-host disease after allogeneic stem cell transplantation. Int J Hematol 2003;78:208–12.

44. Rezvani K, Barrett AJ. Characterizing and optimizing immune responses to leukaemia antigens after allogeneic stem cell transplantation. Best Pract Res Clin Haematol 2008;21:437–53.

45. Kapp M, Stevanovic S, Fick K, et al. CD8+ T-cell responses to tumor-associated antigens correlate with superior relapse-free survival after allo-SCT. Bone Marrow Transplant 2009;43:399–410.

46. Wu CJ, Yang XF, McLaughlin S, et al. Detection of a potent humoral response associated with immune-induced remission of chronic myelogenous leukemia. J Clin Invest 2000;106:705–14.

47. Yang XF, Wu CJ, Chen L, et al. CML28 is a broadly immunogenic antigen, which is overexpressed in tumor cells. Cancer Res 2002;62:5517–22.

48. Hishizawa M, Imada K, Sakai T, et al. Antibody responses associated with the graft-versus-leukemia effect in adult T-cell leukemia. Int J Hematol 2006;83:351–5.

49. Hishizawa M, Imada K, Sakai T, et al. Serological identification of adult T-cell leukaemia-associated antigens. Br J Haematol 2005;130:382–90.

50. Hishizawa M, Imada K, Sakai T, et al. Identification of APOBEC3B as a potential target for the graft-versus-lymphoma effect by SEREX in a patient with mantle cell lymphoma. Br J Haematol 2005;130:418–21.

51. Miklos DB, Kim HT, Miller KH, et al. Antibody responses to H-Y minor histocompatibility antigens correlate with chronic graft-versus-host disease and disease remission. Blood 2005;105:2973–8.

52. Zitvogel L, Apetoh L, Ghiringhelli F, et al. Immunological aspects of cancer chemotherapy. Nat Rev Immunol 2008;8:59–73.

53. Ferrara JL, Cooke KR, Teshima T. The pathophysiology of acute graft-versus-host disease. Int J Hematol 2003;78:181–7.

54. Delisle JS, Gaboury L, Belanger MP, et al. Graft-versus-host disease causes failure of donor hematopoiesis and lymphopoiesis in interferon-gamma receptor-deficient hosts. Blood 2008;112:2111–9.

55. Capitini CM, Herby S, Milliron M, et al. Bone marrow deficient in IFN-{gamma} signaling selectively reverses GVHD-associated immunosuppression and enhances a tumor-specific GVT effect. Blood 2009;113:5002–9.

56. Ruggeri L, Capanni M, Urbani E, et al. Effectiveness of donor natural killer cell alloreactivity in mismatched hematopoietic transplants. Science 2002;295:2097–100.

57. Velardi A, Ruggeri L, Mancusi A, et al. Clinical impact of natural killer cell reconstitution after allogeneic hematopoietic transplantation. Semin Immunopathol 2008;30:489–503.

58. Leung W, Iyengar R, Turner V, et al. Determinants of antileukemia effects of allogeneic NK cells. J Immunol 2004;172:644–50.

59. Lowe EJ, Turner V, Handgretinger R, et al. T-cell alloreactivity dominates natural killer cell alloreactivity in minimally T-cell-depleted HLA-non-identical paediatric bone marrow transplantation. Br J Haematol 2003;123:323–6.

60. Imamura M, Hashino S, Tanaka J. Graft-versus-leukemia effect and its clinical implications. Leuk Lymphoma 1996;23:477–92.

61. Mehta J, Powles R, Kulkarni S, et al. Induction of graft-versus-host disease as immunotherapy of leukemia relapsing after allogeneic transplantation: single-center experience of 32 adult patients. Bone Marrow Transplant 1997;20: 129–35.

62. Porter DL, Roth MS, Lee SJ, et al. Adoptive immunotherapy with donor mononuclear cell infusions to treat relapse of acute leukemia or myelodysplasia after allogeneic bone marrow transplantation. Bone Marrow Transplant 1996;18: 975–80.

63. Porter DL, Connors JM, Van Deerlin VM, et al. Graft-versus-tumor induction with donor leukocyte infusions as primary therapy for patients with malignancies. J Clin Oncol 1999;17:1234.

64. Bertz H, Burger JA, Kunzmann R, et al. Adoptive immunotherapy for relapsed multiple myeloma after allogeneic bone marrow transplantation (BMT): evidence for a graft-versus-myeloma effect. Leukemia 1997;11:281–3.

65. Verdonck LF, Lokhorst HM, Dekker AW, et al. Graft-versus-myeloma effect in two cases. Lancet 1996;347:800–1.

66. Sosman JA, Sondel PM. The graft-vs-leukemia effect. Implications for post-marrow transplant antileukemia treatment. Am J Pediatr Hematol Oncol 1993; 15:185–95.

67. Collins RH Jr, Rogers ZR, Bennett M, et al. Hematologic relapse of chronic myelogenous leukemia following allogeneic bone marrow transplantation: apparent graft-versus-leukemia effect following abrupt discontinuation of immunosuppression. Bone Marrow Transplant 1992;10:391–5.

68. Abraham R, Szer J, Bardy P, et al. Early cyclosporine taper in high-risk sibling allogeneic bone marrow transplants. Bone Marrow Transplant 1997;20:773–7.

69. Mehta J, Powles R, Singhal S, et al. Cytokine-mediated immunotherapy with or without donor leukocytes for poor-risk acute myeloid leukemia relapsing after allogeneic bone marrow transplantation. Bone Marrow Transplant 1995;16: 133–7.

70. Slavin S, Naparstek E, Nagler A, et al. Allogeneic cell therapy with donor peripheral blood cells and recombinant human interleukin-2 to treat leukemia relapse after allogeneic bone marrow transplantation. Blood 1996;87:2195–204.

71. Mehta J, Powles R, Treleaven J, et al. Outcome of acute leukemia relapsing after bone marrow transplantation: utility of second transplants and adoptive immunotherapy. Bone Marrow Transplant 1997;19:709–19.

72. Gardiner N, Lawler M, O'Riordan JM, et al. Monitoring of lineage-specific chimaerism allows early prediction of response following donor lymphocyte infusions for relapsed chronic myeloid leukaemia. Bone Marrow Transplant 1998;21: 711–9.

73. Mackinnon S, Papadopoulos EB, Carabasi MH, et al. Adoptive immunotherapy using donor leukocytes following bone marrow transplantation for chronic

myeloid leukemia: Is T cell dose important in determining biological response? Bone Marrow Transplant 1995;15:591–4.

74. Bacigalupo A, Soracco M, Vassallo F, et al. Donor lymphocyte infusions (DLI) in patients with chronic myeloid leukemia following allogeneic bone marrow transplantation. Bone Marrow Transplant 1997;19:927–32.

75. Pati AR, Godder K, Lamb L, et al. Immunotherapy with donor leukocyte infusions for patients with relapsed acute myeloid leukemia following partially mismatched related donor bone marrow transplantation. Bone Marrow Transplant 1995;15:979–81.

76. Johnson BD, Truitt RL. Delayed infusion of immunocompetent donor cells after bone marrow transplantation breaks graft-host tolerance allows for persistent antileukemic reactivity without severe graft-versus-host disease. Blood 1995; 85:3302–12.

77. van Rhee F, Lin F, Cullis JO, et al. Relapse of chronic myeloid leukemia after allogeneic bone marrow transplant: the case for giving donor leukocyte transfusions before the onset of hematologic relapse. Blood 1994;83:3377–83.

78. Guimond M, Busque L, Baron C, et al. Relapse after bone marrow transplantation: evidence for distinct immunological mechanisms between adult and paediatric populations. Br J Haematol 2000;109:130–7.

79. Barrios M, Jimenez-Velasco A, Roman-Gomez J, et al. Chimerism status is a useful predictor of relapse after allogeneic stem cell transplantation for acute leukemia. Haematologica 2003;88:801–10.

80. Formankova R, Sedlacek P, Krskova L, et al. Chimerism-directed adoptive immunotherapy in prevention and treatment of post-transplant relapse of leukemia in childhood. Haematologica 2003;88:117–8.

81. Gorczynska E, Turkiewicz D, Toporski J, et al. Prompt initiation of immunotherapy in children with an increasing number of autologous cells after allogeneic HCT can induce complete donor-type chimerism: a report of 14 children. Bone Marrow Transplant 2004;33:211–7.

82. Bader P, Niethammer D, Willasch A, et al. How and when should we monitor chimerism after allogeneic stem cell transplantation? Bone Marrow Transplant 2005;35:107–19.

83. Bader P, Kreyenberg H, Hoelle W, et al. Increasing mixed chimerism is an important prognostic factor for unfavorable outcome in children with acute lymphoblastic leukemia after allogeneic stem-cell transplantation: possible role for pre-emptive immunotherapy? J Clin Oncol 2004;22:1696–705.

84. Passweg JR, Tiberghien P, Cahn JY, et al. Graft-versus-leukemia effects in T lineage and B lineage acute lymphoblastic leukemia. Bone Marrow Transplant 1998;21:153–8.

85. Bader P, Stoll K, Huber S, et al. Characterization of lineage-specific chimaerism in patients with acute leukaemia and myelodysplastic syndrome after allogeneic stem cell transplantation before and after relapse. Br J Haematol 2000;108: 761–8.

86. Sykes M, Sachs DH. Bone marrow transplantation as a means of inducing tolerance. Semin Immunol 1990;2:401–17.

87. Nikolic B, Sykes M. Bone marrow chimerism and transplantation tolerance. Curr Opin Immunol. 1997;9:634–40.

88. Roux E, Abdi K, Speiser D, et al. Characterization of mixed chimerism in patients with chronic myeloid leukemia transplanted with T-cell-depleted bone marrow: involvement of different hematologic lineages before and after relapse. Blood 1993;81:243–8.

89. Roux E, Helg C, Chapius B, et al. Mixed chimerism after bone marrow transplantation and the risk of relapse. Blood 1994;84:4385–6.
90. Locatelli F, Zecca M, Rondelli R, et al. Graft versus host disease prophylaxis with low-dose cyclosporine-A reduces the risk of relapse in children with acute leukemia given HLA-identical sibling bone marrow transplantation: results of a randomized trial. Blood 2000;95:1572–9.
91. Kolb HJ. Donor leukocyte transfusions for treatment of leukemic relapse after bone marrow transplantation. EBMT Immunology and Chronic Leukemia Working Parties. Vox Sang 1998;74(Suppl 2):321–9.
92. Kolb HJ, Holler E. Adoptive immunotherapy with donor lymphocyte transfusions. Curr Opin Oncol 1997;9:139–45.
93. Riddell SR, Murata M, Bryant S, et al. T-cell therapy of leukemia. Cancer Control 2002;9:114–22.
94. Luznik L, Fuchs EJ. Donor lymphocyte infusions to treat hematologic malignancies in relapse after allogeneic blood or marrow transplantation. Cancer Control 2002;9:123–37.
95. Bader P, Beck J, Schlegel PG, et al. Additional immunotherapy on the basis of increasing mixed hematopoietic chimerism after allogeneic BMT in children with acute leukemia: is there an option to prevent relapse? Bone Marrow Transplant 1997;20:79–81.
96. Pulsipher MA, Bader P, Klingebiel T, et al. Allogeneic transplantation for pediatric acute lymphoblastic leukemia: the emerging role of peritransplantation minimal residual disease/chimerism monitoring and novel chemotherapeutic, molecular, and immune approaches aimed at preventing relapse. Biol Blood Marrow Transplant 2009;15:62–71.
97. Knechtli CJ, Goulden NJ, Hancock JP, et al. Minimal residual disease status as a predictor of relapse after allogeneic bone marrow transplantation for children with acute lymphoblastic leukaemia. Br J Haematol 1998;102:860–71.
98. Sanchez J, Serrano J, Gomez P, et al. Clinical value of immunological monitoring of minimal residual disease in acute lymphoblastic leukaemia after allogeneic transplantation. Br J Haematol 2002;116:686–94.
99. Spinelli O, Peruta B, Tosi M, et al. Clearance of minimal residual disease after allogeneic stem cell transplantation and the prediction of the clinical outcome of adult patients with high-risk acute lymphoblastic leukemia. Haematologica 2007;92:612–8.
100. Perez-Simon JA, Caballero D, Diez-Campelo M, et al. Chimerism and minimal residual disease monitoring after reduced intensity conditioning (RIC) allogeneic transplantation. Leukemia 2002;16:1423–31.
101. Uzunel M, Jaksch M, Mattsson J, et al. Minimal residual disease detection after allogeneic stem cell transplantation is correlated to relapse in patients with acute lymphoblastic leukaemia. Br J Haematol 2003;122:788–94.
102. Bader P, Kreyenberg H, Henze G, et al. Predictive value of MRD monitoring after allogeneic SCT in relapsed childhood acute lymphoblastic leukaemia: analysis of the ALL-REZ BFM Group. Bone Marrow Transplant 2009;43:40.

T-cell-based Therapies for Malignancy and Infection in Childhood

Nabil Ahmed, MD, MPH[a],*, Helen E. Heslop, MD[b],
Crystal L. Mackall, MD[c]

KEYWORDS

- Hematopoietic stem cell transplantation • Pediatrics
- Adoptive immunotherapy • Tumor vaccines
- Tumor antigens • Lymphopenia
- Immune reconstitution • Chimeric antigen receptor

TUMOR VACCINES

One major advance in T-cell-based immunotherapy in the last 20 years has been the molecular definition of numerous viral and tumor antigens. Immunodominant epitopes have been defined for major viral pathogens, including Epstein-Barr virus (EBV), cytomegalovirus (CMV), adenovirus, human papilloma virus (HPV) and hepatitis B virus (HBV), that can be used to target infections in immunocompromised hosts or tumors that express viral antigens.[1] Many tumor antigens have also been identified in adult cancers, and some of these are expressed in pediatric tumors (**Table 1**). Current concepts in tumor immunology suggest that tumor antigens comprise unique tumor-specific molecules or tumor-associated molecules that are rare on normal tissues but highly expressed on tumors. Unlike viral antigens, which generally induce

N.A. is supported by grants from the Dana Foundation, the V-Foundation for Cancer Research and the American Brain Tumor Association. H.E.H. is the recipient of a Doris Duke Distinguished Clinical Scientist Award and the NIH/NCI P01 CA94237 and SPORE-in Lymphoma. This work was supported, in part, by the Intramural Research Program of the National Cancer Institute (C.L.M.).

[a] Department of Pediatrics, Center for Cell and Gene Therapy, Baylor College of Medicine, 1102 Bates Street, Suite 1770, MC3-3320, Houston, TX 77030, USA
[b] Department of Pediatrics and Medicine, Center for Cell and Gene Therapy, Baylor College of Medicine and The Methodist Hospital, 1102 Bates Street, Suite 1770, MC3-3320, Houston, TX 77030, USA
[c] Center for Cancer Research, National Cancer Institute, NIH, 10-CRC, 1W-3750, 10 Center Drive MSC 1104, Bethesda, MD 20892-1104, USA
* Corresponding author.
E-mail address: nahmed@bcm.edu

Pediatr Clin N Am 57 (2010) 83–96
doi:10.1016/j.pcl.2009.11.002
0031-3955/10/$ – see front matter © 2010 Elsevier Inc. All rights reserved.

pediatric.theclinics.com

Table 1
Antigens expressed on pediatric tumors

Antigen	Pediatric Tumors	References
MAGE-1, -2, -3	Gliomas, medulloblastoma, neuroblastoma, osteosarcoma	2–4
GAGE	Gliomas, medulloblastoma, neuroblastoma, ESFT	2–5
BAGE	AML	2,6
XAGE	ESFT, alveolar rhabdomyosarcoma	7
NY-ESO-1	Synovial sarcoma, osteosarcoma, neuroblastoma	2,8,9
PRAME	AML, Wilms tumor, neuroblastoma	6,10–12
N-Myc	Neuroblastoma	13,14
Proteinase-3	CML, AML, MDS	15,16
WT1	AML, ALL, rhabdomyosarcoma	6,17,18
Survivin	Universal	19–21
Telomerase (hTERT)	Universal	20,22,23
Translocation breakpoints	Synovial sarcoma t(X;18); CML t(9;22), ALL t(12;21), DSRCT t(11;22), alveolar rhabdomyosarcoma t(2;13)	24–27
Mutant p53	Variable across histologies	28,29
HBV and HCV	Hepatocellular carcinoma	30
EBV EBNA2, 3	EBV lymphoproliferative disorder	
EBV EBNA1, LMP1, -2	Hodgkin disease, nasopharyngeal carcinoma, EBV lymphoproliferative disorder, Burkitt lymphoma	31,32

Abbreviations: ALL, acute lymphoblastic leukemia; AML, acute myeloid leukemia; CML, chronic myelogenous leukemia; DSRCT, dermoplastic small round cell tumor; ESFT, Ewing sarcoma family tumor; MDS, myelodysplastic syndrome.

vigorous immune responses in healthy hosts, tumor antigens are not naturally immunogenic as a result of a combination of factors including the immuno-evasive nature of cancer, which diminishes the presentation of antigens to the immune system, and co-expression of tumor-associated antigens on normal tissues, which leads to immune tolerance. The basis of tumor vaccine therapies is that administration of tumor-specific or tumor-associated antigens in the context of immune costimulation induces tumor-specific immunity, resulting in antitumor effects.

Thus far, ample data are available from studies on adult cancer to conclude that tumor vaccines administered as single agents do not reliably induce regression of established tumors.[33] However, tumor burden is 1 critical factor that influences the effectiveness of immunotherapy for cancer. Essentially all animal models of cancer show that minimal residual tumor burdens are more readily treated by the immune system than bulk tumors. In human studies, this is clearly shown in the context of donor leukocyte infusions for chronic myelogenous leukemia (CML), which show an 85% response rate when tumor burdens are low and a <20% response rate in accelerated phase.[34] Therefore, randomized studies are needed to determine whether vaccines administered in the adjuvant setting can prevent tumor recurrence. Indeed, recent results using an antigen-loaded dendritic cell vaccine approach in men with advanced prostate cancer has shown benefit over placebo in a large phase 3 trial (31.7% vs 23% 3-year survival and 25.8 months vs 21.7 months median survival), increasing the prospect that this may be the first cancer vaccine approved for general use by the US Food and Drug Administration.[35] Studies of tumor vaccines in pediatric oncology have largely followed these principles. Several types of vaccines have been administered, all primarily aimed at delivering a tumor antigen (or antigens) in a manner that induces robust immune responses. Many different approaches to tumor-based vaccination are currently used and even within each approach, the choice of appropriate adjuvant, antigen, timing of vaccine, route, and so forth remains under study (**Table 2**). Although essentially all studies of tumor vaccines in pediatric oncology have demonstrated safety, only a few instances of shrinkage of established tumors were observed.[36–39] Thus, as with adult tumors, current efforts in pediatrics are focused on administering tumor vaccines in the setting of minimal residual disease (MRD) or combining vaccines with other cell-based therapies for patients with established disease. This is discussed in the following sections.

ADOPTIVE CELL THERAPIES
Adoptive T-Cell Therapy for Infections

Infections are a major cause of morbidity and mortality in pediatric patients who are immunosuppressed following hematopoietic stem cell transplantation (HSCT).[36] As risk is clearly correlated with impaired virus-specific immunity in the early posttransplant period, there is considerable interest in developing means to adoptively transfer a protective T-cell response to more rapidly reconstitute immunity without transferring alloreactive T cells. Initial studies to evaluate such strategies targeted viruses such as CMV and EBV for which the immune response is well defined and the approach has now been extended to other pathogens such as adenovirus, BK virus and aspergillus.[37–43] The methodology used in these studies has been to generate cytotoxic T cells ex vivo from the transplant donor by repeated stimulation of donor-derived peripheral blood mononuclear cells (PBMCs) with antigen-presenting cells expressing viral antigens (**Fig. 1**). These cells are subsequently administered to the recipient either preemptively to prevent viral infection or to treat documented infections. To identify suitable viral antigens for such immunotherapeutic strategies, it is necessary to know which antigens are required for viral persistence. There must also be a source of the identified viral antigen suitable for clinical use and an appropriate antigen-presenting cell that will effectively present viral antigen and produce the costimulation required to activate an effective T-cell response.

Although the overall incidence of EBV-associated posttransplant lymphoproliferative disease (PTLD) following HSCT is less than 1%, the risk may be much higher in recipients with congenital immune deficiencies or in those who receive highly immunosuppressive conditioning regimens and T-cell–depleted grafts (which are becoming more commonly used as discussed elsewhere in this issue). EBV-PTLD is almost always derived from donor B cells, which express all EBV latency proteins and would normally be eliminated by an EBV-specific immune response. The proliferating cells have the same phenotype and pattern of EBV gene expression as EBV transformed B lymphoblastoid cell lines (LCLs), and these can be readily prepared from any donor by infecting PBMCs with a laboratory strain of EBV. LCLs are excellent antigen-presenting cells (APC) because they present EBV antigens efficiently on the cell surface with robust expression of costimulatory molecules. LCLs have been used after irradiation as effective stimulator cells to generate EBV-specific T cell lines from transplant donors. When EBV-specific cytotoxic T lymphocytes (CTLs) have been administered as prophylaxis or therapy for EBV lymphoma in high-risk HSCT recipients, immunity to EBV has been expanded and reconstituted. In addition, CTLs have been effective in preventing EBV-LPD in high-risk recipients and in treating

Table 2
Current approaches to tumor vaccination

Approach	Antigen	Restrictions	Pros	Cons
Peptide vaccines	9–20 amino acids	HLA allele specific (eg, HLA-A2)	Nontoxic, cheap to produce	Restricted to patients with 1 specific HLA allele, targets only 1 epitope, requires adjuvant
Protein	Whole antigens	None	No restrictions based on HLA type	Expensive to produce, unclear how best to administer
Pox viruses	Whole antigens	Some concern in immunosuppressed hosts	Can also administer costimulatory molecules	Antipox immune response limits repetitive administration
DNA	Whole antigens	None	Relatively simple to produce	May be better at boosting existing immune responses than inducing primary responses
Dendritic cells	Peptides or protein antigens or whole tumor cells	Requires cell harvest, not off the shelf	Individualized therapy, can deliver multiple antigens	Labor intensive, unclear how best to prepare dendritic cells
Genetically engineered tumor cell banks	All antigens expressed by the tumor will be presented	None	Presentation of multiple antigens, can specifically modulate costimulation	Individual cell banks difficult to produce, allogeneic cells banks may or may not be as effective

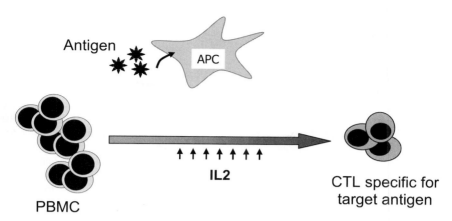

Fig. 1. Generating cytotoxic T lymphocytes (CTLs) by repeated ex vivo stimulation. Low-frequency virus-specific CTLs in a PBMC population are expanded by primary and secondary stimulation with antigen expressed on APCs followed by expansion with IL2. The resulting population is enriched for T cells specific for the viral antigen.

patients who received CTL for established EBV-LPD with sustained response rates of more than 85%.[1,44,45]

The immune response to CMV is also well defined and several studies have transferred donor-derived T cells specific for the immunodominant CMV pp65 protein to HSCT patients and shown that the transferred cells can prevent reactivation and treat CMV reactivation and disease in humans.[43,46,47] In these studies, several sources of antigen were used including purified CMV antigen, CMV-infected cell lysates, and peptides. APCs have included dendritic cells, fibroblasts, and PBMCs. The first studies performed by the Seattle group infused CD8+ CMV-specific T-cell clones, reactive against CMV virion proteins, and showed protection against CMV viremia and disease but long-term persistence only in patients who recovered CD4+ CMV-specific responses.[43] Peggs and colleagues[47] produced CMV-specific CTLs using dendritic cells pulsed with CMV antigens as stimulator cells and after infusion saw rapid expansion and long-term persistence of CMV immunity. Several other groups have confirmed that adoptive transfer of donor-derived CMV-specific T cells reconstitutes immunity to CMV and not only prevents transplant patients from developing CMV infection but also treats active disease.[46]

These approaches target only 1 virus in a patient population that is at risk of infection with many viruses following transplant. Leen and colleagues[40,41] therefore developed an approach to generate CTLs specific for 3 of the viruses that cause morbidity and mortality post transplant: CMV, EBV, and adenovirus. To achieve this they used mononuclear cells transduced with a recombinant adenoviral vector encoding the CMV antigen pp65 for the initial stimulation followed by stimulation with EBV-LCLs transduced with the same vector. Responding T cells were therefore exposed to all 3 antigens. In 2 sequential studies with CMV seropositive and seronegative donors they showed that trivirus (CMV-, EBV- and adenovirus-specific) CTLs could expand in response to viral challenge and clear all 3 viruses in more than 90% of patients with active viral disease. In preclinical studies this approach is being extended to target BK virus.[38]

These methodologies for generating virus-specific CTLs are complex and require considerable time. More rapid selection techniques are therefore being evaluated to provide virus-specific T cells for transplant recipients in a timely manner when they have active infections. Two methodologies to select virus reactive T cells from donor blood have been evaluated in clinical trials. In the first, T cells specific for the CMV-derived antigens were selected from apheresis products obtained from donors by incubating cells with HLA-peptide tetramers (4 joined major histocompatibility complex class I complexes that bind directly to T-cell receptors of a particular specificity) specific for the viral peptides followed by selection with magnetic beads. After infusion, the cells were able to expand by several logs and reconstitute immunity to CMV.[44] A limitation of this approach is that the product has limited specificity for 1 epitope and is only available for some HLA types. A second rapid selection technique is γ-interferon capture assay where donor blood cells are briefly stimulated with antigen and cells are selected that respond to antigenic stimulus based on γ-interferon secretion. Adenovirus-specific donor T cells isolated by this technique were infused into 9 children with systemic adenovirus infection post transplant and responses were seen in 5 of 6 evaluable patients.[40] An alternative to rapid selection is to develop banks of virus-specific cells lines so that the most closely matched product can be accessed rapidly if a patient develops an infection. A recent phase 2 study using banked EBV-specific CTLs to treat PTLD showed a response rate of 64% with no adverse events related to alloreactivity reported.[48] These studies have all targeted viral antigens. However, the T cell immune response may also be important for the clearance of other infections. The Perugia group has generated donor T-cell clones specific for *Aspergillus* and shown it is possible to transfer high-frequency T-cell responses associated with control of *Aspergillus* infections.[46]

Adoptive T-Cell Therapy for Pediatric Malignancies

Development of adoptive T-cell therapies for malignancy presents additional challenges. Although adoptively transferred T cells can in theory be redirected toward antigens that are relatively or absolutely restricted to the cancer cells, as discussed earlier, tumor-specific antigens are not as well defined or as immunogenic as viral antigens. In addition to tumor antigens defined in autologous hosts (see **Table 1**), allo-antigens selectively expressed on hematopoietic cells in the context of allogeneic HSCT are also a potential target and several groups are developing methods for selection of such T cells based on the γ-interferon capture assay.[49] As described earlier, EBV-PTLD has served as a prototype disease for successful targeting of viral antigens in cancer.[50] Other EBV-associated malignancies, such as Hodgkin lymphoma, some types of non-Hodgkin lymphoma (NHL) and nasopharyngeal carcinoma, have also been targeted using this strategy, but show lower response rates compared with EBV-CTL immunotherapy.[51,52] These tumors, which develop in previously immuno-competent individuals, express a more restricted array of EBV-encoded antigens than EBV-PTLD with only the weakly immunogenic EBV antigens (EBNA1, LMP1, and LMP2) being expressed. They also possess a myriad of immune evasion mechanisms that are active in the tumor microenvironment. To overcome these obstacles, investigators have developed ways to tailor CTL specificity to the subdominant tumor antigens expressed in EBV-associated lymphomas by stimulating T cells with latent membrane protein (LMP) antigens transferred to APCs (dendritic cells or LCLs) using adenoviral vectors. The resulting CTLs are enriched for T cells specific for LMP antigens and show increased activity compared with EBV-CTLs when administered to patients with EBV+ Hodgkin disease or NHL, either post transplant or in the setting of relapsed disease.[53]

Although T cells specific for tumor antigens can be identified, most are present at a low frequency, may have receptors with low avidity for the tumor antigens, and are commonly anergic. One strategy to overcome these limitations is to activate T cells ex vivo to circumvent these limitations and to overcome suppressive factors present in vivo thus augmenting the antitumor activity. In 1 study, leukemia reactive T cells derived from an allogeneic donor were selected based on their ability to inhibit in vitro growth of CML progenitor cells, and subsequently expanded to generate CTL lines. When transferred to the recipient they were able to induce remission in a patient with recurrent CML.[54] However, this labor-intensive process is not widely applicable. In a simpler approach, donor lymphocytes activated ex vivo were expanded nonspecifically by incubation with CD3- and CD28-coated beads and administered to 18 patients with relapsed lymphoreticular malignancies after HSCT. Objective responses were seen in 8 patients, 4 of whom had a sustained response at a median 23 months of follow-up.[55] However, such products may also contain alloreactive cells that can induce graft-versus-host disease (GVHD) and thus may be problematic when administered in the context of allogeneic HSCT.

An alternative approach to target tumor antigens is to genetically modify T cells with artificial antigen receptors to redirect their potent effector functions toward tumor cells. This has been achieved by expression of either $\alpha\beta$ T-cell receptor (TCR) heterodimer pairs or tumor antigen-specific chimeric antigen receptors (CAR). High-avidity $\alpha\beta$ TCR heterodimer pairs are either generated by immunizing HLA-A2 transgenic mice with tumor antigen or cloned from human autologous CTL cultures.[56] This approach, albeit attractive, is limited to individuals with a particular HLA type, mostly HLA-A2. Moreover, although $\alpha\beta$ TCR T cells mediate antitumor activities in vitro, their in vivo effector functions may be limited by the inadvertent pairing between the native TCR and the transduced $\alpha\beta$ chains. Such limitations may be overcome by using CARs, which are artificial molecules custom made by fusing an extracellular variable domain derived from a high-affinity monoclonal antibody specific for a tumor-restricted antigen of interest to an intracellular signaling domain usually derived from the ζ-signaling chain of the TCR.[57] On encountering the specific antigen by the extracellular antibody-derived domain, the T-cell–derived signaling domain initiates an intracellular signal that results in T-cell activation. To promote cell activation and survival, investigators have incorporated additional signaling domains from costimulatory molecules to the intracellular portion of the CAR. CARs recognize antigens in an HLA-independent manner (like an antibody), and thus overcoming a major limitation of the $\alpha\beta$ TCR. In addition, the CAR approach circumvents HLA molecule down-regulation, an important mechanism of tumor evasion, and allows for recognition of unprocessed tumor antigens on the surface of the cell.[58] Such artificial molecules can theoretically be designed to target any tumor-restricted or tumor-associated cell surface antigen of interest including those carbohydrate and glycolipid moieties such as the disialoganglioside GD2 in neuroblastoma. Genetically modified T cells have shown promising preclinical effector functions and CARs targeting CD20 and GD2 have already been evaluated in clinical trials in patients with lymphoma and neuroblastoma, respectively.[59,60] Clinical responses were seen in some patients in both studies although the persistence of the transferred T cells was suboptimal. Several trials are currently underway evaluating whether T cells genetically modified with a CAR targeting CD19 have activity in patients with relapsed CD19+ malignancies post transplant.

Among the many hurdles that must be crossed for adoptive T-cell immunotherapy to be successful is the necessity for infused T cells to access the long-term memory pool. There are concerns that excessive ex vivo stimulation can render T cells senescent, and unable to sustain long-term proliferation required of memory T cells.[61] A recent study showed that it may be possible to take advantage of the longevity of virus-specific CTLs and genetically incorporate antitumor specificities onto these cells. Two distinguishable GD2-specific CARs were transferred to EBV-CTL or primary T cells activated with OKT3 and IL2 administered to neuroblastoma patients in a phase 1/2 clinical trial and the EBV-specific CTLs did survive longer than T cells perhaps because of the costimulation received through their native receptor.[59]

HOST FACTORS PLAY AN ESSENTIAL ROLE IN DETERMINING THE EFFECTIVENESS OF T-CELL-BASED IMMUNOTHERAPY

Children with severe viral infection as a result of primary or secondary immunodeficiency and children with cancer are the primary pediatric populations for which T-cell–based immunotherapies are being developed. HSCT is a common cause of secondary immunodeficiency because it induces severe lymphocyte depletion, which typically lasts at least 1 year and may persist for several years following the procedure. Furthermore, common therapies for childhood cancer induce profound lymphocyte depletion and significant immunosuppressive effects result from the cancer itself. Thus, patients receiving T-cell-based immunotherapies have alterations in host immunity that can influence the effectiveness of T-cell-based immunotherapy both positively and negatively. In this section, the changes in immune physiology induced by T-cell depletion are described and the effects that these and other host factors play in enhancing or diminishing the effectiveness of T-cell-based immunotherapies for cancer or viral infection are discussed.

Unlike other marrow-derived populations, B cells and T cells require specialized microenvironments within the bone marrow and thymus, respectively, to recapitulate primary development. The bone marrow microenvironment needed to support B-cell lymphopoiesis remains functional throughout life, however, age-related changes occur within the thymus that limit the capacity for postnatal humans to regenerate T cells.[62] Many investigators have emphasized the importance of puberty and sex steroids in age-associated thymic involution, but from birth onward there is a relatively linear decline in the relative mass and function of the thymus. As a result, adolescents have substantially diminished thymic function compared with younger children,[63] and most patients in the fifth decade of life essentially show a complete inability to recover T cells via thymic-dependent pathways after T-cell depletion.[64] Furthermore, even in very young children, the thymic microenvironment is exquisitely susceptible to damage by various insults, including cytotoxic agents, viral infections, GVHD, and irradiation,[65] thus limiting that capacity for even young children with cancer or immunodeficiency to support thymic-dependent T-cell regeneration.

When thymic-dependent T-cell regeneration is limiting, T lymphocytes can be partially regenerated by thymic-independent homeostatic peripheral expansion. This process substantially increases T cell numbers and immune function, but it does not fully restore immune competence. Briefly, mature T cells (either remaining within the host following the lymphopenia-inducing insult, emerging from a diminished thymus, derived from maternal T cells, or adoptively transferred through a stem cell graft or immunotherapy product) undergo vigorous mitotic expansion, which is dramatically enhanced compared with low level cycling that T cells normally undergo throughout life in the absence of lymphopenia. This cycling represents a combination of enhanced T-cell proliferation toward cognate antigens (eg, viral antigens present during lymphopenia),[66] T-cell proliferation in response to cross-reactive antigens expressed by commensal flora in the gut, and T-cell proliferation toward self-antigens, which do not induce substantial T-cell cycling under lymphoreplete conditions, but can induce marked T-cell proliferation in the setting of lymphopenia.[67] Thus, lymphopenia results in profound increases in global T-cell cycling and increased responsiveness to antigens. These alterations in immune reactivity are driven primarily by interleukin-7 (IL7), a product derived from stromal cells that is a primary regulator of T-cell homeostasis.

IL7 is produced by nonlymphocytes including stroma within lymphoid tissues, and parenchymal cells in the skin, gut, kidney, and so forth. Nearly all T cells express the IL7 receptor and continually use this cytokine for survival.[68] When T cells are depleted, less IL7 is used and IL7 levels increase through accumulatation.[69] Normally, young children maintain serum IL7 levels of 10 to 20 pg/mL, whereas healthy adults maintain IL7 levels of 2 to 8 pg/mL. However, during lymphopenia, IL7 levels increase to as high as 60 pg/mL. Increases in serum IL7 levels associated with lymphopenia in clinical settings have been described following bone marrow transplantation, in human immunodeficiency virus (HIV) infection, following chemotherapy for cancer, and in idiopathic CD4 lymphopenia. The increased availability of IL7 drives the dramatic T-cell cycling that occurs during lymphopenia (termed homeostatic peripheral expansion or HPE). Furthermore, treatment of nonlymphopenic mice, monkeys, and humans[70] with recombinant human IL7 (rhIL7) induces increases in T-cell cycling (and, subsequently, T-cell number) that closely resembles that seen during lymphopenia.

HPE efficiently increases the number of T cells, but does not generate new T-cell specificities from hematopoietic stem cells, and therefore the TCR repertoire of populations generated by this pathway remains limited, especially when depletion is severe. Furthermore, patients reliant on HPE for T-cell regeneration have chronically diminished CD4+ counts, diminished CD4/CD8 ratios, and diminished numbers (but higher proportions) of suppressive CD4+ T cells. Therefore, the changes in immune physiology induced by T-cell depletion enhance T-cell reactivity but also result in chronic immune deficiencies. From an immunotherapist's perspective, these changes are potentially exploitable, especially in the context of adoptive immunotherapy, which requires efficient expansion of adoptively transferred T cells. Indeed, recent nonrandomized studies have suggested that induced lymphocyte depletion may actually enhance the efficacy of adoptive immunotherapy for cancer. Dudley and colleagues[33] administered autologous tumor-infiltrating lymphocytes harvested from patients with melanoma, expanded ex vivo and reinfused with rhIL2 to patients with or without regimens to induce lymphopenia. In sequential nonrandomized trials, they observed progressive increases in tumor response rates associated with increasing degrees of lymphocyte depletion. Similar results were seen in animal studies and in clinical trials wherein monoclonal antibodies targeting CD45 to induce lymphopenia appeared to augment the effectiveness of adoptive immunotherapy for nasopharyngeal carcinoma.[52] Thus, children who experience lymphocyte depletion as a result of congenital or acquired immunodeficiency, HSCT, or dose-intensive chemotherapy for cancer, may be good candidates for T-cell–based therapies because the lymphopenia associated with their underlying disease can serve to increase the effectiveness of adoptive cell therapy.

There are significant short- and long-term toxicities associated with lymphopenia. When the immunotherapy administered incorporates vaccines that rely on endogenous T cells present within the host to mediate immune responses, chronic lymphopenia and limited repertoire diversity induced by T-cell depletion may actually diminish the effectiveness of immune-based therapies. This effect of reduced T-cell number and restricted repertoire has been shown in animal studies in which lymphopenia diminishes the ability to control micrometastatic disease in cancer. Thus, future work seeks to replicate the beneficial aspects of lymphopenia in supporting T-cell–based immunoptherapy but avoiding the detrimental effects. This approach has been effective in animal studies, in which targeted therapies that specifically deplete suppressive T cells and use rhIL7 to replicate the lymphopenic milieu in lymphoreplete hosts resulted in better outcomes following adoptive immunotherapy than when the same therapy was administered to lymphopenic hosts.[71]

There is great interest in incorporating immune-based therapies into existing standard therapies for childhood cancer. Because it is not uncommon for children with high-risk tumors to be rendered free of visible disease using standard multimodality therapy and because such patient populations are also profoundly lymphopenic on completion of dose-intensive therapy, this provides a certain window of opportunity for treating MRD in patients with high-risk cancers. Indeed, consolidative immunotherapy, which combines tumor vaccines with therapies to enhance immune reconstitution has been piloted in patients with high-risk pediatric sarcomas.[72] Briefly, patients with metastatic and recurrent Ewing sarcoma and alveolar rhabdomyosarcoma undergo apheresis for collection of T cells before initiation of therapy. Following treatment with standard dose-intensive chemotherapy and local therapy to attempt to induce a state of MRD, they receive an infusion of autologous T cells as a source for homeostatic peripheral expansion and sequential tumor vaccines using dendritic cells. This approach demonstrated favorable survival using an intent-to-treat analysis, however conclusions regarding its efficacy are hampered by issues of selection bias, and the lack of a randomized control arm. Despite these caveats, the study clearly demonstrated that all immunized patients, regardless of profound lymphopenia present at the time of vaccination, showed the capacity to generate T-cell responses to vaccination within 3 months following chemotherapy, indicating that vaccine-induced T-cell responses can be induced early after cytotoxic chemotherapy when combined with autologous T-cell infusions. A subsequent study targeting patients with metastatic and recurrent pediatric sarcomas is under way with a modified dendritic cell vaccine, which incorporates approaches to deplete regulatory or suppressive CD4+ T cells and rhIL7 to enhance immune reconstitution.

SUMMARY

An increased understanding of the biology of T-cell mediated antiviral responses and tumor/immune interactions have opened up real opportunities to harness T cells for clinical benefit in children with immunodeficiency-associated infections and in children with cancer. Conceptually, the critical elements have been defined and clear proof of principle has been demonstrated. However, substantial work is needed to optimize these therapies, to broaden their applications beyond infection and enhance the effectiveness of tumor-directed therapies, and to simplify their administration so that they can be tested in large, controlled randomized studies. It is clear that if T cells are to be effective therapy for malignancies, CTLs must proliferate in vivo following infusion, while retaining their antitumor activity. Optimal proliferation depends on infusing T cells to an environment that promotes homeostatic expansion. The lymphopenia associated with the post-HSCT environment is similar to that in which autologous immunotherapy has been used. In addition, with the emerging methodologies available to detect relapse following HSCT, an increasing numbers of patients may benefit from these immunotherapeutic approaches instead of or as an adjunct to the nonspecific graft-versus-tumor effect discussed elsewhere in this issue. Furthermore, infectious complications of HSCT are more frequent following T-cell–depleted allografts (also discussed elsewhere in this issue) for which infectious pathogen-specific adoptive therapies play an important role. With increased knowledge of the optimum methodology for generation of T-cell products, and optimization of approaches to enhance the function of adoptively transferred T cells, adoptive immunotherapy strategies may find increasing use to reduce the risk of relapse and prevent and treat infections post transplant.

REFERENCES

1. O'Reilly RJ, Doubrovina E, Trivedi D, et al. Adoptive transfer of antigen-specific T-cells of donor type for immunotherapy of viral infections following allogeneic hematopoietic cell transplants. Immunol Res 2007;38(1–3):237–50.
2. Scanlan MJ, Gure AO, Jungbluth AA, et al. Cancer/testis antigens: an expanding family of targets for cancer immunotherapy. Immunol Rev 2002;188:22–32.
3. Scarcella DL, Chow CW, Gonzales MF, et al. Expression of MAGE and GAGE in high-grade brain tumors: a potential target for specific immunotherapy and diagnostic markers. Clin Cancer Res 1999;5(2):335–41.
4. Sahin U, Koslowski M, Tureci O, et al. Expression of cancer testis genes in human brain tumors. Clin Cancer Res 2000;6(10):3916–22.
5. Cheung IY, Cheung NK. Molecular detection of GAGE expression in peripheral blood and bone marrow: utility as a tumor marker for neuroblastoma. Clin Cancer Res 1997;3(5):821–6.
6. Greiner J, Ringhoffer M, Taniguchi M, et al. mRNA expression of leukemia-associated antigens in patients with acute myeloid leukemia for the development of specific immunotherapies. Int J Cancer 2004;108(5):704–11.
7. Liu XF, Helman LJ, Yeung C, et al. XAGE-1, a new gene that is frequently expressed in Ewing's sarcoma. Cancer Res 2000;60(17):4752–5.
8. Rodolfo M, Luksch R, Stockert E, et al. Antigen-specific immunity in neuroblastoma patients: antibody and T-cell recognition of NY-ESO-1 tumor antigen. Cancer Res 2003;63(20):6948–55.
9. Soling A, Schurr P, Berthold F. Expression and clinical relevance of NY-ESO-1, MAGE-1 and MAGE-3 in neuroblastoma. Anticancer Res 1999;19(3B):2205–9.
10. Li CM, Guo M, Borczuk A, et al. Gene expression in Wilms' tumor mimics the earliest committed stage in the metanephric mesenchymal-epithelial transition. Am J Pathol 2002;160(6):2181–90.
11. Oberthuer A, Hero B, Spitz R, et al. The tumor-associated antigen PRAME is universally expressed in high-stage neuroblastoma and associated with poor outcome. Clin Cancer Res 2004;10(13):4307–13.
12. Steinbach D, Hermann J, Viehmann S, et al. Clinical implications of PRAME gene expression in childhood acute myeloid leukemia. Cancer Genet Cytogenet 2002; 133(2):118–23.
13. Sarkar AK, Nuchtern JG. Lysis of MYCN-amplified neuroblastoma cells by MYCN peptide-specific cytotoxic T lymphocytes. Cancer Res 2000;60(7):1908–13.
14. Sarkar AK, Burlingame SM, Zang YQ, et al. Major histocompatibility complex-restricted lysis of neuroblastoma cells by autologous cytotoxic T lymphocytes. J Immunother 2001;24(4):305–11.
15. Molldrem JJ, Lee PP, Wang C, et al. Evidence that specific T lymphocytes may participate in the elimination of chronic myelogenous leukemia. Nat Med 2000; 6(9):1018–23.
16. Molldrem J. Immune therapy of AML. Cytotherapy 2002;4(5):437–8.
17. Sugiyama H. Cancer immunotherapy targeting WT1 protein. Int J Hematol 2002; 76(2):127–32.
18. Oka Y, Tsuboi A, Elisseeva OA, et al. WT1 as a novel target antigen for cancer immunotherapy. Curr Cancer Drug Targets 2002;2(1):45–54.

19. Andersen MH, Thor SP. Survivin–a universal tumor antigen. Histol Histopathol 2002;17(2):669–75.
20. Gordan JD, Vonderheide RH. Universal tumor antigens as targets for immunotherapy. Cytotherapy 2002;4(4):317–27.
21. Altieri DC. Validating survivin as a cancer therapeutic target. Nat Rev Cancer 2003;3(1):46–54.
22. Vonderheide RH, Hahn WC, Schultze JL, et al. The telomerase catalytic subunit is a widely expressed tumor-associated antigen recognized by cytotoxic T lymphocytes. Immunity 1999;10(6):673–9.
23. Vonderheide RH, Domchek SM, Schultze JL, et al. Vaccination of cancer patients against telomerase induces functional antitumor CD8+ T lymphocytes. Clin Cancer Res 2004;10(3):828–39.
24. Worley BS, van den Broeke LT, Goletz TJ, et al. Antigenicity of fusion proteins from sarcoma-associated chromosomal translocations. Cancer Res 2001; 61(18):6868–75.
25. Yotnda P, Firat H, Garcia-Pons F, et al. Cytotoxic T cell response against the chimeric p210 BCR-ABL protein in patients with chronic myelogenous leukemia. J Clin Invest 1998;101(10):2290–6.
26. Yotnda P, Garcia F, Peuchmaur M, et al. Cytotoxic T cell response against the chimeric ETV6-AML1 protein in childhood acute lymphoblastic leukemia. J Clin Invest 1998;102(2):455–62.
27. van den Broeke LT, Pendleton CD, Mackall C, et al. Identification and epitope enhancement of a PAX-FKHR fusion protein breakpoint epitope in alveolar rhabdomyosarcoma cells created by a tumorigenic chromosomal translocation inducing CTL capable of lysing human tumors. Cancer Res 2006;66(3): 1818–23.
28. Yanuck M, Carbone DP, Pendleton CD, et al. A mutant p53 tumor suppressor protein is a target for peptide-induced CD8+ cytotoxic T cells. Cancer Res 1993;53:3257–61.
29. Maher VE, Worley BS, Contois D, et al. Mutant oncogene and tumor suppressor gene products and fusion proteins created by chromosomal translocations as targets for cancer vaccines. Peptide based cancer vaccines. Austin, TX. Georgetown (TX): Landes Biosciences; 2000. p.17–39.
30. Radvanyi L. Discovery and immunologic validation of new antigens for therapeutic cancer vaccines. Int Arch Allergy Immunol 2004;133(2):179–97.
31. Roskrow MA, Suzuki N, Gan Y, et al. Epstein-Barr virus (EBV)-specific cytotoxic T lymphocytes for the treatment of patients with EBV-positive relapsed Hodgkin's disease. Blood 1998;91(8):2925–34.
32. Bollard CM, Straathof KC, Huls MH, et al. The generation and characterization of LMP2-specific CTLs for use as adoptive transfer from patients with relapsed EBV-positive Hodgkin disease. J Immunother 2004;27(4):317–27.
33. Rosenberg SA, Yang JC, Restifo NP. Cancer immunotherapy: moving beyond current vaccines. Nat Med 2004;10(9):909–15.
34. Dazzi F, Szydlo RM, Goldman JM. Donor lymphocyte infusions for relapse of chronic myeloid leukemia after allogeneic stem cell transplant: where we now stand. Exp Hematol 1999;27(10):1477–86.
35. Finke LH, Wentworth K, Blumenstein B, et al. Lessons from randomized phase III studies with active cancer immunotherapies–outcomes from the 2006 meeting of the Cancer Vaccine Consortium (CVC). Vaccine 2007;25(Suppl 2):B97–109.
36. Kennedy-Nasser AA, Brenner MK. T-cell therapy after hematopoietic stem cell transplantation. Curr Opin Hematol 2007;14(6):616–24.

37. Feuchtinger T, Matthes-Martin S, Richard C, et al. Safe adoptive transfer of virus-specific T-cell immunity for the treatment of systemic adenovirus infection after allogeneic stem cell transplantation. Br J Haematol 2006;134(1):64–76.
38. Gerdemann U, Christin AS, Vera JF, et al. Nucleofection of DCs to generate multi-virus-specific T cells for prevention or treatment of viral infections in the immuno-compromised host. Mol Ther 2009;17(9):1616–25.
39. Heslop HE. How I treat EBV lymphoproliferation. Blood 2009;114(19):4002–8.
40. Leen AM, Christin A, Myers GD, et al. Cytotoxic T lymphocyte therapy with donor T cells prevents and treats adenovirus and Epstein-Barr virus infections after haploi-dentical and matched unrelated stem cell transplant. Blood 2009;114(19):4283–92.
41. Leen AM, Myers GD, Sili U, et al. Monoculture-derived T lymphocytes specific for multiple viruses expand and produce clinically relevant effects in immunocom-promised individuals. Nat Med 2006;12(10):1160–6.
42. Perruccio K, Tosti A, Burchielli E, et al. Transferring functional immune responses to pathogens after haploidentical hematopoietic transplantation. Blood 2005; 106(13):4397–406.
43. Walter EA, Greenberg PD, Gilbert MJ, et al. Reconstitution of cellular immunity against cytomegalovirus in recipients of allogeneic bone marrow by transfer of T-cell clones from the donor. N Engl J Med 1995;333(16):1038–44.
44. Cobbold M, Khan N, Pourgheysari B, et al. Adoptive transfer of cytomegalovirus-specific CTL to stem cell transplant patients after selection by HLA-peptide tetra-mers. J Exp Med 2005;202(3):379–86.
45. Heslop HE SK, Pule MA et al. Long term outcome of EBV specific T-cell infusions to prevent or treat EBV-related lymphoproliferative disease in transplant recipi-ents. Blood. [Epub ahead of print].
46. Einsele H, Roosnek E, Rufer N, et al. Infusion of cytomegalovirus (CMV)-specific T cells for the treatment of CMV infection not responding to antiviral chemo-therapy. Blood 2002;99(11):3916–22.
47. Peggs KS, Verfuerth S, Pizzey A, et al. Adoptive cellular therapy for early cyto-megalovirus infection after allogeneic stem-cell transplantation with virus-specific T-cell lines. Lancet 2003;362(9393):1375–7.
48. Haque T, Wilkie GM, Jones MM, et al. Allogeneic cytotoxic T-cell therapy for EBV-positive post-transplantation lymphoproliferative disease: results of a phase 2 multicenter clinical trial. Blood 2007;110(4):1123–31.
49. Jedema I, Meij P, Steeneveld E, et al. Early detection and rapid isolation of leukemia-reactive donor T cells for adoptive transfer using the IFN-gamma secre-tion assay. Clin Cancer Res 2007;13(2 Pt 1):636–43.
50. Rooney CM, Smith CA, Ng CY, et al. Infusion of cytotoxic T cells for the prevention and treatment of Epstein-Barr virus-induced lymphoma in allogeneic transplant recipients. Blood 1998;92(5):1549–55.
51. Bollard CM, Aguilar L, Straathof KC, et al. Cytotoxic T lymphocyte therapy for Epstein-Barr virus+ Hodgkin's disease. J Exp Med 2004;200(12):1623–33.
52. Louis CU, Straathof K, Bollard CM, et al. Enhancing the in vivo expansion of adoptively transferred EBV-specific CTL with lymphodepleting CD45 monoclonal antibodies in NPC patients. Blood 2009;113(11):2442–50.
53. Bollard CM, Gottschalk S, Leen AM, et al. Complete responses of relapsed lymphoma following genetic modification of tumor-antigen presenting cells and T-lymphocyte transfer. Blood 2007;110(8):2838–45.
54. Falkenburg JH, Wafelman AR, Joosten P, et al. Complete remission of acceler-ated phase chronic myeloid leukemia by treatment with leukemia-reactive cytotoxic T lymphocytes. Blood 1999;94(4):1201–8.

55. Porter DL, Levine BL, Bunin N, et al. A phase 1 trial of donor lymphocyte infusions expanded and activated ex vivo via CD3/CD28 co-stimulation. Blood 2006; 107(4):1325–31.
56. Sadelain M, Riviere I, Brentjens R. Targeting tumours with genetically enhanced T lymphocytes. Nat Rev Cancer 2003;3(1):35–45.
57. Eshhar Z, Waks T, Gross G, et al. Specific activation and targeting of cytotoxic lymphocytes through chimeric single chains consisting of antibody-binding domains and the gamma or zeta subunits of the immunoglobulin and T-cell receptors. Proc Natl Acad Sci U S A 1993;90(2):720–4.
58. Ahmed N, Ratnayake M, Savoldo B, et al. Regression of experimental medulloblastoma following transfer of HER2-specific T cells. Cancer Res 2007;67(12):5957–64.
59. Pule MA, Savoldo B, Myers GD, et al. Virus-specific T cells engineered to coexpress tumor-specific receptors: persistence and anti-tumor activity in individuals with neuroblastoma. Nat Med 2008;14(11):1264–70.
60. Till BG, Jensen MC, Wang J, et al. Adoptive immunotherapy for indolent non-Hodgkin lymphoma and mantle cell lymphoma using genetically modified autologous CD20-specific T cells. Blood 2008;112(6):2261–71.
61. Klebanoff CA, Gattinoni L, Torabi-Parizi P, et al. Central memory self/tumor-reactive CD8+ T cells confer superior antitumor immunity compared with effector memory T cells. Proc Natl Acad Sci U S A 2005;102(27):9571–6.
62. Haynes BF, Sempowski GD, Wells AF, et al. The human thymus during aging. Immunol Res 2000;22(2–3):253–61.
63. Mackall CL, Fleisher TA, Brown MR, et al. Age, thymopoiesis, and CD4+ T-lymphocyte regeneration after intensive chemotherapy. N Engl J Med 1995; 332(3):143–9.
64. Hakim FT, Memon SA, Cepeda R, et al. Age-dependent incidence, time course, and consequences of thymic renewal in adults. J Clin Invest 2005;115(4):930–9.
65. Weinberg K, Blazar BR, Wagner JE, et al. Factors affecting thymic function after allogeneic hematopoietic stem cell transplantation. Blood 2001;97(5):1458–66.
66. Mackall CL, Bare CV, Granger LA, et al. Thymic-independent T cell regeneration occurs via antigen-driven expansion of peripheral T cells resulting in a repertoire that is limited in diversity and prone to skewing. J Immunol 1996;156(12): 4609–16.
67. Surh CD, Sprent J. Regulation of mature T cell homeostasis. Semin Immunol 2005;17(3):183–91.
68. Fry TJ, Mackall CL. The many faces of IL-7: from lymphopoiesis to peripheral T cell maintenance. J Immunol 2005;174(11):6571–6.
69. Guimond M, Veenstra RG, Grindler DJ, et al. Interleukin 7 signaling in dendritic cells regulates the homeostatic proliferation and niche size of CD4+ T cells. Nat Immunol 2009;10(2):149–57.
70. Sportes C, Hakim FT, Memon SA, et al. Administration of rhIL-7 in humans increases in vivo TCR repertoire diversity by preferential expansion of naive T cell subsets. J Exp Med 2008;205(7):1701–14.
71. Cui Y, Zhang H, Meadors J, et al. Harnessing the physiology of lymphopenia to support adoptive immunotherapy in lymphoreplete hosts. Blood 2009.
72. Mackall CL, Rhee EH, Read EJ, et al. A pilot study of consolidative immunotherapy in patients with high-risk pediatric sarcomas. Clin Cancer Res 2008; 14(15):4850–8.

Immunotherapy in the Context of Hematopoietic Stem Cell Transplantation: The Emerging Role of Natural Killer Cells and Mesenchymal Stromal Cells

Arjan C. Lankester, MD, PhD[a],*, Lynne M. Ball, MD, PhD[a],
Peter Lang, MD, PhD[b], Rupert Handgretinger, MD, PhD[b]

KEYWORDS

- Immunotherapy • Hematopoietic stem cell transplantation
- Natural killer cells • Mesenchymal stromal cells

Immunotherapy in the context of hematopoietic stem cell transplantation (HSCT) has been dominated for many years by T cell– and dendritic cell–based treatment modalities. During the last decade, insight into the biology of natural killer (NK) cells and mesenchymal stromal cells (MSC) has rapidly increased and resulted in NK- and MSC-based therapeutic strategies in clinical practice. This article reviews current knowledge of the biology and clinical aspects of NK cells and MSC.

PART 1: NK CELLS
Biology of NK Cells

NK cells were first identified in 1975 in mice as a distinct subpopulation of lymphocytes with the capacity of killing tumor cells without prior sensitization.[1] In humans, NK cells represent about 5% to 20% of peripheral blood lymphocytes and are defined as CD56+CD3− lymphocytes, which often have a granular morphology.[2] Extensive

[a] Department of Pediatrics, Leiden University Medical Centre, Albinusdreef 2, 2300 RC Leiden, The Netherlands
[b] Children's University Hospital, Hoppe-Seyler-Strasse 1, 72076 Tuebingen, Germany
* Corresponding author.
E-mail address: a.lankester@lumc.nl

Pediatr Clin N Am 57 (2010) 97–121
doi:10.1016/j.pcl.2009.12.001
0031-3955/10/$ – see front matter © 2010 Elsevier Inc. All rights reserved.

pediatric.theclinics.com

research has revealed that NK cells are a heterogenous population of cells with various functions in cytokine production and cytotoxicity.[3] In contrast to T-lymphocytes, NK cells do not recognize foreign antigens, but rather detect changes in self-molecules displayed at the surface of autologous cells. Based on initial observations that syngeneic tumor cells with a deficient expression of major histocompatibility complex (MHC) class I molecules are selectively rejected by NK cells, the concept of the "missing-self" recognition was introduced.[4,5] This model provided an explanation why virally infected or malignant cells with decreased MHC class I expression are preferentially lysed by NK cells, whereas autologous cells with normal expression of MHC class I antigens are protected.

NK cells express various surface receptors with inhibitory and activatory functions that play a role in various diseases including cancer.[6] The functional response of NK cells is determined by the activation of these receptors in combination with the signaling of various coreceptors and other surface structures on binding to their cognate ligands.[7] **Fig. 1** presents a schematic overview of the inhibitory, activatory and coreceptors and the various NK receptor ligands. The inhibitory receptors possess different specificities for HLA class I molecules. The 2 main groups are the killer immunoglobulin (Ig)-like receptors (KIRs), which are receptors for human leukocyte antigen (HLA) class I ligands[8] and the CD94-NKG2A/B, which recognize HLA-E.[9] Although HLA-E shows little polymorphism,[10] many inhibitory KIRs are specific for polymorphic domains of MHC class I.[11] KIR2DL1 (CD158a) recognizes HLA-C alleles with lysine in position 80 (C2 specificity, eg, Cw2,4,5,6; group 2), whereas KIR2DL2 and KIR2DL3 (CD158b1/b2) recognize HLA-C alleles with asparagine in position 80 (C1 specificity, eg, Cw1,3,7,8; group 1). KIR 3DL1 (CD158e1) is specific for HLA-B alleles bearing the Bw4 motif and KIR3DL2 (CD158k) recognizes HLA-A epitopes (A3, A11). HLA class I- and KIR-genes are encoded on distinct chromosomes 6p21.3 and 19q13.4, respectively, and inherited independently.[12] KIR genes are encoded by a set of 15 loci and 2 pseudogenes. These KIR genes are closely linked and inherited as a haplotype, and the variability of KIR gene content can be organized into KIR haplotype A and B.[13] Haplotype group A contains a variable number of inhibitory receptor genes, whereas group B haplotype additionally contains several

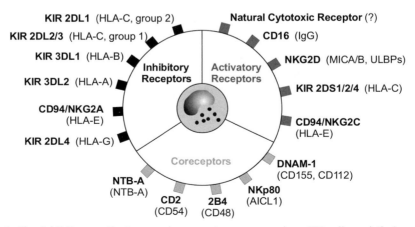

Fig. 1. The inhibitory, activatory, and coreceptors expressed on NK cells and their corresponding ligands in parentheses.

activating receptor genes. Killer activatory Ig-like receptors (KARs) are also triggered by HLA class I alleles,[7] but additional activatory receptors exist, such as NKG2D, the leukocyte adhesion molecule DNAX accessory molecule (DNAM-1; CD226) and natural cytotoxicity receptors NKp46, NKp30, and NKp44, which recognize so far unknown ligands expressed on hematopoietic cells.[7,8,14] The Fc-receptor CD16, binding the Fc portion of IgG, mediates the antibody-dependent cellular cytotoxicity of NK cells. NKD2D and DNAM-1 are receptors for stress-induced ligands, such as MHC class I polypeptide-related sequence A and B (MICA and MICB), UL16-binding proteins, and poliovirus receptor (CD155) and Nectin-2 (CD112), respectively.[15–17] Other surface molecules contribute to the functional status of NK cells, among them the 2B4, NTB-A, and NKp80 coreceptors, CD18/CD11, CD2 adhesion molecules, and Toll-like receptors.[14,18] Incubation of NK cells with various cytokines leads to their stimulation and expression of additional surface and intracellular molecules such as perforin, granzymes, Fas ligand, and tumor necrosis factor-related apoptosis-inducing ligand treatment (TRAIL), which enables them to kill a wide spectrum of tumor cells effectively via induction of necrosis or apoptosis.[19]

In summary, the output signal (ie, the functional status of NK cells) is regulated by various input signals and the large numbers of inhibitory, activatory, and modulating coreceptors allow cross talk of NK cells with other immune or tissue cells.

NK Cells and Cancer

Most evidence for a role of NK cells in tumor surveillance in humans comes from a clinical long-term follow-up study,[20] in which the inherent NK activity of 3625 individuals was measured longitudinally and the results compared with the incidence of cancer. Individuals who had a high spontaneous NK activity had a lower risk of developing cancer, whereas individuals with lower activity had a higher incidence of malignant diseases. It is thought that the main target of NK cell activity is within the hematopoietic system, as shown by the hybrid resistance model, in which NK cells reject allogeneic bone marrow but not skin or solid organs.[21] In patients with leukemia, functional impairment of NK cells has prognostic significance and NK cell–mediated cytotoxicity against autologous blasts tested either in vitro[22–24] or in a xenogeneic in vivo model[25] correlated with the duration of remission. In addition, leukemic blasts can shed MICA, a ligand of the activating NK receptor NKG2D, which can negatively affect the cytotoxicity of NK cells.[26] A decreased number and impaired function of NK cells have also been described in children with acute leukemia at the time of diagnosis and in relapse.[27] The low cytotoxicity of NK cells against autologous leukemic blasts could be restored in vitro after stimulation with interleukin 2 (IL-2).[28,29] The role of NK cells in tumor surveillance of solid tumors is less clear. It has been shown that the infiltration of tumors with NK cells can be a positive prognostic marker in carcinomas.[30,31] In vitro activation of NK cells obtained from children with malignant solid tumors with interferon α (IFN-α) and IL-2 also enhanced their cytotoxicity against solid tumor cell lines.[32] Therefore, strategies to augment the antitumor activity of the NK cell system in the autologous or allogeneic setting could be beneficial in the treatment of pediatric patients with acute leukemia or solid tumors.

NK Cells in the Context of Allogeneic Stem Cell Transplantation

The concept of alloreactive NK cells

This concept is based on the observation that NK cells attack lymphohematopoietic target cells that express HLA class I molecules for which they do not express the corresponding inhibitory receptor as would be predicted based on the missing self model described earlier.[33] As depicted in **Fig. 2A**, NK cells are in a permanent

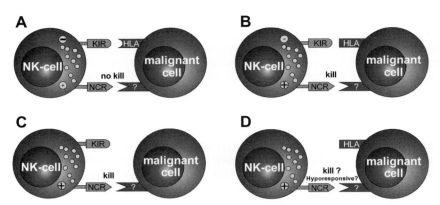

Fig. 2. Possible constellations of the expression of inhibitory receptors (KIR) on NK cells and the expression of KIR-binding or KIR-nonbinding HLA class I molecules on malignant cells (*A–D*), all of which influence the overall cytotoxic activity of NK cells (see text for details). NCR refers to the natural cytotoxicity receptors, for which ligands have not yet been identified.

activated status via binding of natural cytotoxic receptors (NCRs) to their yet unknown ligands expressed on normal or malignant hematopoietic cells. Only in the presence of a corresponding ligand for the inhibitory receptor, such as self HLA-Cw alleles, -Bw4 alleles and some HLA-A alleles, the cytotoxic function of NK cells is inhibited and the target cells are resistant to NK-mediated lysis. In contrast, if the target cell does not express the corresponding inhibitory ligand for the KIR, NK cells lyse their target cells because of the lack of inhibition. This situation is often encountered in HLA-mismatched but also in HLA-matched allogeneic stem cell transplantation because of the disparity of the donors' KIR repertoire and the HLA class I type of the recipients (**Fig. 2**B and discussed earlier). Therefore, the term alloreactive NK cells is used to describe this situation.[34] However, regardless of donor-recipient KIR-HLA matching status (discussed in greater detail later), additional clinical situations can be envisioned, which are shown in **Fig. 2**C and D: Tumor cells can have a reduced expression or complete lack of HLA class I molecules, which can be encountered in leukemic blasts[35] or certain tumors, such as neuroblastoma (**Fig. 2**C).[36] This constellation leads to killing of the tumor cells and the intensity of killing is dependent on the amount of residual HLA molecules expressed on the surface of the target cells.[35] Another situation seen clinically in the early phase of immunoreconstitution of NK cells after pediatric haploidentical transplantation is the absence of killer inhibitory or killer activatory receptors for HLA class I alleles (KIRs or KARs) on the reconstituting NK cells.[37] This situation either results in NK cell killing of their target independent of the expression of the amount, or the specificity of the HLA class I molecules on the tumor target cells, or a hyporesponsive status of NK cells via yet unknown mechanisms (**Fig. 2**D).[38]

What predicts NK alloreactivity between donor and recipient?
Two models have been described to best predict NK alloreactivity in allogeneic transplantation to be used for donor selection: The KIR ligand mismatch model compares the HLA typing of donor and recipient (ligand-ligand model). This model assumes that all NK cells in an individual express at least 1 inhibitory receptor for a self HLA class I molecule to avoid autoimmunity. Based on this assumption, NK alloreactivity between

donor and recipient can be predicted when the donor is mismatched at inhibitory HLA class I antigens in the direction of graft-versus-host disease (GVHD).[39] In **Fig. 3**, the ligand-ligand model is shown in detail. In this example, the patient's HLA type is HLA-Cw1, Cw8 (group 1). If the donor is mismatched at the HLA-C locus in GVHD direction and is for example positive for HLA-Cw2 and Cw8 (groups 1 and 2), the donor's KIR repertoire can be predicted based on the assumption that each NK cell of this mismatched donor should express at least 1 inhibitory receptor for self HLA-Cw2 and Cw8 (KIR2DL1 and KIR2DL2/3, respectively). The donor's NK cells could express single KIRs for self HLA-Cw8. These NK cells would be inhibited by the patient's shared HLA-Cw8 allele (**Fig. 3A**) and thus not be alloreactive. Donor NK cells could also express both KIRs but would still be nonalloreactive because of inhibition by the patient's shared Cw8 allele (**Fig. 3B**). However, donor NK cells expressing single KIR2DL1 receptors cannot be inhibited by the patient's HLA-Cw1 nonshared antigen and the donor NK cells will exert an alloreactive antileukemic effect (**Fig. 3C**). In the case of HLA identity between donor and recipient, alloreactive NK cells

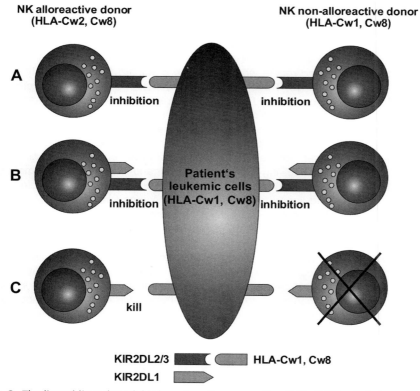

Fig. 3. The ligand-ligand model is based on the assumption that all NK cells have at least 1 KIR for self HLA class I alleles (*A*). In this example (patient's HLA type: HLA-Cw1, Cw8), a donor mismatched at the HLA-Cw allele in GVHD direction (donor HLA-Cw2, patient HLA-Cw1) has NK cells in his repertoire that express at least the inhibitory receptor KIR2DL1 (*B*) (receptor for self HLA-Cw2). These NK cells cannot be inhibited by the patient's HLA-Cw1 allele and the donor is NK alloreactive (depicted in *C*). Because all NK cells should have at least 1 KIR for self HLA class I alleles, NK cells expressing only KIR2DL1 would not be present in an HLA-matched donor's repertoire and the donor is nonalloreactive.

would not be encountered in the KIR repertoire of an HLA-matched donor. Using this model, impressive antileukemic effects based on NK alloreactivity have been reported, especially in adult patients with acute myeloid leukemia (AML).[40]

An alternative model is the missing KIR ligand model (receptor-ligand model).[41] In this model, the HLA type of the donor is not taken into account and only the donor's actual KIR repertoire (as opposed to predicted as in the ligand-ligand model) and the patient's HLA type are considered. The KIR expression on the surface of the donor's NK cells can be determined by flow cytometry or by genotyping.[41,42] Compared with the ligand-ligand model, this model allowed a more accurate prediction of the risk of relapse in children with acute lymphoblastic leukemia after haploidentical stem cell transplantation and, as expected, patients transplanted from a receptor-ligand mismatched haploidentical donor had a lower risk of relapse compared with patients transplanted from a receptor-ligand-matched donor.[41,43] Not all mismatches in these studies were predicted based on the ligand-ligand model. Further comparison of KIR genotyping and phenotyping for selection of the best NK-alloreactive donor showed that genotyping alone may not be sufficient (ie, gene expression does not always determine actual KIR expression) and a simplified algorithm for donor KIR typing has been suggested.[43] The receptor-ligand model has also been applied in patients with AML or myelodysplastic syndrome who received a transplant from HLA-identical siblings and patients lacking HLA ligands for the donors KIRs had significantly less risk of relapse.[44] Because all donor-recipient pairs in this study were HLA-identical siblings, the ligand-ligand model would not have predicted NK alloreactivity in any of the donor-recipient pairs. Therefore, the determination of donor KIR expression among HLA-identical donors may facilitate identification of donors expected to have potent antileukemic activity by alloreactive NK cells. In a large retrospective cohort of more than 2000 unrelated donor transplants,[45] the lack of KIR ligands significantly reduced the risk of relapse in patients with early-stage myeloid cells. However, another study of unrelated donors[46] failed to reveal any differences in leukemia recurrence among patients receiving grafts from KIR-ligand-matched or -mismatched donors. However, KIR-ligand incompatibility in the graft-versus-host direction, according to the ligand-ligand model, improved the outcome after umbilical cord blood transplantation for patients with acute leukemia.[47] The conflicting results in HLA-matched transplantation might be caused by the heterogeneity of the different transplant procedures (conditioning regimen, graft composition, posttransplant immunosuppression) and of the patients (disease, risk category).[48] It has been shown in this context that T cell alloreactivity dominates NK cell alloreactivity in minimally T cell–depleted HLA-nonidentical pediatric bone marrow transplantation.[49] More insights into the complex regulation of the cytotoxicity of NK cells via inhibitory and activatory receptors are necessary to further optimize the donor selection in HLA-matched or-mismatched transplantation.

CLINICAL EXPLOITATION OF NK CELLS AFTER TRANSPLANTATION
Hematological Malignancies

Especially in light of recent findings that AML CD34+CD38– stem cells are susceptible to allorecognition and lysis by single KIR-expressing NK cells,[50] it is foreseeable that NK cells will play an increasingly important role in the KIR-mismatch setting after allogeneic transplantation in the eradication of leukemic blasts. NK cells form the first wave of immunologic recovery after high-dose chemotherapy/radiotherapy and patients with higher numbers of NK cells at 30 days post transplant had a lower risk of relapse and better survival.[51] Although the first NK cells recovering after transplantation are CD94/NKG2A-positive and KIR-negative, patients acquire the donor's KIR repertoire after about 3 months post transplant.[41] A biased early post-transplant NK cell reconstitution toward group C1–specific NK cells and the absence of group 2–specific NK cells was associated with a significantly reduced survival in the presence of C1 ligands.[52] The absence of KIR expression on NK cells in the early phase after transplantation might render these cells cytotoxic against leukemic blasts independent of the patients' inhibitory KIR ligands.[38] Such NK cells might be initially hyporesponsive (for reasons that are unknown), but their cytotoxic function might be induced after stimulation with cytokines and the clinical application of IL-2 post transplant may be considered in patients receiving T cell–depleted grafts.[53]

In addition to their antileukemic properties, it has been shown in mouse models that alloreactive NK cells also facilitate engraftment by the elimination of residual host hematopoiesis,[54] thus increasing the likelihood of donor engraftment following reduced intensity conditioning (RIC) regimens in allogeneic and especially in haploidentical transplantation.[55,56] In addition, recent advances in T cell depletion technologies from mobilized peripheral stem cells allow the coinfusion of large numbers of NK cells.[57] This technology in combination with RIC regimens is associated with a lower transplant-related mortality (TRM) with the same rate of engraftment compared with the previous approach using CD34+ positively selected haploidentical stem cell grafts and fully ablative conditioning regimens.[55]

T cell–depleted and NK cell–enriched grafts can be further activated ex vivo before infusion with cytokines, such as IL-15. This cytokine seems to be more efficient than IL-2 in expanding the NK cells because of promotion of survival and protection of NK cells from activation-induced cell death.[58] Overnight incubation of T cell–depleted mobilized grafts from haploidentical donors led to an increase of their cytotoxicity, and the infusion of such IL-15–activated NK cells was well tolerated in a small series of pediatric patients.[59] In the presence of suitable monoclonal antibodies, such as anti-CD19 or anti-CD20 targeting molecules expressed by the patient's leukemia, engagement of Fc-receptors expressed on NK cells overrides the KIR-mediated inhibition, thus mediating antibody-dependent cytotoxicity and could further increase the antileukemic activity of NK cells.[60,61] Purified alloreactive haploidentical NK cells have been given several days after conditioning and transplantation of purified CD34+ stem cells from the same haploidentical donor.[62] This approach resulted in a long-term remission in a patient with infant leukemia who relapsed after a standard myeloablative allogeneic transplantation and presented with refractory leukemia at time of second haploidentical transplantation. Approaches currently being investigated include posttransplant adoptive transfer of large numbers of ex vivo generated and genetically modified (to enhance function) donor-derived NK cells[63] and large-scale methods have been described that allow the expansion of donor-derived NK cells for clinical application.[64]

Most of the clinical data obtained thus far have been collected in the transplant setting of sustained engraftment of full donor hematopoiesis. Another approach for the exploitation of the antitumor effect of alloreactive NK cells is in a nontransplant setting.[65] With this therapy, patients receive a moderate chemotherapy to induce lymphocyte expansion after infusion of alloreactive IL-2-activated NK cells from an allogeneic KIR-mismatched donor. Additional low-dose IL-2 is administered to the patients to induce and maintain in vivo proliferation of donor NK cells. Transient proliferation of donor NK cells for several weeks has been observed in patients and some impressive tumor responses have been reported. However, this approach does not result in a long-term engraftment of donor NK cells and further long-term follow-up studies are needed.

Solid Tumors

In addition to the studies in leukemia described earlier, the concept of alloreactive NK cells might also apply for the treatment of pediatric metastatic solid tumors.[66] It has been shown that KIR-ligand-mismatched alloreactive NK cells effectively lyse primary solid tumors[67] and tumor cell lines established from melanoma or renal cell carcinoma.[68] In addition, some pediatric tumors, such as neuroblastoma, express no or only low levels of HLA class I molecules on their surface and are therefore susceptible target cells for NK cells (as discussed earlier).[36] Tumor cell lines obtained from and Ewing sarcoma show a variable susceptibility to NK cell-mediated lysis.[69] Based on this concept and similar to the leukemia trials described earlier, clinical protocols using an RIC approach and haploidentical transplantation of CD3/19-depleted and NK cell–enriched stem cell grafts have been initiated in patients with advanced and refractory pediatric malignant solid tumors including neuroblastoma, rhabdomyosarcoma, and Ewing sarcoma.[70]

Summary and Further Directions

New insights into the biology of NK cells have attracted significant interest of researchers and clinicians to exploit this lymphocyte subpopulation for the treatment of patients with malignancies. In the autologous setting, ex vivo induced NK cells have been used with some clinical responses. More convincing evidence exists in the allogeneic transplant setting, in which alloreactive NK cells have been show to exert an antileukemic effect, especially after KIR-ligand mismatched haploidentical transplantation. Increasing insights into the biology of NK cells such as into their ontogeny, the development of the KIR repertoire (especially after transplantation), the cross talk of NK cells with other cells of the immune system, and the interaction of their multiple surface receptors with tumor cells will enable more effective use of this cell population in cancer treatment.

PART 2: MSC
Background to MSC

The bone marrow serves as a reservoir for different classes of stem cells. In addition to hematopoietic stem cells the bone marrow contains a population of marrow stromal or MSC. Stromal stem cells exhibit multilineage differentiation capacity, and are able to generate progenitors with restricted developmental potential, including fibroblasts, osteoblasts, adipocytes, and chondrocyte progenitors.[71] Marrow stromal cells comprise a heterogeneous population of cells, including reticular endothelial cells, fibroblasts, adipocytes, and osteogenic precursor cells, which provide growth factors, cell to cell interactions, and matrix proteins that play a role in the regulation of hematopoiesis.[71] Friedenstein and colleagues[72] originally described a population of adherent cells from the bone marrow that were nonphagocytic and exhibited a fibroblastlike appearance. Following ectopic transplantation under the kidney capsule these cells (colony-forming unit fibroblastoids) gave rise to a broad spectrum of differentiated connective tissues, including bone, cartilage, adipose tissue, and myelosupportive stroma.[72,73] Based on these observations it was proposed that these tissues were derived from a common precursor cell residing in the bone marrow, termed the stromal stem cell, the bone marrow stromal stem cell, the MSC, or the skeletal stem cell.[74] MSC secrete cytokines important for hematopoiesis and promote engraftment of hematopoietic stem cells in experimental animal models, especially when the dose of hematopoietic stem cells is limiting.[75–77] In light of the controversy as to whether MSC at the single cell level truly fulfill the criteria of self-renewal and multilineage differentiation capacity, it was recently proposed to use the term multipotent mesenchymal stromal cells (although not changing the acronym MSC) to describe fibroblastlike plastic adherent cells.[78]

Sources of MSC

Although the bone marrow serves as the primary reservoir for MSC, their presence has been reported in various other tissues. These include periosteum and muscle connective tissue,[79,80] fetal bone marrow, liver, and blood.[81] MSC have been identified in cytokine (granulocyte-specific colony-stimulating factor [G-CSF]) mobilized peripheral blood by some investigators,[82] although other studies have been unable to confirm their presence in peripheral blood.[83] Similarly, initial reports suggested that MSC could be isolated from umbilical cord blood.[84,85] The low frequency of MSC in these sources may explain the initial contradictory findings of different researchers. However, MSC have been successfully isolated from human amniotic fluid.[86] The phenotype of the culture-expanded amniotic fluid-derived cells was similar to that reported for MSC derived from second-trimester fetal tissues and adult bone marrow. It has been reported that the in vivo functions of MSC depend on where they come from, irrespective of the expansion procedure used to obtain them. This finding may have consequences for their future clinical application.[87–89]

Characterization of MSC

No unique phenotype has been identified that allows the reproducible isolation of MSC precursors with predictable developmental potential. The isolation and characterization of stromal cell function therefore still relies primarily on their ability to adhere to plastic and their expansion potential. The capacity of ex vivo expanded MSC to differentiate into multiple mesenchymal lineages, including bone, fat, and cartilage, is presently used as a functional criterion to define MSC.[71]

Similarly, no specific marker or combination of markers is available to identify MSC. Phenotypically, ex vivo expanded MSC express several nonspecific markers, but are devoid of hematopoietic and endothelial markers (**Table 1**).[71]

Expansion for Clinical Use

In recent years, new techniques have become available to isolate and grow mesenchymal progenitors and to manipulate their growth under defined in vitro culture

Table 1	
Characteristic surface markers positively and negatively expressed by MSC	
Marker	**Expression**
HLA-A,B,C	+
HLA-DR	−
CD31, PECAM	−
CD34	−
CD45	−
CD73	+
CD80	−
CD90, Thy-1	+
CD105, SH2	+
CD45	−
CD3	−

conditions. As a result MSC can be rapidly expanded (within 4–6 weeks) to numbers that are required for clinical application. Standard conditions for expansion of MSC include the presence of serum, in most instances fetal bovine serum (FBS), although platelet rich plasma is presently being evaluated as an alternative.[88,90–92]

One of the risks related to in vitro expansion of MSC is of genetic instability and thus the risk of malignant transformation. This genetic instability has been reported during culture of MSC obtained from mice[93] but is believed to be caused by the inherent genetic instability of the species rather than the intrinsic nature of cultured MSC. When human MSC were subjected to prolonged culture conditions, standard karyotypic and genome-based analyses did not demonstrate the acquisition of chromosomal abnormalities, suggesting they remain genetically stable in culture and thus unlikely to induce malignant transformation.[94] However, the addition of exogenous growth factors to the culture medium can induce genetic transformation of expanded human MSC.[93]

In most healthy donors, isolated and expanded MSC display a progressive decrease in proliferative capacity until reaching senescence and cannot be expanded in the long term. Most phase I/II published studies have used bone marrow–derived FBS-expanded MSC, without the addition of exogenous growth factors. It is therefore important to keep in mind that alternatively expanded MSC require extensive clinical testing to establish their efficacy and safety and to determine whether or not they can substitute MSC expanded in FBS.

Immune Modulatory Properties of MSC

Although it is widely accepted that MSC give rise to cells that form the structural network in support and maintenance of normal hematopoiesis, current opinion regarding MSC and their immunosuppressive function is derived from in vitro experiments of expanded MSC. Therefore it is still not known whether they play an important physiologic role in the regulation of immune homeostasis. Although much research has been undertaken to determine the immunomodulatory activities of MSC, the exact mechanisms on how they exert their influence have yet to be fully elucidated.

Experimental models suggest that expanded MSC have potent immunomodulatory effects, primarily through the inhibition of effector functions, thus offering a promising option for treating immune-mediated disorders such as acute GVHD.[95–101] MSC are poor antigen-presenting cells and do not express MHC class II or costimulatory molecules. They were once considered nonimmunogenic but murine studies indicate that MSC can in an immunocompetent host elicit an immune response.[100] Thus, in the clinical setting, especially in those individuals who are not immunosuppressed, MSC should be considered as hypoimmune cells. Human MSC alter the cytokine secretion profile of dendritic cells (DCs), naive and effector T cells (T helper 1 [T_H1] and T helper 2 [T_H2]), and NK cells to induce a more antiinflammatory or tolerant phenotype.[95–99]

T cell interactions

Human bone marrow stromal cells suppress T-lymphocyte proliferation induced by cellular or nonspecific mitogenic stimuli[96] and inhibit the response of naive and memory antigen-specific T cells to their cognate peptide.[96] Accordingly, expanded MSC do not stimulate T cell proliferation in mixed lymphocyte reactions and are able to down-regulate alloreactive T cell responses when added to mixed lymphocyte cultures.[96,97] As this inhibition is not dependent on MHC expression, allogeneic and autologous MSC can induce this effect. MSC do not induce T cell apoptosis but rather promote survival of T cells in a quiescent phase.[102,103] IL-2 stimulation can partially overcome this MSC-mediated effect.[104] MSC-induced inhibition of T cell proliferation is associated with a decreased IFN-γ and an increased IL-4 production, reflecting the induction of an antiinflammatory rather than a proinflammatory state.[98] MSC have also been reported to down-regulate MHC-restricted killing by CD8+ cytotoxic T lymphocytes (CTLs),[105] albeit they themselves are not CTL targets.[106] MSC can influence the generation of T regulatory cells that subsequently suppress activation of the immune system. This process is mediated by the release of IL-10 by plasmacytoid DCs (pDCs) and the release of sHLA-G5 isoform.[95,98]

B cell interactions

Interactions of MSC with B cells are controversial with conflicting reports, which may reflect the variations in experimental procedures.[95] Most reports suggest that in vivo B cell proliferation and differentiation and expression of cytokines are inhibited by MSC.[107,108] Conversely, in vitro data suggest that MSC support proliferation, differentiation, and survival of B cells from healthy individuals and from children with systemic lupus erythematosis.[109,110] As T cells orchestrate B cell function, whatever the ultimate effects are of MSC directly on B cell function, B cells are more likely to be influenced indirectly by MSC-inhibiting T cells.[95]

DC interactions

In vivo experiments have demonstrated that MSC inhibit the maturation of monocytes into dendritic DCs, and skew mature DCs to an immature DC state.[111,112] Incubation of MSC with mature DCs reduces the latter's expression of class II and costimulatory molecules, inhibits tumor necrosis factor α (TNF-α) production, and impairs antigen presentation.[111,113] MSC impair the stimulatory effect of mature DCs on resting NK cells and alter antigen presentation to T cells, preventing proliferation and clonal expansion.

The immune environment may alter the function of MSC. It has been hypothesized that early in the immune response when levels of IFN-γ are low, MSC may behave as nonprofessional antigen-presenting cells. With increasing levels of IFN-γ, MSC are then influenced to switch to their immune-suppressive function.[114]

NK cell interactions

MSC down-regulate the expression of NKp30 and NK group 2, member D (NKG2D) activating receptors involved in NK activation and killing of target cells.[99] Resting NK cells stimulated with either IL-2 or IL-15 in the presence of MSC show markedly reduced proliferation and IFN-γ production, although activated NK cells are more resistant to the effects of MSC.[115]

The lack in MSC of MHC class I expression and the expression of NK-recognized ligands make them a natural target for activated NK cell killing. Cytokine-activated NK cells kill MSC via interaction of NKG2D expressed by NK cells with its ligands UL16-binding protein 3 (ULBP3) or class I polypeptide-related sequence A (MICA) expressed by MSC, and of NK cell–associated DNAM-1 with MSC-associated poliovirus receptor (CD155) or nectin-2 (CD112). This effect can be partially overcome by incubating MSC with IFN-γ, which up-regulates MHC class I expression.[95,99]

It can be postulated that a microenvironment rich in IFN-γ would protect MSC from being attacked and destroyed by NK cells. However, the clinical relevance of these findings has not yet been demonstrated.

In summary, MSC have demonstrated broad immunosuppressive potential in vitro. So far the mode of action in vivo remains unclear.

Potential Mechanisms Involved in MSC-mediated Immunosuppression

Cell to cell contact and soluble factors are believed to be required for the induction of MSC-mediated immunosuppression.[95] Primary contact between MSC and the target cell is initiated by adhesion molecules.[107] Most studies demonstrate that soluble factors are involved, as the separation of MSC and peripheral blood mononuclear cells (PBMCs) by a trans-well permeable membrane does not prevent the inhibition of proliferation of PBMCs.[96,116]

MSC release several soluble molecules either constitutively or following cross talk with other cells.[95] These include the tryptophan-catabolizing enzyme indoleamine 2,3-dioxygenase (IDO)[101] and nitric oxide. Release of IFN-γ by target cells induces the release of IDO by MSC, which in turn depletes tryptophan, an essential amino acid for lymphocyte proliferation.[117,118] IDO is necessary to inhibit proliferation of T_H1 cells and together with prostaglandin E_2 (PGE$_2$) inhibits NK cell function.[95,118]

IFN-γ can, in a murine model with the addition of proinflammatory cytokines, stimulate chemokine production by MSC, resulting in T cell attraction and increased inducible nitric-oxide synthase (i-NOS). T cells are inhibited by the subsequent production of nitrous oxide.[119]

Other soluble factors that have been reported to be released by MSC include transforming growth factor β1 (TGFβ1), heme oxygenase 1, hepatocyte growth factor (HGF), and IL-6.[95,96,98,107,120,121] Cytokines produced by target cells can increase the release of some of these MSC-derived soluble factors.[95] sHLA-G5 released by MSC suppresses T cell proliferation and CD8+ T cell– and NK cell–mediated cytotoxicity.[107,121] Conversely, MSC through the release of sHLA-G5 initiate the up-regulation of CD4+CD25+ Fox P3+ cells (T regulatory immune phenotype),[97,107,121] albeit the depletion of regulatory T cells has no effect on the inhibition of T proliferation by MSC.[98]

The complexity and mechanisms whereby MSC interact with cells, of the adaptive and innate immune system, are summarized in **Fig. 4**.

Despite most of the available understanding of MSC interactions being derived from in vitro experiments, the design of any future clinical studies needs to consider these findings.

Animal Studies

Almeida-Porada and colleagues[116] observed that cotransplantation of human stromal cells into preimmune fetal sheep resulted in an enhancement of long-term engraftment of human cells in the bone marrow and higher levels of donor cells in the circulation during gestation and after birth. Infusion of bone-marrow-derived osteoblasts promoted the engraftment of allogeneic hematopoietic stem cells in mice.[122] Other studies in NOD/SCID mice indicate that cotransplantation of MSC and cord blood enhances engraftment of human hematopoietic cells in the bone marrow of NOD/SCID mice.[123] Coinfusion of MSC derived from fetal lung and CD34$^+$ cells derived from umbilical cord blood promoted the engraftment of myeloid and B-lymphoid cells in the marrow of recipient mice, showing that the engraftment-promoting effect of MSC was not lineage specific.[76] It was also found that enhancement of engraftment might be independent of the homing of MSC to the marrow and might be mediated by the release of cytokines that promote either the homing or proliferation of hematopoietic stem cells. Bartholomew and colleagues[122] demonstrated that MSC infusions can suppress lymphocyte proliferation and prolong skin grafts in a nonhuman primate.

Infusion of allogeneic MSC ameliorated lethal GVHD in mice receiving haploidentical hematopoietic stem cell transplants, but only when MSC were administered early and

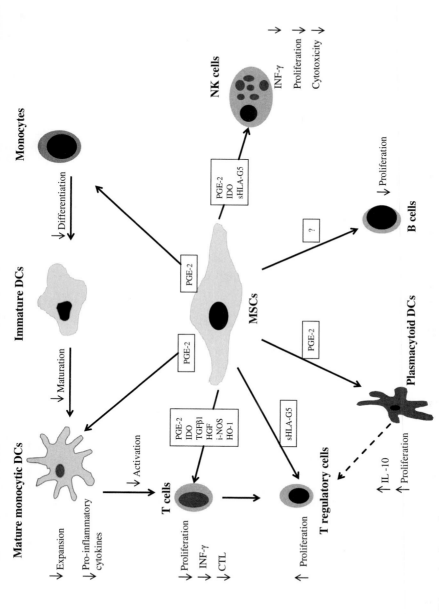

Fig. 4. Possible mechanisms of MSC interactions and cells of the immune system.

repeatedly after transplantation.[123] Effects of MSC have been reported in animal models of autoimmunity, such as amelioration of experimental autoimmune encephalitis in a murine model, raising the possibility of MSC use in autoimmune diseases.[124] However, in a collagen-induced model of rheumatoid arthritis, after infusion of MSC no observed improvement was evident.[125]

The final destination of infused MSC in clinical studies is unknown. It has been difficult to demonstrate engraftment of donor-derived MSC following transplantation. In some studies, gene-marked culture-expanded MSC were infused along with unmodified bone marrow cells and evidence based on the polymerase chain reaction of the presence of marked MSC was found in the marrow several weeks after transplantation.[116,126,127] How long MSC survive after injection and to what extent they are able to target tissues are unknown.[128] In nonhuman primates intravenously administered MSC distribute over a wide range of tissues.[129] Preferential homing to sites of injury has been shown.[128] MSC, like cells of the immune system, can extravasate from blood vessels as a result of expression of adhesion molecules on their surface. MSC display coordinated rolling and adhesion to endothelial cells, dependent on P-selectin and vascular cell adhesion molecule-1.[130] Several chemokines bind to cognate receptors expressed on the cell surface of MSC[131] and facilitate their migration and extravasation.[132]

Also MSC may become trapped in the vasculature, which limits their tissue distribution.[133] In future clinical studies, trafficking of infused MSC needs to be addressed, and consideration given to MSC that remain undifferentiated compared with those that differentiate.[133] Tracking infused MSC will require a suitable labeling method that can be safely administered to patients, without affecting the function of the MSC.

Clinical Results

Animal models may not predict the clinical situation, as the immune modulatory mechanisms between species (eg, murine and human MSC) may differ. Thus far, clinical application of ex vivo expanded MSC therapy in the HSCT setting has exploited their potential immune modulatory properties and their ability to support hematopoietic stem cell proliferation.

Adult HSCT studies

Initial phase I studies involving bone-marrow-derived MSC showed that MSC could be successfully collected, culture expanded ex vivo for 4 to 7 weeks and administered to patients with hematological malignancies in complete remission. The infusions contained up to 50 × 10^6 MSC and were well tolerated without adverse reactions.[82]

In a subsequent phase I/II clinical trial in patients with breast cancer, autologous and expanded MSC were coinfused with autologous peripheral blood progenitor cells.[134] Clonogenic MSC could be detected in venous blood up to 1 hour after infusion in most patients. No toxicities were observed related to the infusion of MSC and hematopoietic reconstitution (defined as time to neutrophil and platelet recovery) was rapid, suggesting some effect of MSC infusion on hematopoietic reconstitution. In another multicenter phase I/II study, allogeneic donor bone-marrow-derived MSC were coinfused with allogeneic hematopoietic stem cells in patients with hematological malignancies undergoing matched-sibling stem cell transplantation.[135] Preliminary data suggest that there was no immediate toxicity following infusion of MSC and that there was more rapid engraftment and a low incidence of acute GVHD in comparison with historical controls.

Pediatric HSCT studies
Correction of inborn errors MSC express high levels of arylsulfatase A and α-L-idur-onidase.[136] The deficiency of these enzymes is associated with specific inborn errors of metabolism. Arylsulfatase A deficiency is the cause of metachromatic leukodystrophy, and α-L-iduronidase deficiency is the cause of Hurler disease, disorders that may be cured by allogeneic HSCT.[137,138] Expanded MSC were administered to patients with metachromatic leukodystrophy and Hurler syndrome, who had previously undergone HSCT but had residual symptoms of their disease.[139] Four of 5 patients with metachromatic leukodystrophy showed improvement in nerve conduction velocity, but no clinical effects were demonstrated in patients with Hurler disease.

MSC have been used to treat bone disease, namely osteogenesis imperfecta.[140] Five children with osteogenesis imperfecta undergoing HSCT had donor osteoblast engraftment, with new bone formation, an increase in total bone mineral content, and an increase in growth velocity and noticeable reduced fracture frequencies.[141] MSC identified by specific gene markers were given to 6 children undergoing HSCT for severe osteogenesis imperfecta.[142] Engraftment of MSC was identified and this was associated with acceleration of growth velocity.

Overcoming graft failure MSC had not been shown to overcome graft rejection, although, given the physiologic role of MSC in hematopoietic stem cell support, it was hypothesized that they could be a valuable adjunct in the haploidentical peripheral blood stem cell transplantation (PBSCT) setting, where graft failure had been reported as a major concern despite large doses of purified CD34+ stem cells being administered. If MSC were to overcome graft failure then there was a considerable opportunity to improve on the historical results of transplantation from HLA-disparate donors.

The feasibility and safety of administering haploidentical bone-marrow-derived expanded MSC to children undergoing haploidentical PBSCT was recently shown.[143] Thirteen patients received haploidentical bone-marrow-derived ex vivo expanded MSC at a dose of 1 to 2×10^6/kg recipient weight. In addition they received haploidentical G-CSF mobilized CD34+ selected peripheral blood stem cells, 4 hours after the infusion of MSC, with a target dose of 20×10^6/kg CD34+. The outcome in feasibility, toxicity, stable engraftment, rates of infection, acute GVHD, and relapse were compared with 52 nonselected historical controls, who received haploidentical PBSCs alone. Epidemiologically there was no difference between the study patients and the historical controls other than the administration of MSC. There was a trend to a statistically significant improvement in sustained engraftment ($P = .06$) without increasing the rate of infections, relapse, or transplant-related toxicities in children receiving MSC compared with controls. Engraftment of infused MSC was less than 1% in serial bone marrow samples up to 1 year post MSC infusion. Despite these encouraging results, the study was limited in that children were assigned to the study in a nonrandomized fashion and compared with historical controls. Since the initial publication, 32 children have been cotransplanted with haploidentical PBSCTs and MSC with no documented graft failure. These results and the fact that posttransplant immune suppression is not required because of the intense T cell depletion suggest that this method may provide a suitable platform for additional cellular therapies.

Treatment of steroid-resistant GVHD Exploiting the immunosuppressive effects of MSC, Le Blanc and colleagues[144] reported the first successful treatment of severe steroid/treatment-resistant grade IV acute GVHD of the gut and liver with haploidentical third-party bone-marrow-derived MSC in a 9-year-old boy.

Subsequently, a phase I/II multicenter trial of 55 patients (30 adults and 25 children) treated with MSC infusions for severe grade II to IV steroid refractory acute GVHD was conducted.[145,146] Patients varied in the time to MSC infusion and the type of previous immunosuppression administered before receiving MSC. Most patients (60%) had received second-line treatments, 25% third-line treatments, and 10% greater than third-line treatments, in addition to steroids, without documented clinical or pathologic response. MSC were expanded according to a common protocol. A median dose of bone-marrow-derived ex vivo expanded MSC of 1.4 (range 0.4–9) $\times$ 10^6 cells/kg was administered. Twenty-seven patients received 1 infusion, 22 patients received 2 infusions, and 6 patients received 3 to 5 infusions. In light of the rapid progression of symptoms necessitating prompt treatment, MSC were mainly derived from third-party HLA-mismatched donors (n = 69), the rest being obtained from either HLA-identical sibling donors (n = 5) or haploidentical donors (n = 18).

No toxicities were documented associated with the infusion of MSC, even in the most seriously ill patients treated. Thirty patients (55%) showed a complete response and 8 showed improvement, resulting in a 69% overall response rate. The response rate was higher in children (80%) than in adults (60%; $P = .28$). Although not significant, the better response of children contributed to the improved overall survival. Patients with a complete response had a lower TRM 1 year after MSC infusion compared with partial or nonresponders (37% vs 72%; $P = .002$) and a higher overall survival 2 years after HSCT (52% vs 16%; $P = .018$). Nearly half the patients survived (n = 21) and 8 patients developed chronic GVHD. The study was hampered because patients were heterogeneous not only in timing of MSC infusions but also because of the variable immune-suppressive regimens administered before MSC. Although compared with historical controls and recent literature the survival rates seem favorable, the efficacy of MSC in the treatment of acute GVHD remains to be confirmed; a European randomized prospective study is under way.

A recent press release by Osiris showed that in a randomized study of third-party MSC used for steroid refractory GVHD MSC proved no better than alternative treatments except in children and severe gastrointestinal GVHD. Publication of this trial is awaited.

In summary, MSC seem to be a promising cellular therapy in children undergoing HSCT to overcome GVHD and graft dysfunction. However, the long-term safety and efficacy have not been proven. Multicenter collaborative studies are needed to determine how and when MSC can be administered most effectively, and determining their in vivo functional capacities. Future studies will also need to address such issues as trafficking of MSC to target tissues and monitoring potential long-term toxicities. These studies may include an increased risk of relapse of underlying malignancies and increased infection risks because of the broad immune-suppressive activities of MSC, together with the risk of malignant transformation of infused expanded MSC.

REFERENCES

1. Kiessling R, Klein E, Pross H, et al. "Natural" killer cells in the mouse. II. Cytotoxic cells with specificity for mouse Moloney leukemia cells. Characteristics of the killer cell. Eur J Immunol 1975;5:117–21.
2. Lanier LL, Phillips JH, Hackett J Jr, et al. Natural killer cells: definition of a cell type rather than a function. J Immunother 1986;137:2735–9.
3. Caligiuri MA. Human natural killer cells. Blood 2008;112:461–9.

4. Ljunggren HG, Karre K. Host resistance directed selectively against H-2-deficient lymphoma variants. Analysis of the mechanism. J Environ Monit 1985; 162:1745–59.
5. Ljunggren HG, Karre K. In search of the 'missing self': MHC molecules and NK cell recognition. Immunol Today 1990;11:237–44.
6. Boyton RJ, Altmann DM. Natural killer cells, killer immunoglobulin-like receptors and human leucocyte antigen class I in disease. Clin Exp Immunol 2007;149: 1–8.
7. Moretta L, Bottino C, Pende D, et al. Different checkpoints in human NK-cell activation. Trends Immunol 2004;25:670–6.
8. Bottino C, Moretta L, Pende D, et al. Learning how to discriminate between friends and enemies, a lesson from Natural Killer cells. Mol Immunol 2004;41: 569–75.
9. Braud VM, Allan DS, O'Callaghan CA, et al. HLA-E binds to natural killer cell receptors CD94/NKG2A, B and C. Nature 1998;391:795–9.
10. Kaiser BK, Barahmand-Pour F, Paulsene W, et al. Interactions between NKG2x immunoreceptors and HLA-E ligands display overlapping affinities and thermodynamics. J Immunother 2005;174:2878–84.
11. Moretta A, Bottino C, Vitale M, et al. Receptors for HLA class-I molecules in human natural killer cells. Annu Rev Immunol 1996;14:619–48.
12. Yokoyama WM, Plougastel BF. Immune functions encoded by the natural killer gene complex. Nat Rev Immunol 2003;3:304–16.
13. Uhrberg M, Valiante NM, Shum BP, et al. Human diversity in killer cell inhibitory receptor genes. Immunity 1997;7:753–63.
14. Trinchieri G. Biology of natural killer cells. Adv Immunol 1989;47:187–376.
15. Pende D, Rivera P, Marcenaro S, et al. Major histocompatibility complex class I-related chain A and UL16-binding protein expression on tumor cell lines of different histotypes: analysis of tumor susceptibility to NKG2D-dependent natural killer cell cytotoxicity. Cancer Res 2002;62:6178–86.
16. Cerwenka A, Lanier LL. NKG2D ligands: unconventional MHC class I-like molecules exploited by viruses and cancer. Tissue Antigens 2003;61:335–43.
17. Pende D, Bottino C, Castriconi R, et al. PVR (CD155) and Nectin-2 (CD112) as ligands of the human DNAM-1 (CD226) activating receptor: involvement in tumor cell lysis. Mol Immunol 2005;42:463–9.
18. Sivori S, Carlomagno S, Moretta L, et al. Comparison of different CpG oligodeoxynucleotide classes for their capability to stimulate human NK cells. Eur J Immunol 2006;36:961–7.
19. Zamai L, Ponti C, Mirandola P, et al. NK cells and cancer. J Immunother 2007; 178:4011–6.
20. Imai K, Matsuyama S, Miyake S, et al. Natural cytotoxic activity of peripheral-blood lymphocytes and cancer incidence: an 11-year follow-up study of a general population. Lancet 2000;356:1795–9.
21. Cudkowicz G, Bennett M. Peculiar immunobiology of bone marrow allografts. II. Rejection of parental grafts by resistant F 1 hybrid mice. J Environ Monit 1971; 134:1513–28.
22. Lowdell MW, Ray N, Craston R, et al. The in vitro detection of anti-leukaemia-specific cytotoxicity after autologous bone marrow transplantation for acute leukaemia. Bone Marrow Transplant 1997;19:891–7.
23. Lowdell MW, Craston R, Samuel D, et al. Evidence that continued remission in patients treated for acute leukaemia is dependent upon autologous natural killer cells. Br J Haematol 2002;117:821–7.

24. Tajima F, Kawatani T, Endo A, et al. Natural killer cell activity and cytokine production as prognostic factors in adult acute leukemia. Leukemia 1996;10: 478–82.
25. Siegler U, Kalberer CP, Nowbakht P, et al. Activated natural killer cells from patients with acute myeloid leukemia are cytotoxic against autologous leukemic blasts in NOD/SCID mice. Leukemia 2005;19:2215–22.
26. Salih HR, Antropius H, Gieseke F, et al. Functional expression and release of ligands for the activating immunoreceptor NKG2D in leukemia. Blood 2003; 102:1389–96.
27. Afify ZA, bdel-Mageed A, Findley HW, et al. Cytotoxicity of purified Leu 19+ cells from the peripheral blood of children with acute lymphocytic leukemia. Cancer 1990;66:469–73.
28. Mageed AA, Findley HW Jr, Franco C, et al. Natural killer cells in children with acute leukemia. The effect of interleukin-2. Cancer 1987;60:2913–8.
29. Findley HW Jr, Abdel MA, Nasr SA, et al. Recombinant interleukin-2 activates peripheral blood lymphocytes from children with acute leukemia to kill autologous leukemic cells. Cancer 1988;62:1928–31.
30. Coca S, Perez-Piqueras J, Martinez D, et al. The prognostic significance of intratumoral natural killer cells in patients with colorectal carcinoma. Cancer 1997;79: 2320–8.
31. Ishigami S, Natsugoe S, Tokuda K, et al. Prognostic value of intratumoral natural killer cells in gastric carcinoma. Cancer 2000;88:577–83.
32. Alvarado CS, Findley HW, Chan WC, et al. Natural killer cells in children with malignant solid tumors. Effect of recombinant interferon-alpha and interleukin-2 on natural killer cell function against tumor cell lines. Cancer 1989; 63:83–9.
33. Velardi A. Role of KIRs and KIR ligands in hematopoietic transplantation. Curr Opin Immunol 2008;20:581–7.
34. Velardi A, Ruggeri L, Mancusi A, et al. Natural killer cell allorecognition of missing self in allogeneic hematopoietic transplantation: a tool for immunotherapy of leukemia. Curr Opin Immunol 2009;21:525–30.
35. Pfeiffer M, Schumm M, Feuchtinger T, et al. Intensity of HLA class I expression and KIR-mismatch determine NK-cell mediated lysis of leukaemic blasts from children with acute lymphatic leukaemia. Br J Haematol 2007;138:97–100.
36. Prigione I, Corrias MV, Airoldi I, et al. Immunogenicity of human neuroblastoma. Ann N Y Acad Sci 2004;1028:69–80.
37. Handgretinger R, Lang P, Schumm M, et al. Immunological aspects of haploidentical stem cell transplantation in children. Ann N Y Acad Sci 2001;938: 340–57 [discussion: 357–8].
38. Feuchtinger T, Pfeiffer M, Pfaffle A, et al. Cytolytic activity of NK cell clones against acute childhood precursor-B-cell leukaemia is influenced by HLA class I expression on blasts and the differential KIR phenotype of NK clones. Bone Marrow Transplant 2009;43:875–81.
39. Ruggeri L, Capanni M, Casucci M, et al. Role of natural killer cell alloreactivity in HLA-mismatched hematopoietic stem cell transplantation. Blood 1999;94: 333–9.
40. Ruggeri L, Mancusi A, Capanni M, et al. Donor natural killer cell allorecognition of missing self in haploidentical hematopoietic transplantation for acute myeloid leukemia: challenging its predictive value. Blood 2007;110:433–40.
41. Leung W, Iyengar R, Turner V, et al. Determinants of antileukemia effects of allogeneic NK cells. J Immunother 2004;172:644–50.

42. Chen X, Knowles J, Barfield RC, et al. A novel approach for quantification of KIR expression in healthy donors and pediatric recipients of hematopoietic SCTs. Bone Marrow Transplant 2009;43:525–32.
43. Leung W, Iyengar R, Triplett B, et al. Comparison of killer Ig-like receptor genotyping and phenotyping for selection of allogeneic blood stem cell donors. J Immunother 2005;174:6540–5.
44. Hsu KC, Keever-Taylor CA, Wilton A, et al. Improved outcome in HLA-identical sibling hematopoietic stem-cell transplantation for acute myelogenous leukemia predicted by KIR and HLA genotypes. Blood 2005;105:4878–84.
45. Miller JS, Cooley S, Parham P, et al. Missing KIR ligands are associated with less relapse and increased graft-versus-host disease (GVHD) following unrelated donor allogeneic HCT. Blood 2007;109:5058–61.
46. Farag SS, Bacigalupo A, Eapen M, et al. The effect of KIR ligand incompatibility on the outcome of unrelated donor transplantation: a report from the center for international blood and marrow transplant research, the European blood and marrow transplant registry, and the Dutch registry. Biol Blood Marrow Transplant 2006;12:876–84.
47. Willemze R, Rodrigues CA, Labopin M, et al. KIR-ligand incompatibility in the graft-versus-host direction improves outcomes after umbilical cord blood transplantation for acute leukemia. Leukemia 2009;23:492–500.
48. Verheyden S, Demanet C. NK cell receptors and their ligands in leukemia. Leukemia 2008;22:249–57.
49. Lowe EJ, Turner V, Handgretinger R, et al. T-cell alloreactivity dominates natural killer cell alloreactivity in minimally T-cell-depleted HLA-non-identical paediatric bone marrow transplantation. Br J Haematol 2003;123:323–6.
50. Langenkamp U, Siegler U, Jorger S, et al. Human acute myeloid leukemia CD34+CD38- stem cells are susceptible to allorecognition and lysis by single KIR-expressing natural killer cells. Haematologica 2009;94:1590–4.
51. Savani BN, Rezvani K, Mielke S, et al. Factors associated with early molecular remission after T cell-depleted allogeneic stem cell transplantation for chronic myelogenous leukemia. Blood 2006;107:1688–95.
52. Fischer JC, Ottinger H, Ferencik S, et al. Relevance of C1 and C2 epitopes for hemopoietic stem cell transplantation: role for sequential acquisition of HLA-C-specific inhibitory killer Ig-like receptor. J Immunother 2007;178:3918–23.
53. Teltschik F, Lang P, Pfeiffer H, et al. Long-term IL2 therapy after transplantation of T-cell depleted stem cells from alternative donors in children [abstract]. Bone Marrow Transplant 2007;39(Suppl 1):S185.
54. Ruggeri L, Capanni M, Urbani E, et al. Effectiveness of donor natural killer cell alloreactivity in mismatched hematopoietic transplants. Science 2002;295:2097–100.
55. Handgretinger R, Chen X, Pfeiffer M, et al. Feasibility and outcome of reduced-intensity conditioning in haploidentical transplantation. Ann N Y Acad Sci 2007; 1106:279–89.
56. Bethge WA, Faul C, Bornhauser M, et al. Haploidentical allogeneic hematopoietic cell transplantation in adults using CD3/CD19 depletion and reduced intensity conditioning: an update. Blood Cells Mol Dis 2008;40:13–9.
57. Barfield RC, Otto M, Houston J, et al. A one-step large-scale method for T- and B-cell depletion of mobilized PBSC for allogeneic transplantation. Cytotherapy 2004;6:1–6.
58. Rodella L, Zamai L, Rezzani R, et al. Interleukin 2 and interleukin 15 differentially predispose natural killer cells to apoptosis mediated by endothelial and tumour cells. Br J Haematol 2001;115:442–50.

59. Pfeiffer M, Lang P, Schumm M, et al. IL-15 activated CD3/10 depleted grafts for haploidentical transplantation in children: strongly increased NK activity in vitro and excellent tolerability in vivo [abstract]. Bone Marrow Transplant 2008;41. S51.

60. Lang P, Barbin K, Feuchtinger T, et al. Chimeric CD19 antibody mediates cytotoxic activity against leukemic blasts with effector cells from pediatric patients who received T-cell-depleted allografts. Blood 2004;103:3982–5.

61. Pfeiffer M, Stanojevic S, Feuchtinger T, et al. Rituximab mediates in vitro antileukemic activity in pediatric patients after allogeneic transplantation. Bone Marrow Transplant 2005;36:91–7.

62. Triplett B, Handgretinger R, Pui CH, et al. KIR-incompatible hematopoietic-cell transplantation for poor prognosis infant acute lymphoblastic leukemia. Blood 2006;107:1238–9.

63. Imai C, Iwamoto S, Campana D. Genetic modification of primary natural killer cells overcomes inhibitory signals and induces specific killing of leukemic cells. Blood 2005;106:376–83.

64. Fujisaki H, Kakuda H, Shimasaki N, et al. Expansion of highly cytotoxic human natural killer cells for cancer cell therapy. Cancer Res 2009;69:4010–7.

65. Miller JS, Soignier Y, Panoskaltsis-Mortari A, et al. Successful adoptive transfer and in vivo expansion of human haploidentical NK cells in patients with cancer. Blood 2005;105:3051–7.

66. Perez-Martinez A, Leung W, Munoz E, et al. KIR-HLA receptor-ligand mismatch associated with a graft-versus-tumor effect in haploidentical stem cell transplantation for pediatric metastatic solid tumors. Pediatr Blood Cancer 2009;53:120–4.

67. Re F, Staudacher C, Zamai L, et al. Killer cell Ig-like receptors ligand-mismatched, alloreactive natural killer cells lyse primary solid tumors. Cancer 2006;107:640–8.

68. Igarashi T, Wynberg J, Srinivasan R, et al. Enhanced cytotoxicity of allogeneic NK cells with killer immunoglobulin-like receptor ligand incompatibility against melanoma and renal cell carcinoma cells. Blood 2004;104:170–7.

69. Verhoeven DH, de Hooge AS, Mooiman EC, et al. NK cells recognize and lyse Ewing sarcoma cells through NKG2D and DNAM-1 receptor dependent pathways. Mol Immunol 2008;45:3917–25.

70. Lang P, Pfeiffer M, Muller I, et al. Haploidentical stem cell transplantation in patients with pediatric solid tumors: preliminary results of a pilot study and analysis of graft versus tumor effects. Klin Padiatr 2006;218:321–6.

71. Fibbe WE, Lazarus HM. Mesenchymal stem cells and hematopoietic stem cell transplantation. In: Atkinson K, Champlin R, Brenner MA, et al, editors. Clinical bone marrow and blood stem cell transplantation. 3rd edition. Cambridge: Cambridge University Press; 2004. p. 67–78.

72. Friedenstein AJ, Deriglasova UF, Kulagina NN, et al. Precursors for fibroblasts in different populations of hematopoietic cells as detected by the in vitro colony assay method. Exp Hematol 1974;2:83–92.

73. Owen M. Marrow stromal stem cells. J Cell Sci Suppl 1988;10:63–76.

74. Prockop DJ. Marrow stromal cells as stem cells for non-hematopoietic tissues. Science 1997;276:71–4.

75. Majumdar MK, Thiede MA, Mosca JD, et al. Phenotypic and functional comparison of cultures of marrow-derived mesenchymal stem cells (MSCs) and stromal cells. J Cell Physiol 1998;176:57–66.

76. Almeida-Porada G, Flake AW, Glimp HA, et al. Cotransplantation of stroma results in enhancement of engraftment and early expression of donor hematopoietic stem cells in utero. Exp Hematol 1999;27:1569–75.

77. In't Anker PS, Noort WA, Kruisselbrink AB, et al. Non expanded primary lung and bone marrow-derived mesenchymal cells promote the engraftment of umbilical cord blood-derived CD34 (+) cells in NOD/SCID mice. Exp Hematol 2003;31:881–9.

78. Horwitz EM, Le Blanc K, Dominici M, et al. Clarification of the nomenclature for MSC: the International Society for Cellular Therapy position statement. Cytotherapy 2005;7:393–5.

79. Nathanson MA. Bone matrix-directed chondrogenesis of muscle in vitro. Clin Orthop 1985;200:142–58.

80. Nakahara H, Dennis JE, Bruder SP, et al. In vitro differentiation of bone and hypertrophic cartilage from periosteal-derived cells. Exp Cell Res 1991;195:492–503.

81. Campagnoli C, Roberts IA, Kumar S, et al. Identification of mesenchymal stem/progenitor cells in human first-trimester fetal blood, liver, and bone marrow. Blood 2001;98:2396–402.

82. Fernandez M, Simon V, Herrera G, et al. Detection of stromal cells in peripheral blood progenitor cell collections from breast cancer patients. Bone Marrow Transplant 1997;20:265–71.

83. Lazarus HM, Haynesworth SE, Gerson SL, et al. Ex vivo expansion and subsequent infusion of human bone marrow-derived stromal progenitor cells (mesenchymal progenitor cells): implications for therapeutic use. Bone Marrow Transplant 1995;16:557–64.

84. Erices A, Conget P, Minguell JJ. Mesenchymal progenitor cells in human umbilical cord blood. Br J Haematol 2000;109:235–42.

85. Bieback K, Kluter H. Mesenchymal stromal cells from umbilical cord blood. Curr Stem Cell Res Ther 2007;2:310–23.

86. In't Anker PS, Scherjon SA, Kleijburg-Van Der Keur C, et al. Amniotic fluid as a novel source of mesenchymal stem cells for therapeutic transplantation. Blood 2003;102:1548–9.

87. Bernardo ME, Emons JA, Karperien M, et al. Human mesenchymal stem cells derived from bone marrow display a better chondrogenic differentiation compared with other sources. Connect Tissue Res 2007;48:132–40.

88. Bernardo ME, Avanzini MA, Perotti C, et al. Optimization of in vitro expansion of human multipotent mesenchymal stromal cells for cell-therapy approaches: further insights in the search for a fetal calf serum substitute. J Cell Physiol 2007;211:121–30.

89. Avanzini MA, Bernardo ME, Cometa AM, et al. Generation of mesenchymal stromal cells in the presence of platelet lysate: a phenotypical and functional comparison between umbilical cord blood- and bone marrow-derived progenitors. Hematologica 2009;94:1649–60.

90. Vogel JP, Szalay K, Geiger F, et al. Platelet-rich plasma improves expansion of human mesenchymal stem cells and retains differentiation capacity and in vivo bone formation in calcium phosphate ceramics. Platelets 2006;17:462–9.

91. Doucet C, Ernou I, Zhang Y, et al. Platelet lysates promote mesenchymal stem cell expansion: a safety substitute for animal serum in cell-based therapy applications. J Cell Physiol 2005;205:228–36.

92. Schallmoser K, Bartmann C, Rohde E, et al. Human platelet lysate can replace fetal bovine serum for clinical-scale expansion of functional mesenchymal stromal cells. Transfusion 2007;47:1436–46.

93. Tolar J, Nauta AJ, Osborn MJ, et al. Sarcoma derived from cultured mesenchymal stem cells. Stem Cells 2007;25:371–9.

94. Bernardo ME, Zaffaroni N, Novara F, et al. Human bone marrow derived mesenchymal stem cells do not undergo transformation after long-term in vitro culture and do not exhibit telomere maintenance mechanisms. Cancer Res 2007;67:9142–9.
95. Uccelli A, Moretta L, Pistoia V. Mesenchymal stem cells in health and disease. Nat Rev Immunol 2008;8:726–36.
96. Di Nicola M, Carlo-Stella C, Magni M, et al. Human bone marrow stromal cells suppress T-lymphocyte proliferation induced by cellular or nonspecific mitogenic stimuli. Blood 2002;99:3838–43.
97. Krampera M, Glennie S, Dyson J, et al. Bone marrow mesenchymal stem cells inhibit the response of naïve and memory antigen-specific T-cells to their cognate peptide. Blood 2004;101:3722–9.
98. Aggarwal S, Pittenger MF. Human mesenchymal stem cells modulate allogeneic immune cell responses. Blood 2005;105:1815–22.
99. Sotiropoulou PA, Perz SA, Gritzapis AD, et al. Interactions between human mesenchymal stem cells and natural killer cells. Stem Cells 2006;24:74–85.
100. Nauta AJ, Westerhuis G, Kruisselbrink AB, et al. Donor-derived mesenchymal stem cells are immunogenic in an allogeneic host and stimulate donor graft rejection in a nonmyeloablative setting. Blood 2006;108:2114–20.
101. Meisel R, Ziber A, Laryea M, et al. Human bone marrow stromal cells inhibit allogeneic responses by indoleamine 2,3 dioxygenase mediated tryptophan degradation. Blood 2004;103:4619–21.
102. Glennie S, Soeiro I, Dyson PJ, et al. Bone marrow mesenchymal stem cells induce division arrest anergy of activated T cells. Blood 2005;105:2821–7.
103. Benvenuto F, Ferrari S, Gerdoni E, et al. Human mesenchymal stem cells promote survival of T cells in a quiescent state. Stem Cells 2007;25:1753–60.
104. Rasmusson I, Ringden O, Sundberg B, et al. Mesenchymal stem cells inhibit lymphocyte proliferation by mitogens and alloantigens by different mechanisms. Exp Cell Res 2005;305:33–41.
105. Rasmusson I, Ringden O, Sundberg B, et al. Mesenchymal stem cells inhibit the formation of cytotoxic T lymphocytes, but not activated cytotoxic T lymphocytes or natural killer cells. Transplantation 2003;76:1208–13.
106. Morandi F, Raffaghello L, Bianchi G, et al. Immunogenicity of human mesenchymal stem cells in HLA-class-I-restricted T-cell responses against viral or tumor-associated antigens. Stem Cells 2008;26:1275–87.
107. Augello A, Tasso R, Negrini SM, et al. Bone marrow mesenchymal progenitor cells inhibit lymphocyte proliferation by activation of the programmed death 1 pathway. Eur J Immunol 2005;35:1482–6.
108. Corcione A, Benvenuto F, Ferretti E, et al. Human mesenchymal stem cells modulate B-cell functions. Blood 2006;107:367–72.
109. Traggiai E, Volpi S, Schena F, et al. Bone marrow-derived mesenchymal stem cells induce both polyclonal expansion and differentiation of B cells isolated from healthy donors and systemic lupus erythematosus patients. Stem Cells 2008;26:562–9.
110. Rasmusson I, Le Blanc K, Sundberg B, et al. Mesenchymal stem cells stimulate antibody secretion in human B cells. Scand J Immunol 2007;65:336–43.
111. Jiang XX, Zhang Y, Liu B, et al. Human mesenchymal stem cells inhibit differentiation and function of monocyte derived dendritic cells. Blood 2005;105:4120–6.
112. Nauta AJ, Kruisselbrink AB, Lurvink E, et al. Mesenchymal stem cells inhibit generation and function of both CD34+-derived and monocyte-derived dendritic cells. J Immunol 2006;177:2080–7.

113. Li YP, Paczesny S, Lauret E, et al. Human mesenchymal stem cells license adult CD34+ hemopoietic progenitor cells to differentiate into regulatory dendritic cells through activation of the Notch pathway. J Immunol 2008;180: 1598–608.

114. Stagg J, Pommey S, Eliopoulos N, et al. Interferon-γ-stimulated marrow stromal cells: a new type of nonhematopoietic antigen-presenting cell. Blood 2006;107: 2570–7.

115. Spaggiari GM, Capobianco A, Becchetti S, et al. Mesenchymal stem cell–natural killer cell interactions: evidence that activated NK cells are capable of killing MSCs, whereas MSCs can inhibit IL-2-induced NK-cell proliferation. Blood 2006;107:1484–90.

116. Almeida-Porada G, Porada CD, Tran N, et al. Co-transplantation of human stromal cell progenitors into pre-immune fetal sheep results in early appearance of human donor cells in circulation and boosts cell levels in bone marrow at later time points after transplantation. Blood 2000;95: 3620–7.

117. Krampera M, Cosmi L, Angeli R, et al. Role for interferon-γ in the immunomodulatory activity of human bone marrow mesenchymal stem cells. Stem Cells 2006;24:386–98.

118. Ryan JM, Barry F, Murphy JM, et al. Interferon-γ does not break, but promotes the immunosuppressive capacity of adult human mesenchymal stem cells. Clin Exp Immunol 2007;149:353–63.

119. Ren G, Zhang L, Zhao X, et al. Mesenchymal stem-cell-mediated immunosuppression occurs via concerted action of chemokines and nitric oxide. Cell Stem Cell 2008;2:141–50.

120. Kogler G, Kögler G, Radke TF, et al. Cytokine production and hematopoiesis supporting activity of cord blood derived unrestricted somatic stem cells. Exp Hematol 2005;33:573–83.

121. Selmani Z, Naji A, Zidi I, et al. Human leukocyte antigen-G5 secretion by human mesenchymal stem cells is required to suppress T lymphocyte and natural killer function and to induce CD4+CD25highFOXP3+ regulatory T cells. Stem Cells 2008;26:212–22.

122. Bartholomew A, Sturgeon C, Siatskas M, et al. Mesenchymal stem cells suppress lymphocyte proliferation in vitro and prolong skin graft survival in vivo. Exp Hematol 2002;30:42–8.

123. Yanez R, Lamana ML, Garcia-Castro J, et al. Adipose tissue-derived mesenchymal stem cells (AD-MSC) have in vivo immunosuppressive properties applicable for the control of graft-versus-host disease (GVHD). Stem Cells 2006;24: 2582–91.

124. Zhang J, Li Y, Chen J, et al. Human bone marrow stromal cell treatment improves neurological functional recovery in EAE mice. Exp Neurol 2005;195: 16–26.

125. Djouad F, Fritz V, Apparailly F, et al. Reversal of the immunosuppressive properties of mesenchymal stem cells by tumor necrosis factor alpha in collagen-induced arthritis. Arthritis Rheum 2005;52:1595–603.

126. Devine SM, Bartholomew AM, Mahmud N, et al. Mesenchymal stem cells are capable of homing to the bone marrow of non-human primates following systemic infusion. Exp Hematol 2001;29:244–55.

127. Noort WA, Kruisselbrink AB, In't Anker PS, et al. Mesenchymol stem cells promote engraftment of human umbilical cord blood-derived CD34(+) cells in NOD/SCID mice. Exp Hematol 2002;30:870–8.

128. Ringden O, Uzunel M, Rasmusson I, et al. Mesenchymal stem cells for treatment of therapy-resistant graft-versus-host disease. Transplantation 2006;81: 1390–7.
129. Devine SM, Cobbs C, Jennings M, et al. Mesenchymal stem cells distribute to a wide range of tissues following systemic infusion into non-human primates. Blood 2003;101:2999–3001.
130. Ruster B, Göttig S, Ludwig RJ, et al. Mesenchymal stem cells display coordinated rolling and adhesion behavior on endothelial cells. Blood 2006;108: 3938–44.
131. Sordi V, Malosio ML, Marchesi F, et al. Bone marrow mesenchymal stem cells express a restricted set of functionally active chemokine receptors capable of promoting migration to pancreatic islets. Blood 2005;106:419–27.
132. Son BR, Marquez-Curtis LA, Kucia M, et al. Migration of bone marrow and cord blood mesenchymal stem cells in vitro is regulated by stromal-derived factor-1–CXCR4 and hepatocyte growth factor–c-Met axes and involves matrix metalloproteinases. Stem Cells 2006;24:1254–64.
133. Karp JM, Teo GSL. Mesenchymal stem cell homing: the devil is in the details. Review Cell Stem Cell 2009;4:206–316.
134. Koc ON, Gerson SL, Cooper BW, et al. Rapid hematopoietic recovery after co-infusion of autologous-blood stem cells and culture-expanded marrow mesenchymal stem cells in advanced breast cancer patients receiving high-dose chemotherapy. J Clin Oncol 2000;18:307–16.
135. Lazarus HM, Curtin P, Devine S, et al. Co-transplantation of HLA-identical sibling culture-expanded mesenchymal stem cells and hematopoietic stem cells in hematologic malignancy patients. Biol Blood Marrow Transplant 2005;11: 389–98.
136. Müller I, Kustermann-Kuhn B, Holzwarth C, et al. In vitro analysis of multipotent mesenchymal stromal cells as potential cellular therapeutics in neurometabolic diseases in pediatric patients. Exp Hematol 2006;34:1413–9.
137. Koc ON, Peters C, Aubourg P, et al. Bone marrow-derived mesenchymal stem cells remain host-derived despite successful hematopoietic engraftment after allogeneic transplantation in patients with lysosomal and peroxisomal storage diseases. Exp Hematol 1999;27:1675–81.
138. Krivit W, Shapiro EG, Lockman LA, et al. Bone marrow transplantation: treatment for globoid cell leukodystrophy, metachromatic leukodystrophy, adrenoleukodystrophy and Hurler syndrome. In: Moser HW, Vinken PJ, Bruyn GW, editors. Handbook of clinical neurology. Amsterdam: Elsevier Science; 1996. p. 87–106.
139. Koc ON, Day J, Nieder M, et al. Allogeneic mesenchymal stem cell infusion for treatment of metachromatic leukodystrophy (MLD) and Hurler syndrome (MPS-IH). Bone Marrow Transplant 2002;30:215–22.
140. Sillence DO, Rimoin DL, Danks DM. Clinical variability in osteogenesis imperfecta-variable expressivity or genetic heterogeneity. Birth Defects Orig Artic Ser 1979;15:113–29.
141. Horwitz EM, Prockop DJ, Gordon PL, et al. Clinical responses to bone marrow transplantation in children with severe osteogenesis imperfecta. Blood 2001; 97:1227–31.
142. Horwitz EM, Gordon PL, Koo WK, et al. Isolated allogeneic bone marrow-derived mesenchymal cells engraft and stimulate growth in children with osteogenesis imperfecta: Implications for cell therapy of bone. Proc Natl Acad Sci U S A 2002;99:8932–7.

143. Ball LM, Bernardo ME, Roelofs H, et al. Co-transplantation of ex vivo expanded mesenchymal stem cells accelerates lymphocyte recovery and may reduce the risk of graft failure in haplo-identical hematopoietic stem cell transplantation. Blood 2007;110:2765–7.

144. Le Blanc K, Rasmusson I, Sundberg B, et al. Treatment of severe acute graft-versus-host disease with third party haploidentical mesenchymal stem cells. Lancet 2004;363:1439–41.

145. Le Blanc K, Frassoni F, Ball LM, et al. Use of bone marrow derived expanded mesenchymal stem cells in the treatment of steroid refractory acute GvHD. Lancet 2008;371:1579–86.

146. Available at: http://investor.osiris.com/releases.cfm.

Current International Perspectives on Hematopoietic Stem Cell Transplantation for Inherited Metabolic Disorders

Jaap J. Boelens, MD, PhD[a], Vinod K. Prasad, MD, MRCP[b],
Jakub Tolar, MD, PhD[c], Robert F. Wynn, MD, MRCP, FRCPath[d],
Charles Peters, MD[e,f,*]

KEYWORDS

- Hematopoietic stem cell transplantation • Pediatrics
- Inherited metabolic disorders • Storage diseases
- Inborn errors of metabolism • Bone marrow transplantation
- Umbilical cord blood transplantation

Inherited metabolic disorders (IMD) or inborn errors of metabolism are a diverse group of diseases arising from genetic defects in lysosomal enzymes or peroxisomal function. Lysosomal enzymes are hydrolytic and are stored in cellular organelles called lysosomes. Peroxisomes are organelles involved in lipid metabolism. These diseases are characterized by devastating systemic processes affecting neurologic and

Contributions: Equally contributing co-first authors listed in alphabetical order: Drs Boelens, Prasad, Tolar, and Wynn. Senior author: Dr Peters.
[a] Department of Pediatrics, Blood and Marrow Transplantation Program, UMC Utrecht, Wilhelmina Children's Hospital, KC.03.063.0, Lundlaan 6, 3584 EA Utrecht, The Netherlands
[b] Department of Pediatrics, Blood and Marrow Transplant Program, Duke University Medical Center, Duke University School of Medicine, 1400 Morreene Road, Durham, NC 27710, USA
[c] Department of Pediatrics, Division of Pediatric Blood and Marrow Transplantation, University of Minnesota School of Medicine, MMC 366, 420 Delaware Street SE, Minneapolis, MN 55455, USA
[d] Blood and Marrow Transplant Programme, Department of Paediatric Haematology and Oncology, Royal Manchester Children's Hospital, Oxford Road, Manchester, M13 OJH, UK
[e] Pediatric Hematology-Oncology, Sanford Children's Hospital, 1600 W. 22nd Street, Sioux Falls, SD 57117, USA
[f] Sanford School of Medicine, The University of South Dakota, Sioux Falls, SD, USA
* Corresponding author.
E-mail address: petersch@sanfordhealth.org

Pediatr Clin N Am 57 (2010) 123–145
doi:10.1016/j.pcl.2009.11.004
0031-3955/10/$ – see front matter © 2010 Elsevier Inc. All rights reserved.

pediatric.theclinics.com

cognitive function, growth and development, and cardiopulmonary status. Onset in infancy or early childhood is typically accompanied by rapid deterioration. Early death is a common outcome.

Timely diagnosis and immediate referral to an IMD specialist are essential steps in management of these disorders. Treatment recommendations are based on the disorder, its phenotype including age at onset and rate of progression, severity of clinical signs and symptoms, family values and expectations, and the risks and benefits associated with available therapies such as allogeneic hematopoietic stem cell transplantation (HSCT). Allogeneic HSCT for IMD is performed using donor cells from bone marrow (BM), umbilical cord blood (CB), or growth factor mobilized peripheral blood (PB). Donor cells are infused into the patient after immunosuppression and myelosuppression with a chemotherapeutic regimen.

The concept of cross-correction of metabolic defects with transferable lysosomal enzymes was described in 1968, when fibroblasts of patients with Hurler (MPS IH) and Hunter (MPS II) syndromes were cocultured in the laboratory.[1] Metabolic correction of lysosomal storage diseases occurs by mannose-6-phosphate receptor-mediated endocytosis of secreted enzyme and by direct transfer of enzyme from adjacent cells.[2,3] Theoretically, both mechanisms should occur after allogeneic HSCT. The mechanism by which HSCT halts cerebral demyelination of the peroxisomal disorder cerebral X-linked adrenoleukodystrophy (X-ALD) is perhaps threefold: immunosuppression, replacement with metabolically competent cell populations, leading to decreased perivascular inflammation and metabolic correction.

Successful transplantation depends on enzyme-replete cells from the donor migrating to and growing in recipient tissues, including the liver (Kupffer cells), lungs (alveolar macrophages), and central nervous system (CNS, microglia). Microglia are a small proportion of nonneuronal cells in the brain and their replacement rate after transplantation is slower than that of Kupffer cells and alveolar macrophages.[4–7] These factors may partially explain the limited ability of HSCT to stabilize neurologic function with rapidly progressing cerebral disorders.[8]

The first allogeneic HSCT for an IMD was performed in 1980, when a 9-month-old boy with MPS IH received BM from his mother. In this child, HSCT led to normal development and intelligence, despite the presence of a homozygous W402X mutation, which is associated with a severe phenotype.[9] In 1982, the first patient with Maroteaux-Lamy (MPS VI) syndrome, a 13-year-old adolescent girl, was successfully transplanted from her human leukocyte antigen (HLA) -matched, enzymatically normal sister, resulting in resolution of hepatosplenomegaly and normalization of cardiopulmonary function.[10] She continues to do well and is able to live independently (Dr W. Krivit, personal communication, 2005). From the late 1980s to the 1990s, successful allogeneic HSCTs were performed for each of the leukodystrophies, including cerebral X-ALD,[11] globoid-cell leukodystrophy (GLD),[12] and metachromatic leukodystrophy (MLD).[13] Currently, bone marrow transplantation (BMT) from an HLA-matched, enzymatically normal related donor and unrelated donor cord blood transplantation (CBT) are the most common modalities of HSCT for IMD. Peripheral blood transplantation (PBT) is rarely performed for these disorders.

Ongoing international collaborative efforts to examine HSCT outcomes began in the late 1980s. Large multi- and single-center reports on the outcomes of HSCT have been published on MPS IH,[14–18] cerebral X-ALD,[19,20] and GLD.[21] In addition, increasing attention is given to outcome analysis by graft source, including PB,[22] BM,[11–15,23] and CB,[16–21,24,25] and the outcomes of combining enzyme replacement therapy (ERT), if available, with HSCT.[26–29] In this review, the indications for HSCT and outcomes of HSCT for selected IMD are discussed. An international perspective on progress, limitations, and future directions is provided.

INDICATIONS FOR HSCT: OVERVIEW

Table 1 identifies the IMD for which allogeneic HSCT is currently indicated or under investigation. HSCT is currently not indicated for selected IMD, including adrenomyeloneuropathy (AMN), Alexander syndrome, Morquio syndrome (MPS IV), vanishing white matter disease, Zellweger syndrome, cerebrotendinous xanthomatosis, Fabry syndrome, Canavan syndrome, and cystinosis.[30] Therefore, these disorders are not included in **Table 1** or the discussion.

HURLER SYNDROME (MPS IH)

Hurler syndrome (MPS IH), the most severe phenotype of α-L-iduronidase deficiency, is an autosomal recessive disorder characterized by progressive accumulation of stored glycosaminoglycans (GAGs). Hurler and other phenotypes of MPS I (Scheie [MPS IS, attenuated] and Hurler-Scheie [MPS IH/S, intermediate]) are a broad, continuous clinical spectrum. Accumulation of GAGs results in progressive, multisystem dysfunction that includes psychomotor retardation, severe skeletal malformations, life-threatening cardiopulmonary complications, and early death.[31] Data from the Center for International Blood and Marrow Transplant Research (CIBMTR) and the European Group for Blood and Marrow Transplant (EBMT) indicate that more than 500 allogeneic HSCTs have been performed worldwide for children with MPS IH since 1980, making it the most commonly transplanted IMD.

HSCT for children with MPS IH is effective, resulting in increased life expectancy and improvement of clinical parameters. To derive maximum long-term benefits in children with MPS IH, allogeneic HSCT must be performed early in the disease course before the onset of irreversible damage. Donor-cell engraftment after HSCT has usually resulted in rapid reduction of obstructive airway symptoms and hepatosplenomegaly. Cardiovascular function benefits from HSCT as certain pathologic conditions before transplant clearly improve. Hearing, vision, and linear growth also improve in many transplanted patients. In addition, hydrocephalus is either prevented or stabilized. Although cerebral damage already present before HSCT seems to be irreversible, successful HSCT is able to prevent progressive psychomotor deterioration and improve cognitive function.[14,15,23,32]

Recent HSCT experience shows significantly improved graft outcomes when compared with earlier results.[16–18,28] It seems that early engrafted survival rates of 25% to 70%[14,15,23] can be attributed to a clinical learning curve, restricted donor availability, graft failure, mixed chimerism, and transplant-related morbidity and mortality.[17] A recent risk analysis showed that graft failures increased with the use of T-cell depleted grafts and reduced intensity conditioning and decreased with the use of dose-adjusted busulfan (BU).[17]

An enzymatically matched normal sibling is the preferred HSCT donor for children with MPS IH. However, in the past decade, unrelated CB has been used with increasing frequency as a graft source for children without a matched sibling donor. CB offers several potential advantages compared with BM or PB for HSCT, including better availability, greater tolerance for HLA mismatch, lower incidence and severity of graft-versus-host disease (GVHD), and reduced likelihood of transmitting viral infections.[16,25,33,34] Laboratory studies suggest that CB stem cells may be capable of transdifferentiation into osteoblasts, chrondoblasts, and neurons.[35–37] Use of CBT for children with MPS

Table 1
IMD for which HSCT may be indicated

Disorder	Enzyme/Protein	HSCT Indication	Comments
Mucopolysaccharidoses			
Hurler (MPS IH)	α-L-Iduronidase	Standard therapy	
Hurler/Scheie (MPS IH/S)	α-L-Iduronidase	Optional	ERT first-line therapy
Scheie (MPS IS)	α-L-Iduronidase	Optional	ERT first-line therapy
Hunter: severe (MPS IIA)	Iduronate-2-sulfatase	Investigational	Only early or asymptomatic
Hunter: attenuated (MPS IIB)	Iduronate-2-sulfatase	Investigational	Only early or asymptomatic
Sanfilippo (MPS IIIA)	Heparan-N-sulfatase	Investigational	Only early or asymptomatic
Sanfilippo (MPS IIIB)	N-Acetylglucosaminidase	Investigational	Only early or asymptomatic
Sanfilippo (MPS IIIC)	AcetylCoA:N-acetyltransferase	Investigational	Only early or asymptomatic
Sanfilippo (MPS IIID)	N-Acetylglucosamine 6-sulfatase	Investigational	Only early or asymptomatic
Maroteaux-Lamy (MPS VI)	Arylsulfatase B	Optional	ERT first-line therapy
Sly (MPS VII)	β-Glucuronidase	Optional	
Leukodystrophies			
X-ALD, cerebral	ALD protein	Standard therapy	Not for advanced disease
MLD: early onset	ARSA	Unknown	Only early or asymptomatic
MLD: late onset	ARSA	Standard therapy	
GLD: early onset	GALC	Standard therapy	Neonate, screening diagnosis, or second case in known family; not for advanced disease
GLD: late onset	GALC	Optional	
Glycoprotein metabolic and miscellaneous disorders			
Fucosidosis	Fucosidase	Optional	
α-Mannosidosis	α-Mannosidase	Optional	

Disorder	Enzyme/defect	Status	Comments
Aspartylglucosaminuria	Aspartylglucosaminidase	Optional	
Farber	Ceraminidase	Optional	
Tay-Sachs: early onset	Hexosaminidase A	Unknown	Neonate, screening diagnosis, or second case in known family
Tay-Sachs: juvenile	Hexosaminidase A	Unknown	
Sandhoff: early onset	Hexosaminidase A & B	Unknown	Neonate, screening diagnosis, or second case in known family
Sandhoff: juvenile	Hexosaminidase A & B	Unknown	
Gaucher 1 (nonneuronopathic)	Glucocerebrosidase	Optional	ERT first-line therapy
Gaucher 2 (acute neuronopathic)	Glucocerebrosidase	Unknown	
Gaucher 3 (subacute neuronopathic)	Glucocerebrosidase	Unknown	Limited benefit of ERT
Gaucher 3 (Norrbottnian)	Glucocerebrosidase	Optional	
Pompe	Glucosidase	Investigational	ERT available
Niemann-Pick: type A	Acid sphingomyelinase	Unknown	
Niemann-Pick: type B	Acid sphingomyelinase	Unknown	ERT in clinical trial
Niemann-Pick: type C	Cholesterol trafficking	Optional for C-2	
Mucolipidosis: type II (I-cell)	N-Acetylglucosamine-1-phosphotransferase	Investigational	Only early or asymptomatic
Wolman syndrome	Acid lipase	Optional	May be viewed as standard
MSD	Sulfatases	Investigational	

Table does not include diseases where HSCT is not indicated. Standard therapy: HSCT applied routinely. Considerable published research evidence from registries and institutions shows efficacy. Delayed diagnosis or advanced disease may preclude transplant for individual patients. Optional: HSCT is effective but other therapy is increasingly considered first choice. Or, insufficient published evidence for HSCT to be considered standard. Investigational: possible a priori reason for HSCT. Further published evidence needed to support the use of HSCT in clinical practice. Unknown: no published evidence that HSCT is beneficial.

IH has been associated with high rates of chimerism, engraftment, and overall survival.[16,25,38,39] Similar results are noted for CBT in other selected IMD.[21,25,39,40]

Because of these data, the EBMT developed transplantation guidelines for patients with MPS IH in 2005. The guidelines are widely used today and include a standardized BU/cyclophosphamide (CY) conditioning regimen, an enzymatically normal matched sibling BM donor if available, and if not, CB as the preferred graft source (http://www.ebmt.org).

Fig. 1 provides a comparison of European survival outcomes for MPS IH patients receiving traditional HSCT (BMT or PBT; 1994–2004) with that of patients who were treated according to the EBMT guidelines (2005–2008). Mixed chimerism, observed in 29% of patients transplanted between 1994 and 2004, declined to 5% of patients transplanted between 2005 and 2008.[17,18]

A recent EUROCORD-Duke University MPS IH collaborative study showed that early transplant (ie, within 4.6 months from diagnosis) with CB and BU/CY conditioning was associated with improved engraftment and overall survival.[18] Furthermore, 94% of engrafted survivors achieved full donor chimerism.

ERT became available for patients with MPS I in 2003. Although ERT is not the primary treatment of MPS IH, it is hypothesized that ERT before HSCT can improve the pretransplant medical condition of the child and decrease the prevalence of HSCT- and MPS IH-related complications.[41] Intravenously administered enzyme does not cross the blood-brain barrier (BBB), so ERT is not able to prevent CNS deterioration.[42,43] ERT trials in patients with attenuated forms of MPS I (Scheie, Hurler-Scheie) have shown reduced organomegaly, decreased sleep apnea/hypopnea, improved pulmonary function, and increased physical ability.[44]

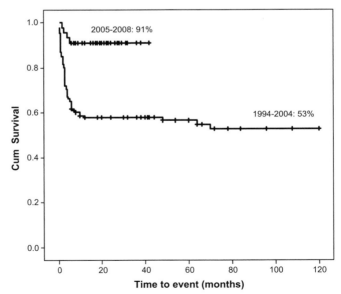

Fig. 1. Event-free survival (defined as alive and engrafted) of MPS IH patients after HSCT, according to the period of transplantation. HSCTs for 1994 to 2004 (n = 146) used various protocols standard for the period. HSCTs for 2005 to 2008 (n = 44) used EBMT protocol of standardized BU/CY conditioning and donor hierarchy of unrelated CB (second only to matched noncarrier sibling). (*Data from* Refs.[18,19])

The combination of ERT and HSCT for MPS IH children has been evaluated in single and multicenter studies. Investigators found that although ERT was well tolerated, the combination of ERT and HSCT did not significantly affect rates of survival, engrafted survival or HSCT-associated morbidity when compared with HSCT alone.[26–29,43,45] However, in the EUROCORD-Duke University study, children receiving HSCT within 4.6 months of diagnosis showed a trend toward significantly higher survival when ERT was used before CBT (n = 23, 83% survival) than when ERT was not used before CBT (n = 70, 63% survival, P = .19).[18] An ongoing CIBMTR comparison study of more than 250 children, including 20% who received ERT with HSCT, may address questions of efficacy and outcome. Currently, many transplant centers administer ERT to MPS IH patients before HSCT and continue this treatment until the patients either start conditioning or achieve donor-derived engraftment.

Despite these areas of success, some disease manifestations persist or can even progress after HSCT. For example, musculoskeletal disorders secondary to the IMD do not resolve following HSCT and often require orthopedic surgical interventions.[46,47] In addition, neurocognitive dysfunction and corneal clouding that developed before HSCT may be irreversible.[32]

The long-term clinical outcome for MPS IH children receiving HSCT seems to be promising, yet variable from child to child. This variability is presumably caused by factors such as genotype, age, and clinical status before HSCT, donor enzyme activity level, donor chimerism (mixed or full), stem-cell source (CB, BM, or PB), and resultant enzyme activity level in the recipient.[32] Neurocognitive outcomes may be enhanced by higher chimerism/enzyme activity levels[15]; however, the impact of these levels on outcomes needs continued evaluation. An international long-term follow-up study involving European and North American centers is under way to evaluate the influence of various patient, donor, and transplant characteristics on HSCT outcomes.

Overall, progress has been made. HSCT for children with MPS IH has become a safer procedure, with recent survival rates exceeding 90%. Quality of life for children with MPS IH following HSCT is also improving. Greater attention is being paid to timely diagnosis, prompt HSCT, and use of better procedures. In the absence of an enzymatically normal matched sibling donor, CBT is now routinely used to foster higher rates of full-donor chimerism and normal enzyme levels. Although HSCT is the procedure of choice for MPS IH, ERT is increasingly used as an adjuvant treatment before HSCT.

OTHER MUCOPOLYSACCHARIDOSIS SYNDROMES

Compared with MPS IH, experience with HSCT for treatment of other MPS disorders is limited. Small numbers and lack of detailed functional outcome data hamper the development of specific therapy guidelines. Conceptually, the basis for the effectiveness of HSCT in these children is the same as those with MPS IH. However, the kinetics of cellular migration, differentiation, distribution, and effective enzyme delivery may differ. Also, there is wide clinical variability within and across specific MPS diseases. As with HSCT for other IMD, important factors in the outcome may be timing of transplant, graft source, and the underlying severity of the phenotype in a given child. To date, most of the published experience is in recipients of BMT.[48–52] Recently, survival has been reported in small cohorts undergoing CBT, but their functional outcomes are not yet published.[25,53,54]

A recent French report on 8 boys with Hunter syndrome (MPS II) treated with BMT (6 matched sibling, 2 unrelated donor) at 3 to 16 years of age and followed for 7 to 17 years showed an excellent survival rate (1 died of unrelated causes), stabilization of cardiovascular problems, resolution of hepatosplenomegaly, improvement in joint stiffness, arrested progression of perceptual hearing defect, and improvement in transmission hearing defects.[50] Neuropsychological outcomes were variable and appeared to be related to the underlying phenotype and severity of symptoms at transplant. Two children with attenuated phenotype achieved adulthood with normal scholastic achievement, social integration, and language, whereas all children with severe phenotype lost ambulation and speech or developed seizures. Lack of neurologic improvement was also described in 3 BMT recipients in a 1999 report.[53] In a recent report of 159 children with IMD treated with unrelated CBT, 6 MPS II boys were included.[25] Their survival was consistent with that of the overall study group, but the study did not examine neurocognitive outcomes.

Despite benefits in the somatic features of the disease, the role of HSCT in MPS II remains controversial because of lack of convincing evidence of neurocognitive benefit. There are no published data on HSCT in very young, early stage, or asymptomatic children with "severe" MPS II phenotype. Limited genotype/phenotype correlation often leads to delays in identifying appropriate candidates for HSCT. However, in families with a known case, prenatal diagnosis and identification of an asymptomatic brother should be possible. ERT is available and likely to benefit some individuals; however, its high cost, lifelong duration, and inability to cross the BBB limit its overall usefulness.

The status of HSCT for Sanfilippo syndrome (MPS III) is similar to that of MPS II with inadequate data and inability to make specific recommendations about timing of transplant, graft source, and potential neurologic benefit. ERT is not currently available to treat children with MPS III. Eleven long-term survivors of BMT have been reported, but all showed decline in neurocognitive function.[55,56] In a study performed by investigators at Duke University, 19 children with MPS III were treated with CBT. After transplant, 12 of 19 survived in the long term.[25] Only the 2 children who were transplanted at less than 2 years of age showed modest gains in cognitive skills, but continue to have overall global developmental delay 3 to 5 years after CBT. Transplanted children seem to have fewer behavioral problems and better sleeping patterns when compared with nontransplanted children. Further evaluation and publication of the neurocognitive and developmental outcomes of patients with MPS III who have undergone CBT is critically important.

Maroteaux-Lamy syndrome (MPS VI) has multiple clinical phenotypes, but generally patients live into the second to fourth decade. In 1984, Krivit and colleagues[10] reported a 13-year-old girl with the severe phenotype who had a matched sibling BMT, leading to normalization of arylsulfatase B activity in peripheral lymphocytes and granulocytes, increased liver enzyme activity, decreased urinary excretion of GAG, decreased hepatosplenomegaly, normalization of cardiopulmonary function, improved visual acuity, and improved joint mobility. In a separate report, BMT in 4 patients (3 with cardiomyopathy, 1 with severe obstructive sleep apnea) led to improvement in cardiopulmonary function, facial features, and quality of life.[57] However, skeletal changes persisted or progressed. Lee and colleagues[58] treated a 5-year-old boy with a severe phenotype with matched sibling CBT, leading to improvement in hepatosplenomegaly, facial features, skin, and joint mobility. In light of these benefits, HSCT can be considered a therapeutic option in patients intolerant to or failing ERT.

ALD

X-ALD is a peroxisomal disorder involving defective β-oxidation of very long chain fatty acids (VLCFA). The affected gene in X-ALD is *ABCD1* and the peroxisomal membrane protein for which it codes is ALDP.[59] More than 500 mutations in the gene are described (http://www.x-ald.nl), but there is almost no relationship between the nature of the mutation and the clinical presentation of illness (no genotype-phenotype correlation).

X-ALD has a variable clinical presentation, and HSCT is indicated only in those individuals with clear evidence of early cerebral inflammatory disease. It is not indicated for asymptomatic individuals who have no cerebral involvement on testing because the risks of HSCT are considered too great. Nor is it indicated for those individuals with advanced cerebral disease because HSCT does not reverse, and may even worsen, established disease. In this illness, judicious timing of the transplant is paramount. Asymptomatic boys should be regularly screened for signs of inflammatory brain disease, a potential donor identified, and HSCT rapidly performed if and when such symptoms appear.

The laboratory diagnosis of X-ALD depends on demonstration of increased VLCFA levels and an *ABCD1* mutation.[60,61] The plasma assay for VLCFA is reliable in males, even in the newborn period, but is less reliable in female carriers, in whom genetic testing should be performed to exclude false-negative plasma assay. Systematic screening of the extended family of affected children is highly recommended because it allows the identification of genetically affected males so that they can be followed for the earliest signs of disease progression, and HSCT can be performed when it has the greatest chance of success.[62] It is particularly important that X-ALD be excluded, using plasma VLCFA assay, in all males presenting with Addison disease.[63]

The pathophysiology of X-ALD is poorly understood. It is unclear how ALDP deficiency leads to the accumulation of VLCFA and how the accumulation of VLCFA leads to clinical manifestations, particularly cerebral X-ALD. Cerebral X-ALD is an inflammatory disease and it is presumed that VLCFA-containing lipids, including CNS gangliosides, act as triggers for an autoimmune inflammatory response.[64] It is also unclear how HSCT corrects the inflammatory cerebral disease. There is no cross-correction of residual enzyme deficiency by secreted enzyme as in lysosomal storage disorders.

At least 4 patterns of clinical presentation can be seen in this illness, but only cerebral inflammatory disease is an indication to transplant.[65] However, it is important to recognize other presentations so that the index case and the wider family can be screened for the earliest evidence of cerebral disease. Factors that influence the clinical presentation are largely unknown, although gender plays a role because heterozygous females do not get CNS disease. Consequently, inflammatory brain disease in a female patient should lead to searching for homozygous mutations.[66] One kindred has been described in which disease always manifested as axonopathy and never as CNS disease.[67]

The 4 X-ALD clinical presentation patterns are:
1. Asymptomatic individual: mutation analysis or elevated plasma VLCFA within known X-ALD kindred.
2. Adrenal insufficiency: affects up to 70% of patients with genetic disease.
3. AMN: noninflammatory axonopathy presenting as progressive paraparesis in young adults, including heterozygous females.[68,69]
4. Cerebral disease: rapidly progressive, intensely inflammatory myelinopathy, which most commonly begins in the splenium of the corpus callosum and typically progresses to the parieto-occipital region.

Cerebral disease may manifest itself during childhood or adolescence. Approximately 40% of genetically affected boys develop childhood cerebral X-ALD. Many of the remainder develop AMN. In 20% of males with AMN, inflammatory brain disease occurs; females with AMN symptoms rarely have CNS disease. Cerebral disease is usually progressive, although clinical stabilization without HSCT can occur.[70,71] Disease progression results in severe disability, dementia, and death in a period of months to years.[72] HSCT is reserved for boys and men who have early yet definitive evidence of cerebral disease as determined by magnetic resonance imaging (MRI).[73] In individuals presenting with neurologic clinical signs, the rapidly progressive nature of the condition precludes a successful transplant outcome in most cases. The presence of brain MRI abnormalities and the presence or absence of enhancement with gadolinium has been shown to be of prognostic value. A 34-point MRI scoring system specific for X-ALD that was designed by Loes and colleagues[74,75] is now used worldwide for patient evaluation and treatment decisions. In patients with typical parietooccipital disease, a mathematical model with variables including age and lesion enhancement predicts progression in severity score, year by year, in untreated disease.

Unaffected boys undergo gadolinium-enhanced brain MRI scans at regular intervals to evaluate cerebral demyelination. An MRI severity score as low as 1 with gadolinium enhancement in a young boy is highly predictive of subsequent progressive demyelination and is an indication for transplant. However, the identification of an HSCT donor for asymptomatic boys should not await MRI anomalies, but be done immediately after diagnosis to prevent delays if a follow-up MRI indicates disease progression.

Review of the literature supports the following statements
1. Most boys have been transplanted from the best available donor using full intensity, chemotherapy-only preparative regimens.[19]
2. Most unrelated donors have been adult BM donors, but some CB donors have been used.[20]
3. Donor-derived engraftment rates seem higher than seen in patients transplanted for MPS IH syndrome (86% of 93 evaluable patients at a median follow-up of 11 months; 93% of related donor transplants; 80% of unrelated donor transplants).[15,19,23]
4. Outcome is affected by disease status, donor source, and HLA matching.[19] The commonest causes of death are progressive cerebral X-ALD disease and GVHD. Transplant-related mortality is approximately 10% in related donors and 18% in unrelated donors. Five-year survival rates for recipients of related donor and unrelated donor transplants have been reported at 64% and 53%, respectively.[19]
5. Survival is clearly affected by disease status at time of transplant as assessed by the number of neurologic deficits and the MRI severity score. In those with 0 or 1 neurologic deficit and MRI score of less than 9, the 5-year survival was 92%; in other patients it was 45%.[19]

The ability of HSCT to alter the natural history of cerebral X-ALD was seminally described by Shapiro and colleagues[76] in 12 boys who were at least 10 years post BMT. MRI abnormalities reversed completely in 2 boys, improved in 1 and were unchanged in 1. In the remaining 8 boys there was early progression and subsequent stabilization of MRI changes. Motor function remained normal or improved in 10, verbal intelligence remained within the normal range in 11 patients, and performance (nonverbal) abilities was improved or stable in 7 patients, and declined and then stabilized in 5. However, in boys with clinical illness and advanced MRI changes at the time of transplant, the disease-specific outcome has been poor, with many patients dying of progressive ALD.[74] For survivors, there are permanent, severe neurologic and neuropsychological sequelae, and life quality is compromised.

It is unclear whether successful transplant for cerebral X-ALD in early life alters the incidence of later AMN as insufficient time has elapsed to allow the survivors of HSCT to be fully assessed for AMN, the onset of which may be beyond the third decade of life. HSCT is not currently offered to asymptomatic boys as prophylaxis against future disease progression. In view of the natural history of the disease such a practice would mean that some boys would undergo HSCT (with its short-term mortality and long-term morbidity risks) who might otherwise have been healthy. There is no evidence yet that HSCT prevents the other neurologic manifestations of the disease. Boys who definitely need HSCT (as identified by MRI lesions) will have a good outcome from HSCT, and this observation underpins current HSCT practice. Recently, peri-transplant antioxidative therapy with N-acetyl-L-cysteine was reported to be protective against fulminant demyelination in advanced cerebral X-ALD. Its role is under continued investigation.[77]

HSCT has no effect on adrenal dysfunction. VLCFA levels decline but remain elevated above the normal range. Adrenal dysfunction may influence cerebral dysfunction and must be monitored closely and managed promptly. Adrenal crisis can precipitate a profound decline in CNS function in these boys, as can significant acute GVHD. Lorenzo's oil is a 4:1 mixture of glycerol trioleate and glyceryl trierucate that normalizes the elevated level of VLCFA. In boys in whom the VLCFA level is significantly lowered, Lorenzo's oil therapy seems to reduce the risk of neurologic progression and so reduce the need for HSCT.[78] However, for those with MRI imaging changes or clinical disease, it has no influence on disease progression. It is therefore of limited interest or relevance to the HSCT team. It may cause thrombocytopenia. In some institutions, Lorenzo's oil is given in the weeks before HSCT to normalize VLCFA, but this is not universal practice and there is no evidence that it is beneficial to HSCT outcomes.

GLD

GLD or Krabbe disease is an autosomal recessive lysosomal storage disorder caused by deficiency of galactocerebrosidase (GALC), an enzyme responsible for degrading β-galactocerebroside, a major component of myelin sheath.[79] GALC deficiency causes defective and decreased myelination and inflammation in the CNS and peripheral nervous system (PNS) from catabolic derivatives of β-galactocerebroside such as psychosine. These changes lead to progressive deterioration in neurologic and cognitive function, resulting in spasticity, mental deterioration, blindness, deafness, seizures, and early death.[79] Prenatal diagnosis is possible by analysis of the gene defect on chromosome 14q31. In the most severe "early-onset or infantile or classic" form, which has an estimated incidence of 1 in 70,000 to 100,000 births, children develop symptoms before 6 months of age and usually do not survive beyond 2 years.[79] In the "late-onset" form, symptoms appear in early to late childhood but only a few children survive into teenage years. Rare cases of "adult-onset" disease have been described. Data on genotype-phenotype correlation are limited and are not likely to help with pretransplant risk assessment.

HSCT is the only available therapy with potential to improve neurocognitive function, increase survival and alter the natural history of the disease. In a 1998 report, Krivit and colleagues[12] described the use of allogeneic HSCT to treat 5 children with GLD. Four of the children received marrow from an HLA-identical sibling and 1 was treated with unrelated CBT from 1 HLA-DR mismatch donor. Two children with late-onset GLD who had substantial neurologic disability, including ataxia, tremors, motor incoordination, and gait dysfunction, showed resolution of their symptoms. Cognition, language, and memory continued to develop normally in 3 children with late-onset disease. Most children had improvement in MRI, cerebrospinal fluid (CSF) protein levels, and all had normalization of enzyme activity. These findings supported the hypothesis that alloge-neic HSCT can be effective in children with GLD. However, many children lack a matched related BM donor, and a suitable unrelated adult donor may not be available in sufficient time for the treatment of rapidly progressive disorders. Publicly banked unrelated donor CB is readily available and can be procured quickly.

In 2005, Escolar and colleagues[21] reported on the safety and efficacy of CBT for the treatment of 25 children with the "infantile or classic" variety of Krabbe disease. Family history in 11 patients led to confirmation of diagnosis in the prenatal or neonatal period. They were transplanted at a median age of 28 days. The remaining 14 children who were the first cases in the family were diagnosed between 4 and 9 months of age and were symptomatic when transplanted at a median age of 7.7 months. All patients received BU, CY, and antithymocyte globulin for conditioning and cyclosporine and steroids for GVHD prophylaxis. All except 1 CB unit were mismatched for either 1 or 2 antigens. The units were tested for GALC activity, and the unit with higher activity was selected. After CBT, all 11 neonates but only 6 of 14 symptomatic infants were surviving at a median of 36 and 41 months, respectively. Survival among neonates was better than either untreated controls ($P = .001$) or symptomatic infants ($P = .01$). In the symptomatic group, 4 infants died of progressive disease. All survivors had normalization of GALC level, high levels of donor chimerism, and low incidence of GVHD. Brain MRI scans after CBT showed normal progression of myelination, with age-appropriate changes in signal intensity in various white-matter sites in all 11 neonates. Improvements were seen in signal intensity in 4 babies who had abnormal hyperintense paraventricular signal consistent with dysmyelination. In contrast, post-CBT MRI scans showed disease progression in 12 of 14 symptomatic patients. Similarly, asymptomatic neonates had better outcomes in visual evoked responses, auditory evoked responses, nerve conduction studies, and electroencephalogram. Clinical seizures developed in all symptomatic but in none of the asymptomatic neonates. Thus, patients who underwent CBT as neonates had neurologic benefits and developmental gains, including preservation of vision, hearing, and cognitive abilities. Deficits in gross motor function became apparent in all children. The report confirmed the clinical usefulness of unrelated donor CBT in neonates with Krabbe disease and showed benefits and low morbidity associated with early intervention. These observations were further substantiated in a series with more patients and longer follow-up.[25]

A clinical staging system based on signs and symptoms of disease was developed and validated for 42 children with infantile Krabbe disease to predict outcomes after CBT and to guide physicians in evaluating, monitoring, and counseling families about treatment outcomes.[80] To identify affected children early, New York State began screening all newborns for Krabbe disease in August 2006 by a rapid and accurate assay of GALC activity.[81] In addition, DNA mutation analysis techniques, standardized clinical evaluation protocol, criteria for CBT for the early infantile phenotype, a clinical registry, and an outcome database were developed.[81] These efforts coupled with studies aimed at decreasing the short-term and long-term complications of CBT may improve outcomes.

MLD

MLD is an autosomal recessive lysosomal disorder arising from deficiency of arylsulfatase A (ARSA) enzyme activity and characterized by increased urinary sulfatides. Documentation of increased sulfatides is of critical importance to confirm the diagnosis because the ARSA pseudodeficiency allele is common in the general population.

Deficiency in ARSA results in defective desulfation of sulfated glycolipids present in myelin sheaths of the CNS and PNS, and to a lesser extent in visceral organs (kidney, gallbladder, liver). Lysosomal accumulation occurs that manifests as metachromatic staining. Deficiency in saposin B can cause MLD also. Furthermore, multiple sulfatase deficiency (MSD) has an overlapping clinical picture with signs of MLD, signs of mucopolysaccharidosis, and icthyosis. Saposin B deficiency and MSD share with MLD: increased CSF protein, slowed nerve conduction velocity (NCV), and increased urinary sulfatides.

The clinical phenotype is a broad continuous spectrum ranging from early-infantile MLD to adult-onset forms. The late-infantile form (onset 0.5–4 years) presents generally in the first or second year of life as a result of loss of motor milestones, including gait disturbance, abnormal speech, loss of neurocognitive skills, optic atrophy, progressive spastic quadriparesis, increased CSF protein, and slowed NCV, culminating in dementia and death within several years. The early-juvenile form (onset 4–6 years) shows gait and postural abnormalities, emotional and behavioral disturbances, optic atrophy, progressive spastic quadriparesis, increased CSF protein, and slowed NCV. The late-juvenile form (onset 6–16 years) exhibits behavioral abnormalities, poor school performance, language regression, gait disturbance, slowly progressive tetraparesis, increased CSF protein, and slowed NCV. The adult form (onset more than 16 years of age) is characterized by mental regression, psychiatric symptoms, incontinence, slowly progressive spastic tetraparesis, normal or increased CSF protein, and normal or slowed NCV.

The first BMT for MLD was performed more than 20 years ago. According to the EBMT and CIBMTR registries, more than 100 transplants have since been performed for this disorder. Despite this number, the lack of graft-outcome and long-term follow-up studies makes it difficult to draw firm conclusions regarding the efficacy of HSCT in MLD. In addition, data (mostly from the last century) suggest that outcomes are less promising than those for MPS IH. Based on these reports and personal communications, all patients transplanted for symptomatic late-infantile MLD seem to have performed poorly in all aspects. Presymptomatic late-infantile MLD patients also seem to perform poorly despite successful HSCT. In late-onset juvenile MLD and perhaps more clearly in adult-onset MLD, CNS disease following HSCT stabilized, although the effect on the PNS has been uncertain.[13,82–89] These results derive from the pioneering years of HSCT in IMD when a significant proportion of children were transplanted at an older age with advanced, irreversible disease. In addition, outdated transplant techniques and the use of carrier donors and mixed chimerism leading to lower enzyme levels may have affected outcomes.

The use of CB grafts (associated with full-donor chimerism and normal enzyme levels) and the development of standardized protocols (eg, HSCT for MPS IH) may result in improved outcomes for MLD. Current preferred practice for HSCT in MLD is to perform transplants only on presymptomatic (or minimally affected older) individuals. At University Medical Center Utrecht (Dr J. Boelens, personal communication, 2009), HSCT was performed in 5 MLD patients (2 early-juvenile, 1 late-juvenile, and 2 adult onset, with 3 asymptomatic and 2 minimally affected) in the past 6 years. All have survived and none has shown disease progression. In a Duke University study, 5-year overall survival in 15 mainly symptomatic MLD patients undergoing unrelated CBT was 58%.[25] Those patients transplanted with advanced disease had worse outcomes. Long-term follow-up and multicenter studies on the efficacy of HSCT for MLD since 2000 are needed.

Recently, an ERT trial for MLD was initiated to examine its effect on the PNS. ERT is not expected to ameliorate CNS disease because of its inability to cross the BBB. The

San Raffaele Institute in Milan is currently developing an MLD gene-therapy trial for patients up to 18 years of age. Use of mesenchymal stromal stem cells (MSC) to correct residual deficits such as PNS abnormalities was investigated by Koç and colleagues,[90] but no clinical improvement was seen, likely because of the inability to obtain sustained engraftment of donor MSC in the PNS.

Outcomes of HSCT for MLD are variable and unclear because no large series have been performed in the last decade. Even after more than 20 years of HSCT for MLD, it is not clear if MLD patients, or which phenotype, might benefit from HSCT. For presymptomatic juvenile- and adult-onset patients there is positive evidence. Improved transplantation techniques and the prompt availability of CB grafts may positively influence long-term outcomes. An international registry would facilitate comparative evaluation of therapeutic options, leading to improved guidelines.

MISCELLANEOUS DISORDERS

In contrast to MPS IH, MPS VI, ALD, GLD, and MLD, other mucopolysaccharidoses, leukodystrophies, and related enzyme deficiencies have a much less uniform treatment history.[91] For example, Wolman disease, caused by deficiency of acid lipase, does respond to early HSCT, and up to 11 years' experience with favorable outcome has been described.[92] This study has shown that lasting correction of hepatic function, normal adrenal function, and normal neurologic outcome are possible after HSCT. Similarly, in α-mannosidosis, stabilization of neurocognitive variables and possibly musculoskeletal features has been observed.[93]

On the other hand, several diseases characterized by GAG accumulation, such as MPS II, MPS III, MPS IV (Morquio syndrome), and MPS VII (Sly syndrome) have all been shown to respond only partially or not at all to HSCT.[52,94,95] The natural history of I-cell disease (mucolipidosis II, deficiency in GlcNAc-I phosphotransferase) can be altered by HSCT, yet significant improvement after HSCT has been rare.[96] Equally disappointing are responses to cellular therapy in GM gangliosidoses (Tay-Sachs disease, Sandhoff disease, and GM1 gangliosidosis), acid-sphingomyelinase-deficient Niemann-Pick disease and in the neuronal ceroid lipofuscinoses.[97–99] There may be some beneficial effect of HSCT when it is performed in a timely and appropriate manner for individuals with the juvenile forms of GM gangliosidoses and possibly Niemann-Pick disease (types B and C2). In the United Kingdom and the Netherlands, these children, and pre- and asymptomatic children with MPS II and MPS III, are receiving CBT. Publication of the outcomes of these experimental procedures will be informative.

Gaucher disease is a glycoprotein metabolic disorder caused by deficient activity of the lysosomal enzyme glucocerebrosidase. It is most common in the Ashkenazi Jewish population. The clinical spectrum includes 3 phenotypes: type 1, nonneuronopathic; type 2, acute neuronopathic; and type 3, subacute neuronopathic. Allogeneic HSCT is effective in treating patients with severe type 1 disease[100,101]; however, most patients in this phenotype group receive ERT.[102] A small subgroup of patients (ie, Norrbottnian) with type 3 disease have been successfully treated by HSCT[103,104] and to a limited extent with ERT.[105]

Despite enormous biochemical variation, the common feature of these neuronopathic metabolic disorders is their progressive nature. Therefore, the ideal time for therapeutic intervention is early in life before damage from substrate accumulation becomes severe and irreversible. Current or planned neonatal screening programs have the potential to change the outcomes for diseases amendable to HSCT or other interventions, such as substrate inhibition, ERT, chaperone therapy, or anti-inflammatory therapy. In addition, conducting clinical trials of novel therapies with well-defined controls and functional end points is necessary for meaningful therapeutic advance. Synthesis of available evidence on successfully and unsuccessfully treated enzymopathies suggests that novel therapeutic approaches with cellular and gene therapy are needed.

NEW DIRECTIONS

An obvious first approach is targeting of the genetic lesion in IMD by gene therapy.[106] There are 2 mechanisms whereby gene therapy can occur. The first is gene replacement, in which a gene of interest is inserted randomly in the genome of the recipient. This procedure results in predictable complications such as dysregulation of the delivered gene at the new genomic site, and a disruption of the gene that is located in the region of insertion. The second mechanism of gene therapy is gene correction, which depends on a process called homologous recombination, whereby the faulty gene is corrected at its original locus. In this way, gene regulation remains intact and no other genomic region is affected by the gene therapy intervention. However, clinically available approaches to accomplish this are not yet available. In the last decade, retroviral, lentiviral, and adenoviral vectors have been shown to be effective in many animal models of human lysosomal storage disease.[107–111] However, it remains unclear whether these observations can be translated into clinical benefits. Two recent gene-therapy trials have focused on MPS VII and X-ALD, but no published data are available. Optimism must be tempered by the development of complications in the first gene-therapy trials, such as insertional mutagenesis leading to development of leukemia in several patients with immune deficiencies.[112] Nevertheless, it remains possible that gene therapy will ultimately offer safer and more effective treatment of IMD.

Equally logical are attempts to improve cellular therapy (the prototype being HSCT, which has benefited patients with selected IMD for several decades). The primary unanswered question is why cross-correction is not equally effective across all IMD. It is possible that cell requirements for sufficient enzyme cross-correction differ for each enzyme and, perhaps, vary from tissue to tissue. Uneven availability of individual enzymes from donor-derived cells may also be contributory. The BBB is an insurmountable hurdle for enzymes elaborated by donor hematopoietic cells.[113] In contrast, some cells, most notably monocytic precursors of microglia, can cross the BBB. This cell-specific brain-specific engraftment can complement, at least partially, some neuronopathic enzymopathies.[5]

An alternative cellular vector could be mesenchymal stromal cells (MSCs). Although the identity and function of MSCs in vivo remains to be elucidated, MSCs can be easily isolated from BM.[114] MSCs have a remarkable capacity to secrete large quantities of proteins, including lysosomal enzymes and to expand rapidly in vitro. Furthermore, their additional functional properties can treat patients with IMD in a disease-specific fashion[90] and patients with GVHD and graft failure.

MSCs are immune modulatory cells that do not elicit alloreactive lymphocyte proliferative response.[115] In that capacity, they are capable of treating GVHD that is resistant to standard therapy.[116] As this form of GVHD is almost uniformly lethal, it is encouraging that a significant number of patients have responded to MSC therapy. In addition, MSCs are closely and functionally associated with blood-forming cells in the BM hematopoietic stem cell niche. In the clinical setting, MSCs enhance engraftment in haploidentical HSCT,[24] which is relevant because graft failure has been a significant obstacle in HSCT for nonmalignant diseases including IMD.

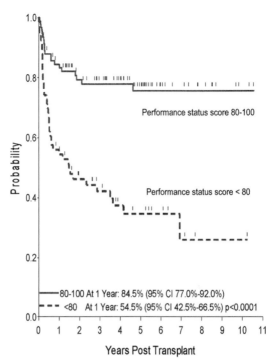

Fig. 2. Probability of overall survival (OS): effect of performance status at transplant. OS following unrelated CBT in 159 patients with IMD treated at Duke University Medical Center and followed in the long-term. Statistically higher (*P*<.0001) survival was seen in patients with a Lansky or Karnofsky score of 80 to 100 at transplant compared with those with less than 80. In patients with high performance status (80–100), the OS at 6 months, 1, 3, and 5 years was 88.4% (95% confidence interval [CI] 79.6%–97.1%), 84.5% (95% CI 77.0%–92.0%), 77.9% (95% CI 69.1%–86.8%), and 75.7% (95% CI 66.1%–85.3%), respectively. These observations reflect survival outcome advantage of transplantation early in the clinical course of disease. (*From* Prasad VK, Mendizabal A, Parikh SH, et al. Unrelated donor umbilical cord blood for inherited metabolic disorders in 159 pediatric patients from a single center: influence of cellular composition of the graft on transplantation outcomes. Blood 2008;112:2982. © American Society of Hematology; with permission.)

Gene and stem-cell therapy can be combined into 1 complementary intervention: stem-cell gene therapy. According to this theoretic concept, autologous gene-corrected hematopoietic or nonhematopoietic stem and progenitor cells would be infused into an enzyme-deficient patient to allow cross-correction with diminished side effects because of the transplantation of autologous rather than allogeneic cells. Safety concerns, including tumorigenesis caused by pluripotency of the cellular vectors or off-target genomic toxicity,[16,25] must be addressed.

Gene therapy, stem-cell therapy, and stem-cell gene therapy are powerful tools that may, in the future, improve care for patients with enzyme deficiencies. Through novel concepts, laboratory experiments, and collaborative clinical trials, care for these patients can be transformed.

SUMMARY

During 3 decades of HSCT for IMD, important lessons have been learned about transplant- and disease-specific factors that affect engraftment, survival, and long-term outcomes. Children with MPS IH have benefited from many advances, including the development of guidelines used worldwide for their evaluation and treatment. The importance of early diagnosis and prompt HSCT for patients with excellent performance scores (ie, 80–100 Karnofsky or Lansky) is clearly documented (**Fig. 2**). Efforts aimed at early diagnosis and treatment have favorably affected all children with IMD, particularly those with cerebral X-ALD, leading to prevention of devastating neurocognitive and neuropsychological sequelae. Developments in newborn screening and therapy will facilitate early diagnosis and direct greater attention to genotype/phenotype correlation.

Twenty years of collaborative international studies have greatly advanced understanding of the benefits and limitations of CBT. Neonatal CBT has led to long-term survival for infants with GLD, but patients with MLD still experience progressive PNS deterioration. CB must be critically examined as a graft source for challenging disorders such as Hunter, Sanfilippo, and Maroteaux-Lamy syndromes, and the gangliosidoses. Similarly, ERT has been found to complement and in some cases supplant HSCT.

The rare nature of these disorders requires a collaborative, multicenter, international, and interdisciplinary research approach. Unrestricted international registries are critical to advancement of the subject in a coordinated and systematic manner. Collaborative longitudinal studies can provide a better understanding of not only survival but also functional ability and quality of life after HSCT.

REFERENCES

1. Fratantoni JC, Hall CW, Neufeld EF. The defect in Hurler and Hunter syndromes. II. Deficiency of specific factors involved in mucopolysaccharide degradation. Proc Natl Acad Sci U S A 1969;64:360–6.
2. Neufeld EF. Lysosomal storage diseases. Annu Rev Biochem 1991;60:257–80.
3. Pfeffer SR. Targeting of proteins to the lysosome. Curr Top Microbiol Immunol 1991;170:43–65.
4. Perry VH, Gordon S. Macrophages and the nervous system. Int Rev Cytol 1991; 125:203–44.
5. Krivit W, Sung JH, Shapiro EG, et al. Microglia: the effector cell for reconstitution of the central nervous system following bone marrow transplantation for lysosomal and peroxisomal storage diseases. Cell Transplant 1995;4:385–92.
6. Giulian D. Ameboid microglia as effectors of inflammation in the central nervous system. J Neurosci Res 1987;18:155–71.
7. Hickey WF. Migration of hematogenous cells through the blood-brain barrier and the initiation of CNS inflammation. Brain Pathol 1991;1:97–105.
8. Kennedy DW, Abkowitz JL. Kinetics of central nervous system microglial and macrophage engraftment: analysis using a transgenic bone marrow transplantation model. Blood 1997;90:986–93.
9. Hobbs JR, Hugh-Jones K, Barrett AJ, et al. Reversal of clinical features of Hurler's disease and biochemical improvement after treatment by bone-marrow transplantation. Lancet 1981;2(8249):709–12.
10. Krivit W, Pierpont ME, Ayaz K, et al. Bone-marrow transplantation in the Maroteaux-Lamy syndrome (mucopolysaccharidosis type VI). N Engl J Med 1984;311:1606–11.
11. Aubourg P, Blanche, Jambaque I, et al. Reversal of early neurologic and neuroradiologic manifestations of X-linked adrenoleukodystrophy by bone marrow transplantation. N Engl J Med 1990;322:1860–6.

12. Krivit W, Shapiro E, Peters C, et al. Hematopoietic stem-cell transplantation in globoid-cell leukodystrophy. N Engl J Med 1998;338:1119–26.
13. Krivit W, Shapiro E, Kennedy W, et al. Treatment of late-infantile metachromatic leukodystrophy by bone marrow transplantation. N Engl J Med 1990;322:28–32.
14. Vellodi A, Young E, Cooper A, et al. Bone marrow transplantation for mucopolysaccharidosis type I: experience of two British centres. Arch Dis Child 1997;76:92–9.
15. Peters C, Shapiro EG, Anderson J, et al. Hurler syndrome. II. Outcome of HLA-genotypically identical sibling and HLA-haploidentical related donor bone marrow transplantation in fifty-four children. The Storage Disease Collaborative Study Group. Blood 1998;91:2601–8.
16. Staba SL, Escolar ML, Poe M, et al. Cord-blood transplants from unrelated donors in patients with Hurler's syndrome. N Engl J Med 2004;350:1960–9.
17. Boelens JJ, Wynn RF, O'Meara A, et al. Outcomes of hematopoietic stem cell transplantation for Hurler's syndrome in Europe: a risk factor analysis for graft failure. Bone Marrow Transplant 2007;40:225–33.
18. Boelens JJ, Rocha V, Aldenhoven M, et al. EUROCORD, Inborn Error Working Party of EBMT and Duke University. Risk factor analysis of outcomes after unrelated cord blood transplantation in patients with Hurler syndrome. Biol Blood Marrow Transplant 2009;15:618–25.
19. Peters C, Charnas LR, Tan Y, et al. Cerebral X-linked adrenoleukodystrophy: the international hematopoietic cell transplantation experience from 1982 to 1999. Blood 2004;104:881–8.
20. Beam D, Poe MD, Provenzale JM, et al. Outcomes of unrelated umbilical cord blood transplantation for X-linked adrenoleukodystrophy. Biol Blood Marrow Transplant 2007;13:665–74.
21. Escolar ML, Poe MD, Provenzale JM, et al. Transplantation of umbilical-cord-blood in babies with infantile Krabbe's disease. N Engl J Med 2005;352:2069–81.
22. Grigull L, Beilken A, Schrappe M, et al. Transplantation of allogeneic CD34-selected stem cells after fludarabine-based conditioning regimen for children with mucopolysaccharidosis IH (M. Hurler). Bone Marrow Transplant 2005;35:265–9.
23. Peters C, Balthazor M, Shapiro EG, et al. Outcome of unrelated donor bone marrow transplantation in 40 children with Hurler syndrome. Blood 1996;87:4894–902.
24. Prasad VK, Kurtzberg J. Emerging trends in transplantation of inherited metabolic diseases. Bone Marrow Transplant 2008;41(2):99–108.
25. Prasad VK, Mendizabal A, Parikh SH, et al. Unrelated donor umbilical cord blood for inherited metabolic disorders in 159 pediatric patients from a single center: influence of cellular composition of the graft on transplantation outcomes. Blood 2008;112:2979–89.
26. Grewal SS, Wynn R, Abdenur JE, et al. Safety and efficacy of enzyme replacement therapy in combination with hematopoietic stem cell transplantation in Hurler syndrome. Genet Med 2005;7:143–6.
27. Cox-Brinkman J, Boelens JJ, Wraith JE, et al. Hematopoietic cell transplantation (HCT) in combination with enzyme replacement therapy (ERT) in patients with Hurler syndrome. Bone Marrow Transplant 2006;38:17–21.
28. Tolar J, Grewal SS, Bjoraker KJ, et al. Combination of enzyme replacement and hematopoietic stem cell transplantation as therapy for Hurler syndrome. Bone Marrow Transplant 2008;41(6):531–5.

29. Wynn RF, Mercer J, Page J, et al. Use of enzyme replacement therapy (Laronidase) before hematopoietic stem cell transplantation for mucopolysaccharidosis I: experience in 18 patients. J Pediatr 2009;154(1):135–9.

30. Peters C. Hematopoietic cell transplantation for storage diseases. In: Appelbaum FR, Forman SJ, Negrin RS, et al, editors. Thomas' hematopoietic cell transplantation. 4th edition. Hoboken (NJ): Wiley-Blackwell; 2009. p. 1136–62.

31. Neufeld EF, Muenzer J. The Mucopolysaccharidosis. In: Scriver C, Beaudet A, Sly W, et al, editors. The metabolic and molecular basis of inherited disease. 8th edition. New York: McGraw-Hill; 2001. p. 3421–52.

32. Aldenhoven M, Boelens JJ, de Koning TJ. The clinical outcome of Hurler syndrome after stem cell transplantation. Biol Blood Marrow Transplant 2008; 14(5):485–98.

33. Boelens JJ. Trends in haematopoietic cell transplantation for inborn errors of metabolism. J Inherit Metab Dis 2006;29(2–3):413–20.

34. Kurtzberg J, Laughlin M, Graham ML, et al. Placental blood as a source of hematopoietic stem cells for transplantation into unrelated recipients. N Engl J Med 1996;335(3):157–66.

35. Chen N, Hudson JE, Walczak P, et al. Human umbilical cord blood progenitors: the potential of these hematopoietic cells to become neural. Stem Cells 2005; 23(10):1560–70.

36. Kogler G, Sensken S, Airey JA, et al. A new human somatic stem cell from placental cord blood with intrinsic pluripotent differentiation potential. J Exp Med 2004;200(2):123–35.

37. Meier C, Middelanis J, Wasielewski B, et al. Spastic paresis after perinatal brain damage in rats is reduced by human cord blood mononuclear cells. Pediatr Res 2006;9(2):244–9.

38. Church H, Tylee K, Cooper A, et al. Biochemical monitoring after haemopoietic stem cell transplant for Hurler syndrome (MPSIH): implications for functional outcome after transplant in metabolic disease. Bone Marrow Transplant 2007; 39(4):207–10.

39. Martin PL, Carter SL, Kernan NA, et al. Results of the cord blood transplantation study (COBLT): outcomes of unrelated donor umbilical cord blood transplantation in pediatric patients with lysosomal and peroxisomal storage diseases. Biol Blood Marrow Transplant 2006;12(2):184–94.

40. Stein J, Zion GB, Dror Y, et al. Successful treatment of Wolman disease by unrelated umbilical cord blood transplantation. Eur J Pediatr 2007;166(7):663–6.

41. Baxter MA, Wynn RF, Schyma L, et al. Marrow stromal cells from patients affected by MPS I differentially support haematopoietic progenitor cell development. J Inherit Metab Dis 2005;28(6):1045–53.

42. Kakkis ED, Muenzer J, Tiller GE, et al. Enzyme-replacement therapy in mucopolysaccharidosis I. N Engl J Med 2001;344(3):182–8.

43. Wraith JE. The first 5 years of clinical experience with laronidase enzyme replacement therapy for mucopolysaccharidosis I. Expert Opin Pharmacother 2005;6(3):489–506.

44. Cimaz R, Vijay S, Haase C, et al. Attenuated type I mucopolysaccharidosis in the differential diagnosis of juvenile idiopathic arthritis: a series of 13 patients with Scheie syndrome. Clin Exp Rheumatol 2006;24(2):196–202.

45. Wraith JE, Beck M, Lane R, et al. Enzyme replacement therapy in patients who have mucopolysaccharidosis I and are younger than 5 years: results of

a multinational study of recombinant human alpha-L-iduronidase (laronidase). Pediatrics 2007;120(1):e37–46.

46. Aldenhoven M, Sakkers R, Boelens J, et al. The musculoskeletal manifestations of lysosomal storage disorders. Ann Rheum Dis 2009;68:1659–65.

47. Manger B, Mengel E, Schaefer RM. Rheumatologic aspects of lysosomal storage diseases. Clin Rheumatol 2007;26(3):335–44.

48. Bergstrom SK, Quinn JJ, Greenstein R, et al. Long-term follow-up of a patient transplanted for Hunter's disease type IIB: a case report and literature review. Bone Marrow Transplant 1994;14(4):653–8.

49. Coppa GV, Gabrielli O, Zampini L, et al. Bone marrow transplantation in Hunter syndrome (mucopolysaccharidosis type II): 2-year follow-up of the first Italian patient and review of the literature. Pediatr Med Chir 1995;17(3): 227–35.

50. Guffon N, Bertrand Y, Forest I, et al. Bone marrow transplantation in children with Hunter syndrome: outcome after 7 to 17 years. J Pediatr 2009;154(5):733–7.

51. Li P, Thompson JN, Hug G, et al. Biochemical and molecular analysis in a patient with the severe form of Hunter syndrome after bone marrow transplantation. Am J Med Genet 1996;64(4):531–5.

52. Peters C, Krivit W. Hematopoietic cell transplantation for mucopolysaccharidosis IIB (Hunter syndrome). Bone Marrow Transplant 2000;25(10):1097–9.

53. Vellodi A, Young E, Cooper A, et al. Long-term follow-up following bone marrow transplantation for Hunter disease. J Inherit Metab Dis 1999;22(5):638–48.

54. Mullen CA, Thompson JN, Richard LA, et al. Unrelated umbilical cord blood transplantation in infancy for mucopolysaccharidosis type IIB (Hunter syndrome) complicated by autoimmune hemolytic anemia. Bone Marrow Transplant 2000;25(10):1093–7.

55. Gungor N, Tuncbilek E. Sanfilippo disease type B. A case report and review of the literature on recent advances in bone marrow transplantation. Turk J Pediatr 1995;37(2):157–63.

56. Vellodi A, Young E, New M, et al. Bone marrow transplantation for Sanfilippo disease type B. J Inherit Metab Dis 1992;15(6):911–8.

57. Herskhovitz E, Young E, Rainer J, et al. Bone marrow transplantation for Maroteaux-Lamy syndrome (MPS VI): long-term follow-up. J Inherit Metab Dis 1999;22(1):50–62.

58. Lee V, Li CK, Shing MM, et al. Umbilical cord blood transplantation for Maroteaux-Lamy syndrome (mucopolysaccharidosis type VI). Bone Marrow Transplant 2000;26(4):455–8.

59. Mosser J, Douar AM, Sarde CO, et al. Putative X-linked adrenoleukodystrophy gene shares unexpected homology with ABC transporters. Nature 1993;361: 726–30.

60. Boehm CD, Cutting GR, Lachtermacher MB, et al. Accurate DNA-based diagnostic and carrier testing for X-linked adrenoleukodystrophy. Mol Genet Metab 1999;66:128–36.

61. Moser AB, Kreiter N, Bezman L, et al. Plasma very long chain fatty acids in 3,000 peroxisome disease patients and 29,000 controls. Ann Neurol 1999;45: 100–10.

62. Bezman L, Moser AB, Raymond GV, et al. Adrenoleukodystrophy: incidence, new mutation rate, and results of extended family screening. Ann Neurol 2001;49:512–7.

63. Aubourg P, Chaussain JL. Adrenoleukodystrophy: the most frequent genetic cause of Addison's disease. Horm Res 2003;59(Suppl 1):104–5.

64. Ito M, Blumberg BM, Mock DJ, et al. Potential environmental and host participants in the early white matter lesion of adreno-leukodystrophy: morphologic evidence for CD8 cytotoxic T cells, cytolysis of oligodendrocytes, and CD1-mediated lipid antigen presentation. J Neuropathol Exp Neurol 2001;60: 1004–119.

65. Moser HW. Adrenoleukodystrophy: phenotype, genetics, pathogenesis and therapy. Brain 1997;120(Pt 8):1485–508.

66. Hershkovitz E, Narkis G, Shorer Z, et al. Cerebral X-linked adrenoleukodystrophy in a girl with Xq27-Ter deletion. Ann Neurol 2002;52:234–7.

67. O'Neill GN, Aoki M, Brown RH Jr. ABCD1 translation-initiator mutation demonstrates genotype-phenotype correlation for AMN. Neurology 2001;57: 1956–62.

68. Powers JM, DeCiero DP, Cox C, et al. The dorsal root ganglia in adrenomyeloneuropathy: neuronal atrophy and abnormal mitochondria. J Neuropathol Exp Neurol 2001;60:493–501.

69. Powers JM, DeCiero DP, Ito M, et al. Adrenomyeloneuropathy: a neuropathologic review featuring its noninflammatory myelopathy. J Neuropathol Exp Neurol 2000;59:89–102.

70. Moser HW, Bergin A, Naidu S, et al. Adrenoleukodystrophy. Endocrinol Metab Clin North Am 1991;20:297–318.

71. Moser HW, Naidu S, Kumar AJ, et al. The adrenoleukodystrophies. Crit Rev Neurobiol 1987;3:29–88.

72. Moser H SK, Watkins P, Powers J, et al. X-linked adrenoleukodystrophy. In: Scriver C, Beaudet B, Sly W, et al, editors. The metabolic and molecular basis of inherited disease. 8th edition. New York: McGraw-Hill; 2001. p. 3257.

73. Peters C, Steward CG. Hematopoietic cell transplantation for inherited metabolic diseases: an overview of outcomes and practice guidelines. Bone Marrow Transplant 2003;31:229–39.

74. Loes DJ, Fatemi A, Melhem ER, et al. Analysis of MRI patterns aids prediction of progression in X-linked adrenoleukodystrophy. Neurology 2003;61:369–74.

75. Loes DJ, Hite S, Moser H, et al. Adrenoleukodystrophy: a scoring method for brain MR observations. AJNR Am J Neuroradiol 1994;15:1761–6.

76. Shapiro E, Krivit W, Lockman L, et al. Long-term effect of bone-marrow transplantation for childhood-onset cerebral X-linked adrenoleukodystrophy. Lancet 2000;356:713–8.

77. Tolar J, Orchard P, Bjoraker K, et al. N-acetyl-L-cysteine improves outcome of advanced adrenoleukodystrophy. Bone Marrow Transplant 2007;39(4):211–5.

78. Moser HW, Raymond GV, Koehler W, et al. Evaluation of the preventive effect of glyceryl trioleate-trierucate ("Lorenzo's oil") therapy in X-linked adrenoleukodystrophy: results of two concurrent trials. Adv Exp Med Biol 2003;544: 369–87.

79. Wenger DA, Suzuki K, Suzuki Y, et al. Galactosylceramide lipidosis: globoid-cell leukodystrophy (Krabbe disease). In: Scriver CR, Beaudet AL, Sly WS, et al, editors. The metabolic and molecular bases of inherited disease. 8th edition. New York: McGraw-Hill; 2001. p. 3669–94.

80. Escolar ML, Poe MD, Martin HR, et al. A staging system for infantile Krabbe disease to predict outcome after unrelated umbilical cord blood transplantation. Pediatrics 2006;118(3):e879–89.

81. Duffner PK, Caggana M, Orsini JJ, et al. Newborn screening for Krabbe disease: the New York State model [comment]. Pediatr Neurol 2009;40(4): 245–52.

82. Stillman AE, Krivit W, Shapiro EG, et al. Serial MR after bone marrow transplantation in two patients with metachromatic leukodystrophy. AJNR Am J Neuroradiol 1994;15:1929–32.
83. Shapiro EG, Lipton ME, Krivit W. White matter dysfunction and its neuropsychological correlates: a longitudinal study of a case of metachromatic leukodystrophy treated with bone marrow transplant. J Clin Exp Neuropsychol 1992; 14:610–24.
84. Pridjian G, Humbert J, Willis J, et al. Pre-symptomatic late-infantile metachromatic leukodystrophy treated with bone marrow transplantation. J Pediatr 1994;125:755–8.
85. Guffon N, Souillet G, Maire I, et al. Juvenile metachromatic leukodystrophy: neurological outcome two years after bone marrow transplantation. J Inherit Metab Dis 1995;18:159–61.
86. Shapiro EG, Lockman LA, Knopman D, et al. Characteristics of the dementia in late-onset metachromatic leukodystrophy. Neurology 1994;44:662–5.
87. Navarro C, Fernandez JM, Dominguez C, et al. Late juvenile metachromatic leukodystrophy treated with bone marrow transplantation: a 4-year follow-up study. Neurology 1996;46:254–6.
88. Kapaun P, Dittmann RW, Granitzny B, et al. Slow progression of juvenile metachromatic leukodystrophy 6 years after bone marrow transplantation. J Child Neurol 1999;14:222–8.
89. Malm G, Ringdén O, Winiarski J, et al. Clinical outcome in four children with metachromatic leukodystrophy treated by bone marrow transplantation. Bone Marrow Transplant 1996;17(6):1003–8.
90. Koç ON, Day J, Nieder M, et al. Allogeneic mesenchymal stem cell infusion for treatment of metachromatic leukodystrophy (MLD) and Hurler syndrome (MPS-IH). Bone Marrow Transplant 2002;30(4):215–22.
91. Orchard PJ, Blazar BR, Wagner J, et al. Hematopoietic cell therapy for metabolic disease. J Pediatr 2007;151:340–6.
92. Tolar J, Petryk A, Khan K, et al. Long-term metabolic, endocrine, and neuropsychological outcome of hematopoietic cell transplantation for Wolman disease. Bone Marrow Transplant 2009;43:21–7.
93. Grewal SS, Shapiro EG, Krivit W, et al. Effective treatment of alpha-mannosidosis by allogeneic hematopoietic stem cell transplantation. J Pediatr 2004;144: 569–73.
94. Yamada Y, Kato K, Sukegawa K, et al. Treatment of MPS VII (Sly disease) by allogeneic BMT in a female with homozygous A619V mutation. Bone Marrow Transplant 1998;21:629–34.
95. Klein KA, Krivit W, Whitley CB, et al. Poor cognitive outcome of eleven children with Sanfilippo syndrome after bone marrow transplantation and successful engraftment. Bone Marrow Transplant 1995;15:S176–81.
96. Grewal S, Shapiro E, Braunlin E, et al. Continued neurocognitive development and prevention of cardiopulmonary complications after successful BMT for I-cell disease: a long-term follow-up report. Bone Marrow Transplant 2003;32:957–60.
97. Bayever E, Kamani N, Ferreira P, et al. Bone marrow transplantation for Niemann-Pick type IA disease. J Inherit Metab Dis 1992;15:919–28.
98. Lake BD, Steward CG, Oakhill A, et al. Bone marrow transplantation in late infantile Batten disease and juvenile Batten disease. Neuropediatrics 1997;28:80–1.
99. Jacobs JF, Willemsen MA, Groot-Loonen JJ, et al. Allogeneic BMT followed by substrate reduction therapy in a child with subacute Tay-Sachs disease. Bone Marrow Transplant 2005;36:925–6.

100. Ringdén O, Groth CG, Erikson A, et al. Longterm follow-up of the first successful bone marrow transplantation in Gaucher disease. Transplantation 1988;46:66–70.

101. Hobbs JR, Jones KH, Shaw PJ, et al. Beneficial effect of pre-transplant splenectomy on displacement bone marrow transplantation for Gaucher's syndrome. Lancet 1987;1:1111–5.

102. Zimran A, Bembi B, Pastores GM. Enzyme replacement therapy for type I Gaucher disease. In: Futerman AH, Zimran A, editors. Gaucher disease. London: Taylor & Francis; 2007. p. 341–54.

103. Erikson A, Groth CG, Månsson JE, et al. Clinical and biochemical outcome of marrow transplantation for Gaucher disease of the Norrbottnian type. Acta Paediatr Scand 1990;79:680–5.

104. Ringdén O, Groth CG, Erikson A, et al. Ten years' experience of bone marrow transplantation for Gaucher disease. Transplantation 1995;59:864–70.

105. Erikson A, Forsberg H, Nilsson M, et al. Ten years' experience of enzyme infusion therapy of Norrbottnian (type 3) Gaucher disease. Acta Paediatr 2006;95:312–7.

106. Porteus MH, Connelly JP, Pruett SM. A look to future directions in gene therapy research for monogenic diseases. PLoS Genet 2006;2. e133.

107. Biffi A, De Palma M, Quattrini A, et al. Correction of metachromatic leukodystrophy in the mouse model by transplantation of genetically modified hematopoietic stem cells. J Clin Invest 2004;113:1118–29.

108. Chung S, Ma X, Liu Y, et al. Effect of neonatal administration of a retroviral vector expressing alpha-L-iduronidase upon lysosomal storage in brain and other organs in mucopolysaccharidosis I mice. Mol Genet Metab 2007;90:181–92.

109. Kobayashi H, Carbonaro D, Pepper K, et al. Neonatal gene therapy of MPS I mice by intravenous injection of a lentiviral vector. Mol Ther 2005;11:776–89.

110. Liu Y, Xu L, Hennig AK, et al. Liver-directed neonatal gene therapy prevents cardiac, bone, ear, and eye disease in mucopolysaccharidosis I mice. Mol Ther 2005;11:35–47.

111. Zheng Y, Rozengurt N, Ryazantsev S, et al. Treatment of the mouse model of mucopolysaccharidosis I with retrovirally transduced bone marrow. Mol Genet Metab 2003;79:233–44.

112. Hacein-Bey-Abina S, Von Kalle C, Schmidt M, et al. LMO2-associated clonal T cell proliferation in two patients after gene therapy for SCID-X1. Science 2003; 302:415–9.

113. Pardridge WM. Molecular biology of the blood-brain barrier. Mol Biotechnol 2005;30:57–70.

114. Phinney DG, Prockop DJ. Concise review: mesenchymal stem/multipotent stromal cells: the state of transdifferentiation and modes of tissue repair–current views. Stem Cells 2007;25:2896–902.

115. Aggarwal S, Pittenger MF. Human mesenchymal stem cells modulate allogeneic immune cell responses. Blood 2005;105:1815–22.

116. Le Blanc K, Rasmusson I, Sundberg B, et al. Treatment of severe acute graft-versus-host disease with third party haploidentical mesenchymal stem cells. Lancet 2004;363:1439–41.

Bone Marrow Transplantation for Inherited Bone Marrow Failure Syndromes

Parinda Mehta, MD[a], Franco Locatelli, MD[b,c], Jan Stary, MD[d], Franklin O. Smith, MD[a,*]

KEYWORDS

- Inherited bone marrow failure syndromes
- Bone marrow transplantation • Gene mutation
- Diagnostic tests

The inherited bone marrow failure (BMF) syndromes are characterized by impaired hematopoiesis and cancer predisposition. Most inherited BMF syndromes are also associated with a range of congenital anomalies. In the past, the diagnosis of these diseases relied on the recognition of characteristic clinical features. With the advent of laboratory and genetic tests for many of these disorders, the understanding of their clinical spectrum has broadened (**Table 1**).[1] Indeed, it is becoming increasingly apparent that patients lacking characteristic physical stigmata may still harbor an inherited BMF syndrome and develop marrow failure or malignancy. Clinical presentation is no longer confined to the pediatric population but may manifest in adults as well. Sensitive and specific diagnostic tests, including identification of mutations in specific genes, are available for many disorders (**Table 2**).[2]

FANCONI ANEMIA

Fanconi anemia (FA) is a genetic disorder characterized by congenital anomalies, progressive BMF, and predisposition to malignancies. Even though this disorder is

[a] Cincinnati Children's Hospital Medical Center and the University of Cincinnati College of Medicine, 3333 Burnet Avenue, Cincinnati, OH 45229, USA
[b] University of Pavia, Ospedale Pediatrico Bambino Gesu, Roma, Italy
[c] Pediatric Haematology/Oncology Fondazione, IRCCS Policlinico San Matteo, 27100-I, Pavia, Italy
[d] Department of Pediatrics Hematology and Oncology, University Hospital Motol, Vúvalu 84, 150 06, Prague 5, Czech Republic
* Corresponding author.
E-mail address: frank.smith@cchmc.org

Pediatr Clin N Am 57 (2010) 147–170
doi:10.1016/j.pcl.2010.01.002
0031-3955/10/$ – see front matter © 2010 Elsevier Inc. All rights reserved.

pediatric.theclinics.com

Table 1
Characteristics of the inherited bone marrow failure syndromes compared with idiopathic aplastic anemia

	FA	DC	SDS	DBA	CAMT	AA
Inheritance pattern	AR, XLR	XLR, AR, AD	AR	AD	AR	?
Somatic abnormalities	Yes	Yes	Yes	Yes	Yes	?
Bone marrow failure	AA (>90%)	AA (~80%)	AA (20%)	RCA[a]	Meg[b]	AA
Short telomeres	Yes	Yes	Yes	Yes	?	Yes
Cancer	Yes	Yes	Yes	Yes	Yes	Yes
Chromosome instability	Yes	Yes	Yes	?	?	Yes
Genes identified	13	4	1	3	1	[c]

Abbreviations: AA, idiopathic aplastic anemia; AD, autosomal dominant; AR, autosomal recessive; CAMT, congenital amegakaryocytic thrombocytopenia; DBA, Diamond-Blackfan anemia; DC, dyskeratosis congenita; FA, Fanconi anemia; SDS, Shwachman-Diamond syndrome; XLR, X-linked recessive.
[a] RCA: red cell aplasia, although some patients can develop global bone marrow failure.
[b] Meg: low megakaryocytes, which can progress to global bone marrow failure.
[c] Heterozygous mutations in TERC and TERT are risk factors for some cases of idiopathic AA.
Data from Dokal I, Vulliamy T. Inherited aplastic anaemias/bone marrow failure syndromes. Blood Rev 2008;22:141–53.

rare, with an incidence of 1 per 100,000 live births, FA represents the most common inherited BMF syndrome. The clinical presentation of FA is highly heterogeneous. Approximately two-thirds of patients present with physical anomalies, which may vary greatly in number and severity. Common congenital abnormalities include short stature, skin pigment abnormalities (eg, café-au-lait spots), radial ray anomalies, genitourinary abnormalities, and microphthalmia.[3–5] It is important to recognize that disease manifestations and severity vary extensively and a subset of patients may lack the characteristic physical stigmata of FA. In addition, patients may first present in adulthood with BMF or malignancy as the primary clinical manifestation of FA. Hence, the possibility of an inherited basis for BMF must be considered for adults as well.

In patients with FA, the risk of developing BMF and hematologic and nonhematologic neoplasms increases with advancing age with a 90%, 33%, and 28% cumulative incidence, respectively, by 40 years of age.[6] The most common malignancies reported include acute myeloid leukemia (AML), myelodysplastic syndrome (MDS), and squamous cell carcinoma (SCC) of the head, neck, vulva and cervix.[6,7] BMF in FA typically presents between the ages of 5 and 10 years,[6,7] and the median age of patients who develop AML is 14 years.[8]

The cellular phenotype of FA is characterized by an abnormally high level of baseline chromosomal breakage along with an increased sensitivity to DNA cross-linking or alkylating agents that block DNA replication and RNA transcription.[9] FA is a complex genetic disorder with 13 complementation groups identified to date.[10] Multiple FA gene products form a nuclear complex believed to function in the DNA damage response and repair pathway.[11–15] Inheritance is mainly autosomal recessive, but is X-linked in a small number of children with biallelic mutations in the *FANCB* gene. Some genotype-phenotype correlation is known and has been reported to affect the transplant outcome.[16,17]

Current treatment of FA involves hematological support in the form of transfusions once advanced marrow failure occurs. Patients with FA do not respond to

Table 2
Genetic and laboratory tests for inherited bone marrow failure syndromes

Syndrome	Inheritance Pattern	Gene	Additional Laboratory Testing
Fanconi anemia	Autosomal recessive	FANCA FANCC FANCD1 FANCD2 FANCE FANCF FANCG FANCI FANCJ FANCL FANCM FANCN	Chromosome breakage
	X-linked recessive	FANCB	
Dyskeratosis congenita	X-linked recessive	DKC1	Telomere length
	Autosomal dominant	TERC TERT TINF2	
	Autosomal recessive	NHP2/NOLA2 NOP10/NOLA3	
Shwachman-Diamond syndrome	Autosomal recessive	SBDS	Serum trypsinogen, pancreatic isoamylase, fecal elastase, pancreatic imaging
Congenital amegakaryocytic thrombocytopenia	Autosomal recessive	C-MPL	
Diamond-Blackfan anemia	Autosomal dominant	RPS19 RPS17 RPS24 RPL35A RPL11	Erythrocyte adenosine deaminase (ADA)

Data from Shimamura A. Clinical approach to marrow failure. In: Gewirtz AM, Keating A, Thompson AA, editors. American Society of Hematology Education Program Book. Washington, DC: American Society of Hematology; 2009. p. 329–37.

antithymocyte globulin (ATG) or cyclosporine (typical treatments for acquired aplastic anemia), but 50% improve with androgen preparations,[16] with a median prolongation of life of 2 years in responders (age from 16 to 18 years at death), although relapses are inevitable.[18] Androgen therapy causes significant liver toxicity, virilization, and risk of hepatic adenoma and carcinoma. Androgens are reported to adversely affect the outcome of subsequent hematopoietic stem cell transplantation (HSCT) in some studies,[16] but not in others.[19] Ultimately, virtually all patients with FA will require treatment with allogeneic HSCT.

Hematopoietic Stem Cell Transplant in Patients with Fanconi Anemia

The definitive treatment for BMF, AML, and MDS associated with FA is allogeneic HSCT. Commonly agreed-upon indications for HSCT in these patients include evidence of severe marrow failure as manifested by an absolute neutrophil count

(ANC) less than 1000/ml^3 with or without granulocyte colony-stimulating factor (G-CSF) support, or hemoglobin less than 8 g/dL, or a platelet count less than 50,000/ml^3, or a requirement for blood product transfusions on a regular basis. In addition, HSCT is indicated for FA patients with evidence of progression to myelodysplasia, as diagnosed by marrow dysplasia or the presence of a cytogenetic clone together with dysplasia. Finally, allogeneic transplantation is indicated for FA patients with AML.

The earliest attempts at transplanting patients with FA in the 1970s and 1980s used the same preparative regimens designed for patients with idiopathic severe aplastic anemia (ie, 50 mg/kg of cyclophosphamide × 4 days). These transplantations had high mortality and morbidity.[20] In one report, only 1 of the 5 FA patients transplanted survived for more than 3 years. Four patients died of severe acute graft-versus-host disease (GVHD) soon after grafting. In addition, all had signs of severe cyclophosphamide toxicity. This study provided the first clinical evidence of a special sensitivity of FA cells to alkylating chemotherapy agents, indicating the need to modify the conditioning regimen in FA patients. Such hypersensitivity was also observed in vitro when FA cells were incubated with alkylating agents.

Gluckman and colleagues[21] were the first to investigate a markedly attenuated conditioning regimen for FA patients. These investigators successfully demonstrated that HSCT could be safely performed using low-dose cyclophosphamide, with long-term survival in 75% of patients with an human leukocyte antigen (HLA)-matched donor. The same group also tested the in vivo radiosensitivity and cell repair after skin contact radiotherapy to calculate the irradiation dose that could be tolerated by patients with FA. The results confirmed the suspected increased radiosensitivity in the majority of patients with FA. Following these results, 4 FA patients were conditioned with low-dose cyclophosphamide (20 mg/kg) in combination with 5 Gy thoracoabdominal irradiation. All engrafted without major complications from the conditioning regimen.[22]

In their long-term follow-up of 50 patients with FA transplanted using this conditioning regimen and a matched sibling donor, Socie and colleagues[23] documented survival estimates of 74.4% at 54 months and 58.5% at 100 months. Acute GVHD (grade II or more) developed in 55% of patients, and 69.9% were diagnosed with chronic GVHD. The survival of patients without chronic GVHD (n = 13) was 100%. In addition to chronic GVHD, 20 or more pretransplant transfusions were shown to have an adverse impact on survival by multivariate analysis (relative risk = 7.08, P = .0003).

Results from 151 matched sibling HSCTs for FA performed between 1978 and 1994 and reported to the International Bone Marrow Transplant Registry (IBMTR) were summarized by Gluckman and colleagues[24] in 1995. The 2-year probability of survival was 66%. The incidence of graft failure was 8%; grade II to IV acute GVHD occurred in 44% of patients, and chronic GVHD in 42%. Also, GVHD prophylaxis with cyclosporine and methotrexate resulted in a decreased incidence of GVHD compared with methotrexate alone. Gluckman and colleagues also noted that the adverse impact of increasing age and lower pretransplant platelet count on transplant outcome favors earlier intervention, especially when there was an HLA-identical sibling donor.

The addition of ATG to the Gluckman regimen was the next important milestone in HSCT of patients with FA. This addition further improved outcomes by decreasing the incidence of both acute and chronic GVHD.[23,25–27] The most recent of these reports[27] showed a 10-year actuarial survival of 89%, with a significant decrease in acute (23%) and chronic (12%) GVHD in 35 patients undergoing matched sibling donor HSCT using peritransplant ATG in combination with low doses of cyclophosphamide and radiation.

Over the last 3 decades, preparative regimens for FA have been modified significantly, with the goal of limiting toxicity while maintaining engraftment and improving outcomes by decreasing GVHD. For those patients with FA who have an HLA-identical related donor, HSCT when severe marrow failure develops is now the first-line treatment of choice, preferably before transfusion dependence develops, to limit the risk of graft failure.

Due to hypersensitivity of FA cells to DNA damage, one of the important goals during HSCT is to use conditioning regimens that minimize the development of treatment-induced secondary malignancies in these patients. A report of the joint Seattle and Paris experience with secondary cancers in patients with aplastic anemia and FA suggested that the risk of secondary cancers was mostly due to radiation. A total of 23 malignancies were reported among 700 patients transplanted for aplastic anemia or FA. At 20 years post transplant, the risk by Kaplan-Meier estimate was 14% for all patients and 42% for patients with FA. A diagnosis FA was an independent risk factor for development of secondary malignancy. Other risk factors included the development of chronic GVHD and the use of radiation in the preparative regimen. Five of the 79 patients with FA developed head and neck SCC.[28] More recent analyses point to the presence of acute or chronic GVHD as a major cause of development of SCC in this patient population.[23,29] Guardiola and colleagues[30] reported a 28% incidence of head and neck cancers 10 years post HSCT in FA patients with a history of acute GVHD versus 0% in those with no such history; this finding points to the importance of minimizing the risk of GVHD.

Investigators from Brazil have returned to the original approach of cyclophosphamide alone as a conditioning regimen for matched sibling donor HSCT. These investigators have systematically reduced the cyclophosphamide dose and have shown an excellent outcome with 93% overall survival (OS), and probabilities of acute and chronic GVHD of 17% and 28.5%, respectively, using a conditioning regimen that uses only 60 mg/kg of cyclophosphamide.[31,32] Ayas and colleagues[33] similarly reported significantly greater OS in patients receiving nonradiation, low-dose cyclophosphamide and ATG regimens compared with those receiving preparative regimens with cyclophosphamide and additional thoracoabdominal radiation (96.9% vs 72.5%; $P = .013$).

In 1997, Kapelushnik and colleagues[34] from Israel published the first case report using a fludarabine-based conditioning regimen for a child with FA in leukemic transformation. This highly immunosuppressive nucleoside analogue is well tolerated by patients with FA and has allowed for the elimination of radiation, with good results.[35–39] Tan and colleagues[36] recently reported an actual OS of 82% in a cohort of 11 patients who underwent a conditioning regimen with low-dose cyclophosphamide, fludarabine, and ATG, followed by transplantation with T-cell–depleted bone marrow or umbilical cord blood stem cells. Transplant-related mortality (TRM) was 9%, and GVHD was minimal. Longer follow-up times are needed to fully evaluate whether this conditioning regimen can reduce the risk of later malignancy after matched related donor HSCT in the FA population.

A recent report by Pasquini and colleagues[40] compared outcomes after radiation and nonradiation regimens in 148 FA patients undergoing matched sibling donor transplant to identify risk factors impacting HSCT outcomes. Hematopoietic recovery, acute and chronic GVHD, and mortality were similar after radiation and nonradiation regimens. In both groups of recipients older than 10 years, prior use of androgens and cytomegalovirus (CMV) seropositivity in either the donor or recipient were associated with higher mortality. With a median follow-up greater than 5 years, the 5-year probability of OS, adjusted for factors impacting overall mortality, was 78% after radiation and 81% after nonradiation regimens ($P = .61$). In view of the high risk of cancer and other radiation-related effects on growth and development, these results support the use of nonradiation conditioning regimens in this population. However, as the peak time for developing solid tumors after HSCT is 8 to 9 years, longer follow-up is required before definitive statements can be made regarding the impact of nonradiation regimens on cancer risk.

Matched Unrelated Donor Transplantation for Patients with Fanconi Anemia

The heritable nature of FA unfortunately reduces the chances of finding an unaffected HLA-matched family donor, which usually leaves matched unrelated donor (MUD) transplantation as the only alternative for most patients with FA who require HSCT. Outcomes of unrelated donor HSCT for FA using unrelated donor stem cells have been inferior to those reported with related donor stem cells. This result is primarily due to high risk of graft failure, acute GVHD, an increased risk of infections, and excessive regimen-related organ toxicity.

In 2000, the results of a retrospective multicenter study of 69 unrelated donor HSCTs for FA facilitated through the European Group for Blood and Marrow Transplantation (EBMT) and the European FA Registry were reported by Guardiola and colleagues.[16] The 3-year probability of survival was 33%. The causes of death were acute GVHD (n = 18), primary or secondary graft failure (n = 13), chronic GVHD (n = 4), infections (n = 7), and veno-occlusive disease of the liver (n = 1). In that study, the presence of 3 or more extramedullary congenital malformations, the use of androgens prior to HSCT, positive recipient CMV serology, and the use of a female donor were independent risk factors associated with poor survival. Because of the high risk of TRM from graft failure and GVHD, unrelated donor transplantation has generally not been recommended until failure of other treatment modalities, such as use of androgens and transfusions.

Graft rejection rates following unrelated donor transplantation has traditionally exceeded 20% in most reported series. This high frequency of graft failure in FA patients contrasts with a lower frequency of approximately 5% in other patient populations receiving unrelated donor HSCT,[16,21,24,41] and seems to be due to reduced doses of radiation and immunosuppressive alkylating chemotherapy agents generally used to reduce regimen-related toxicity associated with excessive sensitivity of FA cells, as discussed earlier. Reduced doses of these agents are typically used in FA patients to avoid excessive toxicity, and the consequence is a high frequency of graft failure due to inadequate peritransplant immune suppression. In an attempt to improve engraftment, MacMillan and colleagues[42] escalated the radiation dose to 600 cGy and added ATG; this decreased the incidence of acute GVHD and chronic GVHD, but did not improve OS. Thus, before the recent introduction of fludarabine in the FA-preparative regimen, OS for unrelated donor transplants was approximately 30%.[16,30]

The introduction of fludarabine-based preparative regimens has resulted in considerable improvements in outcome, with sustained engraftment without significant toxicity. Reported survival rates with fludarabine-containing preparative regimens range from 38% to 96%.[17,19,35,43–45] In a large retrospective study of 98 alternative donor transplantations for FA reported to the IBMTR, Wagner and colleagues[17] reported that fludarabine-containing regimens were associated with improved engraftment, decreased TRM (47% vs 81%), and improved 3-year OS (52% vs 13%, $P<.001$) compared with nonfludarabine regimens (**Fig. 1**).

In the same report, an increased risk of graft failure was confirmed in transplant recipients with mosaicism who underwent transplantation using preparative regimens

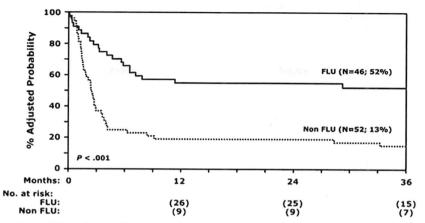

Fig. 1. Probability of overall survival with fludarabine and nonfludarabine regimens after adjusting for prior red blood cell transfusions and CMV serostatus. (*From* Wagner JE, Eapen M, MacMillan ML, et al. Unrelated donor bone marrow transplantation for the treatment of Fanconi anemia. Blood 2007;109(5):2256–62; with permission.)

without fludarabine compared with those using fludarabine-containing regimens. Further, for patients receiving nonfludarabine-containing regimens, the 100-day probability of developing grades 2 to 4 acute GVHD was 70% after the transplantation of non-T-cell–depleted bone marrow and 21% after transplantation with T-cell–depleted bone marrow. The probability of grades 2 to 4 acute GVHD was 16% in patients receiving a fludarabine-containing preparative regimen. Similarly, a reduced incidence of GVHD has been reported in other studies of FA patients using fludarabine, both in the matched related and unrelated donor HSCT settings.[32,36,44] It must be noted that in a study of Japanese patients who received non-T-cell–depleted grafts, the acute GVHD rate was even lower than that for patients who received a T-cell–depleted transplant.[43] Although the numbers of patients and ethnicities in the Japanese and Center for International Blood and Marrow Transplant Research studies are different, these data seem to suggest that, in the presence of fludarabine, T-cell depletion may not be absolutely crucial in abating acute GVHD.

Umbilical Cord Blood Transplantation for Patients with Fanconi Anemia

Umbilical cord blood (UCB) is an attractive source of hematopoietic stem cells for patients who lack an HLA-matched unrelated bone marrow donor. The low incidence of GVHD associated with unrelated UCB HSCT may be particularly advantageous for FA patients, given their increased risk of GVHD. Transplantation of acceptable cell doses can usually be accomplished with UCB HSCT because of the young age and small size of FA patients. The first reported use of UCB as a stem cell source was for a child with FA. Since this initial report, the use of cord blood as a stem cell source for transplanting patients with FA has been increasingly reported.[46,47]

Gluckman and colleagues[48] retrospectively analyzed results of UCB HSCT in 93 FA patients. In 57 patients (61%), the preparative regimen included fludarabine. GVHD prophylaxis consisted mostly of cyclosporine with prednisone. OS was 40% and the incidence of grade II to IV acute and chronic GVHD was 32% and 16%, respectively. As with unrelated bone marrow, patients who received a fludarabine-containing regimen had improved engraftment (72% vs 42%) as well as improved OS (50% vs

25%) compared with those who received other nonfludarabine-containing regimens. These outcomes are very similar to MUD transplants, suggesting that UCB HSCT is a viable stem cell option for patients with FA.

Transplantation for Patients with Fanconi Anemia and Myelodysplasia or Acute Myeloid Leukemia

Allogeneic HSCT can be curative for patients with FA presenting with progressive marrow failure, and excellent disease-free survival (DFS) rates have been documented in different reports. Data are scarce, however, on the ideal management of patients with FA who present with cytogenetic clones, MDS, or AML. FA patients with myelodysplasia or clonal abnormalities are a distinct group that may require more intensive conditioning before HSCT, as the presence of either abnormality may herald the development of AML and hence is considered a marker for an adverse outcome.[5,49] Although very early reports of intensive conditioning for these patients resulted in high TRM,[50] Socie and colleagues[23] reported 5 patients with FA and MDS on presentation who did well; they were prepared with thoracoabdominal irradiation plus cyclophosphamide 40 mg/kg, instead of the 20 mg/kg routinely used for FA patients without myelodysplasia. The study reported an 8-year survival of 75%.

Most recently, groups from Saudi Arabia and New York reported their experience with HSCT of these high-risk FA patients. Ayas and colleagues[51] transplanted a total of 11 patients, 10 patients with MDS and 1 with AML. Ten patients had matched sibling donors and 1 patient was transplanted using a one-antigen mismatched UCB unit. The conditioning regimen included CY (20 mg/kg), ATG (total dose 160 mg/kg of the equine product or 52 mg/kg of the rabbit product), and total body irradiation (TBI) at 450 cGy. Ten patients are currently alive with no evidence of disease, with a median follow-up of almost 4 years. Chaudhury and colleagues[44] similarly reported transplants in 18 high-risk FA patients, with high risk defined as progressive disease with MDS in 22% of patients, 33% with AML, 83% with multiple transfusions, 72% with prior androgen treatment, 77% with prior infections, and 4 patients older than 20 years. A mix of related and unrelated HLA-matched and mismatched donors were used. Cytoreduction included single dose TBI (450 cGy), fludarabine (150 mg/m^2), and CY (40 mg/kg). Immunosuppression included ATG and tacrolimus. Grafts were CD34-selected T-cell–depleted peripheral blood stem cells in 15 patients and T-cell–depleted marrows in 3. All 18 patients engrafted with 100% donor chimerism; only one patient developed GVHD. OS and DFS were 72.2% and 66.6%, respectively, at a median follow-up of 4.2 years, suggesting that this approach might be sufficient to control malignancy in FA.

Patients with FA who present with overt AML pose a further challenge. FA patients have excessive toxicity with chemotherapy regimens used in non-FA AML patients. Given the positive impact of pretransplant chemotherapy in AML on outcome, it is not clear how to best approach FA patients with AML prior to the initiation of the HSCT procedure. Mehta and colleagues[52] recently showed that FA patients can tolerate a reduced-intensity AML chemotherapy regimen as induction chemotherapy before initiation of the HSCT process, with clearance of AML blasts. However, HSCT still remains the only definitive therapy for these patients.

SHWACHMAN-DIAMOND SYNDROME

Shwachman-Diamond syndrome (SDS) is a rare autosomal recessive disorder characterized by exocrine pancreatic insufficiency, skeletal abnormalities in the form of metaphyseal dysostosis, and bone marrow dysfunction manifested as cytopenias.[53–58]

Additional clinical manifestations seen in some patients include short stature, variable immune dysfunction, delayed dentition, and structural and functional abnormalities of the liver.[55,59–61] Patients with SDS are at an increased risk of developing aplastic anemia, MDS, and AML.[55,59,62–66]

Although most patients with SDS have some hematologic abnormalities, most of them do not require HSCT. In the largest reported series, 20% of cases developed pancytopenia and 6% progressed to MDS.[56] Other investigators have reported varying incidences of MDS ranging from 10% to 15% to as high as 44% of cases.[55,59,63,67] The risk of leukemic transformation in SDS patients is significant and increases with age, varying from 5% in childhood to nearly 24% as patients approach adulthood.[67] Although infections and thoracic dystrophy are the leading causes of morbidity and mortality during infancy, the likelihood of long-term survival correlates most closely with the degree of bone marrow dysfunction. Survival is particularly reduced in patients who develop bone marrow aplasia, MDS, or acute leukemia, averaging 14 years in patients with aplastic anemia.[63] The development of acute leukemia portends a poor prognosis as SDS patients do not respond well to chemotherapeutic intervention.

HSCT is the only known curative treatment for bone marrow dysfunction associated with SDS. However, the timing of transplantation remains a subject of controversy, and the apparent lack of genotype-phenotype correlation makes selection of patients for early preemptive HSCT difficult at present. In addition, like FA patients, children with SDS tend to have increased toxicity with intensive conditioning regimens. Tsai and colleagues[61] reported a case of fatal congestive heart failure following a cyclophosphamide-containing conditioning regimen in a patient with SDS. Other investigators have described neurologic complications,[66] pulmonary complications, and multiorgan failure with typical ablative regimens.[68,69]

Overall, the available literature on HSCT in SDS patients is limited and consists mainly of case reports.[70–80] Vibhakar and colleagues[81] recently reviewed the published experience with HSCT in SDS patients and reported a total of 28 patients, including their own. All but 4 patients received myeloablative conditioning regimens containing cyclophosphamide with or without TBI/total lymphoid irradiation (TLI). Most patients received unrelated bone marrow as a source of stem cells, although they reported 3 cases in which UCB was used successfully as a source of stem cells. At the time of reporting, 17 of these patients were alive, although mortality approached 40%. More than 50% of the patients who died succumbed to cardiopulmonary complications in the early posttransplant phase. Similarly, in a recent review of the European experience with HSCT in 26 SDS patients, Cesaro and colleagues[68] reported an overall TRM of 35.5% at 1 year. Interestingly (and reminiscent of the experience in FA), they found a significantly higher mortality rate in patients receiving a TBI-conditioning regimen (67% for TBI vs 20% for non-TBI containing regimen, $P = .03$).

Although the number of patients is very small, the patients who have undergone transplantation for aplasia have been noted to have better outcomes than those who have undergone transplantation for MDS or leukemia.[74] Also, despite the biologic mechanism being unclear, patients with SDS seem to have a predilection for increased cardiac toxicity with cyclophosphamide-containing conditioning regimens.[61,74,79] Savilahti and Rapola[82] reported significant cardiac dysfunction in patients with SDS even without exposure to cyclophosphamide. In their series of 16 Finnish patients, 8 had cardiac abnormalities on necropsy, including cardiac fibrosis and areas of necrosis.

Clinical reports also suggest that patients with SDS are more susceptible to transplant-related toxicity than patients with other disorders like Kostmann syndrome and juvenile myelomonocytic leukemia.[83,84] Dror and Freedman[85] demonstrated that the bone marrow mononuclear cells from patients with SDS show an increased propensity for apoptosis mediated by hyperactivation of the Fas-signaling pathway. The same investigators also reported decreased telomere length in the marrow-derived mononuclear cells from patients with SDS.[86] It is possible, although currently unexplored, that similar mechanisms are important in the increased susceptibility to organ toxicity with intensive conditioning regimens seen in patients with SDS.

Due to significant regimen-related toxicity observed during HSCT for SDS, recent efforts have focused on reduced-intensity preparative regimens that might ameliorate cardiac and pulmonary toxicities. Sauer and colleagues[87] reported 3 patients with SDS and BMF transplanted using a regimen consisting of fludarabine, treosulfan, and melphalan. All 3 patients engrafted rapidly with 100% donor chimerism. Although 2 of the patients tolerated the regimen with minimal toxicity, 1 patient died on day 98 secondary to idiopathic pneumonitis syndrome. The first 2 patients had the common 183-184 TA to CT mutation in the SBDS gene, whereas the third patient who died carried a c.297-300delAAGA deletion, leading the investigators to speculate on whether genotype is predictive of treatment-related toxicity. Attempts have been made to predict the clinical phenotype from the genetic mutation, but no correlation has been found thus far between the hematologic or skeletal manifestations and the genotype in the small numbers of patients that were studied.[88–90]

A recent report from Bhatla and colleagues[91] described the use of a reduced-intensity preparative regimen in 7 patients with SDS associated with aplasia or MDS/AML. The preparative regimen consisted of Campath-1H, fludarabine, and melphalan. Four patients received matched related marrow and 3 received unrelated donor stem cells (2 peripheral blood stem cells [PBSCs] and 1 marrow). All but one donor was 8 of 8 allele-level, HLA matched. All patients established 100% donor-derived hematopoiesis. No patient in this cohort developed grades III to IV GVHD. One patient had grade II acute skin GVHD that responded to systemic corticosteroids and one had grade I acute skin GVHD, treated with topical corticosteroids. Two out of 7 patients developed bacterial infections in the early posttransplant period. Viral infections were seen in 4 of 7 patients and were successfully treated with appropriate antiviral therapy. All 7 patients were alive at the time of the study report, with a median follow-up of 548 days (range, 93–920 days). These preliminary data indicate that HSCT with reduced-intensity conditioning is feasible in patients with SDS and is associated with excellent donor cell engraftment and modest morbidity.

DYSKERATOSIS CONGENITA

Dyskeratosis congenita (DC) is an inherited disorder that usually presents with the clinical triad of abnormal skin pigmentation, nail dystrophy, and mucosal leukoplakia.[92–95] There are also noncutaneous manifestations, including gastrointestinal disorders and pulmonary complications like progressive pulmonary fibrosis. DC is genetically heterogeneous with X-linked, autosomal dominant, and autosomal recessive subtypes recognized. Patients have very short germline telomeres, and at least one-half of patients have mutations in known telomere biology genes. Disease pathology is thought to be a consequence of chromosome instability related to telomerase deficiency due to mutations in DKC1, TERC, and TERT. In patients with DKC1 mutations, defects in ribosomal RNA modification, ribosome biogenesis, translation control, or mRNA splicing may also contribute to disease pathogenesis. The involvement of telomerase complex components in X-linked and autosomal dominant forms and the presence of short telomeres suggest that DC is primarily a disease of defective telomere maintenance.[96]

BMF is the leading cause of early mortality in these patients, with approximately 80% to 90% of patients developing hematopoietic abnormalities by age 30 years.[97,98] Patients with DC are also at increased risk for MDS/AML and solid tumors, especially SCC.[97,99,100] Transient responses to therapy with androgens, prednisone, splenectomy, and hematopoietic growth factors have all been reported.[101–104]

Allogeneic HSCT remains the only curative approach for marrow failure in patients with DC; however, outcomes have been poor due to early and late complications.[105] Langstone and colleagues[106] transplanted 8 patients with marrow failure associated with DC. Six patients received allogeneic marrow grafts from HLA-identical siblings and 2 from HLA-MUDs. Patients who received marrow from HLA-identical siblings were conditioned with CY (140–200 mg/kg), with or without ATG. Patients who received MUD were conditioned with CY (120 mg/kg) and TBI (1200 cGy). Six out of 8 patients who survived for longer than 2 weeks following transplant had hematological evidence of engraftment, and all 3 patients who survived for at least a year following transplant recovered normal hematological function. Three patients died with respiratory failure and pulmonary fibrosis at 70 days, 8 years, and 20 years post transplant. Three patients died of invasive fungal infections during the neutropenic period, one patient died of refractory acute GVHD on day 44, and one patient was alive at 463 days following transplant. The surviving patient underwent surgical resection of a rectal carcinoma diagnosed 14 months post HSCT. Other reports using myeloablative conditioning showed similar results.[105,107–113]

The presence of pulmonary disease in a significant proportion of DC patients prior to HSCT may explain the high incidence of fatal pulmonary complications in the setting of HSCT. More recent studies have used reduced-intensity regimens with encouraging results for successful engraftment with fewer complications, for both related and unrelated allografts.[114–119] However, long-term follow-up data are not available and it remains to be seen how these patients ultimately fare. Regardless of the potential reduction in toxicity associated with these regimens, preexisting conditions characteristic of DC (eg, pulmonary disease) may ultimately limit the effectiveness of HSCT in these patients.[116,120]

CONGENITAL AMEGAKARYOCYTIC THROMBOCYTOPENIA

Congenital amegakaryocytic thrombocytopenia (CAMT) is a rare autosomal recessive disorder characterized by isolated thrombocytopenia at birth due to ineffective megakaryocytopoiesis, and progression to pancytopenia in later childhood. CAMT is usually caused by defective c-mpl expression due to mutations in the thrombopoietin receptor c-MPL.[121] In a recent retrospective review of 20 patients with CAMT, approximately 70% patients developed marrow aplasia and one developed MDS that progressed to acute leukemia.[122] Several therapeutic modalities have been attempted in the treatment of CAMT. Steroids, cyclosporine, and cytokines and hematopoietic growth factors including interleukin-3, interleukin-11, and G-CSF have all been shown to produce only transient responses.[123,124]

HSCT remains the only known curative treatment for CAMT. However, due to the rareness of this disorder, there are only a few reports in the literature describing the role of HSCT in the management of CAMT. Lackner and colleagues[125] reported their experience in 8 patients with CAMT; 5 underwent HSCT from related donors, 2 from unrelated donors, and 1 from a haploidentical mother (T-cell–depleted peripheral stem cells). The preparative regimen was busulfan, cyclophosphamide, and ATG in

6 patients, busulfan and cyclophosphamide in 1 patient, and busulfan and cyclophosphamide with thiotepa in another patient. Both patients receiving MUD transplants died. The remaining 6 patients had normal platelet counts 3 to 27 months post HSCT. Causes of death included bronchiolitis obliterans in one patient and engraftment failure followed by aspergillosis in a second. Recently, King and colleagues[122] reported HSCT outcomes in 15 CAMT patients. Median age at the time of HSCT was 38 months (range 7–89 months). Outcome was good for those who underwent transplantation from HLA-identical family donors (n = 11); in contrast, all of the patients who received HSCT from an unrelated donor (n = 4) died of complications. Similarly, other reports have described mixed results in terms of outcomes following HSCT in CAMT.[126,127]

Steele and colleagues[128] reported on successful unrelated donor HSCT using a reduced-intensity conditioning regimen in a CAMT patient with monosomy 7. The patient underwent a matched unrelated bone marrow transplant at 7.25 years of age. The conditioning regimen consisted of fludarabine (30 mg/m^2/d) from day -10 to day -5, CY (60 mg/kg/d) on day -6 and day -5, and equine ATG (ATGAM, 40 mg/kg/d) from day -4 to day -1. The patient received an 8/8 molecularly matched non-T-cell–depleted bone marrow allograft from a male unrelated donor. GVHD prophylaxis consisted of cyclosporine and steroids. The patient had rapid and durable engraftment with minimal complications, and was alive 24 months post transplantation at the time of the report. Based on this single case report, the possibility exists that reduced-intensity conditioning might be a feasible approach to HSCT in patients with CAMT who do not have a related donor and who are at known increased risk of toxicity from standard conditioning regimens. However, longer follow-up and additional patients are required to completely evaluate the long-term risks and benefits of a reduced-intensity preparative regimen in comparison with myeloablative conditioning.

DIAMOND-BLACKFAN ANEMIA

Diamond-Blackfan anemia (DBA) is a pure red blood cell aplasia of childhood, characterized by normocytic or macrocytic anemia, reticulocytopenia, paucity of bone marrow erythroid precursors and, in more than one-third of patients, somatic abnormalities. Patients also have elevated fetal hemoglobin and erythrocyte adenosine deaminase activity.[129,130] The other hematologic lineages are not generally involved, although slightly abnormal low leukocyte and high platelet counts have been reported at diagnosis.[131,132] Short stature and congenital abnormalities, mainly involving the head, upper limbs, heart, and urogenital system, occur in more than one-third of DBA patients.[133] Information with regard to cancer risk in patients with DBA has been limited primarily to case reports: 29 cases (as well as 3 with MDS who did not develop AML) have been reported among the more than 700 DBA patients in the literature.[3,134]

Recent data show that approximately 40% to 45% of DBA cases are familial with an autosomal dominant inheritance,[135] the remainder being sporadic or familial with seemingly different patterns of inheritance. The genetic basis of DBA is heterogeneous, and approximately 50% of patients are heterozygous for ribosomal protein genes RPS17, RPS19, RPS24, RPL5, RPL11, or RPL35A. All the mutations to date have been found in one allele, resulting in severe loss of function or protein haploinsufficiency. The most common mutation has been found in RPS19. A recent review[136] described more than 60 different RPS19 mutations associated with DBA.[135–143] Overall, DBA is now considered a disorder of ribosome biogenesis or function. There is no clear correlation between the type of *RPS19* mutation and the degree of hematological disease.

Corticosteroids remain the mainstay of treatment for patients with DBA. Approximately 80% of DBA patients respond to an initial course of steroids. Many patients require long-term high-dose steroids, or develop resistance to therapy and require long-term transfusions.[144–146] Although androgens,[147] growth factors (eg, interleukin-3, erythropoietin),[148,149] and cyclosporine[150,151] have been used with temporary success, the main therapeutic options in steroid-resistant patients are chronic red cell transfusions or allogeneic HSCT.

Allogeneic HSCT is a potentially curative treatment option for DBA. However, this approach remains controversial, as most of these patients can achieve long-term survival with supportive therapy alone. However, patients with DBA who are unresponsive to or intolerant of corticosteroids, experience treatment failure with other treatments, develop additional cytopenias or clonal disease, or opt for curative therapy can indeed be treated with allogeneic HSCT. Since the first report in 1976, several investigators have reported successful transplantation for selected patients with DBA.[152–159]

In the largest reported series, Roy and colleagues[160] studied the transplant outcomes of 61 DBA patients whose data were reported to the IBMTR between 1984 and 2000. Forty-one patients (67%) received transplants from an HLA-identical sibling donor, 8 (13%) from a nonsibling family donor, and 12 (20%) from a MUD. All patients but one received conventional, cyclophosphamide-based conditioning regimens. Only 18% of patients received TBI. Cyclosporine and methotrexate were the most frequently used agents for GVHD prophylaxis. Patients who received an alternative donor transplant were more likely to be older (9 vs 5 years; $P = .03$), to have had a longer median time from diagnosis to transplantation (110 vs 58 months; $P = .02$), and to have received TBI as part of the conditioning regimen (45% vs 5%; $P<.001$). The 3-year probability of OS was 64% (range, 50%–74%). Five patients did not achieve neutrophil engraftment. The 100-day mortality was 18% (95% confidence interval [CI], 10%–29%). Grade II to IV acute GVHD occurred in 28% (range, 17%–39%) and chronic GVHD was reported in 26% (range, 15%–39%). In general, more favorable outcomes were seen in patients with a better performance status at the time of transplantation and in recipients of matched sibling donor transplants. The 1- and 3-year probability of OS of patients with a good performance status who received allografts from HLA-identical sibling donors (n = 29) was 83% (95% CI, 67%–94%). Recipients of alternative donor transplants had worse survival compared with HLA-identical sibling donor transplant recipients (76% vs 39%; $P = .005$).

The number of transfusions before transplantation was significantly correlated with the speed of neutrophil and platelet recovery. Patients who received less than 50 transfusions before transplantation were more likely to have neutrophil recovery by day 28 and platelet recovery by day 60 than patients who received 50 transfusions or more. However, this did not affect survival. Of the 38 surviving patients with a median follow-up of 11 years (range, 1–14 years), 37 were reported to have a normal white blood cell count. Of these 38 patients, 25 were known to be red blood cell transfusion independent, while transfusion data were not available for the remaining 13 patients.

Previous studies have reported similar OS rates (66%–87%),[157,158,161] and similar inferior results after alternative donor transplantations compared with matched sibling donor transplants (87% vs 14%).[158] The DBA registry of North America recently reported 36 patients who underwent HSCT, 21 using matched sibling donors and 15 with alternative donors. The majority of HLA-matched sibling transplants were done using a nonirradiation-containing conditioning regimen. The majority of alternative donor transplants was performed using TBI. Sixteen of the 21 matched sibling donor transplants were alive and red cell transfusion independent. Of the 15 alternative donor HSCT, 4 were alive at the time of report. Of note, of the 16 deaths, 15 were related to infection, GVHD, or veno-occlusive disease of the liver, with only 1 death, in the alternative donor group, occurring as a consequence of graft failure. The survival for allogeneic sibling versus alternative donor transplant was 72.7% ± 10.7% versus 19.1% ± 11.9% at greater than 5 years from HSCT (P = .01) (excluding a patient with osteogenic sarcoma diagnosed after SCT) or 17.1% ± 10.8% (including the osteogenic sarcoma patient, P = .012).[162]

Mugishima and colleagues[156] reported their experience with HSCT in 19 Japanese patients with DBA. Stem cell source was bone marrow in 13 (6 HLA-matched siblings, and 6 HLA-matched and 1 HLA-MUDs), UCB in 5 (2 HLA-matched siblings and 3 HLA-mismatched unrelated donors), and peripheral blood from a haploidentical mother in the remaining patient. With regard to the preparative regimen, 13 patients (68%) received cyclophosphamide (60–200 mg/kg) with TBI (3.5–12 Gy)-based conditioning, and 6 patients (32%) received cyclophosphamide without radiation-based conditioning. GVHD prophylaxis included cyclosporine with or without methotrexate and tacrolimus with or without methotrexate. One patient experienced early death from pulmonary bleeding and sepsis on day 10 after a CD34+ cell-selected, peripheral blood stem cell graft from a haploidentical mother. Sixteen of the 18 evaluable patients (88.9%) achieved successful engraftment. Median observation time after transplantation was 89.5 months. Of the 3 patients who received UCB from HLA-MUDs, 1 had complete engraftment but developed grade II acute GVHD and died of EBV-associated lymphoproliferative disease 4 months after UCB HSCT.[163] The other 2 patients experienced graft rejection and returned to being transfusion-dependent. One patient subsequently underwent HSCT from an HLA-one-locus-mismatched father 2 months after the first transplantation. The other patient received bone marrow from an unrelated HLA-matched donor 11 months after the first transplantation. Both patients were reported to be alive 80 months and 63 months after successful second HSCT, respectively. Overall, 15 of 19 DBA patients (79%) survived with successful engraftment after the first HSCT, and 2 patients who initially received an unsuccessful unrelated-donor UCB transplant then received a successful second HSCT as described earlier. The failure-free survival rate of the patients 5 years after HSCT was higher than that after UCB HSCT (100% vs 40%, P = .0019). The OS rate after HSCT (100%) was higher than that after the other types of HSCT (60%, P = .0293) and after unrelated UCB HSCT (67%, P = .0374).

Long-term follow-up of DBA patients has suggested an increased risk of malignancies, including osteosarcoma.[162,164] In this context, reduced doses of radiation or other reduced-intensity preparative regimens are now of interest. Ostronoff and colleagues[165] reported that a 19-month-old patient underwent successful matched sibling donor HSCT following a nonmyeloablative conditioning regimen (2 Gy TBI plus 90 mg/m^2 fludarabine). GVHD prophylaxis included cyclosporine (6 mg/kg/d) and methotrexate on days 1, 3, 6, and 11. The posttransplant course was uneventful. With a follow-up of 10 months, no signs of toxicity or GVHD were observed. The patient had full donor chimerism and was transfusion independent, with a performance status of 100%. In contrast to this successful case report, a matched sibling peripheral blood stem cell transplant after a non-TBI reduced-intensity conditioning regimen led to graft failure in a 4-year-old DBA patient, and to mixed chimerism and chronic GVHD in a 5-year-old with DBA.[166] Thus, although these case reports of successful nonmyeloablative transplantations in DBA are encouraging, further studies with larger patient numbers are needed to critically evaluate its role.

SUMMARY AND FUTURE DIRECTIONS

Progress in improving the outcomes for children with inherited BMF syndromes has been limited by the rarity of these disorders, as well as disease-specific genetic, molecular, cellular, and clinical characteristics that increase the risks of complications associated with HSCT. As a result, the ability to develop innovative transplant approaches to circumvent these problems has been limited. However, recent progress has been made, as best evidenced by the addition of fludarabine to the preparative regimen for children undergoing unrelated donor HSCT for FA. The highly immunosuppressive nature of fludarabine now allows for a high degree of donor engraftment without overlapping toxicities and tissue injury, with further reduction in GVHD. The improvement in outcome with fludarabine has been evident in smaller studies, despite a lack of traditional, large, multicenter clinical trials; this is likely a rare circumstance. The rarity of these diseases coupled with the far more likely incremental improvements that will result from ongoing research will require prospective international clinical trials to improve the outcome for these children.

REFERENCES

1. Dokal I, Vulliamy T. Inherited aplastic anaemias/bone marrow failure syndromes. Blood Rev 2008;22:141–53.
2. Shimamura A. Clinical approach to marrow failure. In: Gewirtz AM, Keating A, Thompson AA, editors. American Society of Hematology Education Program Book. Washington, DC: American Society of Hematology; 2009. p. 329–37.
3. Alter BP. Inherited bone marrow failure syndromes. In: Nathan D, Orkin S, Look A, et al, editors. Hematology of infancy and childhood. Philadelphia: WB Saunders; 2003. p. 280–365.
4. Alter BP. Fanconi's anemia and malignancies. Am J Hematol 1996;53(2):99–110.
5. Tischkowitz M, Dokal I. Fanconi anaemia and leukaemia—clinical and molecular aspects. Br J Haematol 2004;126(2):176–91.
6. Kutler DI, Singh B, Satagopan J, et al. A 20-year perspective on the International Fanconi Anemia Registry (IFAR). Blood 2003;101(4):1249–56.
7. Rosenberg PS, Alter BP, Ebell W. Cancer risks in Fanconi anemia: findings from the German Fanconi Anemia Registry. Haematologica 2008;93(4):511–7.
8. Alter BP. Cancer in Fanconi anemia, 1927-2001. Cancer 2003;97(2):425–40.
9. Auerbach AD, Wolman SR. Susceptibility of Fanconi anaemia fibroblasts to chromosome damage by carcinogens. Nature 1976;261:494.
10. Levitus M, Rooimans MA, Steltenpool J, et al. Heterogeneity in Fanconi anemia: evidence for 2 new genetic subtypes. Blood 2004;103(7):2498–503.
11. Kupfer GM, Naf D, Suliman A, et al. The Fanconi anaemia proteins, FAA and FAC, interact to form a nuclear complex. Nat Genet 1997;17(4):487–90.
12. Naf D, Kupfer GM, Suliman A, et al. Functional activity of the Fanconi anemia protein FAA requires FAC binding and nuclear localization. Mol Cell Biol 1998;18(10):5952–60.
13. Garcia-Higuera I, Kuang Y, Naf D, et al. Fanconi anemia proteins FANCA, FANCC, and FANCG/XRCC9 interact in a functional nuclear complex. Mol Cell Biol 1999;19(7):4866–73.
14. Garcia-Higuera I, Taniguchi T, Ganesan S, et al. Interaction of the Fanconi anemia proteins and BRCA1 in a common pathway. Mol Cell 2001;7(2):249–62.
15. Garcia-Higuera I, Kuang Y, Denham J, et al. The Fanconi anemia proteins FANCA and FANCG stabilize each other and promote the nuclear accumulation of the Fanconi anemia complex. Blood 2000;96(9):3224–30.

16. Guardiola P, Pasquini R, Dokal I, et al. Outcome of 69 allogeneic stem cell transplantations for Fanconi anemia using HLA-matched unrelated donors: a study on behalf of the European Group for Blood and Marrow Transplantation. Blood 2000;95(2):422–9.

17. Wagner JE, Eapen M, MacMillan ML, et al. Unrelated donor bone marrow transplantation for the treatment of Fanconi anemia. Blood 2007;109(5):2256–62.

18. Liu JM, Buchwald M, Walsh CE, et al. Fanconi anemia and novel strategies for therapy. Blood 1994;84(12):3995–4007.

19. de Medeiros CR, Bitencourt MA, Zanis-Neto J, et al. Allogeneic hematopoietic stem cell transplantation from an alternative stem cell source in Fanconi anemia patients: analysis of 47 patients from a single institution. Braz J Med Biol Res 2006;39(10):1297–304.

20. Gluckman E, Devergie A, Schaison G, et al. Bone marrow transplantation in Fanconi anaemia. Br J Haematol 1980;45(4):557–64.

21. Gluckman E. Bone marrow transplantation in Fanconi's anemia. Stem Cells 1993;11(Suppl 2):180–3.

22. Gluckman E, Devergie A, Dutreix J. Radiosensitivity in Fanconi anaemia: application to the conditioning regimen for bone marrow transplantation. Br J Haematol 1983;54(3):431–40.

23. Socie G, Devergie A, Girinski T, et al. Transplantation for Fanconi's anaemia: long-term follow-up of fifty patients transplanted from a sibling donor after low-dose cyclophosphamide and thoraco-abdominal irradiation for conditioning. Br J Haematol 1998;103(1):249–55.

24. Gluckman E, Auerbach AD, Horowitz MM, et al. Bone marrow transplantation for Fanconi anemia. Blood 1995;86(7):2856–62.

25. Ayas M, Solh H, Mustafa MM, et al. Bone marrow transplantation from matched siblings in patients with Fanconi anemia utilizing low-dose cyclophosphamide, thoracoabdominal radiation and antithymocyte globulin. Bone Marrow Transplant 2001;27(2):139–43.

26. Kohli-Kumar M, Morris C, DeLaat C, et al. Bone marrow transplantation in Fanconi anemia using matched sibling donors. Blood 1994;84(6):2050–4.

27. Farzin A, Davies SM, Smith FO, et al. Matched sibling donor haematopoietic stem cell transplantation in Fanconi anaemia: an update of the Cincinnati Children's experience. Br J Haematol 2007;136(4):633–40.

28. Deeg HJ, Socie G, Schoch G, et al. Malignancies after marrow transplantation for aplastic anemia and Fanconi anemia: a joint Seattle and Paris analysis of results in 700 patients. Blood 1996;87(1):386–92.

29. Rosenberg PS, Socie G, Alter BP, et al. Risk of head and neck squamous cell cancer and death in patients with Fanconi anemia who did and did not receive transplants. Blood 2005;105(1):67–73.

30. Guardiola P, Socie G, Li X, et al. Acute graft-versus-host disease in patients with Fanconi anemia or acquired aplastic anemia undergoing bone marrow transplantation from HLA-identical sibling donors: risk factors and influence on outcome. Blood 2004;103(1):73–7.

31. Zanis-Neto J, Flowers ME, Medeiros CR, et al. Low-dose cyclophosphamide conditioning for haematopoietic cell transplantation from HLA-matched related donors in patients with Fanconi anaemia. Br J Haematol 2005; 130(1):99–106.

32. Balci YI, Akdemir Y, Gumruk F, et al. CD-34 selected hematopoietic stem cell transplantation from HLA identical family members for Fanconi anemia. Pediatr Blood Cancer 2008;50(5):1065–7.

33. Ayas M, Al-Jefri A, Al-Seraihi A, et al. Matched-related allogeneic stem cell transplantation in Saudi patients with Fanconi anemia: 10 year's experience. Bone Marrow Transplant 2008;42(Suppl 1):S45–8.

34. Kapelushnik J, Or R, Slavin S, et al. A fludarabine-based protocol for bone marrow transplantation in Fanconi's anemia. Bone Marrow Transplant 1997; 20(12):1109–10.

35. Locatelli F, Zecca M, Pession A, et al. The outcome of children with Fanconi anemia given hematopoietic stem cell transplantation and the influence of fludarabine in the conditioning regimen: a report from the Italian pediatric group. Haematologica 2007;92(10):1381–8.

36. Tan PL, Wagner JE, Auerbach AD, et al. Successful engraftment without radiation after fludarabine-based regimen in Fanconi anemia patients undergoing genotypically identical donor hematopoietic cell transplantation. Pediatr Blood Cancer 2006;46(5):630–6.

37. Bitan M, Or R, Shapira MY, et al. Fludarabine-based reduced intensity conditioning for stem cell transplantation of Fanconi anemia patients from fully matched related and unrelated donors. Biol Blood Marrow Transplant 2006; 12(7):712–8.

38. George B, Mathews V, Shaji RV, et al. Fludarabine-based conditioning for allogeneic stem cell transplantation for multiply transfused patients with Fanconi's anemia. Bone Marrow Transplant 2005;35(4):341–3.

39. de la Fuente J, Reiss S, McCloy M, et al. Non-TBI stem cell transplantation protocol for Fanconi anaemia using HLA-compatible sibling and unrelated donors. Bone Marrow Transplant 2003;32(7):653–6.

40. Pasquini R, Carreras J, Pasquini MC, et al. HLA-matched sibling hematopoietic stem cell transplantation for Fanconi anemia: comparison of irradiation and non-irradiation containing conditioning regimens. Biol Blood Marrow Transplant 2008;14(10):1141–7.

41. Davies SM, Khan S, Wagner JE, et al. Unrelated donor bone marrow transplantation for Fanconi anemia. Bone Marrow Transplant 1996;17(1):43–7.

42. MacMillan ML, Auerbach AD, Davies SM, et al. Haematopoietic cell transplantation in patients with Fanconi anaemia using alternate donors: results of a total body irradiation dose escalation trial. Br J Haematol 2000;109(1): 121–9.

43. Yabe H, Inoue H, Matsumoto M, et al. Allogeneic haematopoietic cell transplantation from alternative donors with a conditioning regimen of low-dose irradiation, fludarabine and cyclophosphamide in Fanconi anaemia. Br J Haematol 2006;134(2):208–12.

44. Chaudhury S, Auerbach AD, Kernan NA, et al. Fludarabine-based cytoreductive regimen and T-cell-depleted grafts from alternative donors for the treatment of high-risk patients with Fanconi anaemia. Br J Haematol 2008;140(6):644–55.

45. Gluckman E, Rocha V, Boyer-Chammard A, et al. Outcome of cord-blood transplantation from related and unrelated donors. Eurocord Transplant Group and the European Blood and Marrow Transplantation Group. N Engl J Med 1997; 337(6):373–81.

46. Auerbach AD, Liu Q, Ghosh R, et al. Prenatal identification of potential donors for umbilical cord blood transplantation for Fanconi anemia. Transfusion 1990; 30(8):682–7.

47. Aker M, Varadi G, Slavin S, et al. Fludarabine-based protocol for human umbilical cord blood transplantation in children with Fanconi anemia. J Pediatr Hematol Oncol 1999;21(3):237–9.

48. Gluckman E, Rocha V, Ionescu I, et al. Results of unrelated cord blood transplant in Fanconi anemia patients: risk factor analysis for engraftment and survival. Biol Blood Marrow Transplant 2007;13(9):1073–82.

49. Alter BP, Caruso JP, Drachtman RA, et al. Fanconi anemia: myelodysplasia as a predictor of outcome. Cancer Genet Cytogenet 2000;117(2):125–31.

50. Flowers ME, Doney KC, Storb R, et al. Marrow transplantation for Fanconi anemia with or without leukemic transformation: an update of the Seattle experience. Bone Marrow Transplant 1992;9(3):167–73.

51. Ayas M, Al-Jefri A, Al-Seraihi A, et al. Allogeneic stem cell transplantation in Fanconi anemia patients presenting with myelodysplasia and/or clonal abnormality: update on the Saudi experience. Bone Marrow Transplant 2008;41(3): 261–5.

52. Mehta PA, Ileri T, Harris RE, et al. Chemotherapy for myeloid malignancy in children with Fanconi anemia. Pediatr Blood Cancer 2007;48(7):668–72.

53. Shwachman H, Diamond LK, Oski FA, et al. The syndrome of pancreatic insufficiency and bone marrow dysfunction. J Pediatr 1964;65:645–63.

54. Bodian M, Sheldon W, Lightwood R. Congenital hypoplasia of the exocrine pancreas. Acta Paediatr 1964;53:282–93.

55. Aggett PJ, Cavanagh NP, Matthew DJ, et al. Shwachman's syndrome. A review of 21 cases. Arch Dis Child 1980;55(5):331–47.

56. Ginzberg H, Shin J, Ellis L, et al. Shwachman syndrome: phenotypic manifestations of sibling sets and isolated cases in a large patient cohort are similar. J Pediatr 1999;135(1):81–8.

57. Berrocal T, Simon MJ, al-Assir I, et al. Shwachman-Diamond syndrome: clinical, radiological and sonographic aspects. Pediatr Radiol 1995;25(4):289–92.

58. Robberecht E, Nachtegaele P, Van Rattinghe R, et al. Pancreatic lipomatosis in the Shwachman-Diamond syndrome. Identification by sonography and CT-scan. Pediatr Radiol 1985;15(5):348–9.

59. Mack DR, Forstner GG, Wilschanski M, et al. Shwachman syndrome: exocrine pancreatic dysfunction and variable phenotypic expression. Gastroenterology 1996;111(6):1593–602.

60. Dror Y, Ginzberg H, Dalal I, et al. Immune function in patients with Shwachman-Diamond syndrome. Br J Haematol 2001;114(3):712–7.

61. Tsai PH, Sahdev I, Herry A, et al. Fatal cyclophosphamide-induced congestive heart failure in a 10-year-old boy with Shwachman-Diamond syndrome and severe bone marrow failure treated with allogeneic bone marrow transplantation. Am J Pediatr Hematol Oncol 1990;12(4):472–6.

62. Huijgens PC, van der Veen EA, Meijer S, et al. Syndrome of Shwachman and leukaemia. Scand J Haematol 1977;18(1):20–4.

63. Smith OP, Hann IM, Chessells JM, et al. Haematological abnormalities in Shwachman-Diamond syndrome. Br J Haematol 1996;94(2):279–84.

64. Dokal I, Rule S, Chen F, et al. Adult onset of acute myeloid leukaemia (M6) in patients with Shwachman-Diamond syndrome. Br J Haematol 1997;99(1): 171–3.

65. Dror Y, Squire J, Durie P, et al. Malignant myeloid transformation with isochromosome 7q in Shwachman-Diamond syndrome. Leukemia 1998;12(10):1591–5.

66. Okcu F, Roberts WM, Chan KW. Bone marrow transplantation in Shwachman-Diamond syndrome: report of two cases and review of the literature. Bone Marrow Transplant 1998;21(8):849–51.

67. Donadieu J, Leblanc T, Bader Meunier B, et al. Analysis of risk factors for myelodysplasias, leukemias and death from infection among patients with

congenital neutropenia. Experience of the French Severe Chronic Neutropenia Study Group. Haematologica 2005;90(1):45–53.

68. Cesaro S, Oneto R, Messina C, et al. Haematopoietic stem cell transplantation for Shwachman-Diamond disease: a study from the European Group for blood and marrow transplantation. Br J Haematol 2005;131(2):231–6.

69. Donadieu J, Michel G, Merlin E, et al. Hematopoietic stem cell transplantation for Shwachman-Diamond syndrome: experience of the French neutropenia registry. Bone Marrow Transplant 2005;36(9):787–92.

70. Barrios N, Kirkpatrick D, Regueira O, et al. Bone marrow transplant in Shwachman Diamond syndrome. Br J Haematol 1991;79(2):337–8.

71. Smith OP, Chan MY, Evans J, et al. Shwachman-Diamond syndrome and matched unrelated donor BMT. Bone Marrow Transplant 1995;16(5):717–8.

72. Arseniev L, Diedrich H, Link H. Allogeneic bone marrow transplantation in a patient with Shwachman-Diamond syndrome. Ann Hematol 1996;72(2): 83–4.

73. Faber J, Lauener R, Wick F, et al. Shwachman-Diamond syndrome: early bone marrow transplantation in a high risk patient and new clues to pathogenesis. Eur J Pediatr 1999;158(12):995–1000.

74. Fleitz J, Rumelhart S, Goldman F, et al. Successful allogeneic hematopoietic stem cell transplantation (HSCT) for Shwachman-Diamond syndrome. Bone Marrow Transplant 2002;29(1):75–9.

75. Cesaro S, Guariso G, Calore E, et al. Successful unrelated bone marrow transplantation for Shwachman-Diamond syndrome. Bone Marrow Transplant 2001; 27(1):97–9.

76. Hsu JW, Vogelsang G, Jones RJ, et al. Bone marrow transplantation in Shwachman-Diamond syndrome. Bone Marrow Transplant 2002;30(4):255–8.

77. Park SY, Chae MB, Kwack YG, et al. Allogeneic bone marrow transplantation in Shwachman-Diamond syndrome with malignant myeloid transformation. A case report. Korean J Intern Med 2002;17(3):204–6.

78. Cunningham J, Sales M, Pearce A, et al. Does isochromosome 7q mandate bone marrow transplant in children with Shwachman-Diamond syndrome? Br J Haematol 2002;119(4):1062–9.

79. Mitsui T, Kawakami T, Sendo D, et al. Successful unrelated donor bone marrow transplantation for Shwachman-Diamond syndrome with leukemia. Int J Hematol 2004;79(2):189–92.

80. Grewal SS, Barker JN, Davies SM, et al. Unrelated donor hematopoietic cell transplantation: marrow or umbilical cord blood? Blood 2003;101(11):4233–44.

81. Vibhakar R, Radhi M, Rumelhart S, et al. Successful unrelated umbilical cord blood transplantation in children with Shwachman-Diamond syndrome. Bone Marrow Transplant 2005;36(10):855–61.

82. Savilahti E, Rapola J. Frequent myocardial lesions in Shwachman syndrome. Eight fatal cases among 16 Finnish patients. Acta Paediatr Scand 1984;73:642–51.

83. Ferry C, Ouachee M, Leblanc T, et al. Hematopoietic stem cell transplantation in severe congenital neutropenia: experience of the French SCN register. Bone Marrow Transplant 2005;35(1):45–50.

84. Donadieu J, Stephan JL, Blanche S, et al. Treatment of juvenile chronic myelomonocytic leukemia by allogeneic bone marrow transplantation. Bone Marrow Transplant 1994;13(6):777–82.

85. Dror Y, Freedman MH. Shwachman-Diamond syndrome marrow cells show abnormally increased apoptosis mediated through the Fas pathway. Blood 2001;97(10):3011–6.

86. Thornley I, Dror Y, Sung L, et al. Abnormal telomere shortening in leucocytes of children with Shwachman-Diamond syndrome. Br J Haematol 2002;117(1): 189–92.
87. Sauer M, Zeidler C, Meissner B, et al. Substitution of cyclophosphamide and busulfan by fludarabine, treosulfan and melphalan in a preparative regimen for children and adolescents with Shwachman-Diamond syndrome. Bone Marrow Transplant 2007;39(3):143–7.
88. Kuijpers TW, Alders M, Tool AT, et al. Hematologic abnormalities in Shwachman Diamond syndrome: lack of genotype-phenotype relationship. Blood 2005; 106(1):356–61.
89. Makitie O, Ellis L, Durie PR, et al. Skeletal phenotype in patients with Shwachman-Diamond syndrome and mutations in SBDS. Clin Genet 2004;65(2): 101–12.
90. Kawakami T, Mitsui T, Kanai M, et al. Genetic analysis of Shwachman-Diamond syndrome: phenotypic heterogeneity in patients carrying identical SBDS mutations. Tohoku J Exp Med 2005;206(3):253–9.
91. Bhatla D, Davies SM, Shenoy S, et al. Reduced-intensity conditioning is effective and safe for transplantation of patients with Shwachman-Diamond syndrome. Bone Marrow Transplant 2008;42(3):159–65.
92. Zinsser F. Atropha cutis reticularis cum pigmentatione, dystrophia unglumet leukoplakia oris. Ikonogr Dermatol (Hyoto) 1906;5:219–23.
93. Engman MF. A unique case of reticular pigmentation of the skin with atrophy. Arch Dermatol Symphiligr 1926;13:685–7.
94. Cole HN, Rauschkollo JC, Toomey J. Dyskeratosis congenital with pigmentation, dystrophia unguis and leukokeratosis oris. Arch Dermatol Symphiligr 1930;21: 71–95.
95. Ogden GR, Connor E, Chisholm DM. Dyskeratosis congenita: report of a case and review of the literature. Oral Surg Oral Med Oral Pathol 1988;65(5):586–91.
96. Mitchell JR, Wood E, Collins K. A telomerase component is defective in the human disease dyskeratosis congenita. Nature 1999;402(6761):551–5.
97. Dokal I. Dyskeratosis congenita in all its forms. Br J Haematol 2000;110(4): 768–79.
98. Knight S, Vulliamy T, Copplestone A, et al. Dyskeratosis Congenita (DC) Registry: identification of new features of DC. Br J Haematol 1998;103(4):990–6.
99. Kirwan M, Dokal I. Dyskeratosis congenita: a genetic disorder of many faces. Clin Genet 2008;73(2):103–12.
100. de la Fuente J, Dokal I. Dyskeratosis congenita: advances in the understanding of the telomerase defect and the role of stem cell transplantation. Pediatr Transplant 2007;11(6):584–94.
101. Smith CM, Ramsay NKC, Branda R, et al. Response to androgens in the constitutional aplastic anemia of dyskeratosis congenita. Pediatr Res 1979;13:441.
102. Russo CL, Glader BE, Israel RJ, et al. Treatment of neutropenia associated with dyskeratosis congenita with granulocyte-macrophage colony-stimulating factor. Lancet 1990;336(8717):751–2.
103. Putterman C, Safadi R, Zlotogora J, et al. Treatment of the hematological manifestations of dyskeratosis congenita. Ann Hematol 1993;66(4):209–12.
104. Alter BP, Gardner FH, Hall RE. Treatment of dyskeratosis congenita with granulocyte colony-stimulating factor and erythropoietin. Br J Haematol 1997;97(2): 309–11.
105. Rocha V, Devergie A, Socie G, et al. Unusual complications after bone marrow transplantation for dyskeratosis congenita. Br J Haematol 1998;103(1):243–8.

106. Langston AA, Sanders JE, Deeg HJ, et al. Allogeneic marrow transplantation for aplastic anaemia associated with dyskeratosis congenita. Br J Haematol 1996; 92(3):758–65.
107. Mahmoud HK, Schaefer UW, Schmidt CG, et al. Marrow transplantation for pancytopenia in dyskeratosis congenita. Blut 1985;51(1):57–60.
108. Berthou C, Devergie A, D'Agay MF, et al. Late vascular complications after bone marrow transplantation for dyskeratosis congenita. Br J Haematol 1991;79(2): 335–6.
109. Dokal I, Bungey J, Williamson P, et al. Dyskeratosis congenita fibroblasts are abnormal and have unbalanced chromosomal rearrangements. Blood 1992; 80(12):3090–6.
110. Lau YL, Ha SY, Chan CF, et al. Bone marrow transplant for dyskeratosis congenita. Br J Haematol 1999;105(2):571.
111. Yabe M, Yabe H, Hattori K, et al. Fatal interstitial pulmonary disease in a patient with dyskeratosis congenita after allogeneic bone marrow transplantation. Bone Marrow Transplant 1997;19(4):389–92.
112. Shaw PH, Haut PR, Olszewski M, et al. Hematopoietic stem-cell transplantation using unrelated cord-blood versus matched sibling marrow in pediatric bone marrow failure syndrome: one center's experience. Pediatr Transplant 1999; 3(4):315–21.
113. Ghavamzadeh A, Alimoghadam K, Nasseri P, et al. Correction of bone marrow failure in dyskeratosis congenita by bone marrow transplantation. Bone Marrow Transplant 1999;23(3):299–301.
114. Nobili B, Rossi G, De Stefano P, et al. Successful umbilical cord blood transplantation in a child with dyskeratosis congenita after a fludarabine-based reduced-intensity conditioning regimen. Br J Haematol 2002;119(2):573–4.
115. Dror Y, Freedman MH, Leaker M, et al. Low-intensity hematopoietic stem-cell transplantation across human leucocyte antigen barriers in dyskeratosis congenita. Bone Marrow Transplant 2003;31(10):847–50.
116. Brazzola P, Duval M, Fournet JC, et al. Fatal diffuse capillaritis after hematopoietic stem-cell transplantation for dyskeratosis congenita despite low-intensity conditioning regimen. Bone Marrow Transplant 2005;36(12):1103–5 [author reply: 1105].
117. Gungor T, Corbacioglu S, Storb R, et al. Nonmyeloablative allogeneic hematopoietic stem cell transplantation for treatment of dyskeratosis congenita. Bone Marrow Transplant 2003;31(5):407–10.
118. Ayas M, Al-Musa A, Al-Jefri A, et al. Allogeneic stem cell transplantation in a patient with dyskeratosis congenita after conditioning with low-dose cyclophosphamide and anti-thymocyte globulin. Pediatr Blood Cancer 2007;49(1): 103–4.
119. Ostronoff F, Ostronoff M, Calixto R, et al. Fludarabine, cyclophosphamide, and antithymocyte globulin for a patient with dyskeratosis congenita and severe bone marrow failure. Biol Blood Marrow Transplant 2007;13(3):366–8.
120. Amarasinghe K, Dalley C, Dokal I, et al. Late death after unrelated-BMT for dyskeratosis congenita following conditioning with alemtuzumab, fludarabine and melphalan. Bone Marrow Transplant 2007;40(9):913–4.
121. Ballmaier M, Germeshausen M, Schulze H, et al. c-mpl mutations are the cause of congenital amegakaryocytic thrombocytopenia. Blood 2001;97(1):139–46.
122. King S, Germeshausen M, Strauss G, et al. Congenital amegakaryocytic thrombocytopenia: a retrospective clinical analysis of 20 patients. Br J Haematol 2005;131(5):636–44.

123. Gillio AP, Gabrilove JL. Cytokine treatment of inherited bone marrow failure syndromes. Blood 1993;81(7):1669–74.
124. Guinan EC, Lee YS, Lopez KD, et al. Effects of interleukin-3 and granulocyte-macrophage colony-stimulating factor on thrombopoiesis in congenital amegakaryocytic thrombocytopenia. Blood 1993;81(7):1691–8.
125. Lackner A, Basu O, Bierings M, et al. Haematopoietic stem cell transplantation for amegakaryocytic thrombocytopenia. Br J Haematol 2000;109(4): 773–5.
126. MacMillan ML, Davies SM, Wagner JE, et al. Engraftment of unrelated donor stem cells in children with familial amegakaryocytic thrombocytopenia. Bone Marrow Transplant 1998;21(7):735–7.
127. Kudo K, Kato K, Matsuyama T, et al. Successful engraftment of unrelated donor stem cells in two children with congenital amegakaryocytic thrombocytopenia. J Pediatr Hematol Oncol 2002;24(1):79–80.
128. Steele M, Hitzler J, Doyle JJ, et al. Reduced intensity hematopoietic stem-cell transplantation across human leukocyte antigen barriers in a patient with congenital amegakaryocytic thrombocytopenia and monosomy 7. Pediatr Blood Cancer 2005;45(2):212–6.
129. Josephs HW. Anaemia of infancy and early childhood. Medicine 1936;15: 307–451.
130. Diamond KL, Blackfan KD. Hypoplastic anemia. Am J Dis Child 1938;56:464–7.
131. Dianzani I, Garelli E, Ramenghi U. Diamond-Blackfan anemia: a congenital defect in erythropoiesis. Haematologica 1996;81(6):560–72.
132. Giri N, Kang E, Tisdale JF, et al. Clinical and laboratory evidence for a trilineage haematopoietic defect in patients with refractory Diamond-Blackfan anaemia. Br J Haematol 2000;108(1):167–75.
133. Willig TN, Gazda H, Sieff CA. Diamond-Blackfan anemia. Curr Opin Hematol 2000;7(2):85–94.
134. Yaris N, Erduran E, Cobanoglu U. Hodgkin lymphoma in a child with Diamond Blackfan anemia. J Pediatr Hematol Oncol 2006;28(4):234–6.
135. Orfali KA, Ohene-Abuakwa Y, Ball SE. Diamond Blackfan anaemia in the UK: clinical and genetic heterogeneity. Br J Haematol 2004;125(2):243–52.
136. Ramenghi U, Campagnoli MF, Garelli E, et al. Diamond-Blackfan anemia: report of seven further mutations in the RPS19 gene and evidence of mutation heterogeneity in the Italian population. Blood Cells Mol Dis 2000;26(5): 417–22.
137. Willig TN, Draptchinskaia N, Dianzani I, et al. Mutations in ribosomal protein S19 gene and Diamond Blackfan anemia: wide variations in phenotypic expression. Blood 1999;94(12):4294–306.
138. Draptchinskaia N, Gustavsson P, Andersson B, et al. The gene encoding ribosomal protein S19 is mutated in Diamond-Blackfan anaemia. Nat Genet 1999; 21(2):169–75.
139. Matsson H, Klar J, Draptchinskaia N, et al. Truncating ribosomal protein S19 mutations and variable clinical expression in Diamond-Blackfan anemia. Hum Genet 1999;105(5):496–500.
140. Cmejla R, Blafkova J, Stopka T, et al. Ribosomal protein S19 gene mutations in patients with Diamond-Blackfan anemia and identification of ribosomal protein S19 pseudogenes. Blood Cells Mol Dis 2000;26(2):124–32.
141. Proust A, Da Costa L, Rince P, et al. Ten novel Diamond-Blackfan anemia mutations and three polymorphisms within the rps19 gene. Hematol J 2003;4(2): 132–6.

142. Campagnoli MF, Garelli E, Quarello P, et al. Molecular basis of Diamond-Blackfan anemia: new findings from the Italian registry and a review of the literature. Haematologica 2004;89(4):480–9.
143. Gazda HT, Zhong R, Long L, et al. RNA and protein evidence for haplo-insufficiency in Diamond-Blackfan anaemia patients with RPS19 mutations. Br J Haematol 2004;127(1):105–13.
144. Young NS, Alter BP. Aplastic anemia: acquired and inherited. Philadelphia: WB Saunders; 1994.
145. Halperin DS, Freedman MH. Diamond-Blackfan anemia: etiology, pathophysiology, and treatment. Am J Pediatr Hematol Oncol 1989;11(4):380–94.
146. Vlachos A, Ball S, Dahl N, et al. Diagnosing and treating Diamond Blackfan anaemia: results of an international clinical consensus conference. Br J Haematol 2008;142(6):859–76.
147. Alter BP. The bone marrow failure syndrome. In: Nathan D, Orkin S, editors. Hematology of infancy and childhood. Philadelphia: WB Saunders; 1998. p. 237–335.
148. Ball SE, Tchernia G, Wranne L, et al. Is there a role for interleukin-3 in Diamond-Blackfan anaemia? Results of a European multicentre study. Br J Haematol 1995;91(2):313–8.
149. Niemeyer CM, Baumgarten E, Holldack J, et al. Treatment trial with recombinant human erythropoietin in children with congenital hypoplastic anemia. Contrib Nephrol 1991;88:276–80 [discussion: 281].
150. Finlay JL, Shahidi NT. Cyclosporine induced remission in Diamond-Blackfan anaemia. Blood 1984;64:104a.
151. Alessandri AJ, Rogers PC, Wadsworth LD, et al. Diamond-Blackfan anemia and cyclosporine therapy revisited. J Pediatr Hematol Oncol 2000;22(2):176–9.
152. August CS, King E, Githens JH, et al. Establishment of erythropoiesis following bone marrow transplantation in a patient with congenital hypoplastic anemia (Diamond-Blackfan syndrome). Blood 1976;48(4):491–8.
153. Iriondo A, Garijo J, Baro J, et al. Complete recovery of hemopoiesis following bone marrow transplant in a patient with unresponsive congenital hypoplastic anemia (Blackfan-Diamond syndrome). Blood 1984;64(2):348–51.
154. Lenarsky C, Weinberg K, Guinan E, et al. Bone marrow transplantation for constitutional pure red cell aplasia. Blood 1988;71(1):226–9.
155. Greinix HT, Storb R, Sanders JE, et al. Long-term survival and cure after marrow transplantation for congenital hypoplastic anaemia (Diamond-Blackfan syndrome). Br J Haematol 1993;84(3):515–20.
156. Mugishima H, Gale RP, Rowlings PA, et al. Bone marrow transplantation for Diamond-Blackfan anemia. Bone Marrow Transplant 1995;15(1):55–8.
157. Alter BP. Bone marrow transplant in Diamond-Blackfan anemia. Bone Marrow Transplant 1998;21(9):965–6.
158. Vlachos A, Federman N, Reyes-Haley C, et al. Hematopoietic stem cell transplantation for Diamond Blackfan anemia: a report from the Diamond Blackfan Anemia Registry. Bone Marrow Transplant 2001;27(4):381–6.
159. Bonno M, Azuma E, Nakano T, et al. Successful hematopoietic reconstitution by transplantation of umbilical cord blood cells in a transfusion-dependent child with Diamond-Blackfan anemia. Bone Marrow Transplant 1997;19(1):83–5.
160. Roy V, Perez WS, Eapen M, et al. Bone marrow transplantation for Diamond-Blackfan anemia. Biol Blood Marrow Transplant 2005;11(8):600–8.
161. Willig TN, Niemeyer CM, Leblanc T, et al. Identification of new prognosis factors from the clinical and epidemiologic analysis of a registry of 229

Diamond-Blackfan anemia patients. DBA group of Societe d'Hematologie et d'Immunologie Pediatrique (SHIP), Gesellschaft fur Padiatrische Onkologie und Hamatologie (GPOH), and the European Society for Pediatric Hematology and Immunology (ESPHI). Pediatr Res 1999;46(5):553–61.

162. Lipton JM, Federman N, Khabbaze Y, et al. Osteogenic sarcoma associated with Diamond-Blackfan anemia: a report from the Diamond-Blackfan Anemia Registry. J Pediatr Hematol Oncol 2001;23(1):39–44.

163. Ohga S, Kanaya Y, Maki H, et al. Epstein-Barr virus-associated lymphoproliferative disease after a cord blood transplant for Diamond-Blackfan anemia. Bone Marrow Transplant 2000;25(2):209–12.

164. Lipton JM, Atsidaftos E, Zyskind I, et al. Improving clinical care and elucidating the pathophysiology of Diamond Blackfan anemia: an update from the Diamond Blackfan Anemia Registry. Pediatr Blood Cancer 2006;46(5):558–64.

165. Ostronoff M, Florencio R, Campos G, et al. Successful nonmyeloablative bone marrow transplantation in a corticosteroid-resistant infant with Diamond-Blackfan anemia. Bone Marrow Transplant 2004;34(4):371–2.

166. Gomez-Almaguer D, Ruiz-Arguelles GJ, Tarin-Arzaga Ldel C, et al. Reduced-intensity stem cell transplantation in children and adolescents: the Mexican experience. Biol Blood Marrow Transplant 2003;9(3):157–61.

Hematopoietic Stem Cell Transplantation for Osteopetrosis

Colin G. Steward, MD, PhD[a,b],*

KEYWORDS

- Osteopetrosis • Hematopoietic transplant • Hypocalcemia
- Pulmonary hypertension

Osteopetrosis (OP) is the generic name for a group of diseases caused by deficient formation or function of osteoclasts (OC), inherited in either autosomal recessive (AR) or dominant (AD) fashion.[1–3] These vary in severity from a disease that may kill infants to an incidental radiological finding in adults. It is increasingly clear that prognosis is governed by which gene is affected, making detailed elucidation of the cause of the disease a critical component of optimal care, including the decision on whether hematopoietic stem cell transplantation (HSCT) is appropriate.[4] HSCT in patients with OP is associated with disease-specific problems that require careful management, including the potential for life-threatening post-transplant hypercalcemia, a high prevalence of pulmonary arterial hypertension (PAH) and, in at least 1 subtype of disease, failure to reverse osteosclerosis despite successful donor cell engraftment.

MAJOR CLINICAL FEATURES OF OP

Aberrant resorption and remodeling of bone caused by defective OC function have many potential clinical consequences. (1) Fractures: bones are under-tubulated so that they break easily. Common fracture sites are long bones of the arms and leg, posterior ribs, and the acromial processes.[5] (2) Central nervous system (CNS) and eye problems: bony overgrowth, or lack of remodeling, results in compression of nerves or blood vessels that pass through bones, especially the optic nerve (resulting in partial or complete visual loss) and, more rarely, the auditory and facial nerves. Arteries or venous sinuses within the skull can also be constricted, as can the foramen magnum. Early fusion of bones may result in craniosynostosis. Some patients have primary neurometabolic (neuronopathic) forms of OP and may have abnormal retinal

---

[a] Department of Cellular & Molecular Medicine, School of Medical Sciences, University of Bristol, University Walk, Bristol, BS8 1TD, UK
[b] BMT Unit, Royal Hospital for Children, Upper Maudlin Street, Bristol, BS2 8BJ, UK
* Corresponding author. BMT Unit, Royal Hospital for Children, Upper Maudlin Street, Bristol, BS2 8BJ, UK.
E-mail address: colin.steward@bristol.ac.uk

Pediatr Clin N Am 57 (2010) 171–180
doi:10.1016/j.pcl.2009.11.006
0031-3955/10/$ – see front matter

pigmentation and cerebral atrophy.[6,7] (3) Cytopenia/pancytopenia: bony encroachment on medullary cavities results in extramedullary hemopoiesis with hepatosplenomegaly and the potential for hypersplenism. Anemia and thrombocytopenia result and blood films often show a markedly leukoerythroblastic picture, with a high white blood cell count and high numbers of circulating stem cells.[8] (4) Growth: most children with OP fall below the tenth percentile on growth charts and some have severe dwarfism.[2,9] (5) Hypocalcemia: defective OC function can disturb calcium homeostasis, which may manifest as symptomatic hypocalcemia in the first few months of life, despite high total body calcium reserves.[2,10] (6) Respiratory compromise: the skull base, choanal bones, and jaw are often severely affected, which produces persistent snuffling, noisy breathing, and upper airway obstruction, and may predispose patients to PAH. Patients often suffer increased ear, nose, and throat infections and respiratory infections.[11] (7) Dentition: tooth eruption is often delayed and tooth quality is poor; osteomyelitis of the jaw can occur.[12] (8) Involvement of other organ systems: the genes involved may have roles in other organs. For example, a small proportion of children have a severe neurometabolic disease and abnormalities of lymphocytes and immunoglobulin production are now recognized in some variants.[4,13]

CLASSIFICATION OF OP

OP is principally classified according to its mode of inheritance: either AR or AD.[4] The most common form of the disease typically presents in adult life and follows AD inheritance. It occurs in 2 forms, autosomal dominant osteopetrosis (ADO) I and II, with most patients having ADO II. ADO often follows a milder and slower progressive pathway than AR disease and has not been treated by HSCT, although some patients are severely compromised by their disease.[14]

Most cases that present in childhood follow AR inheritance; when presenting in infancy this disease has been termed "malignant infantile OP" (MIOP). Typical appearances on presentation are shown in **Fig. 1** and classification is outlined in **Table 1**. Until 2000 only 1 causative gene had been found but since then 8 others have been described.[4] The gene responsible is still not known in approximately 25% of children with autosomal recessive osteopetrosis (ARO) and this cohort of children may yet have many different diseases.

Children presenting beyond 2 years of age often have a slower progressive disease, intermediate AR OP (IRO), characterized by little or no peripheral cytopenia.[16] Such children need particularly careful evaluation as some may have early presentation of ADO (and hence not be candidates for HSCT), whereas others may have mutations that will not produce aggressive disease.

OSTEOCLAST FUNCTION AND GENETIC CONTROL

OC are large multinucleate cells formed by fusion of cells of the monocyte-macrophage line, characterized by expression of several receptors (including receptor activator NF-κB [RANK]) and by production of large quantities of tartrate-resistant acid phosphatase (TRAP), and cathepsin K.[1,4,17]

Their formation is dependent on several proteins produced by adjacent stromal cells and osteoblasts, including receptor activator NF-κB ligand (RANKL). RANKL, which binds to RANK on the surface of OC, seems to be crucial for this process, and deficiency results in OP characterized by the absence of identifiable OC in bone biopsies (osteoclast-poor OP). Because osteoblasts and stromal cells are not replaced to a significant degree by transplantation, patients deficient in RANKL do not respond

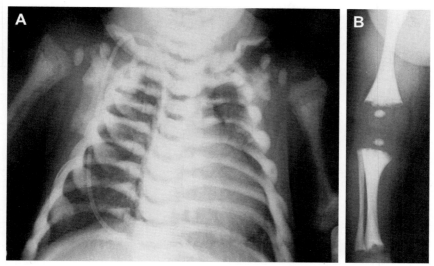

Fig. 1. Characteristic appearances of ARO on presentation. Chest (*A*) and leg (*B*) radiographs from separate patients at presentation of ARO. There is uniform osteosclerosis with no corticomedullary differentiation, bone-within-bone appearance (most marked in the humeri), and rachitic bone ends. Rachitic appearances sometimes cause confusion; in OP they are believed to result from an inability to access the excessive total body calcium stores as a result of OC dysfunction. They are most likely to be found in patients with hypocalcemia, often in ARO caused by TCIRG1 mutations.

to transplantation.[18] Defects in RANK also result in OC-poor OP but these patients do seem to respond to HSCT.[4]

At the resorption site, acidification aids in dissolving the mineralized bone matrix. Therefore hydrogen ions formed by the action of carbonic anhydrase are actively pumped through the OC membrane onto the bone surface and chloride ions follow to maintain electrical neutrality. Defects of this mechanism explain two-thirds of all ARO. Carbonic anhydrase II (CA II) deficiency causes OP complicated by renal tubular acidosis and cerebral calcification. Involvement of the brain suggests that HSCT is not appropriate, although long-term follow-up of several transplanted children is awaited.[15] The *TCIRG1* (formerly *ATP6i*) gene encodes a proton pump; mutations of this gene explain 50% of all cases of ARO. Hypocalcemia and hypogammaglobulinemia are frequently present.[13] The *ClCN7* gene encodes a chloride channel protein. Mutations are responsible for 15% of cases of ARO and all cases of ADO II. In ARO this is caused by loss of function or stop mutations affecting both alleles, whereas in ADO mutation of just 1 allele produces disease through a dominant negative effect. Patients with *ClCN7*-mutated ARO can develop neurologic problems (eg, cerebellar atrophy) despite successful HSCT.[19] Five percent of patients have mutations of the *OSTM1* gene. The function of the Ostm1 protein is not fully elucidated but it must also have an important function in other tissues because patients also have lysosomal storage and neurodegeneration, making OSTM1 disease a contraindication for HSCT.[20]

Mutations affecting the *cathepsin K* gene, CTSK, result in pycnodysostosis (an important differential diagnosis for ARO). Very rarely, patients have been shown to have mutations of 3 other genes: *PLEKHM1*, *Kindlin-3* (with leukocyte adhesion deficiency III) and *NEMO* (NF-κB essential modulator, in a subset of patients with ectodermal dysplasia with immunodeficiency).[4]

Table 1
Classification of OP

Causative Gene/ Protein Product	OC Rich or Poor on Bone Biopsy	Frequency within AR OP (%)	Good Response to HSCT
ATP6i (TCIRG1) (proton pump)	Rich	50	Yes
ClCN7 (chloride channel)	Rich	15	Yes, but contraindicated in neuronopathic forms; late CNS pathology may occur
OSTM1	Rich	5	Contraindicated as neuronopathic disease not alleviated
TNFSF11 (RANKL)	Poor	3	Contraindicated as not caused by an intrinsic osteoclast defect
TNFRSF11A (RANK)	Poor	3	Yes, but long-term neurologic prognosis uncertain
CA2 (carbonic anhydrase II)	Rich	Not reported	Probably contraindicated; neurologic follow-up of patients reported in Ref.[15] awaited
PLEKHM1	Rich	<1	Not needed, mild form of OP
Kindlin-3	Not reported	<1	Not known
NEMO	Rich	<1	Not known
Unknown	Rich or poor	20–25	Not evaluable

Abbreviations: RANK, receptor activator NF-κB; RANKL, receptor activator NF-κB ligand.

Understanding of OC biology in human disease states has advanced rapidly since the late 1990s as a result of the development of in vitro culture systems.[21–23] These studies have become easier with the advent of recombinant RANKL and M-CSF, allowing direct culture of peripheral blood mononuclear cells on devitalized animal bone slices (**Fig. 2**).[17]

MEDICAL AND GENE THERAPY

The main agents that have been used in the management of patients with OP are calcitriol (1,25-hydroxyvitamin D), prednisolone, and γ-interferon.[1] Neither calcitriol nor high-dose steroids has a proven long-term benefit. Low-dose steroids may reduce or abolish transfusion requirements and should be considered in any child who is transfusion dependent. Key and colleagues[24] used γ-interferon after observing defective superoxide production in neutrophils from OP patients and noted a substantial reduction in the rate of infections, together with enhanced bone resorption. With

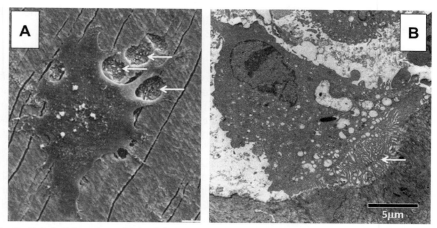

Fig. 2. Detailed imaging of OCs. (*A*) Scanning electron microscope and (*B*) transmission electron microscope images of OCs. (*A*) An OC has been cultured on a dentine slice; resorption pits are clearly seen (*arrowed*). (*B*) OC form ruffled borders (*arrowed*) to increase the surface area of membrane available to resorb bone. (*Courtesy of* Miep Helfrich, John Greenhorn, and Kevin Mackenzie, University of Aberdeen, UK.)

increasing use of HSCT this form of therapy has progressively fallen from favor, especially as the effects are only partial and thrice weekly subcutaneous injections are required.

Retroviral gene therapy resulted in survival of 50% of oc/oc (*TCIRG1*-mutated) mice, with almost complete normalization of skeletal phenotype if 20% of cells were gene corrected.[25] If OC-specific control elements can be introduced into these genes, and transduction or engraftment rates further improved, this is potentially a promising alternative to HSCT.

ANIMAL STUDIES AND FIRST HUMAN TRANSPLANTS

The history of HSCT for OP dates back to a series of seminal experiments performed by Donald Walker.[26] He showed that gray lethal (gl/gl) and microphthalmic (mi/mi) osteopetrotic mouse strains could be cured by temporarily joining the circulations of affected and unaffected mice or by transferring marrow or spleen cells, and that OCs in transplanted animals were of donor origin. These experiments led to the first attempt at unconditioned human bone marrow transplant in France in 1977 in a patient with CA II deficiency, with some transient beneficial effects but no documented donor engraftment.[27]

In 1980, Coccia and colleagues[28] reported successful engraftment of a patient using HLA-identical marrow after cyclophosphamide therapy and modified total body irradiation. Appearances of bone biopsies were completely normalized by 13 weeks after transplant (with male OC but female osteoblasts) and blood and metabolic abnormalities were corrected. Unfortunately, the graft was slowly rejected so that all blood and marrow cells were female by 18 months. This patient has dense bones many years later but no other symptoms of OP. Another patient was later described who had recurrence of osteosclerosis after slow loss of graft but remained free of other signs of OP.[29] This team of investigators, and others, began to report successful transplants during the 1980s from a range of matched and mismatched donors, with busulfan and cyclophosphamide as the backbone of the conditioning protocols to avoid radiotherapy.

LONG-TERM TRANSPLANT RESULTS

Because of the rarity of the disease there are comparatively few published series with long-term follow-up.[9,13,30–32] The largest are reports from the European Group for Blood and Marrow Transplantation (EBMT) on 69 and 122 patients respectively (with considerable overlap).[9,31] Five-year survival is considerably higher after HLA-identical sibling transplant (at 73%–79%) than after HSCT from unrelated or mismatched donors (13%–43%).

These results are comparatively poor for a benign disease, and the reasons seem to be multifactorial. Driessen and colleagues[9] reported post-transplant death in half the patients. Septicemia, pneumonia/pneumonitis, venoocclusive disease (VOD), and aplasia/hemorrhage accounted for 23%, 21%, 13%, and 11% of deaths, respectively. These problems are not surprising in a group of patients prone to ear, nose, and throat/chest infections and airway obstruction, and in whom busulfan has been a mainstay of conditioning therapy. Primary and secondary nonengraftment rates were also high, possibly because of restricted bone marrow cavities and relative hypersplenism compounding donor mismatch. When using non–HLA-identical donors, engraftment was seen in only 63% of patients. Other causes of death were neurologic (mostly in patients with OSTM1-related neuronopathic disease) or post-transplant hypercalcemia.

The high incidence of death caused by respiratory complications is notable in this series and in a large Bedouin kindred affected by *ATP6i* mutations (where acute respiratory distress syndrome or pulmonary hemorrhage caused the death of 5 of 9 patients transplanted).[33] There is reason to think that PAH may have contributed to the high death rates. PAH was recognized late in the time period reported by Driessen and colleagues[9] accounting for 2 deaths in this series and 4 deaths from 12 patients transplanted in the United States and Brazil.[34] In a study of consecutive patients, the incidence of PAH was found to be 29% in 28 patients from 3 European centers.[35] Chest radiographs from patients with PAH often show diffuse interstitial shadowing (suggesting pneumonitis), and right heart failure can produce hepatomegaly and ascites (leading to confusion with VOD). As this complication can respond completely to combinations of nitric oxide, defibrotide, and pulmonary vasodilators,[35] it is vital to consider PAH in any patient with OP who becomes hypoxemic in the first 3 months post-transplant.

Many children have an excellent quality of life after transplantation for OP, particularly if transplantation is performed before serious visual loss occurs. However, there are some important caveats. Vision continues to deteriorate despite technically successful transplantation in 25% of patients, and only a small proportion of children with significant visual loss show any improvement of vision after transplant.[9,33] Very few children grow above the centile that they are on at the time of transplant and some deteriorate further. Some children, particularly a proportion of those with *CICN7* mutation,[19] show neurologic deterioration despite successful HSCT.

RECOMMENDED PRETRANSPLANT WORKUP

Disease-specific components of routine workup should include full blood count, immunoglobulins, peripheral blood lymphocyte immunophenotyping, lactate dehydrogenase, alkaline phosphatase, calcium, phosphate, urine/blood pH (to exclude CA II deficiency). Ideally, serum and cryopreserved blood mononuclear cells should be stored in case more detailed investigations are required. Radiology should include films of 1 limb, the head, and chest. The brain should be imaged by either computed tomography or magnetic resonance imaging. Detailed neurologic, ENT, and ophthalmic examinations are required; an electroencephalogram may be appropriate. An electrocardiogram and an echocardiogram can help to exclude antecedent PAH.[13]

Infants presenting with typical infantile ARO should be investigated immediately for *TCIRG1* and *ClCN7* mutations. Irritable children should be investigated for fractures, but neuronopathic disease must be excluded in those who are hypertonic or irritable despite analgesia. Neuronopathic OP may be caused by *OSTM1* (especially in Arab races) or *ClCN7* mutations; retinal abnormalities are an important indicator (but absence does not exclude neuronopathic OP).

Gene mutation analysis may introduce delay. Serious consideration should therefore be given to an initial closed trephine biopsy from the posterior iliac crest. This is easy to perform and should show normal or increased numbers of OC in most patients with transplantable disease (**Fig. 3**). Patients with reduced or absent OC should be investigated for *RANK* and *RANKL* mutations and discussed with experts, as should patients more than 2 years of age (especially if blood counts are normal).

TCIRG1-mutated patients (50% of cases) should be considered for transplantation as soon as possible, as should those with biallelic mutations of *ClCN7*, although the parents should be counseled about the uncertainty of long-term neurologic outcome in the latter. The decision to transplant should only be taken after careful discussion with the families in those with highly compromised visual ± hearing status or who lack well-matched donors. If vision is failing, a discussion about the role of optic decompression may be appropriate.[7,36] Caution must always be exercised about the prediction of post-transplant visual status.

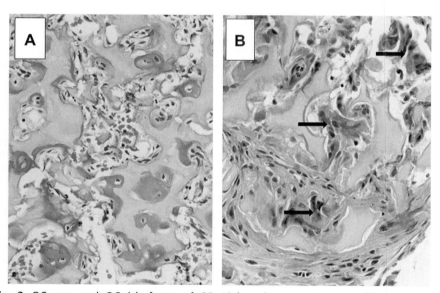

Fig. 3. OC-poor and OC-rich forms of OP. Light microscope images of bone marrow trephines taken percutaneously from the posterior superior iliac spines of patients with (*A*) OC-poor (causative gene unknown) and (*B*) OC-rich (TCIRG1-mutated) forms of OP. Multinucleate OC cannot be identified in (*A*) but are in excess in (*B*), occurring even in clusters (*arrowed*). (*Courtesy of* Pramila Ramani, Royal Infirmary, Bristol, UK.)

Most patients have very high circulating CD34+ lymphocyte counts as part of their leukoerythroblastic blood status. This can allow a backup harvest by limited exchange transfusion, which may be valuable when alternative donor transplantation is to be performed.[8]

DONOR CHOICE AND CONDITIONING THERAPY

Disease-free HLA-identical donors are the optimal choice, followed by phenotypically matched family donors.[9] Bone marrow or peripheral blood stem cells from matched unrelated donors are currently preferred over cord donors, although definitive registry publications on cord transplantation are awaited. Haploidentical transplantation results have improved significantly with use of high-dose CD34 selected peripheral blood stem cells given as an initial infusion followed by a second infusion later in the first month after transplant.[37]

The current preference in Europe is to try to reduce the risk of VOD by using intravenous rather than oral busulfan, to substitute fludarabine for cyclophosphamide (because of lower toxicity profile), and to add thiotepa in nongenoidentical transplants. There is no clear preference for graft-versus-host disease prophylaxis.

POST-TRANSPLANT CARE

Bones often take 12 months or more to progressively normalize on radiographs, even with high-level donor engraftment.[5] Secondary graft rejection may cause recurrence of OP if the level of donor cells becomes less than 10% to 20%. Hypercalcemia is a post-transplant risk, especially in those older than 2 years (60% in 1 series) because of their higher bone mass.[9] Hypercalcemia can occur from engraftment onwards, necessitating careful serial monitoring, and can be treated with bisphosphonates, diuretics, and forced diuresis.[38]

Careful attention should be paid to visual and auditory status, and any requirements for educational or occupational support. Patients should be warned that growth may be compromised despite successful transplantation. Growth hormone deficiency has not been widely reported as a problem and few patients have received radiation therapy. Regular dental review is required.

SUMMARY

OP is a much more complicated disease than was appreciated just a decade ago, caused by a diverse range of genes with differing effects on OC formation and function. Presentation and clinical behavior vary widely even within disease caused by the same gene. HSCT still carries many risks, some unique to this disease, and a high proportion of patients have sequelae of their disease despite transplantation. Careful pretransplant assessment, including a concerted attempt to determine the genetic subtype of the disease, and a low threshold to discussion with experts are critical to determining the appropriateness of transplantation and best management of this complex disease.

REFERENCES

1. Askmyr MK, Fasth A, Richter J. Towards a better understanding and new therapeutics of osteopetrosis. Br J Haematol 2008;140:597–609.
2. Gerritsen EJ, Vossen JM, van Loo IH, et al. Autosomal recessive osteopetrosis: variability of findings at diagnosis and during the natural course. Pediatrics 1994;93:247–53.

3. Wilson CJ, Vellodi A. Autosomal recessive osteopetrosis: diagnosis, management, and outcome. Arch Dis Child 2000;83:449–52.

4. Villa A, Guerrini MM, Cassani B, et al. Infantile malignant, autosomal recessive osteopetrosis: the rich and the poor. Calcif Tissue Int 2009;84:1–12.

5. Cheow HK, Steward CG, Grier DJ. Imaging of malignant infantile osteopetrosis before and after bone marrow transplantation. Pediatr Radiol 2001;31:869–75.

6. Abinun M, Newson T, Rowe PW, et al. Importance of neurological assessment before bone marrow transplantation for osteopetrosis. Arch Dis Child 1999;80: 273–4.

7. Steward CG. Neurological aspects of osteopetrosis. Neuropathol Appl Neurobiol 2003;29:87–97.

8. Steward CG, Blair A, Moppett J, et al. High peripheral blood progenitor cell counts enable autologous backup before stem cell transplantation for malignant infantile osteopetrosis. Biol Blood Marrow Transplant 2005;11:115–21.

9. Driessen GJ, Gerritsen EJ, Fischer A, et al. Long-term outcome of haematopoietic stem cell transplantation in autosomal recessive osteopetrosis: an EBMT report. Bone Marrow Transplant 2003;32:657–63.

10. Srinivasan M, Abinun M, Cant AJ, et al. Malignant infantile osteopetrosis presenting with neonatal hypocalcaemia. Arch Dis Child Fetal Neonatal Ed 2000;83: F21–3.

11. Wong ML, Balkany TJ, Reeves J, et al. Head and neck manifestations of malignant osteopetrosis. Otolaryngology 1978;86:ORL585–94.

12. Luzzi V, Consoli G, Daryanani V, et al. Malignant infantile osteopetrosis: dental effects in paediatric patients. Case reports. Eur J Paediatr Dent 2006;7:39–44.

13. Mazzolari E, Forino C, Razza A, et al. A single-center experience in 20 patients with infantile malignant osteopetrosis. Am J Hematol 2009;84:473–9.

14. Waguespack SG, Hui SL, Dimeglio LA, et al. Autosomal dominant osteopetrosis: clinical severity and natural history of 94 subjects with a chloride channel 7 gene mutation. J Clin Endocrinol Metab 2007;92:771–8.

15. McMahon C, Will A, Hu P, et al. Bone marrow transplantation corrects osteopetrosis in the carbonic anhydrase II deficiency syndrome. Blood 2001;97:1947–50.

16. Del Fattore A, Peruzzi B, Rucci N, et al. Clinical, genetic, and cellular analysis of 49 osteopetrotic patients: implications for diagnosis and treatment. J Med Genet 2006;43:315–25.

17. Flanagan AM, Massey HM, Wilson C, et al. Macrophage colony-stimulating factor and receptor activator NF-kappaB ligand fail to rescue osteoclast-poor human malignant infantile osteopetrosis in vitro. Bone 2002;30:85–90.

18. Sobacchi C, Frattini A, Guerrini MM, et al. Osteoclast-poor human osteopetrosis due to mutations in the gene encoding RANKL. Nat Genet 2007;39:960–2.

19. Frattini A, Pangrazio A, Susani L, et al. Chloride channel ClCN7 mutations are responsible for severe recessive, dominant, and intermediate osteopetrosis. J Bone Miner Res 2003;18:1740–7.

20. Pangrazio A, Poliani PL, Megarbane A, et al. Mutations in OSTM1 (grey lethal) define a particularly severe form of autosomal recessive osteopetrosis with neural involvement. J Bone Miner Res 2006;21:1098–105.

21. Flanagan AM, Sarma U, Steward CG, et al. Study of the nonresorptive phenotype of osteoclast-like cells from patients with malignant osteopetrosis: a new approach to investigating pathogenesis. J Bone Miner Res 2000;15:352–60.

22. Helfrich MH, Gerritsen EJ. Formation of non-resorbing osteoclasts from peripheral blood mononuclear cells of patients with malignant juvenile osteopetrosis. Br J Haematol 2001;112:64–8.

23. Teti A, Migliaccio S, Taranta A, et al. Mechanisms of osteoclast dysfunction in human osteopetrosis: abnormal osteoclastogenesis and lack of osteoclast-specific adhesion structures. J Bone Miner Res 1999;14:2107–17.
24. Key LL Jr, Rodriguiz RM, Willi SM, et al. Long-term treatment of osteopetrosis with recombinant human interferon gamma. N Engl J Med 1995;332:1594–9.
25. Johansson MK, de Vries TJ, Schoenmaker T, et al. Hematopoietic stem cell-targeted neonatal gene therapy reverses lethally progressive osteopetrosis in oc/oc mice. Blood 2007;109:5178–85.
26. Walker DG. Control of bone resorption by hematopoietic tissue. The induction and reversal of congenital osteopetrosis in mice through use of bone marrow and splenic transplants. J Exp Med 1975;142:651–63.
27. Ballet JJ, Griscelli C, Coutris C, et al. Bone-marrow transplantation in osteopetrosis. Lancet 1977;2:1137.
28. Coccia PF, Krivit W, Cervenka J, et al. Successful bone-marrow transplantation for infantile malignant osteopetrosis. N Engl J Med 1980;302:701–8.
29. Coccia PF. Cells that resorb bone. N Engl J Med 1984;310:456–8.
30. Eapen M, Davies SM, Ramsay NK, et al. Hematopoietic stem cell transplantation for infantile osteopetrosis. Bone Marrow Transplant 1998;22:941–6.
31. Gerritsen EJ, Vossen JM, Fasth A, et al. Bone marrow transplantation for autosomal recessive osteopetrosis. A report from the Working Party on Inborn Errors of the European Bone Marrow Transplantation Group. J Pediatr 1994;125:896–902.
32. Solh H, Da Cunha AM, Giri N, et al. Bone marrow transplantation for infantile malignant osteopetrosis. J Pediatr Hematol Oncol 1995;17:350–5.
33. Kapelushnik J, Shalev C, Yaniv I, et al. Osteopetrosis: a single centre experience of stem cell tranisplantation and prenatal diagnosis. Bone Marrow Transplant 2001;27:129–32.
34. Kasow KA, Bonfim C, Asch J, et al. Malignant infantile osteopetrosis and primary pulmonary hypertension: a new combination? Pediatr Blood Cancer 2004;42:190–4.
35. Steward CG, Pellier I, Mahajan A, et al. Severe pulmonary hypertension: a frequent complication of stem cell transplantation for malignant infantile osteopetrosis. Br J Haematol 2004;124:63–71.
36. Cummings TJ, Proia AD. Optic nerve compression in infantile malignant auto-somal recessive osteopetrosis. J Pediatr Ophthalmol Strabismus 2004;41:241–4.
37. Schulz AS, Classen CF, Mihatsch WA, et al. HLA-haploidentical blood progenitor cell transplantation in osteopetrosis. Blood 2002;99:3458–60.
38. Rawlinson PS, Green RH, Coggins AM, et al. Malignant osteopetrosis: hypercal-caemia after bone marrow transplantation. Arch Dis Child 1991;66:638–9.

Hematopoietic Stem Cell Transplantation for Hemoglobinopathies: Current Practice and Emerging Trends

Frans J. Smiers, MD, PhD[a],*, Lakshmanan Krishnamurti, MD[b],
Guido Lucarelli, MD[c]

KEYWORDS

- Hematopoietic stem cell transplantation • HSCT
- Hemoglobinopathies

Hemoglobinopathies are a group of diseases characterized by abnormal function or synthesis of the hemoglobin molecule. The thalassemias and sickle cell disease (SCD) are by far the commonest hemoglobinopathies and represent a significant public health burden. These diseases are characterized by inherited lifelong anemia as a result of hemolysis and dyserythropoiesis. Patients with thalassemia major and a subset of patients with SCD require chronic red cell transfusions and are at risk for complications related to iron overload. In patients with SCD, the consequences of vasoocclusion and chronic vasculopathy contribute to substantial morbidity and premature mortality. Both diseases are associated with significant individual and societal costs, and pose a major burden on the health care system. Advances in managing these patients have substantially improved the quality of life and survival of patients with hemoglobinopathies. However, hematopoietic stem cell transplantation (HSCT) remains for now the only treatment with curative intent.

Results of HSCT using a human leukocyte antigen (HLA)-identical donor are excellent, and all patients with thalassemia major who have an available HLA-identical donor should be considered for HSCT. In addition, HSCT from HLA-identical donors is also being offered to patients with SCD who meet consensually derived criteria of severe disease.

[a] Leiden University Medical Center, Department of Pediatrics, Hematology Oncology and BMT unit, Postbus 9600, 2300 RC, Leiden, The Netherlands
[b] Division of Hematology/Oncology/BoneMarrow Transplantation, Children's Hospital of Pittsburgh of UPMC, One Children's Hospital Drive, 4401 Penn Avenue, Pittsburgh, PA 15224, USA
[c] International Centre for Transplantation in Thalassemia and Sickle Cell Anemia, Mediterranean Institute of Hematology, Corso Vittorio Emanuele II, 14, Rome, 00186, Italy
* Corresponding author.
E-mail address: f.j.smiers@lumc.nl

Pediatr Clin N Am 57 (2010) 181–205
doi:10.1016/j.pcl.2010.01.003
0031-3955/10/$ – see front matter
pediatric.theclinics.com

Existing criteria for recipients and donor selection and transplant procedures for this patient population are being challenged by advances in HLA typing, the development of new and less toxic preparative regimens, improved supportive care, and a better understanding of the natural history of these diseases. This review presents an update of the status and describes emerging trends in HSCT for thalassemia and patients with SCD.

OVERVIEW OF β THALASSEMIA

β thalassemia is an autosomal recessive disease with mutations within the β gene cluster located on chromosome 11. More than 200 different mutations, mostly point mutations and rarely deletions, causing a thalassemic phenotype have been described, with a poor genotype-phenotype correlation.[1] Any of these genetic changes results in a synthesis imbalance between the α and β globin chains and results in an accumulation of excess unpaired α chains leading to oxidative damage of the erythrocyte membrane and hemolysis.[2] The severity of anemia cannot be conferred from the genetic change.[3,4]

Anemia in β thalassemia is the result of 2 pathologic processes: hemolysis and ineffective erythropoiesis. In β thalassemia the patient's excessive erythropoiesis, combined with a high rate of erythroid precursor cell apoptosis, results in a hypercellular bone marrow.[5,6]

Ineffective erythropoiesis can be a result of maturation failure, apoptosis during maturation, or unstable erythrocytes with a severely shortened lifespan. The exact mechanisms leading to ineffective erythropoiesis are elusive.[7–9] Iron metabolism in thalassemia is affected by the level of ineffective erythropoiesis, hypoxia, and the number of transfusions (causing iron overload).[10]

Clinical sequelae of thalassemia include delay in growth and development, deformity of bones because of ectopic marrow expansion, osteopenia, and, most importantly, iron overload. The latter results in serious organ damage[11,12] and can have fatal consequences if not treated adequately with iron-chelating therapy.[13,14] Desferrioxamine has been the mainstay of iron chelation since its introduction in the 1980s. However, patient acceptability and compliance have been limited by the discomfort associated with the need for daily subcutaneous infusions. The introduction of oral iron chelators, deferasirox and deferiprone, has dramatically improved the patients' acceptability of chelation. It remains to be seen whether these will consistently translate into improved compliance and optimal iron chelation.

Treatment is focused on maintaining pretransfusion hemoglobin levels of more than 9 to 10 g/dL to allow normal growth and development and suppress endogenous erythropoiesis, diminish intravascular hemolysis, and therefore lessen the enhanced endogenous iron accumulation. Although the implementation of hypertransfusion regimens has substantially improved the survival and quality of life of patients with thalassemia major, this approach comes at a price. This price includes transfusional hemosiderosis with multiorgan involvement, complications related to exposure to multiple donors (allosensitization, transmission of viruses and other pathogens), cost, discomfort, and inconvenience of a chronic intensive treatment regimen. Another treatment approach is the use of hydroxyurea, an agent that seems to raise hemoglobin F levels, and thereby prolongs the erythrocyte lifespan. In some patients hydroxyurea reduces the need for transfusions dramatically, whereas in others no effect is observed.[15–17] This may be related to the individual's genetic makeup.[18]

Survival in β Thalassemia

Survival in thalassemia is highly correlated with the availability of appropriate medical supportive care. Before 1980, median survival was 17.1 years, with 50% of patients dying before the age of 12 years.[19–21] Regular erythrocyte transfusions combined with iron chelation changed the prognosis of β thalassemia dramatically.[21–23] However, compliance with chelation therapy remains a burden and affects outcome. Compliant patients have a 50% to 60% chance of being alive at age 30 years, whereas noncompliant patients only have a 10% chance of being alive at this age.[21,24,25] The main cause of death is cardiac disease induced by iron overload. New monitoring techniques for cardiac iron accumulation and better compliance with chelation because of the availability of oral iron chelators can potentially result in further improvement of survival and quality of life.[25,26]

OVERVIEW OF SCD

SCD is a hemolytic disease characterized by abnormally sickle-shaped red blood cells (RBCs), which are removed from the circulation and destroyed at increased rates, leading to anemia. Current understanding of the pathophysiology of SCD has been reviewed elsewhere.[27,28] Intravascular hemolysis releases free hemoglobin, which binds with high affinity to nitric oxide, disturbing the normal vascular homeostatic function of nitric oxide. The resulting vasoconstriction further compromises the transit time of erythrocytes and contributes to vasoocclusion.[29–31]

The result of these processes is infarctions of different sizes anywhere in the body with, eventually, destruction of affected organs. Functional asplenia as a result of multiple infarctions has been found before the age of 1 year. At age 5 years 94% of patients with SCD will be asplenic. This condition makes even the young patient with SCD susceptible to encapsulated bacterial infections and sepsis, and this is the most common cause of death in the young patient with SCD.

Bone infarction leads to painful crises, growth disturbance, and high susceptibility to osteomyelitis. Repeated pain crisis has a severely negative effect on quality of life.[32–34] Kidney damage results in uncontrolled loss of proteins and water.[35,36] Vascular damage of the erectile tissue of the penis results in priapism and ultimately erectile dysfunction.[37–40]

Acute chest syndrome (ACS) is a serious and sometimes fatal complication.[41] Chronic pulmonary sequelae include pulmonary fibrosis and pulmonary hypertension, the latter being associated with increased mortality.[42,43]

Stroke in SCD was described more than 75 years ago.[44] The cumulative incidence of stroke ranges from 11% at age 20 years to 24% at age 45 years.[45] Silent infarct identified at age 6 years or older is associated with increased stroke risk.[46] Screening of the cerebral arteries by transcranial Doppler (TCD) ultrasound can identify high-risk patients for stroke.[47–49] Intervention with regular erythrocyte transfusions has been shown to diminish the risk of stroke.[50–55] It is unclear how long these regular transfusions need to be continued, but regular transfusions carry the risk of iron overload, alloimmunization, and hyperhemolysis syndrome.

Hydroxyurea has been used successfully in patients with SCD experiencing recurrent pain crises or ACS.[56,57] Whether hydroxyurea reduces the risk for stroke and could avoid chronic erythrocyte transfusion therapy in high-risk patients is still a matter of debate.[57–61] Short-term toxicity consists of dose-dependent leucopenia. Late effects are becoming more of a concern because spermatogenesis could be severely affected.[58,62–64]

Survival in SCD

Until about 30 years ago, childhood mortality from SCD was high and survival into adulthood uncommon.[65–67] Survival has improved in recent decades and the

Cooperative Study of Sickle Cell Disease (CSSCD) demonstrated 15 years ago that the mean age of death for patients with SCD had increased to 42 years for men and 48 years for women.[41] This still constitutes a 25- to 30-year loss of life expectancy.

HSCT

Despite improvement of supportive care in β thalassemia and SCD, life expectancy remains lower than for those not affected. In addition, quality of life for patients with hemoglobinopathies is usually significantly impaired. Currently, allogeneic HSCT remains the only curative treatment.

In β thalassemia major, results with HSCT are in general better if no iron overload or organ damage is present and the patient has received a minimal number of erythrocyte transfusions. With improved HLA-typing techniques, conditioning regiments, and supportive care, it has become possible to transplant β thalassemia major patients with HLA-identical and unrelated donors. In selected patients haploidentical transplantation in which 1 or both parents serve as stem cell donor, can also be considered.

In patients with SCD, timing of transplantation is more complicated, because the clinical course can be so variable and does not seem linked to specific mutations. Ideally, HSCT is performed before any damage occurs.

HSCT in Thalassemia

Analysis of data on HSCT from HLA-matched family donors in 222 patients with thalassemia aged less than 17 years who were all treated with the same regimen revealed 3 adverse factors: hepatomegaly greater than 2 cm, portal fibrosis, and an irregular chelation history.[68–70] Based on these risk factors, patients were categorized into 3 risk classes. Class 1 patients had no risk factor, class 2 patients had up to 2, and class 3 patients had all 3 risk factors. Pretransplant risk categorization allows adjustment of the preparative regimens, thereby improving outcomes.[71]

Patients with advanced-stage disease (class 3 patients) have a higher incidence of graft failure compared with patients with class 1 or 2 disease. Following graft rejection, there is autologous reconstitution with the thalassemic bone marrow. Occasionally, patients reject donor grafts without recurrence of thalassemia. Unless rescued by a second transplant, such patients will die from the consequences of marrow aplasia. The treatment of patients after graft rejection differs, depending on whether the rejection is accompanied by regeneration of host type hematopoiesis or by marrow aplasia.

RESULTS OF HSCT FROM HLA-MATCHED RELATED DONORS
Historical Experience

Class 1 patients are usually young. Between October 1985 and January 2003, 146 class 1 patients with a median age of 4 years (range 1–16 years) were transplanted following conditioning with busulfan (BU) 3.5 mg/kg/d for 4 consecutive days and cyclophosphamide (CY) 50 mg/kg/d for the subsequent 4 days. Graft-versus-host disease (GVHD) prophylaxis consisted of cyclosporine (CSA) and low-dose methylprednisolone (MP) for all but the last 37 patients who received CSA, MP, and a modified short course of methotrexate (MTX). Overall survival (OS) and thalassemia-free survival were 90% and 87%, respectively. The probability of rejection was 3%.[69,72]

Meanwhile, 315 class 2 patients with a median age of 9 years (range 2–16 years) were transplanted following the same conditioning regimen with an OS and thalassemia-free survival of 87% and 85%, respectively. The probability of rejection was 3%.[69,72]

When class 3 patients less than 17 years of age were transplanted using the same conditioning regimen as used for class 1 and 2 patients, thalassemia-free survival dropped to 53% and OS to 57%.[73] In an attempt to improve outcomes for these patients, new treatment regimens were devised using BU at a total dose of 14 mg/kg and CY at total doses of 160 and 120 mg/kg. Such regimens improved OS from 53% to 79%, but were associated with an increase of rejection probability from 7% to 30%, likely because of inadequate immunosuppression and failure to eradicate the massive erythroid hyperplasia characteristic of these patients.[69,72–74] This experience led to the development of a new preparative regimen (named Protocol 26) for class 3 patients.[71] Protocol 26 was devised on the assumption that preparation with BU 14 mg/kg and CY 160 mg/kg was inadequate to eradicate thalassemic hematopoiesis in class 3 patients less than 17 years of age. The new protocol involved an intensified preparation with 3 mg/kg of azathioprine and 30 mg/kg hydroxyurea daily from day −45 from the transplant, fludarabine (FLU) 20 mg/m^2 from day −17 to day −13, followed by the administration of BU 14 mg/kg total dose and CY 160 mg/kg total dose. GVHD prophylaxis consisted of CSA, low-dose MP, a modified short course of MTX. During HSCT preparation, patients were transfused to keep their hemoglobin levels between 14 and 15 g/dL. They also underwent continuous desferoxamine infusion via a central venous catheter, and received growth factors, granulocyte colony-stimulating factor, and erythropoietin twice weekly to maintain stem cell proliferation in the face of hypertransfusion, thereby facilitating the effect of the hydroxyurea. The probabilities of survival, thalassemia-free survival, rejection, and nonrejection mortality in 33 patients treated on Protocol 26 were 93%, 85%, 8%, and 6%, respectively.[71] This regimen improved the probability of thalassemia-free survival from 58% to 85%, and reduced the probability of rejection from 30% to 8% compared with previous preparative regimens.

Adult patients

Adult patients with thalassemia (age >17 years) have more advanced disease and treatment-related organ complications, mainly because of prolonged exposure to iron overload. Their probabilities of OS, thalassemia-free survival, rejection, and non-rejection mortality were 66%, 62%, 4%, and 37%, respectively.[75,76] Using a slightly modified Protocol 26 (they received CY 90 mg/kg total dose), the probabilities of OS, thalassemia-free survival, rejection, and nonrejection mortality in 15 high-risk adult patients were 65%, 65%, 7%, and 28%, respectively.[77]

CURRENT EXPERIENCE

In 2004, the International Center for Transplantation in Thalassemia and Sickle Cell Anemia was established at the Mediterranean Institute of Hematology in Rome. Since inception, HSCT from HLA-matched related donors have been performed in 18 class 1, 33 class 2, and 44 class 3 patients. The probability of OS, thalassemia-free survival, rejection, and transplant-related mortality in class 1 patients is 94%, 89%, 6%,and 6%, respectively; in class 2 patients 97%, 91%, 6%, and 3%, respectively; and in class 3 patients 86%, 79%, 10%, and 13%, respectively.

Mixed Chimerism

Mixed hematopoietic chimerism (MC) is a common phenomenon after myeloablative transplantation for thalassemia. In a group of 335 patients who were ex-thalassemic the incidence of MC at 2 months was 32.2%.[74] Although none of the 227 patients with complete chimerism at 2 months rejected their grafts, 35 of 108 patients with MC determined at the same time lost the graft, suggesting that MC after HSCT for thalassemia is a risk factor for rejection. The percentages of residual host hematopoietic cells (RHCs) after transplant were predictive for graft rejection with nearly all patients experiencing graft rejection when RHCs exceeded 25%, and only 13% of patients showing rejection when RHCs were less than 10%.[78,79] Patients with RHCs between 10% and 25% had a 41% risk of rejection. MC was shown to occur in all thalassemia patients after HSCT with cord blood,[80] but graft rejection could not be predicted by existence or persistence of MC.

Stable MC can occur after HSCT. Ten percent of patients receiving HSCT for thalassemia following myeloablative conditioning became persistent mixed chimeras and are transfusion-independent, suggesting that few engrafted donor cells might be sufficient for correction of disease phenotype in patients with thalassemia major once a donor-host tolerance has been established. The role of regulatory T cells is intriguing and the focus of important research.[81–83]

Graft Failure or Rejection

Patients with engraftment failure and without functioning marrow have a bleak prospect because an early second transplant with a second course of conditioning is usually not a reasonable option. However, occasionally patients have late graft failure without thalassemia recurrence and, in this situation, second transplant attempts with intensive conditioning may provide the only treatment option for prolonged survival.

Patients who reject their grafts and have a return of host hematopoiesis do not have an urgent need for second transplant. A second HSCT can be delayed until the toxic effects of the conditioning regimen of the first transplants have ameliorated. At least a year should be allowed to elapse between the first and second transplant. Historical data of second transplants for thalassemia show high graft failure and high mortality rates.[84] In 2003 a new conditioning regimen for second transplants in thalassemia was devised. A recent analysis of the results of second transplantation in 16 thalassemia patients treated with this new treatment protocol showed a higher engraftment (94%) and thalassemia-free survival rates (79%).[85]

GVHD

Historical retrospective analysis shows that the probability of grade II to IV acute GVHD (AGVHD) is significantly low (17%) in patients given CSA and a short course of MTX, compared with patients receiving CSA and MP GVHD prophylaxis. However, patients treated with CSA, MP, and MTX have a high incidence of graft failure, and the estimated incidence of AGVHD was probably underestimated. The probability of moderate or severe chronic GVHD in patients with thalassemia was 8% and 2%, respectively.[86]

MANAGEMENT OF PATIENTS WITH THALASSEMIA AFTER SUCCESSFUL TRANSPLANT (EX-THALASSEMIC)

Most patients who are ex-thalassemic still carry the clinical complications acquired during years of transfusion and chelation therapy. Among the issues requiring long-term management are iron overload, chronic hepatitis, liver fibrosis, and endocrine dysfunction. Management of these complications is important. Iron stores after transplantation remain elevated in most patients receiving HSCT in advanced stage of disease (class 2 and class 3 patients).[87] Analysis of the natural history of liver fibrosis following HSCT for thalassemia shows that ion overload and hepatitis C virus (HCV) infection are independent risk factors for liver fibrosis progression.[88] Therefore, the toxic effect of iron overload contributing to progression of already-present organ damage should be avoided as soon as possible using posttransplant iron depletion. Regular phlebotomy or chelation therapy can successfully remove excess iron from the body by normalizing the iron pool, which results in marked improvement in liver and cardiac function.[89–92]

Growth failure and endocrine dysfunction are common in patients with thalassemia major treated by conventional treatment. Although the role of BU-containing regimens on growth velocity after transplant remains controversial, the negative effect of this regimen on gonadal damage is well documented. Children receiving transplant before 8 years of age showed a normal growth rate, whereas older children, class 3 patients, and patients who developed chronic GVHD had impaired growth.[93] Gonadal damage is a common side effect of BU-CY–based conditioning regimens. Approximately one-third of boys and two-thirds of girls failed to spontaneously enter puberty following transplant.[94] Nevertheless, some patients can restore their fertility after transplant, which is supported by the observations of 5 successful pregnancies and 4 spontaneous paternities in patients who are ex-thalassemic (Guido Lucarelli, personal communication, 2009).[95] These data show that patients exposed to BU-CY regimens are not inevitably infertile.

Infection with HCV is common in patients with thalassemia; particularly in those transfused before second generation, enzyme-linked immunosorbent assays (ELISA) became available for detecting HCV in donor blood. In thalassemia, liver damage as a result of HCV infection is exacerbated by iron overload, and liver disease is a recognized cause of mortality and morbidity. Chronic HCV infection and transplant-related complications are probably the only factors that may limit survival in patients who are ex-thalassemic. Thus, avoidance of progression of liver damage to cirrhosis must be a primary goal. Present standard therapy is the peginterferon α/ribavirin combination for adults and children without thalassemia.[96] Concerns about ribavirin-induced hemolysis and worsening of the anemia and iron overload limit the use of this therapy in patients with thalassemia. Patients who are ex-thalassemic with complete donor chimerism and chronic HCV will experience the same side effects as those without thalassemia. Therefore, patients who are ex-thalassemic should be offered treatment with the peginterferon α/ribavirin combination after they have completed their iron-depletion program.

With the increasing number of transplant survivors, there is a risk for secondary malignancies. Patients who received HSCT for thalassemia major and SCD had a low incidence (0.8%) of malignancies (Guido Lucarelli, personal communication, 2009).

INDICATIONS FOR HSCT IN SCD

Indications for HSCT have been empirically determined from prognostic factors derived from studies of the natural history of SCD. **Box 1** describes criteria for transplantation used in the national collaborative study of HSCT for SCD.[97] With improved outcomes for HSCT, advances in other therapeutic options and better understanding of the various complications of SCD, the risk/benefit ratio of HSCT versus conventional treatment, and consequently indications for HSCT, are likely to change. Abnormal TCD, a test that measures the velocity of blood flow through the brain's blood vessels, predicts the risk for stroke. Patients with SCD and abnormal TCD require chronic blood transfusion to prevent stroke.[55] Currently, there is no known safe duration after which chronic transfusion can be discontinued.[98] Further, the natural history of an abnormal TCD following chronic transfusion is unclear. Thus, patients with abnormal TCD are at risk for all the morbidities associated with chronic transfusion and an undefined risk from progression of vasculopathy. It is conceivable

---

Box 1
Indications for HSCT in SCD

Patients 16 years old or younger with SCD with an HLA-identical sibling bone marrow donor with 1 or more of the following:

- Stroke, central nervous system (CNS) hemorrhage or a neurologic event lasting longer than 24 hours or abnormal cerebral magnetic resonance imaging (MRI) scan or cerebral arteriogram or MRI angiographic study and impaired neuropsychological testing

- ACS with a history of recurrent hospitalizations or exchange transfusions

- Recurrent vasoocclusive pain 3 or more episodes per year for 3 years or more or recurrent priapism

- Impaired neuropsychological function and abnormal cerebral MRI scan

- Stage I or II sickle lung disease

- Sickle nephropathy (moderate or severe proteinuria or a glomerular filtration rate [GFR] 30%–50% of the predicted normal value)

- Bilateral proliferative retinopathy and major visual impairment in at least 1 eye

- Osteonecrosis of multiple joints with documented destructive changes

- Requirement for chronic transfusions but with RBC alloimmunization of more than 2 antibodies during long-term transfusion therapy

Data from Walters MC, Patience M, Leisenring W, et al. Bone marrow transplantation for sickle cell disease. N Engl J Med 1996;335(6):369–76.

---

that, in the future, this group of patients will be considered for HSCT. Similarly, pulmonary artery hypertension (PAH) is highly prevalent in adolescents and young adults with SCD and is associated with a high degree of premature mortality.[42] In the future, PAH confirmed by cardiac catheterization may become an indication for HSCT. The availability of oral iron chelation has reduced the pain and complexity of this treatment, although challenges to compliance remain a problem. Efforts to recruit blood donors of minority origin can increase the availability of RBCs matched at minor RBC antigens and decrease the rate of allosensitization. Thus, improved chelation and transfusion practices may make transfusion a more attractive option for some patients and obviate the need for HSCT. The emerging understanding of the rapid progression of disease-related complications and premature mortality in adults is increasingly leading to the consideration of HSCT for this group of patients.[99,100]

ATTITUDES OF PARENTS AND PATIENTS TOWARD ACCEPTABILITY OF HSCT-RELATED RISKS

Consideration of HSCT and its timing has been limited by physicians' concerns regarding the acceptability of morbidity and mortality associated with this therapeutic option. This limitation is shown by the variation in the proportion of patients (0.9%–36%) considered to be eligible for HSCT in various centers participating in a national trial of HSCT for children with SCD.[101] Acceptability of HSCT for this chronic illness is also affected by the attitudes of patients and their parents. In one study, 54% of parents were willing to accept some risk of short-term mortality, 37% were willing to accept at least the 15% short-term mortality risk, 12% were willing to accept a short-term mortality risk of 50% or more, and 13% said they would accept a mortality risk of 15% or more and an additional 15% risk of GVHD.[102] The parents' decisions were not related to the clinical severity of their children's illness. In a study of adult patients with SCD, 63% of patients were willing to accept some short-term risk of mortality in exchange for the certainty of cure, whereas 15% were willing to accept a mortality risk of more than 35%.[103] No differences in patient- or disease-related variables were identified between those accepting risk and those not accepting risk. There was no agreement between the recommendations of health care providers and the risk accepted by patients. Thus, a better understanding of the perspective of patients and their parents on the decision to consider HSCT is critical to the successful application of this therapy for patients with SCD.

RESULTS OF HSCT IN SCD

Allogeneic HSCT after myeloablative therapy has been performed in approximately 250 young (<16 years of age) patients with SCD (**Table 1**). The backbone of the preparative regimens used has consisted of BU (14 to 16 mg/kg) and CY (200 mg/kg). Additional immunosuppressive agents used have included antithymocyte globulin (ATG), rabbit ATG (rATG),[104] antilymphocyte globulin (ALG),[105] or total lymphoid irradiation (TLI).[106] CSA alone or with MP or MTX has been used for posttransplant GVHD prophylaxis.

The outcomes of HSCT for patients with SCD from matched siblings is excellent with an OS of 93% to 97% and an event-free survival (EFS) of 85%.[41,105–119] Stabilization or reversal of organ damage from SCD has been documented after HSCT.[118] In patients who have stable donor engraftment, complications related to SCD resolve, and there are no further episodes of pain, stroke, or ACS. Patients who are successfully allografted do not experience sickle-related CNS complications and have evidence of stabilization of CNS disease by cerebral MRI.[120–125] However, the effect of successful HSCT on reversal of cerebral vasculopathy has been variable.[122–125] HSCT for SCD generally does not cause growth impairment in young children; however, diminished growth may occur if HSCT is performed near or during the adolescent growth spurt.[126] An adverse effect of BU conditioning on ovarian function was reported in 5 of 7 evaluable female patients who are currently at least 13 years of age. None of the 4 male patients tested had elevated serum gonadotropin levels.[118] Radiological improvement of a patient with osteonecrosis of humeral head[127] and correction of splenic reticuloendothelial dysfunction have been reported.[119,128]

ORGAN RECOVERY FOLLOWING TRANSPLANTATION

Stabilization or reversal of organ damage from SCD has been documented after HSCT.[118] Among 59 patients who received HSCT, 55 survived, with 50 free of disease with no further episodes of pain, stroke, or ACS.[118,121] Pulmonary function tests were stable in 22 of 26 patients, worse in 2, and not studied in 2. Seven of 8 patients transplanted for recurrent ACS had stable pulmonary function. Linear growth measured by median height standard deviation score improved from −0.7 before transplantation to −0.2 after transplantation. Patients with SCD who were successfully allografted did not experience sickle-related CNS complications and had evidence of stabilization of CNS disease by cerebral MRI, and in 3 cases that included 2 with stroke, there was evidence of improvement in areas of prior abnormality.[118,121,129] In a blinded examination of MRI and magnetic resonance angiography (MRA) of 8 patients pre- and post-HSCT, no significant changes in the appearance of cerebral arteries or in the luminal diameters were noted after HSCT. Four patients who received allogeneic HSCT were compared with 7 patients who received other therapy and with 13 untreated patients.[130] Quantitative analysis revealed a 10% increase in the measured

Table 1
Results of HSCT for SCD

References	Preparative Regimen	GVHD Prophylaxis	N	Median Age (Range)	Overall Survival	Event-Free Survival/ Follow-up	Complications
Walters et al[118] 2000	BU 14 mg/kg CY 200 mg/kg ATG 90 mg/kg	CsA CsA + MP CsA + MTX	50	9.9 y (3.3–15.9)	94%	84% 2.2 y (0.1–5.6)	Rejection (n = 4) GVHD (n = 1) ICH (n = 1)
Vermylen et al[117] 1998	BU 14–16 mg/kg CY 200 mg/kg ATG/total lymphoid irradiation (TLI)	CsA alone (n = 25) CsA + MTX (n = 25)	50	9.5 y (0.9–23.0)	96%	85% 3.1 y (0.3–6.5)	Rejection (n = 3) GVHD (n = 1)
Bernaudin et al[104,109] 1993, 2002	BU 14–22 mg/kg CY 200–260 mg/kg + rATG	CsA alone (n = 13) CsA + MTX (n = 47)	60	8.8 y (2.2–22)	90%	82% 62 mo (16–138)	Rejection (n = 1) ICH (n = 1) Fatal GVHD (n = 4) Fatal sepsis (n = 1)
Giardini et al[112] 1993	BU 14–16 mg/kg CY120–200 mg/kg ALG	Not described	8	8.0 y (4.0–26.0)	5/8	5/8	GVHD (n = 2) Acute respiratory disease syndrome (ARDS) (n = 1)
Abboud et al[107] 1997	BU 14 mg/kg CY 200 mg/kg	CsA + MTX (n = 8) CsA + MP (n = 2)	10	12.4 y (3.8–19.3)	9/10	9/10	Infection (n = 1)
Ferster et al[105] 1995	BU 14 mg/kg CY 50 mg/kg ALG (in 6 patients)	CsA + MTX	9	8 (2–11)	9/9	6/9 1–3 y	Rejection (n = 3)

Abbreviation: ICH, intracranial hemorrhage.

diameter of 64 vessels (P = .001) following any treatment. Patients who had undergone allogeneic HSCT exhibited a 12% increase in the lumen of 22 vessels (P = .041), whereas patients treated with chronic transfusion or hydroxyurea exhibited an 8% increase in 42 vessels (P = .016). In 2 patients with severe stenosis, the artery normalized after transplantation, and the blood flow rate was reduced in all patients who underwent transplantation. In untreated patients, there was a trend for the size of the arterial lumen to decrease, which is consistent with disease progression.[130] Follow-up studies in 9 children with SCD who successfully underwent HSCT, neurologic examinations, and neuropsychometric tests were stable, but MRI and MRA studies were not.[131] Transient changes occurred early in 2 patients. Persistent changes occurred in 5. Parenchyma lesions occurred in zero of 2 patients without prior lacunae or infarcts and in all 7 with prior lacunae or infarcts (P = .0278).[131] Worsening of cerebral large vessel and stroke has been reported following successful engraftment.[124] Thus, timing of HSCT in relation to the progression of cerebral vasculopathy may be critical to the ultimate CNS outcome, and is worthy of further study.

NOVEL APPROACHES TO HSCT FOR SCD AND THALASSEMIA

Despite the potential for cure, few patients have considered allogeneic HSCT, because of the paucity of suitable donors, restrictions in eligibility requirements, and the risk of early death from regimen-related side effects. Moreover, the acceptance of conventional myeloablative therapy is potentially limited by the associated risk of late effects, including chronic GVHD, sterility, and cancer. Several novel approaches to further improve the safety and applicability of HSCT that aim to decrease the associated toxicity and expand the pool of potential donors promise to improve the safety, applicability, and acceptability of this curative therapy for SCD.

REDUCED-INTENSITY CONDITIONING REGIMEN

Myeloablation for the eradication of host hematopoiesis and host immunosuppression has been considered necessary to create space in the host marrow microenvironment and for the prevention of immunologic rejection of the graft, respectively. However, the observation that, in the immunosuppressed host, the allogeneic marrow graft itself can create its own space by means of a local graft-versus-host reaction has opened up a whole new area of investigation of HSCT following nonmyeloablative preparative regimen.[132–139] Several patients who developed persistent MC after HSCT following myeloablative conditioning experienced a significant amelioration of their clinical phenotype.[79,140] Thus, nonmyeloablative HSCT with the elimination or reduction of myelotoxic therapies and the establishment of partial or complete donor chimerism is an attractive alternative for patients with hemoglobinopathies. Several regimens have been proposed to reduce the toxicity associated with allogeneic HSCT. A truly nonmyeloablative regimen would not eradicate host hematopoiesis and would allow hematopoietic recovery even without donor stem cell infusion. Regimens that produce some myeloablation and require donor marrow infusion for hematopoietic recovery are termed reduced intensity conditioning (RIC).[141] Because of prior chemotherapy, patients with hematologic malignancies may have varying degrees of immunosuppression and decreased marrow reserve before HSCT. In contrast, patients with SCD have received no prior immunosuppressive therapies and may actually have significant marrow hyperplasia. Moreover, there may also be allosensitization as a result of repeated blood transfusion. These factors may be responsible for the 10% to 30% risk of graft rejection after HSCT in patients with hemoglobinopathy.[74,118,142] FLU, a purine analog, is the backbone of most of the nonmyeloablative preparative regimens used. Nonmyeloablative preparative regimens for patients with hemoglobinopathies are based on: (1) RICs consisting of immunosuppressive chemotherapeutic drugs, usually FLU or other purine analogs in combination with an alkylating agent such as BU, CY, or melphalan (MEL)[143–147]; and (2) low-dose total-body irradiation, alone or in combination with FLU.[148–150] **Table 2** describes the current results of nonmyeloablative HSCT for hemoglobinopathies from a matched sibling donor. Duration of myelosuppression in both approaches has been comparable. Although initial engraftment has been achieved in most patients using either approach, sustained engraftment and alleviation of clinical phenotype is better following RIC regimens.[143–147,151] The use of nonmyeloablative conditioning regimens, although well tolerated, has generally not resulted in stable engraftments.[148–150] Engraftment has been an even greater challenge following RIC regimens when an unrelated donor was used as stem cell source. Escalation of immunosuppression in the preparative regimen by the addition of drugs such as alemtuzumab may improve the possibility of engraftment, particularly in patients receiving HSCT from unrelated donors.[146] However, the addition of alemtuzumab comes with an increased risk of delayed immune reconstitution, an increased risk of bacterial and viral infections,[146,152] and increased risk of neurologic complications.[153] In adult patients, severe GVHD has been observed following the use of RIC regimens.[148,153] The proportion of donor chimerism achieved following a nonmyeloablative preparative regimen that is sufficient to achieve stable long-term engraftment has long been the subject of investigation. Murine studies suggest that 100% erythroid chimerism is essential for organ recovery.[154,155] Patients achieving 15% to 100% donor chimerism in unfractionated blood and bone marrow mononuclear cell preparations following an nonmyeloablative regimen eventually lost the graft,[148,154] whereas stable engraftment was achieved following RIC regimens when the observed donor chimerism was greater than 70% and 100% in the mononuclear and erythroid compartments, respectively.[151,156] Thus, rejection of donor marrow is likely to be a challenge in reduced intensity HSCT for SCD. There is a need for further studies before these regimens can become standard for these patients. Ongoing multicenter trials of HSCT for patients with SCD and those with thalassemia using RIC regimens are likely to provide more data to determine the role of these approaches in this patient population.

MATCHED UMBILICAL CORD BLOOD AS STEM CELL SOURCE FOR HSCT

Umbilical cord blood (UCB) from a donor provides a readily available alternate source of stem cells with minimal risk to the donor.[157] Successful HSCTs for patients with SCD from a matched sibling UCB donor have been reported.[111,114,116,157] Matched sibling donor UCB HSCT was performed in 44 patients with hemoglobinopathies (33 thalassemia and 11 SCD).[111,116] Forty-one UCB donors were HLA matched and 3 had 1 HLA-A difference. Median recipient age was 5 years (range 1–20 years) and median follow-up was 27 months (range 1–85 months). The 2-year OS and EFS were 100% and 81%, respectively, for the entire group. The EFS was 90% and 79% for SCD and thalassemia, respectively. In patients with thalassemia, the addition of thiotepa (THIO) to the combination of BU/CY or BU/FLU was associated with a better outcome, with disease-free survival (DFS) for patients who did and did not receive THIO being 94% versus 62%, respectively (*P*<.05). Remote-site collection and directed-donor banking of UCB for sibling recipients with malignancy, SCD, thalassemia major, nonmalignant hematologic conditions, and metabolic errors has been accomplished with a high success rate. Sixteen of 17 UCB allograft recipients had stable engraftment of donor cells.[157] Thus, UCB from a matched sibling donor

Table 2
Results of nonmyeloablative HSCT for hemoglobinopathies

References	Preparative Regimen	GVHD Prophylaxis	N	Age in Years (Range)	Overall Survival	Disease-Free Survival/ Follow-up (Range)	Complications/Comments
Krishnamurti et al[158]	BU 8 mg/kg FLU 175 mg/kg ATG 90 mg/kg TLI 500 cGy	CsA + MMF	7	9.9 y (3.3–18)	7	6/7 (36–102 mo)	AGVHD grade II (n = 1)
Shenoy et al[146]	FLU 150 mg/m² Campath 1H (33/48 mg) Mel 140/70 mg/m²	CsA + prednisone	2	1	2/2	2/2 373 d (293–447)	
Van Besien et al[147]	FLU 14–16 mg/kg Mel 140 mg/m² ATG 200 mg/kg	CsA + MMF	2	9 y (0.9–23.0)	0/2	0/2	Severe fatal GVHD (n = 2)
Slavin et al[159]	BU 8 mg/kg FLU 175 mg/kg ATG 90 mg/kg	CsA + MMF	1		1/1	1/1 >1 y	
Schleuning et al[145]	BU 14–22 mg/kg CY 200–260 mg/kg	CsA + MMF	1	8.6 y (2.2–14.8)	1/1	1/1 1 y	
Iannone et al[149]	FLU 90–150 mg/kg TBI 200 cGy + ATG 90 mg/kg (1 patient)	MMF + CsA/tacrolimus	6	12.4 y (3.8–19.3)	6 of 6	0 of 6	Delayed rejection (n = 6) AGVHD grade II (n = 1)
Horan et al[148]	FLU 90–150 mg/kg rabbit ATG TBI 200 cGy	CsA + MMF	3	(9–30)	3/3	1/3 2 y	1 patient rejected graft and had a stroke
Isola et al[160]	Campath 1H 20 mg/d ×5 + FLU + CY	Campath 1H 20 mg in bag + MMF	3	23 (20–45)	2/3	0/3	0/3

Abbreviation: MMF, mycophenolate mofetil.

provides an acceptable alternative to bone marrow transplantation (BMT), and banking of UCB of siblings of patients with SCD should be offered routinely.

RESULTS OF UNRELATED BMT FOR THALASSEMIA

Results of HSCT from unrelated donors for the treatment of malignant disease have improved steadily, mainly because of the introduction of high-resolution molecular techniques for histocompatibility testing and improvements in the management of posttransplant complications. The excellent results in class 1 and 2 patients with thalassemia with unrelated donors underscore the importance of the timing of transplantation. In the first published results of BMT from extended haplotype-matched volunteer unrelated donors in 32 patients with thalassemia major who received BU-CY with or without THIO regimen, thalassemia-free survival was 66% and mortality was 25%. Patients sharing at least 1 extended haplotype had a better survival.[81,161]

Results are significantly better if patients belong to Pesaro class 1 or 2 with OS 96% and thalassemia-free survival 80%.[162] Compared with HLA-identical donor transplantation of mixed class 1 to 2 and class 3 patients, OS was 92% and 82% with thalassemia-free survival of 82% versus 71%.[163] Conditioning regimens were all BU based.

Although a small number of patients have been transplanted so far, these data show that unrelated marrow transplantation with well-selected donors, not only in younger low-risk patients but also in class 3 high-risk patients, may offer a success rate similar to those obtained from HLA-identical sibling transplantation.

The main limitation of the experience with unrelated HSCT for thalassemia is that, using such stringent criteria, only about one-third of patients with thalassemia who started the search found a suitable donor in a median time of 3 to 4 months. One possibility to increase the donor pool could be adopting less stringent criteria of HLA matching for selection donors with 1 or 2 allelic disparity, but the results of such transplants remain to be determined.

Recently, results on haploidentical HSCT were published showing a 90% OS and 61% EFS.[164] Haploidentical HSCT offers the advantage of having a high chance of donor availability, reduced risk for GVHD, and potential for posttransplant cellular therapy. However, because of increased risk for rejection, significantly delayed immune recovery, and concomitant high risk for lethal viral reactivation or infection, the general applicability of this transplant option is limited.

HSCT FROM UNRELATED DONORS FOR SCD

Although young patients without advanced disease who have received HSCT from a matched sibling have an excellent outcome, the applicability of HSCT for these conditions is limited because fewer than one-third of these patients will find a suitable HLA-matched related donor.[101] In the past, HSCT from unrelated donors has not been offered to patients with hemoglobinopathies. Because these diseases may be associated with prolonged survival, the increased regimen-related toxicity of unrelated-donor HSCT was considered unacceptable. The advent of novel strategies to reduce regimen-related toxicity, including the use of nonmyeloablative preparative regimens,[144,145] and the improvement in outcomes of unrelated-donor HSCT,[165] has sparked fresh interest in the consideration of unrelated-donor HSCT for patients with hemoglobinopathies. Experience with alternative donor transplants remains limited for SCD.[119,166] General applicability of unrelated-donor HSCT remains limited because of a regimen-related mortality of 30% and a high incidence of chronic GVHD (27%).[161] This must be compared with a 90% survival probability to age 20 years,[100] with a subsequent 20 to 30 years shortened lifespan because of cumulative morbidity and sudden death in adulthood,[42] and overall loss of 20 to 30 years' life expectancy. Therefore, efforts to reduce regimen-related toxicity and the long-term sequelae of unrelated-donor HSCT are needed to make the option of unrelated-donor HSCT more attractive. Concerns have been expressed about the availability of matched unrelated hematopoietic stem cell donors for patients with SCD, because minorities are usually underrepresented in national donor registries. Actual searches suggest that most patients with SCD will find at least 1 bone marrow donor matched at 5 of 6 HLA loci[167] and, if the patient weighs 40 kg or less, UCB units matching at 4 or more of 6 HLA loci at acceptable cell doses.[168] Availability of units matched at 6 HLA loci is more limited.[167,168] However, because more than 30% of potential donors are not available or decline to donate at key decision points in the donation process, the actual availability of bone marrow donors may be lower.[169] The effect of HLA mismatches on outcomes of HSCT from unrelated donors for various diseases suggests that mismatches at HLA-A, -B, -C, and -DRB1 each had similar adverse effects on mortality.[170] This suggests that matching for HLA-C should be incorporated into algorithms for unrelated-donor selection. However, the likelihood of identifying unrelated-donor bone marrow or UCB for patients with SCD that match at 8 of 8 or 10 of 10 HLA loci is low. Although applicability of UCB in adult patients is limited by recipient weight, the encouraging data with the use of multiple UCB units[171] offer the possibility of offering this source of stem cells for adult patients with hemoglobin-opathy. An ongoing multicenter clinical trial sponsored by the BMT Clinical Trials Network is likely to generate data regarding the role of unrelated-donor HSCT for patients with SCD. Thus, although progress made is encouraging, the role of unre-lated-donor HSCT for SCD is yet to be established.

Future Directions

Development of less toxic, nonmyeloablative conditioning regimens has the potential to reduce procedure-related mortality to even lower levels and improve applicability of HSCT to patients for whom it is currently unavailable. Improvement in the risk/benefit ratio would also affect the indications for HSCT, particularly for SCD. There may be differences in the recommendations made by different health care providers, and differences in accepting the risks associated with HSCT by patients or parents.[102] Most parents and patients are willing to accept some mortality risk. Further studies are indicated to study the effect of parental beliefs and preferences on selection of patients for HSCT. Selection criteria currently in use were empirically derived and require the patient to manifest features of severe disease or involvement of the target organ. A risk prediction model may potentially offer objective criteria for the selection of patients with SCD for HSCT.[172] Additional studies are required to validate such or similar models. A better understanding of the effect of HSCT on the natural history of vasculopathy and organ damage may also influence decision making. Expansion of the donor pool by use of unrelated matched donors awaits further improvement in outcomes of unrelated-donor HSCT. The representation of minorities in donor regis-tries and the availability of potential HLA-matched donors for patients with hemoglo-binopathy have improved.[167] However, there remain several limitations to the possibility of finding fully HLA-matched donors. Implementation of strategies for improved minority donor registration and retention is critical to the development of this therapeutic option for patients with hemoglobinopathies. UCB offers the possi-bility of reduced complications such as severe GVHD. Ex vivo expansion of UCB cells or the use of multiple UCB units also offers the possibility of offering this source of stem cells for adult patients with hemoglobinopathy.[171,173]

REFERENCES

1. Giardine B, van BS, Kaimakis P, et al. HbVar database of human hemoglobin variants and thalassemia mutations: 2007 update. Hum Mutat 2007;28(2): 206.
2. Pootrakul P, Sirankapracha P, Hemsorach S, et al. A correlation of erythrokinetics, ineffective erythropoiesis, and erythroid precursor apoptosis in Thai patients with thalassemia. Blood 2000;96(7):2606–12.
3. Weatherall DJ. Phenotype-genotype relationships in monogenic disease: lessons from the thalassaemias. Nat Rev Genet 2001;2(4):245–55.
4. Kong Y, Zhou S, Kihm AJ, et al. Loss of alpha-hemoglobin-stabilizing protein impairs erythropoiesis and exacerbates beta-thalassemia. J Clin Invest 2004; 114(10):1457–66.
5. Centis F, Tabellini L, Lucarelli G, et al. The importance of erythroid expansion in determining the extent of apoptosis in erythroid precursors in patients with beta-thalassemia major. Blood 2000;96(10):3624–9.
6. Mathias LA, Fisher TC, Zeng L, et al. Ineffective erythropoiesis in beta-thalassemia major is due to apoptosis at the polychromatophilic normoblast stage. Exp Hematol 2000;28(12):1343–53.
7. Rivella S. Ineffective erythropoiesis and thalassemias. Curr Opin Hematol 2009; 16(3):187–94.
8. Chen JJ. Regulation of protein synthesis by the heme-regulated eIF2alpha kinase: relevance to anemias. Blood 2007;109(7):2693–9.
9. Libani IV, Guy EC, Melchiori L, et al. Decreased differentiation of erythroid cells exacerbates ineffective erythropoiesis in beta-thalassemia. Blood 2008;112(3): 875–85.
10. Finch C. Regulators of iron balance in humans. Blood 1994;84(6):1697–702.
11. Cunningham MJ, Macklin EA, Neufeld EJ, et al. Complications of beta-thalassemia major in North America. Blood 2004;104(1):34–9.
12. Vogiatzi MG, Macklin EA, Fung EB, et al. Bone disease in thalassemia: a frequent and still unresolved problem. J Bone Miner Res 2009;24(3):543–57.
13. Olivieri NF, Brittenham GM. Iron-chelating therapy and the treatment of thalassemia. Blood 1997;89(3):739–61.
14. Olivieri NF, Brittenham GM, McLaren CE, et al. Long-term safety and effectiveness of iron-chelation therapy with deferiprone for thalassemia major. N Engl J Med 1998;339(7):417–23.
15. Koren A, Levin C, Dgany O, et al. Response to hydroxyurea therapy in beta-thalassemia. Am J Hematol 2008;83(5):366–70.
16. Zamani F, Shakeri R, Eslami SM, et al. Hydroxyurea therapy in 49 patients with major beta-thalassemia. Arch Iran Med 2009;12(3):295–7.
17. Olivieri NF, Rees DC, Ginder GD, et al. Elimination of transfusions through induction of fetal hemoglobin synthesis in Cooley's anemia. Ann N Y Acad Sci 1998; 850:100–9.
18. Yavarian M, Karimi M, Bakker E, et al. Response to hydroxyurea treatment in Iranian transfusion-dependent beta-thalassemia patients. Haematologica 2004;89(10):1172–8.
19. Borgna-Pignatti C, Cappellini MD, De SP, et al. Survival and complications in thalassemia. Ann N Y Acad Sci 2005;1054:40–7.
20. Borgna-Pignatti C, Cappellini MD, De SP, et al. Cardiac morbidity and mortality in deferoxamine- or deferiprone-treated patients with thalassemia major. Blood 2006;107(9):3733–7.

21. Ehlers KH, Giardina PJ, Lesser ML, et al. Prolonged survival in patients with beta-thalassemia major treated with deferoxamine. J Pediatr 1991;118(4 Pt 1): 540–5.

22. Brittenham GM, Griffith PM, Nienhuis AW, et al. Efficacy of deferoxamine in preventing complications of iron overload in patients with thalassemia major. N Engl J Med 1994;331(9):567–73.

23. Modell B, Letsky EA, Flynn DM, et al. Survival and desferrioxamine in thalassaemia major. Br Med J (Clin Res Ed) 1982;284(6322):1081–4.

24. Modell B, Khan M, Darlison M. Survival in beta-thalassaemia major in the UK: data from the UK Thalassaemia register. Lancet 2000;355(9220):2051–2.

25. Delea TE, Edelsberg J, Sofrygin O, et al. Consequences and costs of noncompliance with iron chelation therapy in patients with transfusion-dependent thalassemia: a literature review. Transfusion 2007;47(10):1919–29.

26. Anderson LJ, Holden S, Davis B, et al. Cardiovascular T2-star (T2*) magnetic resonance for the early diagnosis of myocardial iron overload. Eur Heart J 2001;22(23):2171–9.

27. Bunn HF. Pathogenesis and treatment of sickle cell disease. N Engl J Med 1997; 337(11):762–9.

28. Stuart MJ, Nagel RL. Sickle-cell disease. Lancet 2004;364(9442):1343–60.

29. Reiter CD, Wang X, Tanus-Santos JE, et al. Cell-free hemoglobin limits nitric oxide bioavailability in sickle-cell disease. Nat Med 2002;8(12):1383–9.

30. Wang X, Tanus-Santos JE, Reiter CD, et al. Biological activity of nitric oxide in the plasmatic compartment. Proc Natl Acad Sci U S A 2004;101(31):11477–82.

31. Belhassen L, Pelle G, Sediame S, et al. Endothelial dysfunction in patients with sickle cell disease is related to selective impairment of shear stress-mediated vasodilation. Blood 2001;97(6):1584–9.

32. Bakare MO, Omigbodun OO, Kuteyi OB, et al. Psychological complications of childhood chronic physical illness in Nigerian children and their mothers: the implication for developing pediatric liaison services. Child Adolesc Psychiatry Ment Health 2008;2(1):34.

33. Benton TD, Ifeagwu JA, Smith-Whitley K. Anxiety and depression in children and adolescents with sickle cell disease. Curr Psychiatry Rep 2007;9(2):114–21.

34. Levenson JL, McClish DK, Dahman BA, et al. Depression and anxiety in adults with sickle cell disease: the PiSCES project. Psychosom Med 2008;70(2):192–6.

35. Pham PT, Pham PC, Wilkinson AH, et al. Renal abnormalities in sickle cell disease. Kidney Int 2000;57(1):1–8.

36. Wigfall DR, Ware RE, Burchinal MR, et al. Prevalence and clinical correlates of glomerulopathy in children with sickle cell disease. J Pediatr 2000;136(6): 749–53.

37. Bruno D, Wigfall DR, Zimmerman SA, et al. Genitourinary complications of sickle cell disease. J Urol 2001;166(3):803–11.

38. Fowler JE Jr, Koshy M, Strub M, et al. Priapism associated with the sickle cell hemoglobinopathies: prevalence, natural history and sequelae. J Urol 1991; 145(1):65–8.

39. Mantadakis E, Cavender JD, Rogers ZR, et al. Prevalence of priapism in children and adolescents with sickle cell anemia. J Pediatr Hematol Oncol 1999; 21(6):518–22.

40. Miller ST, Rao SP, Dunn EK, et al. Priapism in children with sickle cell disease. J Urol 1995;154(2 Pt 2):844–7.

41. Platt OS, Brambilla DJ, Rosse WF, et al. Mortality in sickle cell disease. Life expectancy and risk factors for early death. N Engl J Med 1994;330(23):1639–44.

42. Gladwin MT, Sachdev V, Jison ML, et al. Pulmonary hypertension as a risk factor for death in patients with sickle cell disease. N Engl J Med 2004; 350(9):886–95.
43. Machado RF, Gladwin MT. Chronic sickle cell lung disease: new insights into the diagnosis, pathogenesis and treatment of pulmonary hypertension. Br J Haematol 2005;129(4):449–64.
44. Bridges W. Cerebral vascular disease accompanying sickle cell anemia. Am J Pathol 1939;15:353–60.
45. Ohene-Frempong K, Weiner SJ, Sleeper LA, et al. Cerebrovascular accidents in sickle cell disease: rates and risk factors. Blood 1998;91(1):288–94.
46. Miller ST, Macklin EA, Pegelow CH, et al. Silent infarction as a risk factor for overt stroke in children with sickle cell anemia: a report from the Cooperative Study of Sickle Cell Disease. J Pediatr 2001;139(3):385–90.
47. Kugler S, Anderson B, Cross D, et al. Abnormal cranial magnetic resonance imaging scans in sickle-cell disease. Neurological correlates and clinical implications. Arch Neurol 1993;50(6):629–35.
48. Seibert JJ, Miller SF, Kirby RS, et al. Cerebrovascular disease in symptomatic and asymptomatic patients with sickle cell anemia: screening with duplex transcranial Doppler US–correlation with MR imaging and MR angiography. Radiology 1993;189(2):457–66.
49. Seibert JJ, Glasier CM, Kirby RS, et al. Transcranial Doppler, MRA, and MRI as a screening examination for cerebrovascular disease in patients with sickle cell anemia: an 8-year study. Pediatr Radiol 1998;28(3):138–42.
50. Adams R, McKie V, Nichols F, et al. The use of transcranial ultrasonography to predict stroke in sickle cell disease. N Engl J Med 1992;326(9):605–10.
51. Adams RJ, Nichols FT, Figueroa R, et al. Transcranial Doppler correlation with cerebral angiography in sickle cell disease. Stroke 1992;23(8):1073–7.
52. Adams RJ, McKie VC, Carl EM, et al. Long-term stroke risk in children with sickle cell disease screened with transcranial Doppler. Ann Neurol 1997;42(5): 699–704.
53. Adams RJ, McKie VC, Brambilla D, et al. Stroke prevention trial in sickle cell anemia. Control Clin Trials 1998;19(1):110–29.
54. Adams RJ, McKie VC, Hsu L, et al. Prevention of a first stroke by transfusions in children with sickle cell anemia and abnormal results on transcranial Doppler ultrasonography. N Engl J Med 1998;339(1):5–11.
55. Adams RJ. Stroke prevention in sickle cell disease. Curr Opin Hematol 2000; 7(2):101–5.
56. Charache S, Terrin ML, Moore RD, et al. Effect of hydroxyurea on the frequency of painful crises in sickle cell anemia. Investigators of the Multicenter Study of Hydroxyurea in Sickle Cell Anemia. N Engl J Med 1995;332(20):1317–22.
57. Ferster A, Tahriri P, Vermylen C, et al. Five years of experience with hydroxyurea in children and young adults with sickle cell disease. Blood 2001;97(11): 3628–32.
58. Hankins JS, Ware RE, Rogers ZR, et al. Long-term hydroxyurea therapy for infants with sickle cell anemia: the HUSOFT extension study. Blood 2005; 106(7):2269–75.
59. Sumoza A, de BR, Sumoza D, et al. Hydroxyurea (HU) for prevention of recurrent stroke in sickle cell anemia (SCA). Am J Hematol 2002;71(3):161–5.
60. Ware RE, Zimmerman SA, Schultz WH. Hydroxyurea as an alternative to blood transfusions for the prevention of recurrent stroke in children with sickle cell disease. Blood 1999;94(9):3022–6.

61. Ware RE, Zimmerman SA, Sylvestre PB, et al. Prevention of secondary stroke and resolution of transfusional iron overload in children with sickle cell anemia using hydroxyurea and phlebotomy. J Pediatr 2004;145(3):346–52.

62. Berthaut I, Guignedoux G, Kirsch-Noir F, et al. Influence of sickle cell disease and treatment with hydroxyurea on sperm parameters and fertility of human males. Haematologica 2008;93(7):988–93.

63. Jones KM, Niaz MS, Brooks CM, et al. Adverse effects of a clinically relevant dose of hydroxyurea used for the treatment of sickle cell disease on male fertility endpoints. Int J Environ Res Public Health 2009;6(3):1124–44.

64. Lukusa AK, Vermylen C, Vanabelle B, et al. Bone marrow transplantation or hydroxyurea for sickle cell anemia: long-term effects on semen variables and hormone profiles. Pediatr Hematol Oncol 2009;26(4):186–94.

65. Quinn CT, Rogers ZR, Buchanan GR. Survival of children with sickle cell disease. Blood 2004;103(11):4023–7.

66. Serjeant GR. Sickle-cell disease. Lancet 1997;350(9079):725–30.

67. Gill FM, Sleeper LA, Weiner SJ, et al. Clinical events in the first decade in a cohort of infants with sickle cell disease. Cooperative Study of Sickle Cell Disease. Blood 1995;86(2):776–83.

68. Giardini C, Lucarelli G. Bone marrow transplantation for beta-thalassemia. Hematol Oncol Clin North Am 1999;13(5):1059–64, viii.

69. Lucarelli G, Galimberti M, Polchi P, et al. Bone marrow transplantation in patients with thalassemia. N Engl J Med 1990;322(7):417–21.

70. Lucarelli G, Galimberti M, Polchi P, et al. Bone marrow transplantation in thalassemia. Hematol Oncol Clin North Am 1991;5(3):549–56.

71. Sodani P, Gaziev D, Polchi P, et al. New approach for bone marrow transplantation in patients with class 3 thalassemia aged younger than 17 years. Blood 2004;104(4):1201–3.

72. Lucarelli G, Galimberti M, Polchi P, et al. Marrow transplantation in patients with thalassemia responsive to iron chelation therapy. N Engl J Med 1993;329(12):840–4.

73. Lucarelli G, Clift RA, Galimberti M, et al. Marrow transplantation for patients with thalassemia: results in class 3 patients. Blood 1996;87(5):2082–8.

74. Lucarelli G, Andreani M, Angelucci E. The cure of thalassemia by bone marrow transplantation. Blood Rev 2002;16(2):81–5.

75. Lucarelli G, Galimberti M, Polchi P, et al. Bone marrow transplantation in adult thalassemia. Blood 1992;80(6):1603–7.

76. Lucarelli G, Clift RA, Galimberti M, et al. Bone marrow transplantation in adult thalassemic patients. Blood 1999;93(4):1164–7.

77. Gaziev J, Sodani P, Polchi P, et al. Bone marrow transplantation in adults with thalassemia: treatment and long-term follow-up. Ann N Y Acad Sci 2005;1054: 196–205.

78. Andreani M, Manna M, Lucarelli G, et al. Persistence of mixed chimerism in patients transplanted for the treatment of thalassemia. Blood 1996;87(8): 3494–9.

79. Andreani M, Nesci S, Lucarelli G, et al. Long-term survival of ex-thalassemic patients with persistent mixed chimerism after bone marrow transplantation. Bone Marrow Transplant 2000;25(4):401–4.

80. Lisini D, Zecca M, Giorgiani G, et al. Donor/recipient mixed chimerism does not predict graft failure in children with beta-thalassemia given an allogeneic cord blood transplant from an HLA-identical sibling. Haematologica 2008;93(12): 1859–67.

81. Locatelli F. Tolerance: pregnancy matters. Blood 2009;114(11):2208–9.

82. Serafini G, Andreani M, Testi M, et al. Type 1 regulatory T cells are associated with persistent split erythroid/lymphoid chimerism after allogeneic hematopoietic stem cell transplantation for thalassemia. Haematologica 2009;94(10): 1415–26.

83. van Halteren AG, Jankowska-Gan E, Joosten A, et al. Naturally acquired tolerance and sensitization to minor histocompatibility antigens in healthy family members. Blood 2009;114(11):2263–72.

84. Gaziev D, Polchi P, Lucarelli G, et al. Second marrow transplants for graft failure in patients with thalassemia. Bone Marrow Transplant 1999;24(12):1299–306.

85. Gaziev J, Sodani P, Lucarelli G, et al. Second hematopoietic SCT in patients with thalassemia recurrence following rejection of the first graft. Bone Marrow Transplant 2008;42(6):397–404.

86. Gaziev D, Polchi P, Galimberti M, et al. Graft-versus-host disease after bone marrow transplantation for thalassemia: an analysis of incidence and risk factors. Transplantation 1997;63(6):854–60.

87. Lucarelli G, Angelucci E, Giardini C, et al. Fate of iron stores in thalassaemia after bone-marrow transplantation. Lancet 1993;342(8884):1388–91.

88. Angelucci E, Muretto P, Nicolucci A, et al. Effects of iron overload and hepatitis C virus positivity in determining progression of liver fibrosis in thalassemia following bone marrow transplantation. Blood 2002;100(1):17–21.

89. Angelucci E, Muretto P, Lucarelli G, et al. Phlebotomy to reduce iron overload in patients cured of thalassemia by bone marrow transplantation. Italian Cooperative Group for Phlebotomy Treatment of Transplanted Thalassemia Patients. Blood 1997;90(3):994–8.

90. Angelucci E, Muretto P, Lucarelli G, et al. Treatment of iron overload in the "ex-thalassemic". Report from the phlebotomy program. Ann N Y Acad Sci 1998; 850:288–93.

91. Giardini C, Galimberti M, Lucarelli G, et al. Desferrioxamine therapy accelerates clearance of iron deposits after bone marrow transplantation for thalassaemia. Br J Haematol 1995;89(4):868–73.

92. Mariotti E, Angelucci E, Agostini A, et al. Evaluation of cardiac status in iron-loaded thalassaemia patients following bone marrow transplantation: improvement in cardiac function during reduction in body iron burden. Br J Haematol 1998;103(4):916–21.

93. Gaziev J, Galimberti M, Giardini C, et al. Growth in children after bone marrow transplantation for thalassemia. Bone Marrow Transplant 1993;12(Suppl 1): 100–1.

94. De Sanctis V, Galimberti M, Lucarelli G, et al. Growth and development in ex-thalassemic patients. Bone Marrow Transplant 1997;19(Suppl 2):126–7.

95. Borgna-Pignatti C, Marradi P, Rugolotto S, et al. Successful pregnancy after bone marrow transplantation for thalassaemia. Bone Marrow Transplant 1996; 18(1):235–6.

96. Strader DB, Wright T, Thomas DL, et al. Diagnosis, management, and treatment of hepatitis C. Hepatology 2004;39(4):1147–71.

97. Walters MC, Patience M, Leisenring W, et al. Bone marrow transplantation for sickle cell disease. N Engl J Med 1996;335(6):369–76.

98. Adams RJ, Brambilla D. Discontinuing prophylactic transfusions used to prevent stroke in sickle cell disease. N Engl J Med 2005;353(26):2769–78.

99. Aduloju S, Palmer S, Eckman J. Mortality in sickle cell patient transitioning from pediatric to adult program: 10 years Grady comprehensive sickle cell center experience [abstract 1426]. Blood 2008;112.

100. Powars DR, Chan LS, Hiti A, et al. Outcome of sickle cell anemia: a 4-decade observational study of 1056 patients. Medicine (Baltimore) 2005;84(6):363–76.
101. Walters MC, Patience M, Leisenring W, et al. Barriers to bone marrow transplantation for sickle cell anemia. Biol Blood Marrow Transplant 1996;2(2):100–4.
102. Kodish E, Lantos J, Stocking C, et al. Bone marrow transplantation for sickle cell disease. A study of parents' decisions. N Engl J Med 1991;325(19):1349–53.
103. van Besien K, Koshy M, nderson-Shaw L, et al. Allogeneic stem cell transplantation for sickle cell disease. A study of patients' decisions. Bone Marrow Transplant 2001;28(6):545–9.
104. Bernaudin F, Vernant JP, Vilmer E, et al. Results of allogeneic stem cell transplant for severe sickle cell disease (SCD) in France and consideration about conditioning regimen and indications in 2002. 30th Anniversary of the National Sickle Cell Disease Program National Heart, Lung, and Blood Institute National Institutes of Health and the Sickle Cell Association of America Inc, Washington Hilton and Towers, Washington, DC 2002;33.
105. Ferster A, Corazza F, Vertongen F, et al. Transplanted sickle-cell disease patients with autologous bone marrow recovery after graft failure develop increased levels of fetal haemoglobin which corrects disease severity. Br J Haematol 1995;90(4):804–8.
106. Vermylen C, Fernandez RE, Ninane J, et al. Bone marrow transplantation in five children with sickle cell anaemia. Lancet 1988;1(8600):1427–8.
107. Abboud M, Kletzl M, Miller S, et al. Bone marrow transplantation for sickle cell disease. Blood 1997;90:229a.
108. Abboud MR, Jackson SM, Barredo J, et al. Bone marrow transplantation for sickle cell anemia. Am J Pediatr Hematol Oncol 1994;16(1):86–9.
109. Bernaudin F, Souillet G, Vannier JP, et al. Bone marrow transplantation (BMT) in 14 children with severe sickle cell disease (SCD): the French experience. GEGMO. Bone Marrow Transplant 1993;12(Suppl 1):118–21.
110. Bernaudin F. [Results and current indications of bone marrow allograft in sickle cell disease]. Pathol Biol (Paris) 1999;47(1):59–64 [in French].
111. Brichard B, Vermylen C, Ninane J, et al. Persistence of fetal hemoglobin production after successful transplantation of cord blood stem cells in a patient with sickle cell anemia. J Pediatr 1996;128(2):241–3.
112. Giardini C, Galimberti M, Lucarelli G, et al. Bone marrow transplantation in sickle-cell anemia in Pesaro. Bone Marrow Transplant 1993;12(Suppl 1):122–3.
113. Golden F. The sickle-cell kid. An experimental transplant succeeds, giving a brave little boy the best Christmas present he can imagine. Times 1999; 154(25):92.
114. Gore L, Lane PA, Quinones RR, et al. Successful cord blood transplantation for sickle cell anemia from a sibling who is human leukocyte antigen-identical: implications for comprehensive care. J Pediatr Hematol Oncol 2000;22(5): 437–40.
115. Hoppe CC, Walters MC. Bone marrow transplantation in sickle cell anemia. Curr Opin Oncol 2001;13(2):85–90.
116. Locatelli F, Rocha V, Reed W, et al. Related umbilical cord blood transplantation in patients with thalassemia and sickle cell disease. Blood 2003;101(6):2137–43.
117. Vermylen C, Cornu G, Ferster A, et al. Haematopoietic stem cell transplantation for sickle cell anaemia: the first 50 patients transplanted in Belgium. Bone Marrow Transplant 1998;22(1):1–6.
118. Walters MC, Storb R, Patience M, et al. Impact of bone marrow transplantation for symptomatic sickle cell disease: an interim report. Multicenter investigation

of bone marrow transplantation for sickle cell disease. Blood 2000;95(6): 1918–24.

119. Werner E, Yanovich S, Rubinstein P, et al. Unrelated placental cord blood transplantation in a patient with sickle cell disease and acute non-lymphocytic leukemia. Blood 1997;90:4542, 399b.

120. Bernaudin F, Socie G, Kuentz M, et al. Long-term results of related myeloablative stem-cell transplantation to cure sickle cell disease. Blood 2007;110(7):2749–56.

121. Walters MC, Patience M, Leisenring W, et al. Updated results of bone marrow transplantation (BMT) for sickle cell disease (SCD): impact on CNS disease. Blood 2002;100(46):160, p45a.

122. Adamkiewicz T, Chiang KY, Haight A, et al. Significant progression of large central nervous system (CNS) vessel disease following G Full matched sibling marrow engraftment in a child with hemoglobin SS. 30th Anniversary of the National Sickle Cell Disease Program National Heart, Lung, and Blood Institute. National Institutes of Health and the Sickle Cell Disease Association of America Inc, Washington Hilton and Towers, Washington, DC 2002;(1).

123. Horan j, Liesveld J, Fenton P, et al. Hematopoietic stem cell transplantation for sickle cell disease and thalassemia after low dos TBI, Fludarabine and rabbit ATG. 30th Anniversary of the National Sickle Cell Disease Program National Heart, Lung and Blood Institute. National Institutes of Health and the Sickle Cell Disease Association of America Inc, Washington Hilton and Towers, Washington, DC, 2002;34.

124. Kalinyak KA, Morris C, Ball WS, et al. Bone marrow transplantation in a young child with sickle cell anemia. Am J Hematol 1995;48(4):256–61.

125. Steen RG, Helton KJ, Horwitz EM, et al. Improved cerebrovascular patency following therapy in patients with sickle cell disease: initial results in 4 patients who received HLA-identical hematopoietic stem cell allografts. Ann Neurol 2001;49(2):222–9.

126. Eggleston B, Patience M, Edwards S, et al. Effect of myeloablative bone marrow transplantation on growth in children with sickle cell anaemia: results of the multicenter study of haematopoietic cell transplantation for sickle cell anaemia. Br J Haematol 2007;136(4):673–6.

127. Hernigou P, Bernaudin F, Reinert P, et al. Bone-marrow transplantation in sickle-cell disease. Effect on osteonecrosis: a case report with a four-year follow-up. J Bone Joint Surg Am 1997;79(11):1726–30.

128. Ferster A, Bujan W, Corazza F, et al. Bone marrow transplantation corrects the splenic reticuloendothelial dysfunction in sickle cell anemia. Blood 1993;81(4): 1102–5.

129. Walters MC. Sickle cell anemia and hematopoietic cell transplantation: When is a pound of cure worth more than an ounce of prevention? Pediatr Transplant 2004;8(Suppl 5):33–8.

130. Steen RG, Emudianughe T, Hankins GM, et al. Brain imaging findings in pediatric patients with sickle cell disease. Radiology 2003;228(1):216–25.

131. Woodard P, Helton KJ, Khan RB, et al. Brain parenchymal damage after haematopoietic stem cell transplantation for severe sickle cell disease. Br J Haematol 2005;129(4):550–2.

132. Baron F, Sandmaier BM. Current status of hematopoietic stem cell transplantation after nonmyeloablative conditioning. Curr Opin Hematol 2005;12(6):435–43.

133. Champlin R, Khouri I, Anderlini P, et al. Nonmyeloablative preparative regimens for allogeneic hematopoietic transplantation. Biology and current indications. Oncology (Williston Park) 2003;17(1):94–100.

134. Chao NJ, Liu CX, Rooney B, et al. Nonmyeloablative regimen preserves "niches" allowing for peripheral expansion of donor T-cells. Biol Blood Marrow Transplant 2002;8(5):249–56.
135. Mielcarek M, Sandmaier BM, Maloney DG, et al. Nonmyeloablative hematopoietic cell transplantation: status quo and future perspectives. J Clin Immunol 2002;22(2):70–4.
136. Resnick IB, Shapira MY, Slavin S. Nonmyeloablative stem cell transplantation and cell therapy for malignant and non-malignant diseases. Transpl Immunol 2005;14(3-4):207–19.
137. Shimoni A, Nagler A. Nonmyeloablative stem cell transplantation: lessons from the first decade of clinical experience. Curr Hematol Rep 2004;3(4):242–8.
138. Slavin S, Or R, Aker M, et al. Nonmyeloablative stem cell transplantation for the treatment of cancer and life-threatening nonmalignant disorders: past accomplishments and future goals. Cancer Chemother Pharmacol 2001;48(Suppl 1): S79–84.
139. Storb RF, Lucarelli G, McSweeney PA, et al. Hematopoietic cell transplantation for benign hematological disorders and solid tumors. Hematology Am Soc Hematol Educ Program 2003;372–97.
140. Walters MC, Patience M, Leisenring W, et al. Stable mixed hematopoietic chimerism after bone marrow transplantation for sickle cell anemia. Biol Blood Marrow Transplant 2001;7(12):665–73.
141. Storb RF, Champlin R, Riddell SR, et al. Non-myeloablative transplants for malignant disease. Hematology Am Soc Hematol Educ Program 2001;375–91.
142. Miniero R, Rocha V, Saracco P, et al. Cord blood transplantation (CBT) in hemoglobinopathies. Eurocord. Bone Marrow Transplant 1998;22(Suppl 1):S78–9.
143. Hongeng S, Chuansumrit A, Hathirat P, et al. Full chimerism in nonmyeloablative stem cell transplantation in a beta-thalassemia major patient (class 3 Lucarelli). Bone Marrow Transplant 2002;30(6):409–10.
144. Krishnamurti L, Blazar BR, Wagner JE. Bone marrow transplantation without myeloablation for sickle cell disease. N Engl J Med 2001;344(1):68.
145. Schleuning M, Stoetzer O, Waterhouse C, et al. Hematopoietic stem cell transplantation after reduced-intensity conditioning as treatment of sickle cell disease. Exp Hematol 2002;30(1):7–10.
146. Shenoy S, Grossman WJ, DiPersio J, et al. A novel reduced-intensity stem cell transplant regimen for nonmalignant disorders. Bone Marrow Transplant 2005; 35(4):345–52.
147. van Besien K, Bartholomew A, Stock W, et al. Fludarabine-based conditioning for allogeneic transplantation in adults with sickle cell disease. Bone Marrow Transplant 2000;26(4):445–9.
148. Horan JT, Liesveld JL, Fenton P, et al. Hematopoietic stem cell transplantation for multiply transfused patients with sickle cell disease and thalassemia after low-dose total body irradiation, fludarabine, and rabbit anti-thymocyte globulin. Bone Marrow Transplant 2005;35(2):171–7.
149. Iannone R, Casella JF, Fuchs EJ, et al. Results of minimally toxic nonmyeloablative transplantation in patients with sickle cell anemia and beta-thalassemia. Biol Blood Marrow Transplant 2003;9(8):519–28.
150. Woolfrey AE, Pulsipher MA, Storb R. Non-myeloablative hematopoietic cell transplant for treatment of nonmalignant disorders in children. Int J Hematol 2002;76(Suppl 2):271–7.
151. Krishnamurti L, Wu CJ, Baker KS, et al. Matched sibling donor hematopoietic cell transplantation for sickle cell disease using a reduced intensity conditioning

regimen can lead to stable long term engraftment [abstract 3172]. Blood 2005; 106.

152. Dodero A, Carrabba M, Milani R, et al. Reduced-intensity conditioning containing low-dose alemtuzumab before allogeneic peripheral blood stem cell transplantation: graft-versus-host disease is decreased but T-cell reconstitution is delayed. Exp Hematol 2005;33(8):920–7.

153. Avivi I, Chakrabarti S, Kottaridis P, et al. Neurological complications following alemtuzumab-based reduced-intensity allogeneic transplantation. Bone Marrow Transplant 2004;34(2):137–42.

154. Iannone R, Luznik L, Engstrom LW, et al. Effects of mixed hematopoietic chimerism in a mouse model of bone marrow transplantation for sickle cell anemia. Blood 2001;97(12):3960–5.

155. Kean LS, Manci EA, Perry J, et al. Chimerism and cure: hematologic and pathologic correction of murine sickle cell disease. Blood 2003;102(13):4582–93.

156. Wu CJ, Krishnamurti L, Kutok JL, et al. Evidence for ineffective erythropoiesis in severe sickle cell disease. Blood 2005;106(10):3639–45.

157. Reed W, Smith R, Dekovic F, et al. Comprehensive banking of sibling donor cord blood for children with malignant and nonmalignant disease. Blood 2003;101(1): 351–7.

158. Krishnamurti L, Bunn HF, Williams AM, et al. Hematopoietic cell transplantation for hemoglobinopathies. Curr Probl Pediatr Adolesc Health Care 2008;38(1):6–18.

159. Slavin S, Nagler A, Naparstek E, et al. Nonmyeloablative stem cell transplantation and cell therapy as an alternative to conventional bone marrow transplantation with lethal cytoreduction for the treatment of malignant and nonmalignant hematologic diseases. Blood 1998;91(3):756–63.

160. Isola LM, Chao NJ, Weinberg RS, et al. Donor chimerism after T-cell depleted (TCD)-non-myeloablative allogeneic SCT (NST) in hemoglobinopathies. Blood 2002;100(11):part 2.

161. La NG, Giardini C, Argiolu F, et al. Unrelated donor bone marrow transplantation for thalassemia: the effect of extended haplotypes. Blood 2002;99(12):4350–6.

162. La NG, Argiolu F, Giardini C, et al. Unrelated bone marrow transplantation for beta-thalassemia patients: the experience of the Italian Bone Marrow Transplant Group. Ann N Y Acad Sci 2005;1054:186–95.

163. Hongeng S, Pakakasama S, Chuansumrit A, et al. Outcomes of transplantation with related- and unrelated-donor stem cells in children with severe thalassemia. Biol Blood Marrow Transplant 2006;12(6):683–7.

164. Sodani P, Isgro A, Gaziev J, et al. Purified T-depleted, CD34+ peripheral blood and bone marrow cell transplantation from haploidentical mother to child with thalassemia. Blood 2009 [Epub ahead of print].

165. Chakraverty R, Peggs K, Chopra R, et al. Limiting transplantation-related mortality following unrelated donor stem cell transplantation by using a nonmyeloablative conditioning regimen. Blood 2002;99(3):1071–8.

166. Adamkiewicz T, Mehta PS, Boyer MW, et al. Transplantation of unrelated placental blood cells in children with high-risk sickle cell disease. Bone Marrow Transplant 2004;34(5):405–11.

167. Krishnamurti L, Abel S, Maiers M, et al. Availability of unrelated donors for hematopoietic stem cell transplantation for hemoglobinopathies. Bone Marrow Transplant 2003;31(7):547–50.

168. Adamkiewicz T, Boyer MW, Bray R, et al. Identification of unrelated cord blood units for hematopoietic stem cell transplantation in children with sickle cell disease. J Pediatr Hematol Oncol 2006;28(1):29–32.

169. Myaskovsky L, Switzer GE, Dew MA, et al. The association of donor center characteristics with attrition from the national marrow donor registry. Transplantation 2004;77(6):874–80.

170. Flomenberg N, Baxter-Lowe LA, Confer D, et al. Impact of HLA class I and class II high-resolution matching on outcomes of unrelated donor bone marrow transplantation: HLA-C mismatching is associated with a strong adverse effect on transplantation outcome. Blood 2004;104(7):1923–30.

171. Barker JN, Weisdorf DJ, Wagner JE. Creation of a double chimera after the transplantation of umbilical-cord blood from two partially matched unrelated donors. N Engl J Med 2001;344(24):1870–1.

172. Miller ST, Sleeper LA, Pegelow CH, et al. Prediction of adverse outcomes in children with sickle cell disease. N Engl J Med 2000;342(2):83–9.

173. Shpall EJ, Quinones R, Giller R, et al. Transplantation of ex vivo expanded cord blood. Biol Blood Marrow Transplant 2002;8(7):368–76.

Bone Marrow Transplantation for Primary Immunodeficiency Diseases

Paul Szabolcs, MD[a,b,*], Marina Cavazzana-Calvo, MD, PhD[c,d], Alain Fischer, MD, PhD[e], Paul Veys, MBBS, FRCP, FRCPath, FRCPCH[f]

KEYWORDS

- Primary immunodeficiency diseases
- Hematopoietic stem cell transplantation
- Bone marrow transplantation
- Reduced intensity conditioning

Hematopoietic stem cell transplantation (HSCT) has emerged over the past 50 years as a life-saving therapy for many human diseases. Most recipients of allogeneic HSCT suffer from acquired disorders: leukemia, lymphoma, or aplastic anemia. From the beginning of HSCT use, however, it became apparent that adoptive transfer of healthy marrow and the progeny of donor bone marrow–derived hematopoietic stem cells lead to full reconstitution of the immune system. This recognition led to the use of HSCT for treatment of severe forms of inherited cellular immunodeficiencies. As early as 1968, only a year after the discovery of the human major histocompatibility complex (MHC) locus,[1] a child with severe combined immunodeficiency (SCID)[2] and another with Wiskott-Aldrich syndrome (WAS)[3] were transplanted successfully from their histocompatible siblings. The infant boy transplanted for SCID is the first long-term survivor of

[a] Department of Pediatrics, Pediatric Blood and Marrow Transplant Program, Box 3350, Duke University Medical Center, Durham, NC 27705, USA
[b] Department of Immunology, Duke University, Durham, NC, USA
[c] Department of Biotherapy, Hôpital Necker Enfants-Malades, Assistance Publique – Hôpitaux de Paris, Université Paris Descartes, Paris, France
[d] Clinical Investigation Center in Biotherapy, Groupe Hospitalier Ouest, Assistance Publique – Hôpitaux de Paris and INSERM, Paris, France
[e] Department of Pediatrics, Immunology & Hematology Unit, Hôpital Necker Enfants-Malades, Assistance Publique – Hôpitaux de Paris, Université Paris Descartes, Paris, France
[f] Department of BMT, Great Ormond Street Hospital for Children NHS Trust, London, UK
* Corresponding author. Department of Pediatrics, Pediatric Blood and Marrow Transplant Program, Box 3350, Duke University Medical Center, Durham, NC 27705.
E-mail address: szabo001@mc.duke.edu

Pediatr Clin N Am 57 (2010) 207–237
doi:10.1016/j.pcl.2009.12.004
0031-3955/10/$ – see front matter
pediatric.theclinics.com

HSCT.[4] SCID and WAS represent two common forms of the so-called primary immuno-deficiency diseases (PIDs). Rapid advances in molecular immunology over the past 15 years have led to a breathtaking expansion of recognized PIDs.[5–9] In most cases, PIDs are inherited as a result of monogenic defects with more than 120 disease-related genes recognized to date that manifest in more than 150 distinct clinical entities.[8]

Currently, up to 10 new genetic defects of PID are recognized each year,[9] requiring regular adjustment to the incidence of PIDs. A recent telephone survey of 10,000 households with nearly 27,000 household members by the United States Immunode-ficiency Network suggests a population prevalence of diagnosed PID in the United States at approximately 1 in approximately 1200 persons, rendering this diagnosis more common than previously suggested.[10]

The classical and severe forms of PID manifest with life-threatening infections during the first years of life as a result of blockage in T-lymphocyte (SCID) or B-lymphocyte (X-linked agammaglobulinemia) development. Antibody deficiencies due to abnormal B cell numbers or function can be effectively treated by replacement intravenous (IV) immunoglobulin infusions to prevent the recurrent bacterial respiratory tract infections. This is in contrast to T-lymphocyte defects that generally cannot be corrected without HSCT. This review does not discuss the promising results and associated challenges of gene therapy and thymus transplantation but rather focuses on the scientific and clinical advances in HSCT for the more common and severe forms of PID (**Table 1**).

Several challenges and controversies face clinical immunologists deciding when or whether or not to refer patients for transplantation and when facing transplanters choosing between sources of grafts and conditioning regimens. Until the late 1990s, almost all HSCT was performed after myeloablative conditioning (MAC) regimens with busulfan and cyclophosphamide or no chemotherapy conditioning at all. Over the past 10 years, however, reduced intensity conditioning (RIC) protocols have been introduced to reduce transplant-related mortality (TRM) and morbidity for children already experiencing liver, lung, and gastrointestinal complications of their underlying PID but nevertheless capable of rejecting a graft with residual natural killer (NK) cells and T lymphocytes. HLA MSDs remain the gold standard to which all alternative grafts are compared, but careful selection of donor sources and preparatory regimens has improved outcome with alternative donors. Some centers of excellence have already reported data for several PID syndromes WAS, hemophagocytic lymphohistiocytosis ([HLH], and leukocyte adhesion deficiency [LAD]) demonstrating that matched unrelated donor (MUD) recipients have comparable outcomes to those receiving MSD marrow grafts. Nevertheless, significant differences will likely remain between centers based on their expertise and preferences when deciding between alternative donor grafts, in their use or avoidance of T cell depletion and even in graft-versus-host disease (GVHD) prophylaxis. Recent advances in unrelated cord blood (UCB) transplantation have made it possible for virtually all children with PID to find a suitable graft donor.[11,12] The newly formed Primary Immune Deficiency Transplant Consortium recently surveyed 34 pediatric transplant centers in North America and reported that more than 1000 children have received allogeneic HSCT for one of three common PID syndromes: SCID, WAS, and chronic granulomatous disease (CGD).[13] Significantly, approximately 750 of these children are alive.[13]

SEVERE COMBINED IMMUNODEFICIENCY SYNDROMES

SCIDs constitute a heterogeneous group of genetically determined diseases impairing the T-cell differentiation program. Overall, the incidence of typical SCIDs is estimated to be 1 in 500,000. Fifteen distinct SCID conditions have been fully

Table 1
Primary immunodeficiency diseases treatable with hematopoietic stem cell transplantation

Classical SCID syndromes	
Nonclassical "leaky" SCID/CID syndromes	BLS
	OS
	CHH
	PNP deficiency
	ZAP70 deficiency
Other well-defined non-SCID/CID syndromes	WAS
	HIGM
Congenital defects of phagocyte numbers/function	CGD
	LADs
	MSMD
	Schwachman-Diamond syndrome
	SCN
Diseases of immune dysregulation	HLH
	Griscelli syndrome
	X-linked LPD
	CHS
	ALPS syndrome
	IPEX syndrome

described by genetic and molecular analysis to date and this will likely increase.[14] Even though all SCID patients experience an intrinsic impairment in T-cell development, there is marked heterogeneity due to variable differentiation of other hematopoietic cell lineages (ie, NK lymphocytes, B-lymphocytes, and neutrophils). In addition, in some of the diseases, developmental defects, such as microcephaly, deafness, neurologic abnormalities, and intestinal atresia, can be associated, raising specific issues in therapy. The absence of adaptive immunity is responsible for a fairly uniform clinical presentation, however, characterized by broad-spectrum susceptibility to pathogens and vulnerability to several opportunistic microorganisms that occur 3 to 12 months post birth. The exception to this paradigm is reticular dysgenesis (RD), in which the absence of neutrophils and T cells results in an earlier disease onset (ie, approximately 2 weeks after birth) characterized by septic episodes.[15] The severity of the clinical manifestations implies that SCIDs are medical emergencies. Untreated patients typically do not live beyond the age of 6 to 12 months. The lack of T cells and the correspondingly severe outcome explains why SCID was the first condition to be successfully treated by allogeneic HSCT more than 40 years ago.[2] Independent of the cell type used (ie, allogeneic HLA genocompatible or partially incompatible HSCT), dissection of the problems raised by HSCT in these settings has contributed to its development in the treatment of other genetic and acquired disorders of hematopoiesis.

Six Main Causes of Severe Combined Immunodeficiency and Consequences for Hematopoietic Stem Cell Transplantation

1. Defective survival differentiation of T-cell and neutrophil precursor (RD).
2. Premature cell death caused by the accumulation of purine metabolites (adenosine deaminase [ADA] deficiency).
3. Defective cytokine-dependent survival signaling in T-cell precursors (and sometimes in NK-cell precursors). This mechanism accounts for more than approximately 50% of SCID cases. Impairment in the expression or function of the γ

common (γc) cytokine receptor subunit (shared by the receptors for interleukin [IL]-2, IL-4, IL-7, IL-9, IL-15, and IL-21) causes the X-linked form of SCID, which is characterized by the complete absence of T and NK lymphocytes.[16] Deficiency in JAK3 (which normally binds to the cytoplasmic region of γc) results in an identical phenotype that displays AR inheritance. Deficiency in IL-7Rα results in T-cell deficiency but normal NK cell development and is inherited in an AR fashion.

4. Defective V(D)J rearrangements of the T-cell receptor (TCR) and B-cell receptor genes. In the Paris experience, this group accounts for 30% of SCID cases, contrasting with the Duke University series of 174 children, where it was identified in less than 5%.[17] Deficiency in RAG1 or RAG2 (the lymphoid-specific recombination initiating elements) or Artemis (a factor involved in the nonhomologous end-joining repair pathway) leads to defective V(D)J rearrangements and thereby thymocyte and pre–B-cell death.

5. Defective pre-TCR and TCR signaling. Pure T-cell deficiencies are caused by defects in a CD3 subunit (such as CD3-δ, -ϵ, or -ζ)[18–20] or the CD45 tyrosine phosphatase—both of which are key proteins involved in pre-TCR or TCR signaling at the positive selection stage.[21]

6. Defective egress of thymocytes from the thymus.[22]

The relative frequencies of the different genetic types of SCID are different in Europe from those observed in the United States.[23] In particular, frequencies of V(D)J rearrangement defects are approximately 30% in Europe and only 4.2 in the United States. Furthermore, ADA and cytokine-dependent survival signaling defects account for 80% of all SCID forms in the United States and 60% in Europe. This difference in frequency has to be kept in mind when trying to compare HSCT clinical results in these two continents, taking into account the influence of the SCID form on the long-term outcome of these patients.[24,25]

Some researchers include other T-cell immunodeficiencies in the SCID group, such as ZAP70 deficiency,[26] CD3-γ deficiencies,[27] HLA class II expression deficiency,[28] purine nucleoside phosphorylase (PNP) deficiency,[29] ligase IV and Cernunnos deficiencies,[30,31] and Omenn syndrome (OS).[32] Because these conditions are characterized by the presence of residual mature (although functionally defective) T cells, they are discussed later.

Allogeneic Hematopoietic Stem Cell Transplantation

The easiest situation: hematopoietic stem cell transplantation from an HLA identical sibling

Since the pioneering experiment in 1968, hundreds of SCID patients worldwide have undergone HSCT.[4,24,33–35] At present, HSCT from an HLA MSD confers a 90% chance of a cure. For patients without pre-existing infections (such as neonates with SCID), the outcome is even better.[36,37] This setting does not require myeloablative therapy to enable donor cell engraftment and is associated with an extremely infrequent occurrence of GVHD, for reasons that are not clear. The second favorable aspect of HLA-identical HSCT is the fast rate of T-cell recovery because of the homeostatic- and also antigen-driven expansion of the mature/memory donor T cells present in the graft. In HLA-identical HSCT, T cells can be observed as early as 10 to 15 days after transplantation and reach normal levels within 1 to 2 months. Later on (usually 3 to 4 months after transplantation), the peripheral detection of naïve T cells indicates that neothymopoiesis is also taking place. The rapid restoration of the T cell compartment and the quasi-absence of GVHD explain the excellent prognosis for HLA-identical HSCT.

Matched unrelated donors
This source of hematopoietic stem cells generally can provide results close to a HLA genoidentical-related HSCT, rendering this graft source theoretically preferable for SCID patients. Grunebaum and colleagues[35] have recently reported good clinical results in SCID patients (80.5% survival) treated with MUD grafts. The overall European experience is slightly different. In the 2000–2005 period, the survival rates for MUD and related HLA mismatched treated patients were 69% and 66%, respectively.[38] The major obstacle to the routine use of this HSC source is the median time that can be required from diagnosis to MUD HSCT, which is 4 to 6 months. This delay can be detrimental to infected patients as it increases the risk of clinical deterioration in patients with poorly treatable infection (for instance, severe respiratory viruses). Thus, in order to more accurately evaluate the role of MUD source for SCID patients, a comparison should be made assessing patients in similar clinical conditions as "intention to treat." This type of comparison is not available today. Likely, the use of a MUD requiring several weeks or months for transplantation to be organized should be restricted to SCID patients in good clinical condition or for atypical SCID patients over the age of 2 with residual T-cell immunity.

The most difficult situation: hematopoietic stem cell transplantation from an HLA partially matched familial donor or umbilical cord blood
Haploidentical HSCT was introduced in this setting in 1982 to 1983, when techniques were developed to efficiently deplete contaminating donor mature T cells in the graft.[39] Substantial numbers of SCID patients have received transplants across the major HLA barrier, and it seems that this type of donor provides a more favorable outcome in SCID than results generally reported for other clinical settings treated with haploidentical transplantation.[33,40] Taking into account the obstacles raised by haploidentical HSCT, the question can be raised of the value of cord blood–derived HSC in this particular setting. The preliminary results of an international survey comparing the outcome of haploidentical versus cord blood HSCT in primary immunodeficiencies seem to indicate that event-free survival is essentially the same in both groups. This emphasizes the importance of the transplantation center's expertise (rather than the donor source) in the HSCT outcome.[41]

More than 40 years' experience has provided essential information that may enable building up a la carte treatments for the four main groups of SCID patients. The defective cytokine-dependent survival signaling in T cell precursors (and sometimes NK-cell precursors) represents the most favorable situation—even for haploidentical HSCT. The combination of a lack of NK cells (in γc and JAK3 deficiencies) and a very early block in T-cell precursors completely abolishes graft rejection, resulting in high engraftment rates in the absence of any conditioning. The immediate consequence is greater than 70% survival rate in these patients, as long as severe, pre-existing, OIs are not present,[38] a result similar to that reported by Buckley for X-linked SCID transplanted patients.[23] In the absence of a myeloablative regimen, characteristic split chimerism is observed in this condition, characterized by the detection of donor T cells and host B cells in most cases.[42,43] Despite the use of immunoglobulin substitution therapy, the absence of B-cell engraftment is responsible for recurrent respiratory tract infections more than 10 years after HSCT in some of the patients.[24] In addition to these infectious episodes, the long-term prognosis of such patients is hampered by the occurrence in up to 30% of severe human papilloma virus infections, probably related to the nonhematopoietic consequences of γc and JAK3 deficiencies.[44]

The poorest prognosis is observed in *ADA*-deficient patients transplanted with an HLA partially compatible donor. The toxic accumulation of ADA metabolites in organs, such as lung and thymus, and the high toxicity of the required conditioning regimen to achieve engraftment are responsible for this poorer outcome. As a result, stem cell transplantation using a haploidentical donor is not recommended for this particular SCID form, except for neonates.

Patients affected by defective V(D)J rearrangements of the TCR and B-cell receptor genes and transplanted with an HLA partially incompatible donor exhibit an intermediate outcome. The presence of functional NK cells potentially able to reject the graft and the occupation of the stromal niches by double-negative T-precursors in Rag 1 or Rag 2 or Artemis deficiencies diminish the likelihood of adequate engraftment in the absence of an appropriate conditioning regimen.

Impact of immune reconstitution and graft-versus-host disease on outcome

SCID patients with faster and better immune reconstitution have more successful outcomes. In a survey of 90 patients transplanted in Paris at Hôpital Necker, it has been clearly demonstrated that the 1- and 2-year post-HSCT event-free survival rates of patients with low CD4+ T-cell counts were significantly lower than for patients with normal CD4+ T-cell counts.[24] The occurrence of acute GVHD (aGVHD) and chronic GVHD (cGVHD) is strongly associated with poor immune reconstitution, so GVHD prevention is mandatory in this setting. The results of this long-term outcome of a single-center cohort is difficult to compare with the survey reported by the team at Duke University on the long-term immune reconstitution in 128 transplanted SCID patients.[25] There are significant differences between these two large cohorts, largely due to the different prevalence of genetic subsets. In Sarzotti-Kelsoe and colleagues' survey, 86 of 128 patients have a defect in the cytokine signaling pathway and only seven presented with SCID due to a V(D)J rearrangement defect and only one with Artemis deficiency. Nevertheless, the Sarzotti-Kelsoe and colleagues' analysis clearly indicates that the ADA and Rag-deficient patients are not as healthy as those with the other molecular types of SCID in line with their lower T-cell numbers, function, and thymic output after transplantation.[25] In the survey from Paris,[24] the same number of cytokine-dependent signaling defect and V(D)J recombination defects have been analyzed (n = 38), thus sufficiently powering the analysis to conclude that the poorest prognosis is for patients with an Artemis deficiency SCID form. Artemis is a protein ubiquitously expressed and is a key element of the nonhomologous end-joining process involved in double-stand DNA break repair. Thus, in the group of patients with this defective DNA repair pathway,[24] there was a higher incidence of long-term complications, such as persistent aGVHD, auto-immunity/inflammation, requirement for some form of long-term nutritional support, opportunistic infection, and growth failure. These results indicate that further efforts should be made to design more tailored regimens in the future for these two different SCID forms.

Poor or slow immune reconstitution can result from thymic damage. In these patients, the latter is the sum of (1) the profound abnormalities in the distribution and function of cortical and medullary thymic epithelial cells (TECs) and thymic dendritic cells caused by genetic defects and thymic damage due to infection prior to transplant, (2) GVHD-induced thymic dysplasia, and (3) possibly toxicity of conditioning regimen. These conditions can profoundly affect the mechanisms of central tolerance and likely contribute to the autoimmune/inflammatory complications observed in mismatched related donor (MMRD) HSCT transplant recipients.[45] The specific contribution of each of these mechanisms to the long-lasting immune reconstitution is difficult to determine. Clave and colleagues[46] recently reported that in patients with grade I aGVHD, the median naïve positive TCR excision circles T-cell count was closer to that of patients with grades II–IV GVHD than that of patients with no detectable aGVHD. Subclinical, GVHD-mediated thymic lesions may thus play an important role in persistent immunodeficiency. Hence, any factor or cell therapy approach able to improve post-HSCT immune reconstitution is highly warranted. For example, it may be worth investigating the use of an anti–interferon (IFN)-γ antibody to prevent the thymic damage due to alloreactivity. Fibroblast growth factor 7 (also known as keratinocyte growth factor) is a potent epithelial cell mitogen and is able to protect against radiotherapy- and chemotherapy-induced damage and could improve TEC recovery after HSCT. Another strategy for speeding up immune reconstitution in this setting involves providing recipients with mature T cells devoid of specific antihost alloreactivity or pathogen-specific mature donor T cells.[47–49] Other potentially feasible approaches include the use of Notch ligands to preferentially expand lymphoid progenitors. Thus, understanding of the precise mechanisms underlying de novo thymus-dependent generation of T cells serves as a basis for new strategies aimed at improving T-cell reconstitution; anticytokine antibodies, growth factors, and Notch-based culture systems are currently under investigation.

COMBINED IMMUNODEFICIENCY SYNDROMES

The heterogeneous collection of nonclassical SCID syndromes—bare lymphocyte syndrome (BLS), OS, cartilage hair hypoplasia (CHH), PNP deficiency, ZAP70 defects, and other yet uncharacterized PID—are variably described as leaky SCID or CID syndromes. They are characterized by the presence of some mature T lymphocytes in the circulation (>10% of normal) associated with measurable T-cell function, typically exhibiting at least 10% or higher mitogen-induced proliferation in response to phytohemagglutinin. Despite the measurable T-cell numbers and function, these values are typically less than 25% of age-matched normal. There is a wide range of genetic defects leading to numeric deficits and functional defects as a result of low protein expression or a hypomorphic mutation in a known SCID disease gene. As a result of residual T-cell function, children with CID syndromes have a life expectancy typically beyond the first year of life. Nevertheless, children afflicted by one of the CID/nonclassical SCID syndromes usually die during childhood as a result of insufficient cellular immunity against opportunistic infections (OIs). CID syndromes almost invariably require chemotherapy-based conditioning to prevent host NK- or T-cell–mediated rejection of the graft. Because of the frequent pulmonary and other comorbidities, however, CID syndromes have become the ideal patient population to explore, in rigorous clinical trials, the benefits of non-MAC (discussed later).[50]

Omenn Syndrome

OS is a prototypical leaky SCID/CID syndrome with AR inheritance. Young infants with OS typically present with the triad of lymphadenopathy, hepatosplenomegaly, and erythroderma with many also demonstrating alopecia and failure to thrive due to chronic diarrhea. The clinical symptoms reflect the tissue infiltration of oligoclonal, autoreactive T cells that have likely escaped negative selection in the thymus. Although eosinophilia is the most striking laboratory feature, most cases also present with hypogammaglobulinemia, elevated serum IgE, and defective antibody production. Hypomorphic mutations in the Rag 1 or Rag 2 genes leading to partial VDJ recombination activity, autoimmune regulator (AIRE) deficiency,[51] and mutation in DNA ligase IV[52] have been all described to lead to OS. OS is inevitably fatal if untreated and HSCT is the only potentially curative option. Initial reports suggested that survival after HSCT was poor for children with OS, mainly as a result of graft failure, infections, and metabolic complications.[53,54] More recently, however, survival rates of greater than 80% have been reported with the use of HLA-haploidentical parental and unrelated donor (UD) graft.[55,56] Although most children successfully transplanted so far have received MAC, there are reports of full donor chimerism even after RIC that typically also include serotherapy with antithymocyte globulin (ATG).[57,58]

Bare Lymphocyte Syndrome

BLS is caused by defective expression of class II MHC molecules arising from at least four well-defined gene defects.[28] Any of these results in defective maturation and activation of CD4+ T cells, impaired antigen presentation by B cells, and dendritic cells. These patients develop severe infections in the first months of life. Despite normal mitogenic T-cell responses, antigen-specific responses are impaired.[5] Fungal, viral, and bacterial pathogens cause life-threatening meningoencephalitis and recurrent, unremitting liver and respiratory tract infections. More than 10% of nonclassical SCID patents transplanted in Europe had BLS.[33] Due to the high incidence of graft failure and infectious complications, survival has been dismal in most transplant series ranging between 20% and 40%.[33,59–61] Even in successfully engrafted cases of MSD transplantation there is concern of altered immune recovery manifesting in reduced MHC class II antigen expression and a restricted TCR repertoire on T-cell activation.[62] These donor T-cell defects are likely caused by a host environment that continues to lack MHC class II even after HSCT.

Purine Nucleoside Phosphorylase Deficiency

PNP deficiency is a rare CID syndrome characterized by T-cell immunodeficiency, hypouricemia, and profound lymphopenia.[63] Unlike ADA deficiency, uric acid levels in serum and urine are low because PNP is necessary to form the urate precursors, hypoxanthine and xanthine. Genetic analysis of the PNP gene reveals several recurring mutations.[64] A significant proportion of patients develop autoimmune syndromes with cytopenias, systemic lupus erythematosus–like syndromes, and up to two-thirds display neurologic deficits ranging from ataxia to spasticity and even mental retardation. PNP syndrome represented onlyapproximately 1% of all transplants among 444 non-SCID patients transplanted between 1968 and 1999 in Europe.[33] After donor-cell engraftment, lymphocyte function and numbers rapidly improve in concert with PNP activity and rising uric acid levels[65]; however, it remains unclear whether or not CNS deficits progress or possibly improve.[66,67]

Zap-70 Deficiency

The TCR ζ chain–associated protein tyrosine kinase 70 defect (also known as ZAP70 deficiency) leads to profound and isolated CD8+ T-cell lymphopenia and a few cases of this rare PID have been transplanted succesfully.[35,68] Although CD4+ T-cell numbers are within normal range, they fail to respond in vitro to mitogens or allogeneic stimulators. In contrast to the T cell defects, B- and NK-cell numbers and function seem normal.[5,26]

Cartilage Hair Hypoplasia

CHH is a recessively inherited pleiotropic syndrome with metaphyseal chondrodysplasia manifesting as short-limbed dwarfism, hypoplastic hair growth, and impaired cell-mediated immunity and is sometimes associated with severe anemia and Hirschsprung disease. The syndrome is exceptionally prevalent among the Finns (carrier frequency approximately 1:76) and among the Amish in the United States, and sporadic cases have been reported from other countries.[69] CHH is caused by mutations in the ribonuclease mitochondrial RNA processing (MRP) gene, encoding the

RNA component of the ribonuclease complex, RNase MRP.[70] The spectrum of immune defects in CHH range from SCID-like severity to mild reduction in T-cell–mediated immunity, although IgA and IgG subclass defects and autoimmune cytopenias have also been described.[71] HSCT has been highly successful in correcting the more severe cases of immunodeficiency and anemia, whereas bone growth may also improve.[72,73]

OTHER WELL-DEFINED NON–SEVERE COMBINED IMMUNODEFICIENCY/COMBINED IMMUNODEFICIENCY SYNDROMES
Wiskott-Aldrich Syndrome

WAS is an X-linked disorder with an incidence of four per million live male births; it has a broad range of clinical phenotypes,[74] but is characterized by thrombocytopenia with small platelets, eczema, progressive immunodeficiency, and an increased risk of autoimmune disorders and cancers.[75] The disorder is caused by mutations in the WASP gene at Xp11.22,[76] which encodes for a cytoplasmic protein, primarily expressed in hematopoietic cells, and is involved in the regulation of cytoskeletal reorganization.

Without HSCT, WAS patients have a poor prognosis with the major causes of death being infection, bleeding, and lymphoproliferative disease (LPD). Splenectomy usually increases platelet count and reduces the risk of significant hemorrhage but the risk of death from sepsis is increased.[77] In 1968, Bach and associates[3] reported partial correction of WAS after transplantation with high-dose cyclophosphamide and HLA-matched related donor (MRD) bone marrow. The recipient initially only recovered donor-derived T-cell immunity and required retransplant with MAC secondary to clinically significant thrombocytopenia and has since died at age 36 years, secondary to complications of aGVHD and cGVHD. Since that first transplant, HSCT from a matched sibling donor (MSD) has become standard of care. A worldwide review from 1968 through 1995 reported long-term survival in 57 of 65 (88%) children with WAS undergoing MSD bone marrow transplantation (BMT), and HLA MSD grafts administered after MAC remain the treatment of choice for this disorder. In the absence of a MRD, impressive results have been reported from the Center for International Blood and Marrow Transplant Research (CIBMTR) with 71% of patients surviving after matched UD HSCT.[78] The prognosis seems better when HSCT was performed below the age of 5 years (89% cure vs 30%) with significant problems from GVHD in older children.

Between 1968 and 2000, 103 patients undergoing HSCT for WAS (with a minimum follow-up of 6 months) were reported to the Stem Cell Transplantation for Immunodeficiency in Europe (SCETIDE) registry from 37 centers in 18 European countries.[33] Thirty-three patients received HSCT from a MSD, five from other HLA MRDs, 45 from a MMRD, and 20 patients from an UD (some of these patients were also reported in the CIBMTR database). The 3-year overall survival for the whole group was 62%. The outcome for MSD HSCT was 81%, the outcome of UD HSCT (75% of which were fully HLA matched) was analyzed together with other non-SCID immunodeficiencies because of small numbers but did not differ significantly from that of MSD HSCT (59% vs 71%).

A more current analysis from the CIBMTR comparing 113 recipients of UD bone marrow to 65 patients who received UCB transplants between 1995 and 2005 shows equivalent survival 3 years post transplant for recipients under 5 years of age at the time of the procedure (73% and 75%).[79] Similarly good recent results have also been reported from a Japanese group using unrelated cord blood transplantation, with 80% survival in 15 children with WAS.[80] Recent results from a single center show further improvement: at Cincinnati Children's Hospital Medical Center 33 boys have been treated for WAS since 2000. All 21 boys treated under 5 years of age (19 using UD grafts) are alive and hematologically reconstituted, although during the first year post UD HSCT, approximately half of the boys experienced some degree of aGVHD or immune cytopenias.[79]

For patients who lack a closely matched HLA identical donor, therapeutic options are limited. Results of haplotyped-MMRDs are significantly poorer than related identical donors (45% vs 81% survival)[33] and (52% vs 87% survival),[78] with failures due to graft rejection, Epstein-Barr virus (EBV)-associated LPD, and GVHD. Splenectomy, if appropriate, and supportive care may be the preferred approach until alternative therapies (eg, gene therapy) become available.

A recent study from multiple European centers examined the long-term outcome of 96 WAS patients who underwent HSCT after a MAC regimen between 1979 and 2001 and who survived at least 2 years after HSCT.[81] Overall, the 7-year event-free survival was 75% and was significantly influenced by donor group: MSD HSCT—88%, UD HSCT—71% (P = .03), and MMRD—55% (P = .003). cGVHD-independent autoimmunity in 20% of patients was strongly associated with MC or split (donor T-cell, host myeloid, and B-cell) chimerism status suggesting that residual host cells can moderate autoimmune disease despite coexistence of donor cells. The overall incidence of autoimmunity was 8% in patients with full donor chimerism and 71% in patients with mixed/split chimerism (P = .001). Autoimmune manifestations were more frequent in recipients of UDs (28%) and MMRD (26%) transplants than MSD HSCT (11%). A more detailed analysis of chimerism performed on different cell lineages based primarily on WASP expression should provide further insight into which host-cell lineages could provoke autoimmunity, and further follow-up is required to understand the significance of mixed/split chimerism. Infectious complications related to splenectomy were significant in this study, suggesting that splenectomy should be avoided in patients with WAS who are candidates for HSCT or who have already undergone HSCT. These findings, if confirmed, may have important implications for reduced intensity HSCT in WAS where the incidence of mixed chimerism (MC) may be increased (discussed later).[82]

Hyper IgM Syndrome

HIGM syndrome can result from a growing number of distinct molecular defects, each manifesting with impaired immunoglobulin class-switch recombination, associated with abnormal/absent germinal center formation and low/undetectable levels of IgA, IgE, and IgG accompanied by normal or elevated IgM levels. The most common form, type 1 X-linked HIGM syndrome (HIGM1), is caused by mutations in the gene encoding the CD154 protein, also known as CD40 ligand (CD40L). CD40L is a key signaling molecule between dendritic cells, B cells, and T lymphocytes and is critical in initiating immunoglobulin class switching.[7,9,83] Affected boys commonly present with *Pneumocystis jiroveci* pneumonia, recurrent viral and bacterial sinopulmonary infections, the uniquely common gastroenteritis caused by *Cryptosporidium parvum* that advances in many cases to sclerosing cholangitis, and cirrhosis in more than 15% of all patients. Neutropenia and autoimmune disease are also common. Other clinically related but genetically distinct HIGM syndromes are characterized by severe class-switch recombination deficiency. HIGM2 is characterized by defects in the master regulator called activation-induced cytidine deaminase gene resulting in no somatic hypermutation (SHM), an essential mutation process for selection of higher-affinity antibodies over time. In HIGM3, the uracil-DNA-glycosylate enzyme deficiency leads to a biased SHM pattern, whereas patients with HIGM4 exhibit normal SHM due to the C-terminal mutation of activation-induced cytidine deaminase. There is a wealth of data on the efficacy of HSCT, in particular for HIGM1, including case reports,[84] registry data,[33,58] and an expansive European retrospective survey that analyzed outcome between 1993 and 2003 in 38 patients with CD40L deficiency.[85] Despite significant comorbidities, two-thirds of these patients were alive and well at the time of publication and 22 of 38 (58%) were cured, all expressing CD40L appropriately. Survival was not inferior when comparing MSD to UD grafts. Engraftment was noted in approximately 90% regardless of T-cell depletion practices and even in four of six patients who received RIC regimens. Despite sclerosing cholangitis or cirrhosis in 20 patients, venoocclusive disease (VOD) occurred only in four. Pre-existing lung disease was the most important adverse risk factor and all 12 patients who failed to survive died of infections related to cryptosporidiosis, cytomegalovirus (CMV), and *Aspergillus* infection.[85]

CONGENITAL DEFECTS OF PHAGOCYTE NUMBERS OR FUNCTION
Chronic Granulomatous Disease

CGD is a prototypic PID characterized by abnormal phagocytic function with low prevalence (approximately 1:250,000) due to a mutation in one of the four subunits of the NADPH oxidase enzyme complex. Regardless of X-linked or autosomal recessive (AR) inheritance, affected children lack a "respiratory burst," essential for the clearance of phagocytosed microorganisms predisposing them to life-threatening infections (suppurative lung disease, osteomyelitis, and brain and other abscesses) and granuloma formation anywhere in the gastrointestinal tract and urinary bladder.[86–88] Inflammatory complications, most notably inflammatory bowel disease, are not uncommon.[86–88] Recurrent bacterial and fungal infections are typically caused by a relatively narrow spectrum, including *Staphylococcus*, *Aspergillus*, and atypical mycobacteria. Seger reported in 2002 the largest survey from a combined European Group for Blood and Marrow Transplantation (EBMT) /European Society for Immunodeficiencies (ESID) registry analyzing 15 years experience with an OS of 23 of 27 patients and 22 cured of CGD.[89] In addition, seven of nine MUD recipients are survivors in a recent series from Ulm,[90] and 18 of 20 transplanted in Newcastle (median follow-up of 51 months) survived with most patients achieving normal neutrophil function, remission of colitis, and catch-up growth after MSD (n = 10) or MUD (n = 10) transplantation.[91] In the latter series, most, 16 of 20, received busulfan-based MAC regimens (discussed later).

Leukocyte Adhesion Deficiency

LAD is a rare AR PID reported in approximately 300 patients worldwide. Its most common form, LAD-I, is caused by defects in the ITGB2 gene encoding CD18, the β2 integrin subunit essential for leukocyte adhesion and migration when combining with one of three α integrin subunits to form leukocyte function-associated antigen 1 (LFA1). Extreme leukocytosis, recurrent bacterial and fungal infections, impaired pus formation, and slow wound healing resulting in disfiguring scars characterize this disorder.[92] The recently described LAD variant syndromes have intact CD18 but display defective functions of selectin ligands or have defects in adaptor proteins required for integrin signaling (discussed later).[93]

Mendelian Susceptibility to Mycobacterial Disease

MSMD is often treated as isolated refractory mycobacterial infections or CGD; however, the spectrum of disease extends from early-onset overwhelming mycobacterial infection to adult-onset localized disease and tuberculosis.[94] Although genetically different, these conditions are immunologically related, as all result in impaired IL-12/23–IFN-γ–mediated immunity. These disorders have been diagnosed in more than 220 patients from more than 43 countries worldwide.[95,96] There are six MSMD-causing genes, including one X-linked gene (nuclear factor κB-essential modulator [*NEMO*]) and five autosomal genes (IFN-γ receptors 1 and 2 [*IFNGR1, IFNGR2*], signal transducer and activator of transcription 1 [*STAT1*], IL-12 p40 subunit [*IL12P40*], and IL-12 receptor β-subunit [*IL12RB1*]).[95] Most patients are ideal candidates for cytokine therapy; nevertheless, HSCT has been successfully performed.[97,98] Graft failure and poorly controlled mycobacterial infections were the major cause of failure in children with complete *IFNGR1* deficiency.[97]

Severe Congenital Neutropenia

In 1956, Kostmann first described a disorder that is part of the heterogeneous marrow failure syndrome called severe congenital neutropenia (SCN). SCN includes a variety of hematologic disorders characterized by severe neutropenia and systemic bacterial infections from early infancy (reviewed by Welte and colleagues).[99,100] Data on more than 600 patients with SCN collected by the Severe Chronic Neutropenia International Registry demonstrate that, regardless of the particular congenital neutropenia (CN) subtype, more than 95% of these patients respond to recombinant human granulocyte colony-stimulating factor (G-CSF) maintaining absolute neutrophil count (ANC) above $1.0 \times 10(9)/L$.[100] Nevertheless, allogeneic HSCT is the only cure for SCN, and the emerging data on the risk for myelodysplastic syndromes or acute leukemia in high-risk SCN subsets, such as neutrophil elastase mutations,[101] justify HSCT.[102] A recent review analyzed 374 SCN and 29 SDS patients receiving long-term G-CSF.[103] In G-CSF less-responsive patients, the cumulative incidence of adverse events was highest: after 10 years, 40% developed myelodysplastic syndromes/acute myelogenous leukemia and 14% died of sepsis. Although several successful cases have been described with variable graft and preparatory regimens, including RIC, outcomes of HSCT have been poor when leukemic transformation has already taken place.[104–106]

Schwachmann-Diamond Syndrome

SDS is an AR disorder characterized by exocrine pancreas insufficiency, metaphyseal dysostosis, and bone marrow dysfunction. Recurrent severe bacterial infections leading to bronchiectasis and susceptibility to leukemia are the major causes of morbidity and mortality occurring preferentially in patients with pancytopenia and myelodysplastic features. Allogeneic HSCT has clearly demonstrated efficacy using marrow[19] and UCB[107] (reviewed by Myers and Davies).[108] As reported by Bhatla and colleagues,[109] RIC regimen with fludarabine/melphalan/alemtuzumab (Campath-1H) (FMC) conditioning led to 100% survival in eight patients (discussed later).

DISEASES OF IMMUNE DYSREGULATION
Hemophagocytic Lymphohistiocytosis

HLH constitutes a rare but severe syndrome that can be primary (with a genetic etiology) or secondary (associated with malignancies, autoimmune diseases, or infections).[110] Infections associated with hemophagocytic syndrome are most frequently caused by viruses, in particular EBV. Inherited primary HLH, also called familial HLH, presents during infancy with fever, pancytopenia, hypofibrinogenemia, elevated ferritin, and triglyceride levels associated with hemophagocytosis in bone marrow aspirates. CNS involvement is frequent. HLH may present in association with other immunodeficiencies, mostly with Chediak-Higashi syndrome (CHS) 1, Griscelli syndrome 2, and

X-linked lymphoproliferative (XLP) syndrome. HLH is caused by genetic defects that impair T-cell–mediated and natural cytotoxicity resulting in persistent antigen-driven T-cell activation along with sustained macrophage activation and tissue infiltration. During active HLH there is massive production of inflammatory cytokines (granulo-cyte-macrophage colony-stimulating factor, IFN-γ, IL-6, and IL-8) that perpetuate the clinical symptoms. Allogeneic HSCT after induction with immuno/chemotherapy remains the only curative option (reviewed by Jordan and Filipovich).[111] A recently completed multicenter trial, HLH-94, reported 64% event-free survival at 3 years in 86 children.[112] Remarkably, event-free survival was similar, with greater than 70% using MSD or MUD donors, whereas survival with partially MMRDs was inferior. The outcome of MUD recipients on HLH-94 surpassed registry results of 91 MUD patients from an older era, spanning 1989 to 2005.[113] Patients who responded well to initial pre-transplant induction therapy fared best, similar to those in the report summarizing 48 patients transplanted over 2 decades in Paris,[56] who also demonstrated that donor chimerism of at least 20% was associated with clinical remission (discussed later).[113]

Chediak-Higashi Syndrome

Eapen and colleagues reported the international experience on transplant outcomes for CHS.[114] With a median follow-up of 6.5 years, the 5-year probability of overall survival was 62% among 35 children. Children with CHS manifest with oculocutane-ous albinism, recurrent infections, mild coagulation defects, and varying neurologic problems.[115] The hematologic hallmark of CHS is the presence of huge cytoplasmic peroxidase-positive granules in circulating granulocytes and many other cell types. Mutations in the lysosomal trafficking regulator gene, called *CHS1/LYST*, impair chemotaxis, bactericidal activity, and NK-cell function.[115]

Autoimmune Lyphoproliferative Syndrome

Autoimmune lyphoproliferative syndrome (ALPS) was previously called Canale-Smith syndrome after their description of the constellation of lymphadenopathy, spleno-megaly, and autoimmune cytopenias in 1967.[116] The molecular defects responsible for defective lymphocyte apoptosis that lead to an increase in CD4−/CD8− double-negative T cells range from mutations first discovered in CD95/FAS (ALPS Ia) to those impairing CD95 ligand (ALPS Ib) and caspase-8 and caspase-10 (ALPS IIa and IIb).[9] ALPS I and II patients share with the Fas-independent (ALPS III) patients the patho-gnomonic features of nonmalignant lymphoproliferation and autoimmune abnormali-ties and most will likely not need HSCT unless they have the rare homozygous form of Fas-deficiency.[117]

Immune Dysregulation, Polyendocrinopathy, Enteropathy, X-Linked Syndrome

Immune dysregulation, polyendocrinopathy, enteropathy, X-linked syndrome (IPEX) results from mutations of a unique DNA-binding protein gene, FOXP3, that is highly expressed in CD4+/CD25+ naturally occurring regulatory T cells (reviewed by Ben-nett and Ochs).[118] Loss of functional regulatory T cells leads to fatal autoimmunity unless lifelong immunosuppression is administered to control debilitating colitis and food allergies. The first case of HSCT for IPEX was reported in 2001[119] and since then the RIC approach has also been successfully employed.[120]

MODIFIED CONDITIONING/REDUCED INTENSITY CONDITIONING

Many children with PID have significant comorbidities at the time of HSCT and conventional MAC may therefore result in significant treatment-related toxicity and long-term sequelae. Over the past decade, the use of reduced intensity transplantation has become a well-established approach in adult patients with malignant disease, extending curative HSCT to older individuals and patients with comorbidities otherwise ineligible for myeloablative procedures.[121–123] Because pediatric patients generally tolerate more intensive transplant approaches, MAC regimens have continued to be preferred in childhood malignancies. However, as there is no requirement for high-dose chemotherapy to eradicate malignancy in children undergoing HSCT, for non-malignant disorders, the use of reduced intensity regimens has become an attractive option, and may be particularly suitable in those with PID as variable immunodeficiency reduces the chance of rejection.

Two general approaches have been used to develop less toxic regimens.[50,124] Terminology may be confusing but so-called RIC protocols (**Fig. 1**) have been developed by replacing myeloablative agents with more immunosuppressive and less myelosuppressive properties.[125,126] Such protocols still contain agents capable of ablating stem cells (eg, busulfan or melphalan) but at a reduced dose compared to conventional HSCT. In contrast, regimens with minimal toxicity or minimal intensity conditioning (MIC) (see **Fig. 1**) are truly nonmyeloablative and contain only immunosuppressive agents.

A truly nonmyeloablative/MIC regimen should not eradicate host hematopoiesis and should allow relatively prompt autologous hematopoietic recovery without a transplant but be sufficient to enable at least partial donor engraftment to occur post HSCT.[127] In this setting, initial chimerism is often mixed. In contrast, RIC regimens require HSCT for prompt hematologic recovery and if the graft is rejected, prolonged aplasia may occur. Initial chimerism after RIC HSCT is frequently 100% donor but may decline thereafter in the absence of graft versus marrow, as autologous hematopoiesis recovers.

Reduced Intensity Conditioning Protocols for Primary Immunodeficiency

Fludarabine/melphalan

The combination of fludarabine, melphalan, and ATG (FMA) was first reported by Amrolia and colleagues[128] from London, in eight patients with SCID and non-SCID

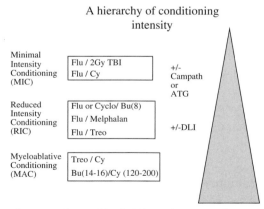

Fig. 1. A hierarchy of commonly used MIC, RIC, and MAC regimens in PID patients. BU8, busulfan (8 mg/kg); BU14-16, busulfan (14–16 mg/kg); cyclo, cyclophosphamide; CY120-200, cyclophosphamide (120–200 mg/kg); Flu, fludarabine; Gy, gray. (*From* Satwani P, Cooper N, Rao K, et al. Reduced intensity conditioning and allogeneic stem cell transplantation in childhood malignant and nonmalignant diseases. Bone Marrow Transplant 2008;41(2):174; with permission.)

immunodeficiencies; despite significant comorbidities prior to HSCT, seven of eight were surviving with donor cell engraftment 8 to 17 months after transplant. The same investigators recently updated their series, reporting 113 patients with PID who had undergone HSCT preceded by RIC between 1998 and 2006.[50] The majority of patients (93/113) received a FMC-RIC regimen consisting of Campath-1H (1 mg/kg), fludarabine (150 mg/m^2), and melphalan (140 mg/m^2), whereas the remaining 20 patients received MIC HSCT. Donor source was mainly unrelated (81/113). With a median follow-up of 2.9 years (range 2 months to 8 years) the overall survival (OS) for these patients was 82% (93/113), and 91/133 (81%) had stable donor engraftment. Fourteen patients (12%) had or were likely to require additional procedures, including second HSCT, marrow infusion, additional CD34+ cells, or gene therapy. The survival curve for each disease is shown in **Fig. 2**.

There are no prospective randomized studies comparing RIC to conventional MAC conditioning in PID; however, Rao and colleagues[82] from the same London group retrospectively compared the results in children with PID transplanted from UDs using a FMC-RIC regimen versus a MAC regimen used in an earlier time cohort and showed a decreased overall mortality (2/33 RIC compared to 4/19 MAC, P<.01). There was no difference in the incidence of aGVHD, and immune reconstitution with RIC was similar to that seen after conventional intensity conditioning. There was an increase in viral infections/reactivations in the RIC cohort (29% for RIC compared to 21% after MAC, P = .02); viral infections included CMV (n = 3), adenovirus (n = 5), and EBV (n = 10) in those receiving RIC. There was also an increased rate of MC when compared to MAC HSCT (45% MC of which 13% had low-level donor chimerism for RIC vs 36% MC and 0% low-level donor chimerism for MAC); however, in general, MC after RIC seemed to stabilize or improve with withdrawal of immunosuppression and there were low rates of recurrent disease (2/23 patients). OS was improved in the RIC group, mainly through improved survival in patients with non-SCID

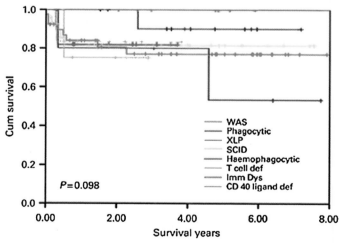

Fig. 2. Overall survival of pediatric patients undergoing RIC-SCT for PID/HLH stratified by disease. Phagocytic, neutrophil phagocytic defect; Imm Dys, immunodysregulatory disorders; CD40 ligand def, CD40 ligand deficiency. T cell def, T-cell immunodeficiencies; XLP, X-linked lymphoproliferative disorder. (*From* Satwani P, Cooper N, Rao K, et al. Reduced intensity conditioning and allogeneic stem cell transplantation in childhood malignant and nonmalignant diseases. Bone Marrow Transplant 2008;41(2):176; with permission.)

immunodeficiency (**Fig. 3**). To assess the potential effects of the different time cohorts in this study the outcome of a larger cohort of PID patients undergoing RIC HSCT from the London group was compared with that of PID patients undergoing largely MAC HSCT and reported from European centers to the SCETIDE database. In this comparison (**Fig. 4**), the improvement in RIC HSCT seems to be largely confined to children with T-cell deficiencies.

Some of the outcomes associated with FMC/FMA-RIC HSCT in PID have been studied further. Higher levels of viral reactivation,[129] in particular EBV, have been noted. The increased incidence of EBV viremia is thought to reflect the profound immunosuppression after RIC HSCT, together with the incomplete ablation of recipient-derived B cells.[130] Nevertheless, the combination of pre-emptive rituximab and EBV-specific cytotoxic T-lymphocytes was successful in curing all eight patients with EBV-driven LPD complicating PID and immunodysregulatory syndromes, after FMC-type RIC regimen.[131] This suggests that close monitoring of EBV by polymerase chain reaction and pre-emptive therapy, mainly with rituximab, can overcome complications associated with EBV viremia after RIC HSCT. In adult patients, a high incidence of CMV reactivation has been described after FMC-RIC HSCT.[132]

Shenoy and colleagues[133] used FMC-RIC HSCT in 16 patients with nonmalignant disorders, including two PID patients. These investigators administered Campath-1H

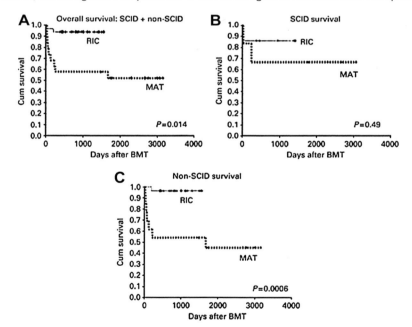

Fig. 3. Kaplan-Meier analysis comparing OS in children with primary immunodeficiences receiving RIC or conventional conditioning (MAC or MAT) stem cell transplantation. (*A*) OS in all patients was significantly better in patients who received RIC (94% OS) compared to MAC (53% OS). When divided into disease type, the improved survival after RIC was particularly marked in patients with non-SCID (who had a 54% death rate after MAC compared to a 30% death rate after MAC for SCID). (*B*) OS after RIC or MAC in patients with SCID. (*C*) OS after RIC or MAC in patients with non-SCID. (*Reproduced from* Satwani P, Cooper N, Rao K, et al. Reduced intensity conditioning and allogeneic stem cell transplantation in childhood malignant and nonmalignant diseases. Bone Marrow Transplant 2008;41(2):178; with permission.)

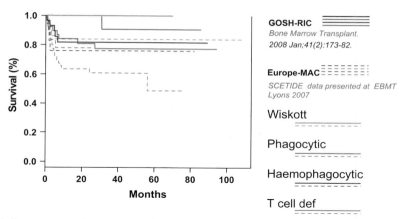

Fig. 4. Improvement in outcome of stem cell transplantation for T-cell immunodeficiency. def, deficiency; Europe-MAC, myeloablative HSCT performed in European centers; GOSH-RIC, Great Ormond Street Hospital RIC HSCT.

(33 or 48 mg total dose) early pre-HSCT from day −21 to day −19. The study included sibling bone marrow (n = 5), sibling peripheral blood stem cell (PBSC) (n = 5), unrelated bone marrow (n = 3), and unrelated CB (n = 3). All 14 evaluable patients had complete or high level (>50%) donor chimerism in all lineages, suggesting that lower doses or administration of Campath-1H away from the graft may increase donor chimerism in the HLA-matched setting.

The benefit from FMC-RIC HSCT was most evident in children over 1 year of age. For SCID patients under 1 year, TRM remained high even with RIC HSCT (28% in the London series).[16] Occasionally very young patients seem to develop a fatal melphalan shock syndrome with massive capillary leak within hours of receiving melphalan (Rao K, MD, personal observation, 2008), although the mechanism of this is not understood. An alternative RIC or MIC protocol (discussed later) might be preferable for this group of patients.

Fludarabine/busulfan

Jacobsohn and colleagues[134] reported the outcome of RIC HSCT in patients with nonmalignant disorders, using fludarabine, busulfan, and ATG (FBA) modeled after Slavin and colleagues.[126] Six children with PID underwent MSD PBSC (n = 2), MUD PBSC (n = 2), and unrelated CB (n = 2) HSCT. Patients received fludarabine (180 mg/m²) and busulfan (IV 6.4 mg/kg) in 8 doses on days −5 to −4 or pharmacokinetic monitoring to achieve an area under the curve of 3800 to 4200 μmol × minute with single daily dosing of busulfan on days −5 and −4. Two patients with X-linked HIGM were phenotypically cured, off IV immunoglobulin, and had reversal of cholangiopathy. One had full donor and one 30% donor chimerism. One patient with XLP syndrome was also alive and well, with 98% donor chimerism. One patient with SCID was too early to evaluate and two patients, one with CGD and one with OS, died within 100 days of HSCT. There was little aGVHD or cGvHD in evaluable patients.

Horn and colleagues[135] also reported the use of FBA in six children with PID. The conditioning regimen consisted of IV busulfan, fludarabine, and rabbit ATG (thymoglobulin). Donors were MUD bone marrow (n = 3), MRD bone marrow (n = 2), and UCB. Three patients achieved greater than 95% donor chimerism and three, MC. One patient with WAS died of CMV pneumonitis; the others are alive and disease-free.

There were 13 other non-PID patients included in the study and overall MC was more common with bone marrow was a stem cell source and graft rejection was more common in patients receiving mismatched UDs (MMUDs). Four patients experienced graft failure; all four patients underwent second HSCT; and three-quarters of them are alive and disease-free, illustrating how second HSCT after failed first RIC-HSCT is well tolerated and frequently successful. A similar protocol was used in five other children with PID.[136] All are alive and disease-free—one patient has CGD required donor lymphocyte infusion (DLI) for low-level donor chimerism and the others have stable MC, except one patient with complete donor chimerism who experienced significant aGVHD and cGVHD. In this study investigators prolonged immunosuppression for MC rather than tailing it as the usual course of action; this did not seem to increase graft rejection although it might have reduced donor chimerism in this group. Further work may establish an area under the curve for IV busulfan that is tailored to disease, donor type, and stem cell source in order to achieve lineage specific donor engraftment with the minimum amount of acute and long-term toxicity.

Fluttarabine/treosulfan

Fludarabine/treosulfan

Another approach to reduced intensity transplants (RIT) in PID has been to replace busulfan with treosulfan. Treosulfan (L-treitol-1,4-bis-methanesulphonate) is the pro-drug of L-epoxybutane, an alkylating agent with myeloablative and immunosuppressive properties.[137] Recent reports in adult patients have suggested that regimens containing treosulfan provide effective HSCT conditioning with reduced risk of VOD when compared to busulfan.[138,139] In addition, there is no need for prophylactic anticonvulsant treatment and unlike with busulfan, it is not necessary to measure drug levels. Phase 1 studies have suggested stable linear pharmacokinetics of treosulfan up to the clinically effective dose of 42 g/m^2.[138] Eighteen patients with PID with a mean age of less than 1 year underwent HSCT with a variety of donors and stem cell sources, using treosulfan (14 g^2) × 3 days + fludarabine (30 mg/m^2) × 5 days with Campath-1H (FTC) (n = 14) or ATG (FTA) (n = 2).[139] One patient received cyclophosphamide (50 mg/m^2) × 4 days and ATG. Although the latter is considered modified conditioning it should probably be classified as MAC rather than RIC (see **Fig. 1**). Thirteen patients achieved 100% donor chimerism, which remained stable in 10 patients. Three achieved stable MC: 90% to 99% donor (n = 2); 30% donor in peripheral blood; and 80% donor T cells (n = 1), which was sufficient to cure the underlying disease. Two patients achieved low-level donor chimerism (<50%) and are under consideration of second HSCT. Toxicity was tolerable particularly given such a young group of patients and may be preferable to FMC-RIC in this cohort.

Minimal Intensity Conditioning

Minimal Intensity Conditioning

Fludarabine/low-dose total body irradiation

Fludarabine/low-dose total body irradiation

Burroughs and colleagues[140] in Seattle investigated a MIC regimen in 14 patients (12 children and 2 adults) with PID and coexisting infections, organ toxicity, or other factors precluding conventional HSCT. The majority of patients received 200 cGy total body irradiation plus fludarabine (30 mg/m^2 per day ×3 days, days −4 to −2) as conditioning and all patients received HLA-matched grafts with intensive postgraft immunosuppression with cyclosporine A and mycophenolate mofetil. No serotherapy was given. Thirteen patients established MC (n = 5) or full (n = 8) donor chimerism and one rejected the graft. OS at 3 years was 62% with a TRM of 23%. Eight of ten evaluable patients had correction of immunodeficiency with stable donor engraftment. There was a high rate of GVHD, however, with 11 of 14 developing significant aGVHD (mostly grade II) and extensive cGVHD in eight patients, reflecting the use of peripheral blood as the stem cell source and the absence of serotherapy. This approach was associated with a lower incidence of viral infections/reactivations, notably EBV, than RIC regimens utilizing serotherapy; however, the high incidence of cGVHD would be a significant obstacle to broader use of this regimen in children with nonmalignant disorders.

Fludarabine/cyclophosphamide/monoclonal antibodies

The London group has explored a MIC protocol combining fludarabine (30 mg/m^2 × 5 days, days −8 to −4) and low-dose cyclophosphamide (300 mg/m^2 × 4 doses on days −7 to −4) with two rat anti-CD45 monoclonal antibodies, YTH 24.5/YTH 54.12 for additional myelosuppression and serotherapy with Campath-1H (0.6 mg/kg or 0.3 mg/kg) with UD or MSD, respectively.[141] Patients were at particularly high risk from HSCT-related toxicity even with RIC protocols due to severe pre-existing organ toxicity, age less than 1 year, or the presence of DNA/telomere repair disorders. In total, 16 patients underwent MIC HSCT from MSD (five), MUD (nine), and MMUD (two). Conditioning was well tolerated with only two cases of grade 3 and no grade 4 toxicity. Six out of 16 patients (38%) developed significant aGVHD (three grade II skin and three grade III skin/gut). Five of 16 patients (31%) developed cGVHD (limited in three and extensive in two), which has resolved in all cases. The incidence of GVHD was reduced when bone marrow was used as stem cell source (2/10 bone marrow recipients compared with 4/4 evaluable PBSC recipients developed aGVHD >grade II). Similarly, the incidence of cGVHD was lower in recipients of bone marrow (2/10) as compared to PBSC (3/4). At a median of 9.5 days (range 1–15), 16 of 16 patients had a neutrophil count greater than 0.5 × 10^9/L. One patient failed to engraft and had autologous recovery and one patient who received a mismatched CB engrafted with stable MC after an extended period. Donor chimerism was 100% in three-fourths PBSC recipients with one PBSC recipient rejecting the graft. Three of 10 bone marrow recipients achieved 100% donor chimerism, three achieved stable high-level MC in mononuclear and granulocyte lineages, and three achieved donor T-cell chimerism without sustained myeloid chimerism. One achieved very low-level donor chimerism and required a second stem cell transplantation. At a median of 37 months post HSCT, 13 of 16 patients in this high-risk cohort were alive and cured from their underlying disease. In terms of OS, SCID patients less than 1 year of age seemed to gain particular benefit from this MIC HSCT protocol (**Fig. 5**).

Stem Cell Source

The use of PBSCs as opposed to bone marrow in HSCT preceded by RIC seems to be associated with improved donor chimerism in recipients with PID[129,140,141] but at the cost of increased rates of GVHD; in this setting, OS seems similar between the two groups. The balance of host versus graft and graft versus host/graft versus marrow reflects the complex interactions of stem cell source with disease type, conditioning regimen, serotherapy, graft content (CD34+, CD3+, NK–killer-cell immunoglobulin-like receptor alloreactivity), and GVHD prophylaxis and is more finely balanced in RIT than MAC HSCT. The optimal combinations for PID remain to be determined. Regardless, there is likely to remain a risk of rejection with RIC. Recipient chimerism status in NK cells on day +28,[142] or increasing presence of host cells greater than 30%,[136] may represent early warning signs of future graft rejection that could allow timely intervention by withdrawal of immune suppression or pre-emptive administration of DLI.

There is less experience using UCB and RIT in PID. Bradley and colleagues[143] described the outcome of 21 children, median age 9 years (range 0.33–20 years), with malignant (n = 14) and nonmalignant conditions (n = 7) transplanted using heterogeneous RIC-MIC regimens. Five patients—HLH (n = 2), SCID (n = 2), and

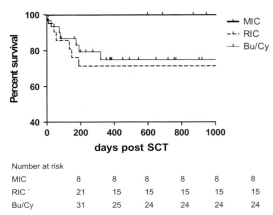

Fig. 5. Comparison of disease-free survival of SCID patients less than 1 year of age transplanted using anti-CD45 monoclonal antibody–based MIC, fludarabine/melphalan– based RIC, and busulfan/cyclophosphamide conditioning. Kaplan-Meier curves showing disease-free survival (days) of SCID patients age less than 1 year conditioned with (1) CD45 monoclonal antibody–based MIC regimen (n = 8, DFS 100%), (2) fludarabine/melphalan–based RIC regimen (n = 21, DFS 71.4%), and (3) busulfan/cyclophosphamide–based conditioning (n = 31, DFS 77.4%). The cohort conditioned with CD45-based MIC was transplanted between 2003 and 2007 (donor source 63% MUD, 25% MMUD, 13% MSD, and 37% B[neg] phenotype); the cohort conditioned with fludarabine/melphalan was transplanted between 1999 and 2003 (donor source 81% MUD, 19% MMUD, and 57% B[neg] phenotype); and the cohort transplanted with busulfan/cyclophosphamide was transplanted between 2003 and 2005 (donor source 57% MUD, 30% MSD, 13% MFD, and 46% B[neg] phenotype).

WAS—received four to six of six HLA-matched UCB after MIC conditioning with fludarabine, cyclophosphamide, and ATG. The HLH patients received additional VP16, but both rejected; one underwent a successful second MAC HSCT. Two of the three remaining patients died from viral pneumonitis and GVHD-related complications. The London group transplanted three patients with PID using a MIC protocol as described by Barker and colleagues.[144] Only one out of three survived; one died from disseminated cryptosporidiosis and the other from idiopathic pneumonitis (Rao K, MD personal communication, 2003). Based on few patients, therefore, the combination of MIC and UCB does not initially seem to offer any survival advantage to PID patients. More intensive regimens that qualify as RIC could be effective, however. Two centers in the United Kingdom (London and Newcastle) have performed 13 RIC-UCB HSCTs using fludarabine plus melphalan or fludarabine plus treosulfan with 11 of 13 patients surviving with donor engraftment (Rao K, MD, and Gennery A, MD, personal communication, 2009). Similarly, six of six patients with nonmalignant conditions at Duke survived beyond 5 months with a RIC approach that is based on a modified FMC backbone (Parikh S, MD, and Szabolcs P, MD, personal communication, 2009). Nevertheless, host cell recovery or MC will likely remain associated with this approach that might be prevented by careful selection of appropriate patients and high-quality/ cell dose UCB grafts to ensure donor cell chimerism. A prospective trial is under way.

Reduced Intensity Transplants in Specific Primary Immunodeficiency Diseases

Hemophagocytic lymphohistiocytosis
Patients with HLH often have significant pretransplant comorbidities and require intensive cardiorespiratory support pre-HSCT. This toxicity results in a high TRM with

conventional MAC, mostly from noninfectious pulmonary toxicity and VOD. The use of RIT has, therefore, been examined closely in HLH.[145,146] Twenty-five consecutive patients with primary HLH underwent RIT in London using MUD (n = 8), MMUD (n = 11), MFD (n = 2), and haploidentical (n = 4) donors. Most patients were conditioned with fludarabine (30 mg/m² × 5, days −7 to −3), melphalan (140 mg/m², day −2) and Campath-1H (0.2 mg/kg × 5, days −8 to −4). After RIC, 21 of 25 (84%) children are alive and in CR at a median of 36 months from transplant (range 2–105 months) with Lansky scores of 90% to 100%. The overall survival data compare favorably with historical data, particularly for patients receiving mismatched HSCT. In the RIC group, seven of eight patients (87%) transplanted from a MUD and 9 of 11 (82%) transplanted from an HLA-mismatched donor survive in CR, compared with corresponding figures of 70% and 54% using MAC HSCT in the HLH-94 study.[30]

Further published studies of RIC HSCT in patients with HLH are limited; however, an abstract presented at the Histiocyte Society annual meeting in 2007[147] describes 100% survival in 10 children with HLH (n = 7) or XLP syndrome (n = 3) treated with FMC-RIC HSCT. Six patients developed MC, with four receiving repeated T-cell infusions. All 10 are alive and well and remain in remission at a median of 10 months. RIC HSCT, therefore, seems a promising approach for children with HLH with 34 of 38 patients surviving in initial studies.

Wiskottt-Aldrich syndrome

The finding that MC post HSCT for WAS might be associated with an increased incidence of autoimmunity[81] might deter the use of RIC in WAS. Conversely, WAS patients older than 5 years old who have accumulated more comorbidities have a poor outcome after MAC HSCT, and RIT may offer some advantages in this setting.[78] Investigators in London have explored the use of RIC HSCT in WAS as updated from a previous report.[79] Between 1995 and 2007, 17 patients with WAS with a median age of 27 months underwent MSD (n = 5) or UD HSCT (n = 12). MAC (busulfan/cyclophosphamide) was used in six patients and RIC HSCT in 11: treosulfan/fludarabine (n = 5), fludarabine/melphalan (n = 6). In the 11 patients receiving RIC, 10 had WAS and one X-linked thrombocytopenia. The mean age in this group was 70 months (15–194 months) and the mean Ochs score was 4.8. Donor source was MUD (n = 10) and MMUD (n = 1). Eight patients received bone marrow and three patients PBSCs. All patients survive with a median follow-up of 4 years. Five of the 17 patients have MC/split chimerism, all after UD HSCT: one of two after MAC UD HSCT, and 4 of 11 (36%) after RIC UD HSCT, all of whom received in vivo T-cell depletion with Campath-1H (1 mg/kg total dose) days −8 to −4. Only one of these RIC patients has so far developed definite autoimmune disease. Three subsequent patients underwent UD-RIC HSCT with reduced Campath-1H (0.6 mg/kg total dose, days −8 to day −6), and all achieved 100% donor chimerism with only one patient experiencing aGVHD grade 2 skin. Three of four patients with MC developed aGVHD greater than grade II, as opposed to 3 of 15 with full donor chimerism (P<.05). Comparative incidence of MC/split chimerism after MAC HSCT in other studies is 28%[81] and 38%.[148] RIC-HSCT protocols may be suitable for UD HSCT in WAS, particularly in older children with comorbidities; however, some graft-versus-marrow reaction is required to secure 100% donor chimerism in all patients.

Chronic granulomatous disease

Horwitz and colleagues[149] reported 10 patients with CGD who underwent MIC HSCT comprising cyclophosphamide (120 mg/kg), fludarabine (125 mg/m²), and ATG (160 mg/kg) followed by transplant of CD34+-selected PBSCs from MSDs. Delayed DLI was given at intervals of 30 or more days to increase the level of donor chimerism. After a median follow-up of 17 months. donor myeloid chimerism in 8 of 10 patients ranged from 33% to 100%, a level that could be expected to provide normal host defense. Graft rejection occurred in two patients. Significant aGHVD developed in three of four adult patients with engraftment, one of whom subsequently had extensive cGVHD. Seven patients were reported to have survived from 16 to 26 months. Two patients died of transplant-related complications and one patient who rejected the graft died after a second HSCT.

As a comparison, RIC HSCT using FBA (busulfan [8 to 10 mg/kg] (adjusted with busulfan kinetics in pediatric patients), fludarabine [180 mg/m^2], and ATG [40 mg/kg]) and matched donors (MSD = 5 and MUD = 3) in eight high-risk CGD patients led to 90% to 100% donor chimerism in all cases at a median follow-up of 26 months.[150,151] This is despite the use of bone marrow in seven of eight cases. Seven patients are alive and well and all active inflammatory and infectious foci are cured. One adult patient who had received PBSC from a CMV negative MUD died on day +150 of CMV pneumonitis. Another type of RIC HSCT (4 Gy of total body irradiation, cyclophosphamide [50 mg/kg] and fludarabine 200 [mg/m^2]) followed by two mismatched unrelated CB units in a single adult McLeod phenotype CGD patient with invasive aspergillosis also resulted in full donor engraftment and cure.[152] All five CGD patients who received FMC-RIC HSCT survived but sustained donor engraftment was achieved in only two of five (Gungor T, MD, personal communication, 2007). RIC HSCT using the FBA combination may be particularly suitable for high-risk patients with CGD.[87]

Leukocyte adhesion deficiency

The worldwide transplant experience for 36 children with LAD undertaken at 14 centers between 1993 and 2007 was recently surveyed.[153] At a median follow-up of 62 months, OS was 75%. MAC was used in 28 patients, and the remaining eight patients received RIC (FMC = 5, FTC/FTA = 2). Survival after MFD and UD transplants was similar, with 11 of 14 MFD and 12 of 14 UD recipients surviving; mortality was greatest after haploidentical HSCT, where four of eight children did not survive. Full donor chimerism was achieved in 17 of the survivors, mixed multilineage chimerism in seven patients, and mononuclear cell–restricted chimerism in a further three cases. Causes of death in the nine patients who died included pneumonitis (n = 2), infection (n = 5), VOD (n = 3), and malignancy (n = 1) (some had >1 contributing factor) and all had received MAC HSCT. Overall, the use of RIC regimens seemed to be associated with reduced toxicity, with all eight patients surviving, although two patients have low-level donor chimerism not requiring second HSCT to date.

Fertility and Late Effects

One major impetus for choosing RIC regimens in children is the avoidance or reduction of long-term sequleae associated with MAC regimens. The toxicities, which are discussed extensively in this issue, include growth failure, gonadal failure, secondary malignancies, and myelodysplasia.[50] Whether or not RIC regimens are less toxic in that regard is unknown. Their true incidence, particularly in children with PID, awaits well-planed and well-executed follow-up studies as the first cohorts of survivors approach adulthood. Intact fertility and uncomplicated pregnancies have been reported in dogs with canine LAD after MIC HSCT.[154] There have been several reports of successful pregnancies in adults after FMC- and FBA-RIC protocols for malignant disease; one adult CGD patient fathered a child after FBA HSCT[154]; however, the impact of the same drugs on the pediatric gonadal and endocrine systems may be different.

SUMMARY

Studies so far indicate that RIT may have an important role in treating patents with PID. Unlike more standard approaches, such regimens can be used without severe toxicity in patients with severe pulmonary or hepatic disease. In the absence of prospective or larger registry studies, it is not possible to prove superiority of RIT in more stable PID patients; however, RIT does offer the advantage that long-term sequelae, such as infertility and growth retardation, may be avoided or reduced. Currently, RIC HSCT using UDs may offer a survival advantage in T-cell deficiencies, HLH, WAS (>5 years), and CGD patients with ongoing inflammatory or infective complications. MIC HSCT may be particularly suited to UD HSCT in young SCID patients with significant comorbidities. Caution is required when using RIT for MSD HSCT in PID, due to the increased incidence of low-level donor chimerism. After RIT, a second HSCT or DLI may be required more frequently than after conventional HSCT, but the second procedure is well tolerated and frequently successful.

REFERENCES

1. Bach FH, Amos DB. Hu-1: major histocompatibility locus in man. Science 1967; 156:1506–8.
2. Gatti RA, Meuwissen HJ, Allen HD, et al. Immunological reconstitution of sex-linked lymphopenic immunological deficiency. Lancet 1968;2:1366–9.
3. Bach FH, Albertini RJ, Joo P, et al. Bone-marrow transplantation in a patient with the Wiskott-Aldrich syndrome. Lancet 1968;2:1364–6.
4. Buckley RH. A historical review of bone marrow transplantation for immunodeficiencies. J Allergy Clin Immunol 2004;113:793–800.
5. Buckley RH. Primary cellular immunodeficiencies. J Allergy Clin Immunol 2002; 109:747–57.
6. Buckley RH. Primary immunodeficiency diseases due to defects in lymphocytes. N Engl J Med 2000;343:1313–24.
7. Fischer A. Human primary immunodeficiency diseases: a perspective. Nat Immunol 2004;5:23–30.
8. Geha RS, Notarangelo LD, Casanova JL, et al. Primary immunodeficiency diseases: an update from the International Union of Immunological Societies Primary Immunodeficiency Diseases Classification Committee. J Allergy Clin Immunol 2007;120:776–94.
9. Marodi L, Notarangelo LD. Immunological and genetic bases of new primary immunodeficiencies. Nat Rev Immunol 2007;7:851–61.
10. Boyle JM, Buckley RH. Population prevalence of diagnosed primary immunodeficiency diseases in the United States. J Clin Immunol 2007;27: 497–502.
11. Gluckman E, Rocha V. Cord blood transplantation: state of the art. Haematologica 2009;94:451–4.
12. Kurtzberg J. Update on umbilical cord blood transplantation. Curr Opin Pediatr 2009;21:22–9.
13. Griffith LM, Cowan MJ, Kohn DB, et al. Allogeneic hematopoietic cell transplantation for primary immune deficiency diseases: current status and critical needs. J Allergy Clin Immunol 2008;122:1087–96.
14. Pessach I, Walter J, Notarangelo LD. Recent advances in primary immunodeficiencies: identification of novel genetic defects and unanticipated phenotypes. Pediatr Res 2009;65(5 Pt 2):3R–12R.

15. Lagresle-Peyrou C, Six EM, Picard C, et al. Human adenylate kinase 2 deficiency causes a profound hematopoietic defect associated with sensorineural deafness. Nat Genet 2009;41:106–11.
16. Notarangelo LD, Giliani S, Mazza C, et al. Of genes and phenotypes: the immunological and molecular spectrum of combined immune deficiency. Defects of the gamma(c)-JAK3 signaling pathway as a model. Immunol Rev 2000;178: 39–48.
17. Buckley RH. The multiple causes of human SCID. J Clin Invest 2004;114: 1409–11.
18. Dadi HK, Simon AJ, Roifman CM. Effect of CD3delta deficiency on maturation of alpha/beta and gamma/delta T-cell lineages in severe combined immunodeficiency. N Engl J Med 2003;349:1821–8.
19. de Saint Basile G, Geissmann F, Flori E, et al. Severe combined immunodeficiency caused by deficiency in either the delta or the epsilon subunit of CD3. J Clin Invest 2004;114:1512–7.
20. Rieux-Laucat F, Hivroz C, Lim A, et al. Inherited and somatic CD3zeta mutations in a patient with T-cell deficiency. N Engl J Med 2006;354:1913–21.
21. Kung C, Pingel JT, Heikinheimo M, et al. Mutations in the tyrosine phosphatase CD45 gene in a child with severe combined immunodeficiency disease. Nat Med 2000;6:343–5.
22. Shiow LR, Roadcap DW, Paris K, et al. The actin regulator coronin 1A is mutant in a thymic egress-deficient mouse strain and in a patient with severe combined immunodeficiency. Nat Immunol 2008;9:1307–15.
23. Buckley RH. Molecular defects in human severe combined immunodeficiency and approaches to immune reconstitution. Annu Rev Immunol 2004;22:625–55.
24. Neven B, Leroy S, Decaluwe H, et al. Long-term outcome after hematopoietic stem cell transplantation of a single-center cohort of 90 patients with severe combined immunodeficiency. Blood 2009;113:4114–24.
25. Sarzotti-Kelsoe M, Win CM, Parrott RE, et al. Thymic output, T-cell diversity, and T-cell function in long-term human SCID chimeras. Blood 2009;114:1445–53.
26. Elder ME, Hope TJ, Parslow TG, et al. Severe combined immunodeficiency with absence of peripheral blood CD8+ T cells due to ZAP-70 deficiency. Cell Immunol 1995;165:110–7.
27. Arnaiz-Villena A, Timon M, Corell A, et al. Brief report: primary immunodeficiency caused by mutations in the gene encoding the CD3-gamma subunit of the T-lymphocyte receptor. N Engl J Med 1992;327:529–33.
28. Villard J, Masternak K, Lisowska-Grospierre B, et al. MHC class II deficiency: a disease of gene regulation. Medicine (Baltimore) 2001;80:405–18.
29. Dror Y, Grunebaum E, Hitzler J, et al. Purine nucleoside phosphorylase deficiency associated with a dysplastic marrow morphology. Pediatr Res 2004;55: 472–7.
30. Buck D, Malivert L, de Chasseval R, et al. Cernunnos, a novel nonhomologous end-joining factor, is mutated in human immunodeficiency with microcephaly. Cell 2006;124:287–99.
31. Buck D, Moshous D, de Chasseval R, et al. Severe combined immunodeficiency and microcephaly in siblings with hypomorphic mutations in DNA ligase IV. Eur J Immunol 2006;36:224–35.
32. Villa A, Sobacchi C, Notarangelo LD, et al. V(D)J recombination defects in lymphocytes due to RAG mutations: severe immunodeficiency with a spectrum of clinical presentations. Blood 2001;97:81–8.

33. Antoine C, Muller S, Cant A, et al. Long-term survival and transplantation of hae-mopoietic stem cells for immunodeficiencies: report of the European experience 1968-99. Lancet 2003;361:553–60.
34. Gaspar HB, Aiuti A, Porta F, et al. How I treat ADA deficiency. Blood 2009; 114(17):3524–32.
35. Grunebaum E, Mazzolari E, Porta F, et al. Bone marrow transplantation for severe combined immune deficiency. JAMA 2006;295:508–18.
36. Kane L, Gennery AR, Crooks BN, et al. Neonatal bone marrow transplantation for severe combined immunodeficiency. Arch Dis Child Fetal Neonatal Ed 2001;85:F110–3.
37. Myers LA, Patel DD, Puck JM, et al. Hematopoietic stem cell transplantation for severe combined immunodeficiency in the neonatal period leads to superior thymic output and improved survival. Blood 2002;99:872–8.
38. Gennery AR, Slatter MA, Grandin L, et al. Transplantation of haemato-poietic stem cells and long term survival for primary immunodeficiencies in Europe: entering a new century, can we do better? submitted for publication.
39. Reisner Y, Kapoor N, Kirkpatrick D, et al. Transplantation for acute leukaemia with HLA-A and B nonidentical parental marrow cells fractionated with soybean agglutinin and sheep red blood cells. Lancet 1981;2:327–31.
40. Ciceri F, Labopin M, Aversa F, et al. A survey of fully haploidentical hematopoi-etic stem cell transplantation in adults with high-risk acute leukemia: a risk factor analysis of outcomes for patients in remission at transplantation. Blood 2008; 112:3574–81.
41. Fernandes JFRV, Labopin M, et al. Comparison of outcomes of mismatched related stem cell and unrelated cord blood transplants in children with severe T-cell deficiencies. In Blood, Suppl; Abstract; 51st Annual meeting of the Amer-ican Society of Hematology, New Orleans, LA, 2009.
42. Cavazzana-Calvo M, Carlier F, Le Deist F, et al. Long-term T-cell reconstitution after hematopoietic stem-cell transplantation in primary T-cell-immunodeficient patients is associated with myeloid chimerism and possibly the primary disease phenotype. Blood 2007;109:4575–81.
43. Haddad E, Landais P, Friedrich W, et al. Long-term immune reconstitution and outcome after HLA-nonidentical T-cell-depleted bone marrow transplantation for severe combined immunodeficiency: a European retrospective study of 116 patients. Blood 1998;91:3646–53.
44. Laffort C, Le Deist F, Favre M, et al. Severe cutaneous papillomavirus disease after haemopoietic stem-cell transplantation in patients with severe combined immune deficiency caused by common gammac cytokine receptor subunit or JAK-3 deficiency. Lancet 2004;363:2051–4.
45. Krenger W, Hollander GA. The immunopathology of thymic GVHD. Semin Immu-nopathol 2008;30:439–56.
46. Clave E, Busson M, Douay C, et al. Acute graft-versus-host disease transiently impairs thymic output in young patients after allogeneic hematopoietic stem cell transplantation. Blood 2009;113:6477–84.
47. Amrolia PJ, Muccioli-Casadei G, Huls H, et al. Adoptive immunotherapy with al-lodepleted donor T-cells improves immune reconstitution after haploidentical stem cell transplantation. Blood 2006;108:1797–808.
48. Andre-Schmutz I, Le Deist F, Hacein-Bey-Abina S, et al. Immune reconstitution without graft-versus-host disease after haemopoietic stem-cell transplantation: a phase 1/2 study. Lancet 2002;360:130–7.

49. Li Pira G, Kapp M, Manca F, et al. Pathogen specific T-lymphocytes for the reconstitution of the immunocompromised host. Curr Opin Immunol 2009;21: 549–56.

50. Satwani P, Cooper N, Rao K, et al. Reduced intensity conditioning and allogeneic stem cell transplantation in childhood malignant and nonmalignant diseases. Bone Marrow Transplant 2008;41:173–82.

51. Cavadini P, Vermi W, Facchetti F, et al. AIRE deficiency in thymus of 2 patients with Omenn syndrome. J Clin Invest 2005;115:728–32.

52. Grunebaum E, Bates A, Roifman CM. Omenn syndrome is associated with mutations in DNA ligase IV. J Allergy Clin Immunol 2008;122:1219–20.

53. Loechelt BJ, Shapiro RS, Jyonouchi H, et al. Mismatched bone marrow transplantation for Omenn syndrome: a variant of severe combined immunodeficiency. Bone Marrow Transplant 1995;16:381–5.

54. Gomez L, Le Deist F, Blanche S, et al. Treatment of Omenn syndrome by bone marrow transplantation. J Pediatr 1995;127:76–81.

55. Mazzolari E, Moshous D, Forino C, et al. Hematopoietic stem cell transplantation in Omenn syndrome: a single-center experience. Bone Marrow Transplant 2005; 36:107–14.

56. Nahum A, Reid B, Grunebaum E, et al. Matched unrelated bone marrow transplant for Omenn syndrome. Immunol Res 2009;44:25–34.

57. Rossi G, Zecca M, Giorgiani G, et al. Non-myeloablative stem cell transplantation for severe combined immunodeficiency—Omenn syndrome. Br J Haematol 2004;125:406–7.

58. Tsuji Y, Imai K, Kajiwara M, et al. Hematopoietic stem cell transplantation for 30 patients with primary immunodeficiency diseases: 20 years experience of a single team. Bone Marrow Transplant 2006;37:469–77.

59. Jabado N, Le Deist F, Cant A, et al. Bone marrow transplantation from genetically HLA-nonidentical donors in children with fatal inherited disorders excluding severe combined immunodeficiencies: use of two monoclonal antibodies to prevent graft rejection. Pediatrics 1996;98:420–8.

60. Klein C, Cavazzana-Calvo M, Le Deist F, et al. Bone marrow transplantation in major histocompatibility complex class II deficiency: a single-center study of 19 patients. Blood 1995;85:580–7.

61. Saleem MA, Arkwright PD, Davies EG, et al. Clinical course of patients with major histocompatibility complex class II deficiency. Arch Dis Child 2000;83: 356–9.

62. Godthelp BC, van Eggermond MC, Peijnenburg A, et al. Incomplete T-cell immune reconstitution in two major histocompatibility complex class II-deficiency/bare lymphocyte syndrome patients after HLA-identical sibling bone marrow transplantation. Blood 1999;94:348–58.

63. Markert ML. Purine nucleoside phosphorylase deficiency. Immunodefic Rev 1991;3:45–81.

64. Grunebaum E, Zhang J, Roifman CM. Novel mutations and hot-spots in patients with purine nucleoside phosphorylase deficiency. Nucleosides Nucleotides Nucleic Acids 2004;23:1411–5.

65. Carpenter PA, Ziegler JB, Vowels MR. Late diagnosis and correction of purine nucleoside phosphorylase deficiency with allogeneic bone marrow transplantation. Bone Marrow Transplant 1996;17:121–4.

66. Baguette C, Vermylen C, Brichard B, et al. Persistent developmental delay despite successful bone marrow transplantation for purine nucleoside phosphorylase deficiency. J Pediatr Hematol Oncol 2002;24:69–71.

67. Delicou S, Kitra-Roussou V, Peristeri J, et al. Successful HLA-identical hematopoietic stem cell transplantation in a patient with purine nucleoside phosphorylase deficiency. Pediatr Transplant 2007;11:799–803.

68. Fagioli F, Biasin E, Berger M, et al. Successful unrelated cord blood transplantation in two children with severe combined immunodeficiency syndrome. Bone Marrow Transplant 2003;31:133–6.

69. Makitie O. Cartilage-hair hypoplasia in Finland: epidemiological and genetic aspects of 107 patients. J Med Genet 1992;29:652–5.

70. Ridanpaa M, van Eenennaam H, Pelin K, et al. Mutations in the RNA component of RNase MRP cause a pleiotropic human disease, cartilage-hair hypoplasia. Cell 2001;104:195–203.

71. Notarangelo LD, Roifman CM, Giliani S. Cartilage-hair hypoplasia: molecular basis and heterogeneity of the immunological phenotype. Curr Opin Allergy Clin Immunol 2008;8:534–9.

72. Berthet F, Siegrist CA, Ozsahin H, et al. Bone marrow transplantation in cartilage-hair hypoplasia: correction of the immunodeficiency but not of the chondrodysplasia. Eur J Pediatr 1996;155:286–90.

73. Guggenheim R, Somech R, Grunebaum E, et al. Bone marrow transplantation for cartilage-hair-hypoplasia. Bone Marrow Transplant 2006;38:751–6.

74. Notarangelo LD, Miao CH, Ochs HD. Wiskott-Aldrich syndrome. Curr Opin Hematol 2008;15:30–6.

75. Aldrich RA, Steinberg AG, Campbell DC. Pedigree demonstrating a sex-linked recessive condition characterized by draining ears, eczematoid dermatitis and bloody diarrhea. Pediatrics 1954;13:133–9.

76. Derry JM, Ochs HD, Francke U. Isolation of a novel gene mutated in Wiskott-Aldrich syndrome. Cell 1994;79:922.

77. Lum LG, Tubergen DG, Corash L, et al. Splenectomy in the management of the thrombocytopenia of the Wiskott-Aldrich syndrome. N Engl J Med 1980;302:892–6.

78. Filipovich AH, Stone JV, Tomany SC, et al. Impact of donor type on outcome of bone marrow transplantation for Wiskott-Aldrich syndrome: collaborative study of the International Bone Marrow Transplant Registry and the National Marrow Donor Program. Blood 2001;97:1598–603.

79. Ochs HD, Filipovich AH, Veys P, et al. Wiskott-Aldrich syndrome: diagnosis, clinical and laboratory manifestations, and treatment. Biol Blood Marrow Transplant 2008;15:84–90.

80. Kobayashi R, Ariga T, Nonoyama S, et al. Outcome in patients with Wiskott-Aldrich syndrome following stem cell transplantation: an analysis of 57 patients in Japan. Br J Haematol 2006;135:362–6.

81. Ozsahin H, Cavazzana-Calvo M, Notarangelo LD, et al. Long-term outcome following hematopoietic stem-cell transplantation in Wiskott-Aldrich syndrome: collaborative study of the European Society for Immunodeficiencies and European Group for Blood and Marrow Transplantation. Blood 2008;111:439–45.

82. Rao K, Amrolia PJ, Jones A, et al. Improved survival after unrelated donor bone marrow transplantation in children with primary immunodeficiency using a reduced-intensity conditioning regimen. Blood 2005;105:879–85.

83. Manis JP, Alt FW. Novel antibody switching defects in human patients. J Clin Invest 2003;112:19–22.

84. Fasth A. Bone marrow transplantation for hyper-IgM syndrome. Immunodeficiency 1993;4:323.

85. Gennery AR, Khawaja K, Veys P, et al. Treatment of CD40 ligand deficiency by hematopoietic stem cell transplantation: a survey of the European experience, 1993-2002. Blood 2004;103:1152–7.
86. Holland SM. Chronic granulomatous disease. Clin Rev Allergy Immunol 2010; 38(1):3–10.
87. Seger RA. Modern management of chronic granulomatous disease. Br J Haematol 2008;140:255–66.
88. van den Berg JM, van Koppen E, Ahlin A, et al. Chronic granulomatous disease: the European experience. PLoS One 2009;4:e5234.
89. Seger RA, Gungor T, Belohradsky BH, et al. Treatment of chronic granulomatous disease with myeloablative conditioning and an unmodified hemopoietic allograft: a survey of the European experience, 1985-2000. Blood 2002;100: 4344–50.
90. Schuetz C, Hoenig M, Gatz S, et al. Hematopoietic stem cell transplantation from matched unrelated donors in chronic granulomatous disease. Immunol Res 2009;44:35–41.
91. Soncini E, Slatter MA, Jones LB, et al. Unrelated donor and HLA-identical sibling haematopoietic stem cell transplantation cure chronic granulomatous disease with good long-term outcome and growth. Br J Haematol 2009;145:73–83.
92. Bunting M, Harris ES, McIntyre TM, et al. Leukocyte adhesion deficiency syndromes: adhesion and tethering defects involving beta 2 integrins and selectin ligands. Curr Opin Hematol 2002;9:30–5.
93. Zimmerman GA. LAD syndromes: FERMT3 kindles the signal. Blood 2009;113: 4485–6.
94. Holland SM. Treatment of infections in the patient with Mendelian susceptibility to mycobacterial infection. Microbes Infect 2000;2:1579–90.
95. Al-Muhsen S, Casanova JL. The genetic heterogeneity of mendelian susceptibility to mycobacterial diseases. J Allergy Clin Immunol 2008;122:1043–51 [quiz 1043–51]
96. Filipe-Santos O, Bustamante J, Chapgier A, et al. Inborn errors of IL-12/23- and IFN-gamma-mediated immunity: molecular, cellular, and clinical features. Semin Immunol 2006;18:347–61.
97. Roesler J, Horwitz ME, Picard C, et al. Hematopoietic stem cell transplantation for complete IFN-gamma receptor 1 deficiency: a multi-institutional survey. J Pediatr 2004;145:806–12.
98. Roesler J, Kofink B, Wendisch J, et al. Listeria monocytogenes and recurrent mycobacterial infections in a child with complete interferon-gamma-receptor (IFNgammaR1) deficiency: mutational analysis and evaluation of therapeutic options. Exp Hematol 1999;27:1368–74.
99. Welte K, Zeidler C. Severe congenital neutropenia. Hematol Oncol Clin North Am 2009;23:307–20.
100. Welte K, Zeidler C, Dale DC. Severe congenital neutropenia. Semin Hematol 2006;43:189–95.
101. Rosenberg PS, Alter BP, Link DC, et al. Neutrophil elastase mutations and risk of leukaemia in severe congenital neutropenia. Br J Haematol 2008;140:210–3.
102. Elhasid R, Rowe JM. Hematopoetic stem cell transplantation in neutrophil disorders: severe congenital neutropenia, leukocyte adhesion deficiency and chronic granulomatous disease. Clin Rev Allergy Immunol 2010;38(1):61–7.
103. Rosenberg PS, Alter BP, Bolyard AA, et al. The incidence of leukemia and mortality from sepsis in patients with severe congenital neutropenia receiving long-term G-CSF therapy. Blood 2006;107:4628–35.

104. Choi SW, Boxer LA, Pulsipher MA, et al. Stem cell transplantation in patients with severe congenital neutropenia with evidence of leukemic transformation. Bone Marrow Transplant 2005;35:473–7.

105. Ferry C, Ouachee M, Leblanc T, et al. Hematopoietic stem cell transplantation in severe congenital neutropenia: experience of the French SCN register. Bone Marrow Transplant 2005;35:45–50.

106. Zeidler C, Welte K, Barak Y, et al. Stem cell transplantation in patients with severe congenital neutropenia without evidence of leukemic transformation. Blood 2000;95:1195–8.

107. Vibhakar R, Radhi M, Rumelhart S, et al. Successful unrelated umbilical cord blood transplantation in children with Shwachman-Diamond syndrome. Bone Marrow Transplant 2005;36:855–61.

108. Myers KC, Davies SM. Hematopoietic stem cell transplantation for bone marrow failure syndromes in children. Biol Blood Marrow Transplant 2009;15:279–92.

109. Bhatla D, Davies SM, Shenoy S, et al. Reduced-intensity conditioning is effective and safe for transplantation of patients with Shwachman-Diamond syndrome. Bone Marrow Transplant 2008;42:159–65.

110. Janka GE. Familial and acquired hemophagocytic lymphohistiocytosis. Eur J Pediatr 2007;166:95–109.

111. Jordan MB, Filipovich AH. Hematopoietic cell transplantation for hemophagocytic lymphohistiocytosis: a journey of a thousand miles begins with a single (big) step. Bone Marrow Transplant 2008;42:433–7.

112. Horne A, Janka G, Maarten Egeler R, et al. Haematopoietic stem cell transplantation in haemophagocytic lymphohistiocytosis. Br J Haematol 2005;129: 622–30.

113. Baker KS, Filipovich AH, Gross TG, et al. Unrelated donor hematopoietic cell transplantation for hemophagocytic lymphohistiocytosis. Bone Marrow Transplant 2008;42:175–80.

114. Eapen M, DeLaat CA, Baker KS, et al. Hematopoietic cell transplantation for Chediak-Higashi syndrome. Bone Marrow Transplant 2007;39:411–5.

115. Kaplan J, De Domenico I, Ward DM. Chediak-Higashi syndrome. Curr Opin Hematol 2008;15:22–9.

116. Worth A, Thrasher AJ, Gaspar HB. Autoimmune lymphoproliferative syndrome: molecular basis of disease and clinical phenotype. Br J Haematol 2006;133: 124–40.

117. Sleight BJ, Prasad VS, DeLaat C, et al. Correction of autoimmune lymphoproliferative syndrome by bone marrow transplantation. Bone Marrow Transplant 1998;22:375–80.

118. Bennett CL, Ochs HD. IPEX is a unique X-linked syndrome characterized by immune dysfunction, polyendocrinopathy, enteropathy, and a variety of autoimmune phenomena. Curr Opin Pediatr 2001;13:533–8.

119. Baud O, Goulet O, Canioni D, et al. Treatment of the immune dysregulation, polyendocrinopathy, enteropathy, X-linked syndrome (IPEX) by allogeneic bone marrow transplantation. N Engl J Med 2001;344:1758–62.

120. Rao A, Kamani N, Filipovich A, et al. Successful bone marrow transplantation for IPEX syndrome after reduced-intensity conditioning. Blood 2007;109:383–5.

121. Alousi A, de Lima M. Reduced-intensity conditioning allogeneic hematopoietic stem cell transplantation. Clin Adv Hematol Oncol 2007;5:560–70.

122. Barrett AJ, Savani BN. Stem cell transplantation with reduced-intensity conditioning regimens: a review of ten years experience with new transplant concepts and new therapeutic agents. Leukemia 2006;20:1661–72.

123. Rezvani AR, Storb R. Using allogeneic stem cell/T-cell grafts to cure hematologic malignancies. Expert Opin Biol Ther 2008;8:161–79.
124. Woolfrey A, Pulsipher MA, Storb R. Nonmyeloablative hematopoietic cell transplant for treatment of immune deficiency. Curr Opin Pediatr 2001;13:539–45.
125. Champlin R, Khouri I, Shimoni A, et al. Harnessing graft-versus-malignancy: non-myeloablative preparative regimens for allogeneic haematopoietic transplantation, an evolving strategy for adoptive immunotherapy. Br J Haematol 2000;111:18–29.
126. Slavin S, Nagler A, Naparstek E, et al. Nonmyeloablative stem cell transplantation and cell therapy as an alternative to conventional bone marrow transplantation with lethal cytoreduction for the treatment of malignant and nonmalignant hematologic diseases. Blood 1998;91:756–63.
127. Giralt S, Estey E, Albitar M, et al. Engraftment of allogeneic hematopoietic progenitor cells with purine analog-containing chemotherapy: harnessing graft-versus-leukemia without myeloablative therapy. Blood 1997;89:4531–6.
128. Amrolia P, Gaspar HB, Hassan A, et al. Nonmyeloablative stem cell transplantation for congenital immunodeficiencies. Blood 2000;96:1239–46.
129. Veys P, Rao K, Amrolia P. Stem cell transplantation for congenital immunodeficiencies using reduced-intensity conditioning. Bone Marrow Transplant 2005; 35(Suppl 1):S45–7.
130. Cohen J, Gandhi M, Naik P, et al. Increased incidence of EBV-related disease following paediatric stem cell transplantation with reduced-intensity conditioning. Br J Haematol 2005;129:229–39.
131. Cohen JM, Sebire NJ, Harvey J, et al. Successful treatment of lymphoproliferative disease complicating primary immunodeficiency/immunodysregulatory disorders with reduced-intensity allogeneic stem-cell transplantation. Blood 2007;110:2209–14.
132. Chakrabarti S, Mackinnon S, Chopra R, et al. High incidence of cytomegalovirus infection after nonmyeloablative stem cell transplantation: potential role of Campath-1H in delaying immune reconstitution. Blood 2002;99:4357–63.
133. Shenoy S, Grossman WJ, DiPersio J, et al. A novel reduced-intensity stem cell transplant regimen for nonmalignant disorders. Bone Marrow Transplant 2005; 35:345–52.
134. Jacobsohn DA, Duerst R, Tse W, et al. Reduced intensity haemopoietic stem-cell transplantation for treatment of non-malignant diseases in children. Lancet 2004;364:156–62.
135. Horn B, Baxter-Lowe LA, Englert L, et al. Reduced intensity conditioning using intravenous busulfan, fludarabine and rabbit ATG for children with nonmalignant disorders and CML. Bone Marrow Transplant 2006;37:263–9.
136. Ozyurek E, Cowan MJ, Koerper MA, et al. Increasing mixed chimerism and the risk of graft loss in children undergoing allogeneic hematopoietic stem cell transplantation for non-malignant disorders. Bone Marrow Transplant 2008;42:83–91.
137. Greystoke B, Bonanomi S, Carr TF, et al. Treosulfan-containing regimens achieve high rates of engraftment associated with low transplant morbidity and mortality in children with non-malignant disease and significant co-morbidities. Br J Haematol 2008;142:257–62.
138. Beelen DW, Trenschel R, Casper J, et al. Dose-escalated treosulphan in combination with cyclophosphamide as a new preparative regimen for allogeneic haematopoietic stem cell transplantation in patients with an increased risk for regimen-related complications. Bone Marrow Transplant 2005;35:233–41.

139. Casper J, Knauf W, Kiefer T, et al. Treosulfan and fludarabine: a new toxicity-reduced conditioning regimen for allogeneic hematopoietic stem cell transplantation. Blood 2004;103:725–31.
140. Burroughs LM, Storb R, Leisenring WM, et al. Intensive postgrafting immune suppression combined with nonmyeloablative conditioning for transplantation of HLA-identical hematopoietic cell grafts: results of a pilot study for treatment of primary immunodeficiency disorders. Bone Marrow Transplant 2007;40:633–42.
141. Straathof KC, Rao K, Eyrich M, et al. Haemopoietic stem-cell transplantation with antibody-based minimal-intensity conditioning: a phase 1/2 study. Lancet 2009; 374:912–20.
142. Matthes-Martin S, Lion T, Haas OA, et al. Lineage-specific chimaerism after stem cell transplantation in children following reduced intensity conditioning: potential predictive value of NK cell chimaerism for late graft rejection. Leukemia 2003;17:1934–42.
143. Bradley MB, Satwani P, Baldinger L, et al. Reduced intensity allogeneic umbilical cord blood transplantation in children and adolescent recipients with malignant and non-malignant diseases. Bone Marrow Transplant 2007;40:621–31.
144. Barker JN, Weisdorf DJ, DeFor TE, et al. Rapid and complete donor chimerism in adult recipients of unrelated donor umbilical cord blood transplantation after reduced-intensity conditioning. Blood 2003;102:1915–9.
145. Cooper N, Rao K, Gilmour K, et al. Stem cell transplantation with reduced-intensity conditioning for hemophagocytic lymphohistiocytosis. Blood 2006;107:1233–6.
146. Cooper N, Rao K, Goulden N, et al. The use of reduced-intensity stem cell transplantation in haemophagocytic lymphohistiocytosis and Langerhans cell histiocytosis. Bone Marrow Transplant 2008;42(Suppl 2):S47–50.
147. Vaughn GBJ, Jordan M, Marsh R. Hematopoietic cell transplantation with reduced intensity conditioning (RIC HCT) for hemophagocytic lymphohistiocytosis (HLH) and X-linked lymphoproliferative syndrome. In: Histiocyte Society Meeting. Cambridge; 2007. p. 20.
148. Pai SY, DeMartiis D, Forino C, et al. Stem cell transplantation for the Wiskott-Aldrich syndrome: a single-center experience confirms efficacy of matched unrelated donor transplantation. Bone Marrow Transplant 2006;38:671–9.
149. Horwitz ME, Barrett AJ, Brown MR, et al. Treatment of chronic granulomatous disease with nonmyeloablative conditioning and a T-cell-depleted hematopoietic allograft. N Engl J Med 2001;344:881–8.
150. Gungor T, Halter J, Klink A, et al. Successful low toxicity hematopoietic stem cell transplantation for high-risk adult chronic granulomatous disease patients. Transplantation 2005;79:1596–606.
151. Gungor T, Halter J, Stussi G, et al. Successful busulphan-based reduced intensity conditioning in high-risk paediatric and adult chronic granulomatous disease-The Swiss experience [abstract]. Bone Marrow Transplant 2009;43:S75.
152. Suzuki N, Hatakeyama N, Yamamoto M, et al. Treatment of McLeod phenotype chronic granulomatous disease with reduced-intensity conditioning and unrelated-donor umbilical cord blood transplantation. Int J Hematol 2007;85:70–2.
153. Qasim W, Cavazzana-Calvo M, Davies EG, et al. Allogeneic hematopoietic stem-cell transplantation for leukocyte adhesion deficiency. Pediatrics 2009; 123:836–40.
154. Burkholder TH, Colenda L, Tuschong LM, et al. Reproductive capability in dogs with canine leukocyte adhesion deficiency treated with nonmyeloablative conditioning prior to allogeneic hematopoietic stem cell transplantation. Blood 2006; 108:1767–9.

Autologous Hematopoietic Stem Cell Transplantation for Childhood Autoimmune Disease

Francesca Milanetti, MD[a,b], Mario Abinun, MD, PhD, FRCPCH, FRCP[c,d], Julio C. Voltarelli, MD, PhD[e], Richard K. Burt, MD[a,*]

KEYWORDS

- Autoimmune diseases • Rheumatic diseases
- Pediatric • Hematopoietic transplant

Autologous and allogeneic hematopoietic stem cell transplantation (HSCT) can be used in the management of patients with autoimmune disorders. Because the experience with allogeneic HSCT is limited, this review focuses on the use of autologous HSCT. This treatment modality began as salvage therapy for end-stage treatment refractory autoimmune diseases using myeloablative regimens before stem cell transplantation. Experience gained in recent decades, mostly in adults, has helped to better define the conditioning regimens required and appropriate selection of patients who are most likely to benefit from autologous HSCT. Specifically, the field has been shifting toward the use of safer and less intense nonmyeloablative regimens used earlier in the disease course before patients accumulate extensive irreversible organ damage.

---

[a] Division of Immunotherapy, Department of Medicine, Northwestern University Feinberg School of Medicine, 750 North Lake Shore Drive, Chicago, IL 60611, USA
[b] Division of Rheumatology and Clinical Immunology, Department of Medicine, Sapienza Università di Roma, II Facoltà di Medicina e Chirurgia, A.O.S. Andrea, Via di Grottarossa 1035-39, 00189 Roma, Italy
[c] Children's BMT Unit, Department of Paediatrics, Newcastle upon Tyne Hospitals NHS Foundation Trust, Newcastle General Hospital, Westgate Road, Newcastle upon Tyne, NE4 6BE, UK
[d] Institute of Cellular Medicine, Medical School, Newcastle University, Framlington Place, Newcastle upon Tyne, NE2 4HH, UK
[e] Department of Clinical Medicine, Bone Marrow Transplantation Unit, School of Medicine of Ribeirão Preto, University of São Paulo, Hemocentro-RP, Campus USP, CEP (ZIP) 14051-140, Ribeirão Preto, Brazil
* Corresponding author.
E-mail address: rburt@northwestern.edu

Pediatr Clin N Am 57 (2010) 239–271
doi:10.1016/j.pcl.2009.12.003
0031-3955/10/$ – see front matter © 2010 Elsevier Inc. All rights reserved.

pediatric.theclinics.com

AUTOLOGOUS HSCT FOR AUTOIMMUNE DISEASES
Introduction and Rationale

Autologous HSCT, although a well-accepted term, is believed to be a misnomer by some, because there is no transplant, only infusion of an autologous blood product (the patient's own stem cells). These stem cells collected from the patient's own blood by leukapheresis (or from the bone marrow) are by convention called hematopoietic stem cells (HSCs). HSCs are multipotent stem cells that give rise to blood, immune, and endothelial cells and, for the purpose of autoimmune diseases, are more appropriately viewed as immune stem cells. The therapeutic effect and in particular toxicity from autologous HSCT arises not from the infused autologous stem cells but rather from the immunosuppressive conditioning used to suppress the autoreactive immune system before infusion of HSCs.

The goal of conditioning regimens before HSC infusion in patients with autoimmune diseases is not to use cancer drugs that destroy the entire bone marrow compartment but rather to combine or dose escalate standard immune-suppressive medications to lymphoablate transiently, not myeloablate permanently, the immune system. This lymphoablation allows immune regeneration and a resetting of immune self-tolerance from the multipotent HSCs. For autoimmune diseases nonmyeloablative regimens are safer and less toxic than myeloablative regimens. In particular myeloablative regimens based on total body irradiation (TBI), which are associated with a high rate of growth retardation, infertility, and late cancers, are not indicated for patients with autoimmune disorders. TBI causes approximately a 10% incidence of myelodysplastic syndrome (MDS)/leukemia between 2 and 5 years after transplantation and beginning 8 to 10 years after treatment; the incidence of solid tumors for the remainder of the exposed individual's life increases linearly.[1]

The most common nonmyeloablative regimen for autoimmune diseases is cyclophosphamide (Cy) combined with rabbit antithymocyte globulin (rATG), a regimen commonly used as a conditioning regimen for patients with aplastic anemia. Another nonmyeloablative regimen used for autologous HSCT of autoimmune diseases is Cy combined with alemtuzumab instead of rATG. However, this regimen is complicated by late autoimmune cytopenias including potentially life-threatening immune thrombocytopenia pupura, autoimmune hemolytic anemia, or immune-mediated neutropenia. Hence, alemtuzumab should not be used in an autologous conditioning regimen for autoimmune diseases.[2] Immune-mediated cytopenias associated with alemtuzumab have generally not been reported when maintenance immunosuppression continues after transplantation, for example, in patients receiving allogeneic HSCT for leukemias or patients receiving immunosuppression following solid organ transplant. Another nonmyeloablative regimen used in autologous HSCT for autoimmune diseases is termed rituximab sandwich, in which 1 dose of rituximab is given before and after the traditional Cy/rATG regimen. The currently preferred conditioning regimen used for juvenile idiopathic arthritis (JIA) is a nonmyeloablative regimen of Cy, rATG, and fludarabine (Flu) (see JIA section).

Special attention should be given to minimize the risk of regimen-related infertility, a side effect that may occur after high-dose Cy, the backbone of nonmyeloablative regimens. In an analysis of 212 patients undergoing allogeneic (not autologous) HSCT for aplastic anemia treated with 200 mg/kg of Cy (the same dose used in HSCT for autoimmune diseases) and ATG, 50% of patients who developed graft-versus-host disease (GVHD) fathered children, versus 62% who did not develop GVHD.[3] This analysis did not document what percentage of patients did not wish to father children. Therefore it could be speculated that the actual fertility rate is higher than 62% because patients receiving an autologous HSCT do not develop GVHD. Although the use of Cy results in significantly less infertility than the use of TBI,[4] a more thorough analysis of pre- and posttransplant fertility (sperm count, motility, morphology, ultrasound-guided antral follicle count, follicle-stimulating hormone, luteinizing hormone, estradiol, testosterone, antimüllerian hormone, inhibin B levels, and referral to reproductive endocrinology) should be considered for patients with an autoimmune disease undergoing HSCT.

It remains unclear whether the collected peripheral blood stem cells (or bone marrow) should be lymphocyte depleted (usually by means of a commercially available instrument that positively selects for CD34+ progenitor cells) before reinfusion of the autograft. T-cell depletion (TCD) of the autograft does increase the risk of late opportunistic infections, especially life-threatening viral infections such as cytomegalovirus (CMV) and Epstein-Barr virus (EBV).[5] The argument in favor of TCD is that it minimizes reinfusion of autoreactive lymphocytes that could lead to early relapse. The argument against taking the increased infectious risk from a TCD graft is that complete lymphoablation may not be necessary. Immune reset occurs from re-establishing the immune regulatory networks and tolerance as a result of conditioning regimen-induced neutropenia/lymphopenia and thymic-derived rebound of nonspecific regulatory cells (CD4+CD25+Foxp3+) and antigen-specific suppressor T cells (discussed in the systemic lupus erythematosus [SLE] section). Whether or not lymphocytes should be depleted from the autograft requires future randomized disease-specific and conditioning regimen-specific protocols. Most autologous HSCT so far reported in children have been T cell depleted, while the center with the largest world-wide experience in HSCT for adult autoimmune diseases, Northwestern University, performs most transplants without ex vivo TCD. Before HSCT, mild in vivo TCD and disease amelioration is obtained by means of mobilization of stem cells with Cy (2.0 g/m^2) and granulocyte colony-stimulating factor (G-CSF). In patients not heavily pretreated with immune-suppressive medications, the subsequent transplants have been easily tolerated without life-threatening infections.

This article reviews the experience gained with using autologous HSCT in treating the most common childhood autoimmune and rheumatic diseases, primarily JIA, SLE, and diabetes mellitus.

JIA

The most common chronic rheumatic condition in children with a prevalence of between 16 and 150/100,000, is defined as persistent arthritis in 1 or more joints lasting at least 6 weeks in a child or adolescent less than 16 years old, after excluding other causes. Consequently, JIA refers to a group of clinically heterogonous conditions. The current International League of Association of Rheumatologists recognizes 7 different disease categories: systemic, persistent oligoarticular, extended oligoarticular, polyarticular rheumatoid factor (RF) negative, polyarticular RF positive, enthesitis-related arthritis, and psoriatic.[6]

The cause and pathogenesis of JIA are still poorly understood. There is increasing evidence that environmental and genetic factors play a role[7] in influencing crucial mediators of the inflammatory process, such as cytokines tumor necrosis factor α (TNF-α), interleukin 1 (IL-1), and IL-6.[8,9] Together with involvement of the innate and adaptive immune system,[6] there is emerging evidence that altered immune system function, in particular that of T-cell regulation, plays a major role in the pathogenesis of joint damage and the disease progression.[10,11]

The most common form is the early onset (before age 6 years) oligo- (or mono-)articular JIA, with 1 to 4 asymmetrical joints affected, high frequency of positive antinuclear antibodies (ANA), and high risk (in 30%) of chronic uveitis. The subsequent disease course is either persistent to the affected joint(s), when treatment with intra-articular steroids and physiotherapy may be all that is needed and the prognosis is good, or progressing to more than 4 joints during the first 6 months, resembling the RF-negative polyarticular form with not such a good prognosis and need for systemic long-term antiiflammatory treatment.[6]

Polyarticular JIA, with more than 4 joints affected at onset, is either RF positive when it resembles the disease in adults, or RF-negative. Bone erosion is present in 75% of these children after 5 years' follow-up and polyarticular onset and polyarticular disease course are significant risk factors for disability.

Systemic-onset JIA is distinct from other subtypes, associated with features of systemic inflammatory reaction. In about half of patients the disease course is monocyclic or intermittent, with favorable long-term outcome; however, the other half has an unremitting disease course with polyarthritis; ongoing active systemic disease at 6 months is a bad prognostic sign. Some of these children (<10%) develop the life-threatening complication of hemophagocytic lymphohystiocytosis, also known as macrophage activation syndrome (MAS).[6]

Most children with JIA never achieve long-term remission. Three recent reviews summarized the experience and current approach to treatment.[6,12,13] The introduction of methotrexate with its effect on bone erosion prevention has been a major progress over the last 2 decades, aside from the use of intra-articular and systemic steroids for short-term disease control, and the emergence of a new generation of disease-modifying drugs, the biologic response modifiers such as blocking agents of inflammatory cytokine functions (TNF-α, IL-1, IL-6), or of costimulatory molecules expressed on cells of the immune system, in particular activated T cells (eg, CD28) or B cells (eg, CD20).

Despite the recent progress in treatment options, JIA causes significant morbidity and despite good prognosis for the majority, more than one-third of children have ongoing active disease into adulthood with sequelae from chronic inflammation. Children with systemic and polyarticular onset, and particularly those with polyarticular course of disease, tend to have worse prognosis, even with the early use of disease-modifying antirheumatic drugs such as methotrexate and the biologic response modifiers mentioned earlier. Such patients experience considerable morbidity from joint damage, osteoporosis, growth retardation, psychosocial morbidity, reduced quality of life, and educational or employment disadvantage.[6] For this minority of children with JIA who do not respond to, or who develop significant side effects from the currently used combined immunosuppressive and antiinflammatory treatments, the option of autologous HSCT has been reserved as salvage therapy, that is the last option (in heavily pretreated patients).

AUTOLOGOUS HSCT FOR JIA

Most of the experience regarding the effects and complications of HSCT comes from a pioneering clinical trial in children with severe JIA from the Netherlands. Following their initial report[14] and based on the conclusions from the First Workshop on Autologous Stem Cell Transplantation in Rheumatic Diseases of Childhood (Utrecht, the Netherlands, May 1998),[15] a multicenter trial of TCD auto-HSCT was initiated by the European Group for Blood and Marrow Transplantation (EBMT) Working Party, with defined guidelines and inclusion criteria.[16] These criteria were refined during subsequent international American-European workshops.[17,18] In the United Kingdom, the

2 national centers already experienced in TCD HSCT procedures for children with primary immunodeficiencies were approved and funded by the Department of Health and the National Health Service in 2000. After the experience with the first 2 successful procedures, and in line with the evolving international protocols,[16–20] guidelines were developed,[21] which have recently been updated.[22] These guidelines address the specific issues relevant to referral pathways in the United Kingdom, such as the role of the independent assessors appointed by the British Society for Pediatric and Adolescent Rheumatology, and liaison with the EBMT Working Party.

The original rationale for the strategy of autologous TCD HSCT was based on the removal of the presumed autoaggressive lymphocyte clones by immunosuppressive conditioning and TCD, and the hypothesis that the newly developing lymphocyte population may lead to resetting of the immune system (ie, self-tolerance). Initial analysis of the multicenter cohort outcome was promising: of 34 children with severe JIA followed for 12 to 60 months post autologous TCD HSCT, 53% showed complete, drug-free remission (CR), 18% partial response (PR), whereas 21% failed the procedure.[19,23] The evidence suggests disease improvement is a 2-step process. Clinically, the immediate improvement of acute inflammation observed in all patients is often a dramatic melting away of the active synovitis, caused by the immunosuppressive conditioning regimen.[19] Subsequent improvement, including achievement of CR in more than half of patients, is believed to be the result of the immunomodulatory effect of TCD auto-HSCT. After TCD of the graft, new T-cell clones emerge during immune reconstitution, suggestive of new thymic rearrangements.[24] The posttransplant T-cell immunodeficiency state allows an opportunity for the re-establishment of immune tolerance and resetting the adaptive immune system.[23,25] Recent emerging evidence suggests a crucial role for CD4+CD25+Foxp3+ T-regulatory cells in reinstating the immune balance.[10,11]

Further analysis of a subset of 22 patients from the original multicenter cohort after a longer follow-up (52–104 months; median 80 months) reported relapse in 1 patient 7 years post transplant.[26] The most recent follow-up reported another relapse in a patient 9 years post HSCT.[27] Data from a UK cohort of 9 transplanted children are similar: 5 children are in CR, including the 2 previously reported as part of the original multicenter cohort[19,23] who are now 9 years post transplant (see video clips online within this article at http://www.pediatric.theclinics.com/) and 2 relapsed,[28] (M Abinun, unpublished data, 2009). These data suggest that, despite long-term complete remission (9 years), it is premature to consider autologous HSCT a definitive cure.[19,23,26–29] However, the extended significantly improved quality of life for transplanted patients in CR is beneficial. During CR, most such patients do not experience disease manifestations, do not require any antiinflammatory treatments (ie, drug-free remission) and experience catch-up growth.[23,26–28] As expected, already damaged joints do not improve during post-HSCT CR; however, no further progression was observed either. Children remain with reduced exercise tolerance years post transplant.[30] Most children achieving PR respond well (ie, better than before the transplant) to subsequent treatment with combination of conventional and new disease-modifying agents.[27]

HSCT itself carries a significant risk of morbidity, as up to now it has been performed as salvage therapy in heavily pretreated patients. Approximately 70% of transplanted patients develop mainly viral infection or reactivation: CMV, EBV, varicella zoster virus (VZV), herpes simplex virus.[19,23,26–28] This is believed to be a direct consequence of severe and prolonged T-cell immunodeficiency caused by prior chronic immune suppression, the immunosuppressive conditioning regimen, and ex vivo TCD.[29] The original myeloablative conditioning regimen included TBI, ATG, and Cy.[14] When the interim data review showed no added benefit from TBI,[19] the use of a nonmyeloablative protocol with ATG, Cy, and Flu was explored,[23] and subsequently proven to be effective in achieving and maintaining long-term CR.[27,28] In contrast, protocols including only ATG and Cy[23,28,31–33] have been associated with relapses.[26,28,33] Although some patients who relapse can be managed with different immunosuppressive and immunomodulatory agents, others have a poor prognosis with progressive disease and significant morbidity and mortality.

Two patients from the Dutch group who were treated with further aggressive immunosuppression post HSCT relapse died of EBV and VZV (re)infections,[23,26,27] and another 2 patients underwent a second (allogeneic) HSCT.[28,33] Of the latter 2, 1 child died of CMV infection following a haploidentical umbilical cord blood transplant,[33] whereas the other initially achieved remission following a well-matched unrelated donor peripheral blood HSCT preceded by reduced intensity conditioning (alemtuzumab, Flu, melphalan). The posttransplant period was complicated by adenovirus and EBV reactivation and severe liver and gut GVHD.[28] This patient died a year post second (allogeneic) transplant during hip replacement surgery (Paul Veys, personal communication, 2009). At this stage the authors recommend that an allogeneic HSCT as salvage therapy after a failed autologous HSCT should be performed only as part of a carefully monitored clinical trial.

The transplant-related mortality (TRM) in patients with JIA who undergo TCD autologous HSCT is high at 12% (5 deaths of 43 patients),[23,28] (M Abinun, unpublished data). The initial transplant-related deaths in 1999 of 3 children were from infection (EBV, toxoplasma, or coagulase-negative staphylococcus) induced haemophagocytic syndrome[34] or MAS.[23,31,35,36]

Factors recognized to significantly influence the development of MAS at the time of transplant are clinical features of active systemic disease with raised inflammatory markers, with evidence of active or ongoing infection.[16–18] The initial observation that too stringent TCD (ie, $<1 \times 10^5$/kg vs $1–5 \times 10^5$/kg CD3+ T cells) is a major factor predisposing to MAS[17] remains controversial.[26] Nevertheless, there seem to be less severe and less frequent cases of MAS when using a less intense nonmyeloablative (ATG/Cy/Flu) conditioning protocol with less intense ex vivo TCD (ie, only CD34 positive selection).[37]

In patients with systemic-onset JIA, achieving clinical control of active disease before starting pre-HSCT conditioning is essential to proceed with TCD autologous HSCT.[16,18] Unlike patients with other autoimmune diseases, patients with systemic-onset JIA are temporarily treated with corticosteroids or cyclosporine after autologous transplantation to prevent T-cell–driven MAS. For those patients with systemic-onset JIA or a history of previous MAS, inclusion of cyclosporin A (CsA) prophylaxis during the conditioning regimen and throughout the engraftment period and slow tapering of maintenance steroids is strongly recommended.[27,28] Despite this approach, the risks of HSCT remain high, with 2 patients dying of multiorgan failure: 1 on day +100 from disseminated adenovirus infection/reactivation,[28] the other on day +45, associated with α-hemolytic streptococcus central venous catheter infection (M Abinun, unpublished data). Before transplant, both patients had received long-term combined disease-modifying agents (corticosteroids and methotrexate) and several biologic response modifiers (TNF and IL-1 blocking agents; anti-CD20 monoclonal antibody).

Aside from the immunosuppression and TCD induced by the conditioning regimen, other risk factors, such as patient selection, disease activity, and extent and duration of prior immunosuppression,[29] contribute to the increased incidence of serious infectious complications post HSCT.

In summary, in patients with JIA, performing HSCT with a nonmyeloablative regimen and less intense TCD reduces the morbidity and mortality of the procedure considerably. If performed before the patient has received multiple immune suppressive agents and before the onset of permanent joint destruction, HSCT is likely to reverse what would otherwise become permanent disabilities.

SLE

SLE is a chronic systemic autoimmune disease that results in inflammation and eventual damage in a broad range of organ systems (**Table 1**). SLE is a rare disease in childhood, with estimated incidence ranging from 10 to 20 per 100,000 children, depending on the ethnic population. Onset of SLE before the age of 18 years (juvenile-onset SLE) accounts for 15% to 20% of total cases[38]; children and adolescents generally have a more severe disease presentation, develop disease damage more

Table 1
Frequency of organ-specific clinical manifestations in SLE

Clinical Manifestations/Frequency (%)	
Cutaneous	**Pulmonary** (5–77)
Malar rash (44–74)	Pleuritis (40–60)
Oral ulcers (26–48)	Pneumonitis (1–4)
Vasculitis (16–52)	Pulmonary hypertension (5–14)
Photosensitivity (16–40)	Diffuse interstitial disease (3–8)
Alopecia (7–48)	Pulmonary hemorrhage (2)
Discoid lesions (10–19)	Pulmonary embolism (30)
Raynaud phenomenon (39–49)	Shrinking lung syndrome
Arthritis (74–90)	BOOP (rare)
Ocular (20–35)	**Cardiac**
Keratoconjunctivitis sicca	Pericarditis (5–26)
Conjunctivitis	Myocarditis
Uveitis	Valvular disease
Episcleritis/scleritis	Coronary artery disease
Keratitis	Silent abnormalities (16–42)
Optic neuritis	**Renal** (30–80)
Ischemic optic neuropathy	Glomerulonephritis
Ophthalmoplegia	WHO class I (7.5–8)
Retinal disease	WHO class II (14–21)
Gastrointestinal (8–40)	WHO class III (2–36)
Rectitis	WHO class IV (40–65)
Duodenitis	WHO class V (5–20)
Gastritis	**Neuropsychiatric** (20–95)
Esophagus dysmotility	Headache (43–72)
Cholecystitis	Seizures (26–51)
Chronic intestinal pseudo-obstruction	Psychosis (10–12)
Enteritis	Peripheral neuropathy (15–16)
Ischemic bowel disease	Transverse myelitis (1)
Ascites	Cerebral vascular disease (12)
Pancreatitis	Cognitive disorder (55)
Autoimmune hepatitis	Mood disorder (57)
Hematological 39	Movement disorder (7–9)
Thrombocytopenia (8–74)	
Leukopenia (27–52)	
Lymphopenia (30–59)	
Anemia (72–84)	
Antiphospholipid syndrome (19–87)	

Abbreviations: BOOP, bronchiolitis obliterans organizing pneumonia; WHO, World Health Organization.

Data from Stichweh D, Arce E, Pascual, V. Update on pediatric systemic lupus erythematosus. Curr Opin Rheumatol 2004;16(5):577–87.

quickly than adults with SLE, and have a higher overall burden of disease throughout their lifetimes. Children receive more intensive drug therapy to achieve disease control and accrue more damage, related to the disease and to its treatment (eg, steroid toxicity).[39–44] In general, the prevalence of involvement of the internal organs in infants is more severe than in other age groups. Prepubertal patients have an intermediate disease severity and no gender predilection; postpubertal patients have a strong female preponderance and more specific signs of disease at onset.[45]

In the past 2 decades, there has been a marked improvement of prognosis in juvenile-onset SLE, caused by earlier diagnosis and better approaches to treatment. For all age groups, 5-year survival rates have improved from 59% to 93% in the 1980s to 94% to 100% in the late 1990s.[46] The increase in all-cause mortality that results from SLE is highest in patients aged less than 24 years (almost 8 times > the average for all patients with SLE).[47] Children and adolescents with SLE enter adult life with considerable morbidity, which is secondary to the sequelae of disease activity, side effects of medications, and comorbid conditions. This morbidity may affect their quality of life, raising problems related to physical and psychological adaptation to a chronic illness.[48]

The concordance rate for lupus is approximately 25% to 50% among monozygotic twins and around 2% among dizygotic twins, highlighting the relevance of environmental exposure and genetic contribution.[49] Environmental factors, especially sun exposure, are disease triggers. However, the exact cause is not well understood. Immune abnormalities in patients with SLE include defects in macrophage phagocytosis,[50] complement abnormalities,[51] reduction in the number or function of regulatory T cells,[52,53] presence of autoantibodies,[54] and loss of T-cell tolerance to histone peptides within nucleosomes.[55]

More than 100 different autoantibodies have been described in patients with SLE (**Box 1**). These include autoantibodies that target antigens within the nucleus, cytoplasm, cell membrane, phospholipid-associated antigens, blood cells, endothelial cells, central nervous system, plasma proteins, matrix proteins, and miscellaneous antigens.[54] Autoantibodies have been associated with specific clinical features of adult-onset SLE[56]: the strongest associations were reported for antidouble-stranded DNA (dsDNA), antinucleosome, and anti-SSA(Ro) with skin and kidney disease; anti-α-actinin, anti-complement 1q (anti-C1q) and anti-Smith (anti-Sm) with lupus nephritis; anti-N-methyl-D-aspartate receptor with brain disease; and antiphospholipid antibodies with thromboembolic events.[57]

To date, there have been few studies of autoantibody associations with clinical disease in pediatric-onset SLE: dsDNA correlating with active disease, arthritis and rash[58]; anticardiolipin antibodies (ACLA) with neurologic involvement[59]; anti-Ro/SS-A and anti-La/SS-B with cardiac conduction abnormalities[60]; anti-ribosomal P protein and anti-dsDNA association with disease activity and nephritis[61,62]; and ACLA with thrombotic events.[63]

The clinical course is usually characterized by the alternation of periods of disease activity and quiescence. It may involve any organ system and the range of disease severity is wide. The diagnosis of SLE, whether affecting an adult or a child, is made based on a combination of clinical and laboratory features. The diagnosis of SLE is likely if 4 of the 11 revised American College of Rheumatology (ACR) criteria are present in a patient simultaneously or over time.[64] The 11 ACR criteria are: (1) malar rash, (2) discoid rash, (3) photosensitivity, (4) oral ulcers, (5) arthritis, (6) serositis, (7) renal proteinuria, cellular casts, (8) neurologic (seizures, psychosis), (9) hematologic (hemolytic anemia, leukopenia, thrombocytopenia, lymphopenia), (10) antinuclear antibody, or (11) other immunologic abnormalities (anti-DNA, anti-Sm, false-positive syphilis test, positive antiphospholipid antibody).

Box 1
Autoantibodies and their target antigens in SLE

Autoantibodies that target nuclear antigens: autoantibodies to chromatin-associated antigens, DNA-binding proteins, and proteins that participate in DNA transcription

ANA, nucleosomes

DNA: dsDNA, single-stranded (denatured) DNA (ssDNA), Z-DNA

Telomeres, nucleosides, nucleotides, histones, DNA-dependent adenosine triphosphatase, DNA polymerase-α, replication protein A, Ku, poly(adenosine diphosphate [ADP]-ribose) polymerase, poly(ADP-ribose), high mobility group protein (HMG) 17, DEK oncoprotein, centromere proteins, anti-sense to the excision repair cross complementing 1 DNA excision repair enzyme gene, proliferating cell nuclear antigen, RNA polymerase I- II-III, transcription factor TFIIF, transcription factor TFIIB, protein kinase NII

Autoantibodies that target nuclear antigens: autoantibodies to antigens that bind to RNA, participate in RNA processing, and to nucleolar antigens

Ro (SS-A), La (SS-B), nuclear poly(A) polymerase, nucleolar RNA helicase (Gu) protein, SR proteins, Alu RNA-protein complex, small nuclear ribonucleoprotein particles spliceosomal (U and Sm), nonspliceosomal P ribonuclease, heterogeneous nuclear ribonucleoprotein particles, nucleolin, B23/nucleophosmin, 90 kDa protein of the nucleolus organizer region/human upstream binding factor, interferon-inducible protein IFI 16

Autoantibodies that target nuclear antigens: autoantibodies to miscellaneous nuclear antigens

Mitotic spindle apparatus: type 1 nuclear mitotic apparatus protein (NuMA-1, MA-I), spindle kinesinlike protein HsEg5 (NuMA-2, MA-II), Ki-67, p53, c-myc oncogene product, proteins phosphorylated during apoptosis, Ki, nuclear lamins B-type lamins B1 and B2, Su, prothymosin α, DA1, DA2, Me

Autoantibodies that target cytoplasmic antigens

Outer ring subunit HC9 (α3) of 20S proteasome, ribosomal P proteins, ribosomal protein S10, ribosomal protein L12, 28S ribosomal RNA, JA, eukaryotic protein L7, Golgi apparatus proteins, transfer RNA, cytoskeletal antibodies microfilaments, calpastatin, follistatin-related protein, heat-shock protein 90 (HSP 90), FK506 binding protein 12, carbonic anhydrase (CA) I-II, pyruvate dehydrogenase (M2 type), profilaggrin (perinuclear factor)

Autoantibodies to cell membrane antigens

CD45, CD4, FcγR I-II-III, insulin receptor, gangliosides, galactocerebrosides, cell membrane associated DNA, cell membrane DNA binding protein, lipocortin-1, β 2-microglobulin

Autoantibodies to phospholipid-associated antigens

Lupus anticoagulant, anionic phospholipids, cardiolipin, phosphatidylinositol, phosphatidylserine , phosphatidate, Zwitterionic phospholipids phosphatidylethanolamine, phosphatidylcholine, platelet activating factor, β2-glycoprotein I, prothrombin (factor II), annexins IV-V-XI, protein S, protein C, thrombomodulin, factor XII, tissue type plasminogen activator, bound to fibrin, high and low molecular weight kininogens, kininogen binding proteins, factor XI and prekallikrein, thromboplastin (tissue factor), vascular heparan sulfate proteoglycan, oxidized low-density lipoprotein, malonaldehyde-modified lipoprotein (a), antimitochondrial antibodies of M5 type, lysophosphatidylcholine

Autoantibodies that target blood cells, endothelial cells, and nervous system

Platelets: Glycoprotein IIb-IIIa GPIb-IX CD36 (GPIV)

Antineutrophil cytoplasmic antibodies (ANCA): with cytoplasmic staining pattern proteinase 3 (PR3), ANCA with perinuclear staining pattern (pANCA), myeloperoxidase (MPO), ANCA with specificity other than MPO and PR3 lactoferrin, cathepsin G

High mobility group proteins: HMG1, HMG2, lysozyme, elastase, α-enolase

Endothelial cells: candidate antigens: ribosomal P protein P0, endothelial cell specific plasminogen activator inhibitor, ribosomal protein L6, elongation factor 1α, adenyl cyclase associated protein, DNA replication licensing factor, profilin II, tubulin, vimentin human endothelial associated putative lupus antigens HEAPLA 1, HEAPLA 2, nervous system (neuronal antibodies) gangliosides galactocerebrosides 50 kDa antigen 97 kDa antigen, ribosomal P protein, neurofilaments

Lymphocytes, T cells, B cells: CD45, CD4, T-cell receptor, major histocompatibility complex class I and II antigens, ribosomal antigens including P protein, red blood cells warm autoantibodies, Rh family antigens p34 and gp37–55, glycophorin A, band 3 anion transporter, other blood group system antigens Wrb, LW, U, K, Kpb, K13, Fy, cold autoantibodies

Autoantibodies to plasma protein antigens

Collagenlike region of C1q, C1 inhibitor, erythropoietin, idiotypes anti-DNA 16/6 Id, anti-idiotypic antibodies, calreticulin, prolactin, RF, Von Willebrand factor, factor VIII, apolipoprotein A1

Acute-phase proteins: C-reactive protein, ceruloplasmin, α1-antitrypsin

Autoantibodies to matrix protein antigens

Collagen (C) type I, II, III, IV, V, VI, laminins, fibronectin

Autoantibodies to miscellaneous antigens

PL 4, corpus luteum, retroviruses: endogenous (ERV), human T lymphotropic virus type 1-related endogenous sequence, ERV-9 envelope C-terminal surface glycoprotein, human ERV- H derived human transmembrane sequence clones 1-1 peptide, human immunodeficiency virus 1, glycoprotein gp24, gp41, gp120, citrullinated peptide

Poly(amino acids): polyhistidine, polyproline

Nerve growth factor, entactin (nidofen)

Data from Sherer Y, Gorstein A, Fritzler MJ, et al. Autoantibody explosion in systemic lupus erythematosus: more than 100 different antibodies found in SLE patients. Semin Arthritis Rheum 2004;34(2):501–37.

The common symptoms of SLE in children and adolescents include fever, fatigue, weight loss, arthritis, rash, and renal disease.[65] Lupus nephritis is 1 of the main clinical presentations (up to 80%) of pediatric SLE, and it determines the course and outcome of the disease because kidney damage is a major threat to long-term survival.[66] The outcome of nephritis is dependent on the severity of the lesion on renal biopsy. The risk of progression to end-stage renal disease is greatest in patients with diffuse proliferative glomerulonephritis (class IV).

Neuropsychiatric SLE syndromes (NPSLE) affecting peripheral and central nervous systems are also prevalent in pediatric lupus populations and often pose diagnostic and therapeutic challenges. NPSLE syndromes affect 20% to 95% of pediatric SLE patients and are associated with significant morbidity and higher mortality.[67] Neurocognitive impairment is believed to affect as many as 59% of children and adolescents with SLE.[68]

Cardiac disease is now being recognized as a significant cause of morbidity and mortality in children with SLE. Although its prevalence and natural history are largely unknown, as there are no published longitudinal studies, the spectrum of cardiac disease in children mirrors that of adult SLE, and silent cardiac abnormalities are a common finding. Accelerated atherosclerosis is observed in SLE patients, and ischemic disease occurs in up to 16% of asymptomatic children. Various factors that contribute to the development of atherosclerosis have been identified, including traditional risk factors and additional factors that are likely to be the result of the basic immune pathogenesis of SLE that makes SLE itself a potent, independent, cardiovascular risk factor.[69] SLE may also cause endocarditis (Lieberman-Sachs) and pericarditis that may be complicated by tamponade or constriction.

The lung is involved in 5% to 77% of children with SLE, and pulmonary function studies are abnormal in the majority, with the most frequent alteration being restrictive disease even if infrequently associated with the development of clinical interstitial lung disease. Pleural disease is the most frequent finding.[70] Other pulmonary manifestations include: pleural effusions, alveolar hemorrhage, shrinking lung syndrome, bronchiolitis obliterans, interstitial fibrosis, and pulmonary emboli.

Lupus has no cure, and up to 90% of patients require corticosteroids for disease control. More than half of patients with SLE have permanent organ damage, much of which is either directly caused by or increased by corticosteroids.[71] Immunosuppressants are also a cause of significant transient or permanent toxicity (**Table 2**). In the past 50 years, only 3 drug treatments have been approved by the US Food and Drug Administration (FDA) for lupus: corticosteroids, hydroxychloroquine, and aspirin.

Overall, children and adult patients with SLE receive similar treatments depending on the clinical manifestations and the presence/absence of major organ involvement. Most children with mild disease, with symptoms limited to arthralgias, rash, or photosensitivity receive corticosteroids and hydroxycloroquine as the first line of treatment. Immunosuppressive drugs such as Cy or mycophenolate mofetil (MMF) are added when there is major organ involvement. Intravenous Cy, because of its potential toxicity, is reserved for the most severe manifestations of pediatric SLE, including diffuse proliferative glomerulonephritis, severe neuropsychiatric lupus, significant interstitial lung disease, and pulmonary hemorrhage.

Few prospective studies on immunosuppressants addressing specifically the pediatric population have been conducted. Most of the evidence for treatment derives from studies performed in adults: a series of randomized controlled trials conducted at the US National Institutes of Health have indicated that combination high-dose Cy ($0.5–1.0 \, g/m^2$) and methylprednisolone intravenous pulse therapy is the most effective at improving patient and renal outcomes,[72–74] and it is considered the standard of care for American patients with lupus and severe organ involvement. Nevertheless, high-dose intravenous Cy has been shown to have no effect on survival, to be less effective in Black patients, and to have many side effects.[75] Moreover, failure to achieve remission, which is associated with an increased rate of progression to renal failure, is reported in 18% to 57% of patients who received Cy.[74,76–78] In view of these limitations, there is a continuous search to develop therapies equally effective but with less toxic side effects.

The Euro-Lupus Nephritis Trial found that low-dose intravenous Cy could be used as an alternative to a high-dose regimen and was associated with half as many severe infections.[79] New studies and meta-analyses comparing MMF with Cy have confirmed the efficacy of the former for induction and maintenance therapy with a favorable toxicity profile[80] However, the Aspreva Lupus Management Study (ALMS) trial, a recent large international randomized controlled trial comparing intravenous Cy

Table 2
Side effects of immunosuppressive medications used in SLE

Medication	Toxicities
Glucocorticoids	Weight gain, growth retardation, striae rubrae, effects on body image, sleep disruption, affective disorders, psychosis, hypertension, dyslipidemia, impaired glucose tolerance, immunosuppression, inadequate gain of bone mass, avascular necrosis, myopathy, gastrointestinal irritation, cataracts, glaucoma
Hydroxychloroquine	Retinal toxicity Rare: hepatitis, neuromyopathy, cardiomyopathy
NSAIDs	Headache, aseptic meningitis, fatigue, change in personality or school performance, gastrointestinal irritation/ulcer, constipation, hepatitis, renal toxicity, possible cardiovascular risk
Methotrexate	Nausea, diarrhea, immunosuppression, bone marrow suppression, hepatotoxicity Rare: pulmonary toxicity, possible malignancy risk
MMF	Nausea, diarrhea, immunosuppression, bone marrow suppression, hepatotoxicity
Cy	Nausea, immunosuppression, bone marrow suppression, hemorrhagic cystitis (particularly with oral Cy), gonadal failure, hair loss, malignancy (bladder and hematologic cancers)
Azathioprine	Bone marrow suppression, hepatotoxicity Rare: possible malignancy risk
Cyclosporin	Hirsutism, hypertension, renal toxicity, dyslipidemia, seizures
Rituximab	Fatal infusion reactions, severe mucocutaneous reactions, progressive multifocal leukoencephalopathy

Abbreviations: Cy, cyclophosphamide; MMF, mycophenolate mofetil; NSAID, nonsteroidal antiinflammatory drug.
Data from Ardoin SP, Schanberg LE. The management of pediatric systemic lupus erythematosus. Nat Clin Pract Rheumatol 2005;1(2):82–92.

(IVCy) and MMF in a 24-week induction study for active lupus nephritis, did not meet its primary objective of showing that MMF was superior to IVCy as an induction treatment of lupus nephritis. Furthermore, significant differences between the MMF and IVCy groups with regard to rates of adverse events, serious adverse events, or infections were not detected.[81] Whether MMF is better than azathioprine for the maintenance of remission will be addressed in the MAINTAIN Nephritis Trial and in the maintenance phase of the ALMS trial.

Rituximab given with or without Cy seems to offer some benefit with an acceptable toxicity profile. It has been studied for treating lupus in several open-label studies that altogether have included more than 400 patients. In early studies, nearly 80% of treated patients entered at least partial remission, and 25% to 50% are still in remission more than 12 months later.[82–85] However, the results of the first randomized controlled trial of rituximab versus placebo (EXPLORER trial), presented at the 2008 ACR meeting in Boston, did not show significant differences between rituximab and placebo in major or partial clinical response at 12 months in 257 patients with moderately to severely active extrarenal SLE. Moreover, recently Genentech announced that the second randomized controlled trial of rituximab plus MMF and corticosteroids versus placebo in 144 patients with class III or IV lupus nephritis did not meet its primary end point of significantly reducing disease activity at 52 weeks.[86]

Abatacept, a fusion protein of immunoglobulin and extracellular CTLA-4, is designed to inhibit T-cell costimulation. As with the rituximab trial, in the first 12-month study to assess the safety and efficacy of abatacept, there was no significant difference between those treated with the drug and those receiving placebo (ACR meeting, 2008). There is currently no evidence that anti-TNF molecules may be beneficial in lupus, above all for lupus nephritis.[87] A randomized controlled trial is ongoing in patients with class V renal nephritis who are being randomized to azathioprine plus either 4 infusions of infliximab or placebo (http://www.ClinicalTrials.gov Identifier: NCT00368264). Drugs that inhibit inflammatory cytokines, particularly interferon α are also being tested in clinical trials (http://www.ClinicalTrials.gov Identifier: NCT00541749). A list of randomized controlled trials on SLE therapy conducted so far is presented in **Table 3**.

AUTOLOGOUS HSCT FOR SLE

Two large nonrandomized trials of autologous HSCT for SLE have been reported and were conducted predominately in adults with refractory disease: a European multicenter trial with 53 patients[108] and an American single-center trial with 50 patients[109] (**Table 4**). The European and American studies were salvage trials for patients with severe disease failing multiple standard immune-suppressive regimens. The European and American trials had similar 5-year disease-free survival: 55% and 50%, respectively.

The major difference between the 2 studies was in mortality. The European study was an analysis from a composite of diverse myeloablative and nonmyeloablative regimens with and without TCD of the autograft, involving 23 different centers with an overall mortality of 23% and treatment-related mortality of 13%. The American study was a single-center study using a single nonmyeloablative regimen and CD34 selection of the autograft with overall mortality of 16% and disease-related mortality of 4%. The difference in treatment-related mortality between the European and American trials (13% vs 4%, respectively) is likely caused by a center effect in experience and supportive care and use of diverse regimens including myeloablative regimens in the European study.

The risk of transplant could also be minimized by treating patients earlier in disease instead of applying transplant as a salvage therapy for heavily and chronically immune-suppressed patients with end-stage treatment refractory disease.

Including the 2 predominately adult SLE HSCT trials mentioned earlier, approximately 20 children with severe juvenile SLE have undergone auto-HSCT. Seventeen children were reported as part of the European multicenter cohort of 53 patients described earlier.[108] Four children have been reported separately in detail,[110,111] all showing remarkable decrease of disease activity and marked improvement in the quality of life, with follow-up from 9 months to 4 years; 1 experienced relapse with thrombocytopenia.[111]

It has previously been demonstrated that an immune reset with regeneration of thymic-derived naive T cells occurs after autologous HSCT for autoimmune diseases such as multiple sclerosis.[112] For patients with lupus, investigators at Northwestern University (Chicago) have focused on studying pre- and posttransplant T cells reactive to nucleosome histone peptides and on pre- and posttransplant T regulatory (CD4+CD25highFoxP3+) and T suppressor (CD8+FoxP3+) cells. These investigators found that CD4+CD25highFoxP3+ (Treg), and an unusual CD8+FoxP3+ T-suppressor subset return in posttransplant patients, accompanied by almost

Table 3
Randomized controlled trials in SLE

First Author/Year of Publication	Number of Patients/Follow-up (months)	Regimen	Outcome
Austin III 1986[72]	107/84	Oral pred versus IV Cy in LN	Renal: Cy superior ($P = .027$)
Canadian HCQ study group 1998[88,89]	47/42	HCQ versus placebo in clinically stable SLE	Prevention of flares: HCQ superior at 6 mo ($P = .02$), n.s. at 42 mo
Boumpas 1992[73]	65/36	IV MP versus IV Cy mo versus IV Cy mo/quarterly for LN	Renal: long-course Cy superior ($P<.04$ and $P<.01$)
Gourley 1996[74]	82/62	IV MP versus IV Cy mo/quarterly versus their combination for LN	Renal: combination treatment superior to MP alone ($P<.057$ and $P<.028$)
Chan 2000[90]	42/12	MMF + pred versus oral Cy + pred/AZA for LN	Renal: equal efficacy
Chan 2005[91]	64/63	As above	Renal: equal efficacy MMF fewer infections ($P = .013$)
Houssiau 2002, 2004[79,92]	90/73	IV Cy mo/quarterly + AZA versus IV Cy mo + AZA for LN	Renal: equal efficacy No differences in adverse events
Yee 2004[93]	32/44	Cy (IV + oral) + MP (IV + oral) versus oral Cy/AZA + pred for LN	Renal: equal efficacy n.s. differences in adverse events
Tam 2004[94]	12/6	Leflunomide	Disease activity (SLE DAI): Leflunomide superior to placebo ($P = .026$)

Study	n	Comparison	Results
Contreras 2004[95]	59/72	Quarterly IV Cy versus AZA versus MMF for LN	Renal: MMF superior (P = .02) MMF or AZA safer (P = .05 and P = .009)
Barile-Fabris 2005[96]	32/12	IV MP + either IV Cy mo/quarterly versus IV MP mo/quarterly	NPSLE: Cy superior (P<.03)
Ginzler 2005[97]	140/6	MMF versus IV Cy for LN	Renal: MMF superior
Ong 2005[98]	44/6	MMF versus IV Cy for LN	Renal: equal efficacy n.s. differences in adverse events
Bezerra 2005[99]	33/6	CFZ versus CDP for cutaneous SLE	Cutaneous: equal efficacy
Grootscholten 2007[100,101]	87/68	AZA/IV MP + oral pred versus IV Cy + oral pred for LN	Renal: equal efficacy Chronicity index: Cy superior (P<.05)
Tseng 2006[102]	154/18	Pred oral versus placebo in SACS SLE	Prevention of flares: pred superior (P<.007)
Moroni 2006[103]	75/48	CsA versus AZA for LN	Renal: equal efficacy n.s. differences in adverse events
Wang 2007[104]	20/6	MMF versus IV Cy or LN	Renal: MMF superior (P = .026)
Fortin 2008[105]	86/12	MTX versus placebo	Steroid sparing effect: MTX superior
Cardiel 2008[106]	317/22	Abetimus versus placebo	Renal: no difference with placebo
Appel 2009[81]	370/12	IV Cy + oral pred versus MMF + oral pred for LN	Renal: equal efficacy n.s. differences in adverse events
Austin III 2009[107]	42/12	CsA or IV Cy versus oral pred alone for membranous LN	Renal: IV Cy and CsA superior to pred in inducing remissions of proteinuria

Abbreviations: AZA, azathioprine; CDP, chloroquine diphosphate; CFZ, clofazimine; Cy, cyclophosphamide; HCQ, hydroxychloroquine; IV, intravenous; LN, lupus nephritis; MMF, mycophenolate mofetil; mo, monthly; MP, methylprednisolone; MTX, methotrexate; n.s., not significant; Pred, prednisone; SACS, serologically active clinically stable.

Table 4
Autologous HSCT in SLE

First Author/ Year	Number of Patients	Mean Age (years)	Mean Follow-up (months)	CD34 (%)	Mobilization	Conditioning	Overall Mortality/ TRM (%)	Survival (%)
Jayne 2004[108]	53	29	26	42	Cy + G-CSF (93%)	Cy (84%) ATG (76%,) TBI (22%) Other (27%) Cy + ATG (48%)	21/12	84 at 12 mo 62 at 48 mo
Burt 2006[109]	50	30	29	100	Cy + G-CSF	Cy + eATG	16/4	84 at 5 y

Abbreviations: CD34, graft T cell depleted by CD34+ selection; Cy, cyclophosphamide; eATG, equine antithymocyte globulin; G-CSF, granulocyte colony stimulating factor; TBI, total body irradiation.

complete inhibition of pathogenic CD8 T-cell response to histone peptide autoepitopes from nucleosomes, the major lupus autoantigen derived from apoptotic cells.[113]

In addition to the 2 nonrandomized trials mentioned earlier, 2 randomized trials were developed for HSCT of SLE: 1 in Europe (Autologous Stem Cell Transplant International Lupus, ASTIL) and 1 in America (Lupus Immune Suppression vs Stem Cell Transplant, LIST). Both trials were subsequently closed because of impractical design. Given the lack of any new FDA-approved therapy for SLE in decades, and the promising response of autologous HSCT in refractory disease[108,109] and immune studies indicating an immunologic remission following transplant,[113,114] something never before demonstrated, renewed interest exists to develop a randomized trial of autologous HSCT for SLE. Based on transplant experience with patients early after disease onset for relapsing-remitting multiple sclerosis[115] and for type 1 diabetes mellitus,[116,117] consideration is being given to randomize SLE patients early after onset of major visceral organ involvement to either autologous HSCT or conventional therapy (protocol in development, Burt and colleagues).

TYPE 1 DIABETES MELLITUS

Type 1 diabetes mellitus (T1DM) is the most common autoimmune disorder in childhood,[118] but the disease may become manifest at any age. The incidence of T1DM has increased considerably among children less than the age of 15 years in most developed countries since World War II.[119] The clinical diagnosis is made when the residual pancreatic β cells are not able to secrete enough insulin to maintain glucose homeostasis. This effect usually occurs after approximately 60% to 80% of the β cells have been destroyed.[120] T1DM represents only 5% to 10% of all diabetic causes but is associated with a high frequency of vascular complications and compromises quality and expectancy of life.[121,122]

T1DM results from a chronic autoimmune process toward pancreatic β cells leading to their progressive destruction. The subclinical prodromal period is characterized by selective loss of insulin-producing β cells in the pancreatic islet in genetically susceptible subjects. There are 2 major haplotypes conferring disease-susceptibility (DR3-DQ2 and DR4-DQ8), and in addition 10 other genes or genetic regions have been observed to be associated with T1DM.[123]

The issue whether there is any primary autoantigen in T1DM has remained controversial. So far, the most relevant antigenic targets identified are native insulin, the 65-KDa form of glutamic acid decarboxylase (GAD$_{65}$), and insulinoma antigen 2 (IA-2). Islet cell, anti-insulin, anti-GAD$_{65}$, and anti-IA-2 autoantibodies are detected with variable frequency in serum of diabetic patients, showing different sensibility, specificity, and predictive value of disease manifestation.[124] Selective autoantibody titer to a single CC chemokine named CCL3 has been recently suggested as a more reliable biomarker than each of those mentioned earlier alone, including for diagnosis of T1DM at its preclinical stage.[125]

The appearance of autoantibodies is the first detectable sign of emerging β-cell autoimmunity. The number of detectable autoantibodies is unequivocally related to the risk of progression to overt T1DM. In family studies positivity for 3 to 4 autoantibodies is associated with a risk of developing clinical T1DM in the range of 60% to 100% over the next 5 to 10 years.[126] Humoral β-cell autoimmunity is dynamic in the first year after the appearance of the first autoantibodies including epitope spreading and isotype spreading and switching, suggesting that this period would be the optimal interval for any immune intervention. It has, however, been shown that most of the infiltrating cells into the islets are CD8 T cells, strongly supporting the view that β-cell

Table 5
Trials of immunomodulatory therapy in type 1 diabetes

Study	Number Patients/ Time from Diagnosis	Therapy	Mean Follow-up (mo)	Outcome
Raz 2001[152]	35/< 6 mo	DiaPep277	10	Insulin use lower at 10 mo ($P = .042$).
Schloot 2007[153]	50 adults + 49 children/ < 3 mo	DiaPep277	18	C-peptide: n.s. Insulin use: n.s. HbA1c: n.s.
Ludvigsson 2008[154]	70/< 18 mo	GAD-alum	30	C-peptide AUC declined from baseline less ($P = .04$) Insulin use: n.s. HbA1c n.s.
Herold 2002[149]	42 /< 6 weeks	Anti-CD3	24	C-peptide AUC increase ($P<.02$) HbA1c lower ($P<.05$) at 6 and 18 mo Insulin use lower at 6–24 mo ($P<.01$) versus control group
Keymeulen 2005 (phase II)[150]	80/< 6 months	Anti-CD3	18	C-peptide release increase 6–18 mo ($P<.01$) Insulin use lower at 6–18 mo ($P<.05$ at 18) HbA1c: n.s. Versus control group
Buckingham 2000[155]	10/< 11 days	MTX	36	Islet failure earlier in patients receiving MTX ($P<.02$)
Feutren 1986[142]	122/< 6 mo	CsA	9	At 9 mo CR in 24.1% CsA versus 5.8% placebo ($P<.01$)

Bougneres 1988[143]	40/<3 mo	CsA	12	27/40 insulin free at 4 mo; 12/40 insulin free at 1 year
Canadian-European RCT group 1988[144]	188/< 14 weeks	CsA	12	NIR state > in the treated group ($P<.09$ at 12 mo) HbA1c n.s.
Assan 1990[147]	219/3.4 mo mean	CsA	24	Insulin use lower at 12 and 24 mo ($P<.01$ at 12 mo and <0.05 at 24 mo)
De Filippo 1996[148]	130/<3 months	CsA	72	Plasma C-peptide higher ($P<.02$) HbA1c lower. ($P<.02$) Insulin use lower ($P<.02$) Versus control group more than 4 y
Harrison 1985[139]	24/< 12 weeks	AZA	36	At 12 mo 7/13 remission in the treated group versus 1/11 in the untreated group
Silverstein 1988[141]	46/< 2 weeks insulin therapy	Pred +AZA	12	Insulin use lower at 12 mo ($P<.001$) Versus control
Cook 1989[140]	49/newly diagnosed	AZA	12	Fasting plasma C-peptide higher in treated group at 3 and 6 mo ($P<.04$) n.s. at 12 mo
Saudek 2004[151]	17/< 4 weeks	rATG 18 mg/kg	12	Insulin use lower at 12 mo ($P = .01$) versus control

Abbreviations: AUC, area under curve; AZA, azathioprine; CR, complete remission; CsA, cyclosporine A; Diapep277, diabetes peptide 277; Gad-alum, alum-formulated glutamic acid decarboxylase; MTX, methotrexate; NIR, not insulin requiring; n.s., not significant; Pred, Prednisolone; rATG, rabbit anti-thymocyte globulin.

destruction is a cytotoxic T-cell–mediated disease, followed by macrophages, CD4 T cells, and B lymphocytes.[127]

Patients with T1DM depend on exogenous insulin administration for survival and for control of long-term complications. The gold standard for therapy is tight control of blood glucose by intensive insulin therapy (IIT), achieved by multiple daily injections or continuous subcutaneous insulin infusion. Both forms of IIT have shown evidence of better metabolic control than traditional insulin therapy with 1 to 2 injections per day.[128,129] IIT reduces the risk of retinopathy, nephropathy, and neuropathy by 35% to 90% and results in reduction in their progression from 39% to 60% when compared with conventional therapy with 1 to 2 injections per day.[130,131] IIT is, however, complicated by lack of patient acceptance/compliance, and it cannot fully prevent chronic complications related to diabetes. It is associated with a threefold increase in severe hypoglycemia.[132]

Reconstitution of organ function by pancreas transplantation or by replacement of insulin-producing β cells is another therapeutic option but is limited by risks of the procedure, limited organ or islet cell availability, and requirement of chronic immunosuppression. Organ or islet cell transplant is usually limited to brittle diabetic patients or patients with renal failure and diabetes. Because graft survival when pancreas transplant is combined with kidney transplant is superior to pancreas transplant alone, whole-organ pancreas transplantation is an accepted therapeutic option for uremic patients with T1DM, in which it is frequently performed at the same time as kidney transplantation (simultaneous pancreas-kidney transplantation) or after kidney transplantation (pancreas-after-kidney). The number of solitary pancreas transplants (pancreas transplant alone) performed in nonuremic T1DM patients continues to increase.[133] Five-year graft survival of solitary pancreas and simultaneous kidney-pancreas transplantation is 55% and 70%, respectively.[133]

An alternative approach to replace insulin-producing cells is the portal vein implantation of allogeneic pancreatic islet cells. The long-term graft function depends on multiple parameters, including the preparation of high-quality islets, and immunosuppressive regimen (avoidance of corticosteroids). Islet allotransplantation can restore endogenous insulin production and stability of blood glucose levels, but insulin independence is frequently not sustainable. The 5-year insulin independence after islet cell transplant of approximately 20%[134] is less than after whole-organ transplant (55% to 70%). Large-scale application of pancreatic islet transplantation is currently limited by a lack of organs, and, similarly to whole-organ pancreas transplantation, long-term graft function is also influenced by side effects of the current immunosuppressive regimens. Currently, the American Diabetes Association recommends that islet transplantation be performed only within the setting of controlled research studies.[135]

PRESERVING AUTOLOGOUS ISLET CELL MASS

Subgroup analysis of the Diabetes Control and Complications Trial showed that patients with a larger β-cell reserve demonstrable by serum C-peptide levels presented a slower decline of these levels during the study and experienced fewer microvascular complications than patients with low or undetectable C-peptide concentrations. Even modest residual insulin secretion, with stimulated C-peptide levels greater than 0.2 nmol/L (0.6 ng/mL), has been reported to provide clinically meaningful benefits in reducing long-term complications[136] Therefore, β-cell preservation is another important target in the management of T1DM and in the prevention of its related complications.[137]

To preserve islet cells, many clinical trials have evaluated the role of immunointervention in preventing residual β-cell loss by blocking the autoimmune response with prednisone,[138] azathioprine,[139,140] prednisone plus azathioprine,[141] cyclosporine,[142–148] antibodies against CD3,[149,150] and rATG.[151] These therapies were shown to induce a slower decline or some improvement in C-peptide levels when compared with placebo groups. However, almost all patients continued to require exogenous insulin. Decreased insulin requirements after immune suppression usually was restricted to patients treated within 12 weeks of diagnosis. The results achieved using immunosuppressive therapy in T1DM are presented in **Table 5**. As an alternative to immunosuppression, autoantigens have been tried in an attempt to induce immunologic tolerance. The 65-kDa isoform of GAD and the 60-kDa hsp60 are known target autoantigens in patients with T1DM. These peptide-based therapies have been proven effective in preventing diabetes and saving residual β function in nonobese diabetic mice but showed disappointing results in humans.[152–154]

AUTOLOGOUS HSCT FOR T1DM

Autologous HSCT, a technique that allows brief but intense immune suppression, is also an approach to preserve islet cell mass in patients with T1DM. As already mentioned, standard immune-suppressive drugs, although unable to achieve insulin independence, diminished insulin requirements but only if treatment was initiated within the first 12 weeks of T1DM onset. For this reason, a recent study restricted HSCT to patients with new-onset T1DM, that is, within 6 weeks of disease diagnosis.

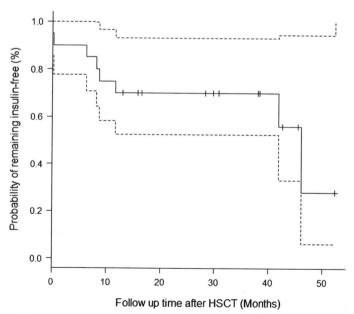

Fig. 1. Probability of remaining insulin free over time after HSCT in type 1 diabetes. The 95% confidence intervals are represented by the dashed lines. Because the number of patients with longer follow-up diminishes with time, the 95% confidence intervals widen with time post transplant. (*Reproduced from* Voltarelli JC, Martinez EZ, Burt RK. Autologous nonmyeloablative hematopoietic stem cell transplantation in newly diagnosed type 1 diabetes mellitus—Reply. JAMA 2009;302(6):625; with permission.)

Moreover, the study included only adults and teenagers, excluding children. To confirm the clinical diagnosis of T1DM, eligibility required presence of autoantibodies to islet cell antigens including anti-GAD.

The initial protocol used a standard nonmyeloablative approach of peripheral blood stem cell mobilization with Cy and G-CSF, conditioning with Cy and rATG, and transplant using an unmanipulated graft without ex vivo TCD. It is routine to infuse solumedrol before each dose of rATG to minimize febrile reactions. However, corticosteroids, although also immune-suppressive, induce islet cell apoptosis and could induce suicide of the remaining islet cells. Two patients who received corticosteroids did not respond. Subsequently, to avoid corticosteroid prophylaxis, the antihistamine dexchlorpheniramine was given to prevent rATG side effects.

Of the first 15 patients undergoing HSCT for T1DM, 14 who had not received corticosteroids became insulin free, with the longest ongoing continuous insulin-free interval with normal glycosylated hemoglobin (HbA1c) being more than 3 years.[116] Most patients achieved insulin independence before hospital discharge but in 2 patients insulin independence occurred at only 12 and 22 months, respectively. This study demonstrated for the first time that patients with T1DM can become insulin

Table 6
Autologous HSCT for childhood autoimmune/rheumatic diseases

Number of Children	Outcome	Follow-up	References
JIA ~50			
34	CR>50%	1–9 y	[23]
22[a]	PR ~20%		[26]
9 2[a]	Failed ~20%		[28] (MA)
19[a]	TRM ~12%		[27]
1	CR	1.5 y	[32]
3	2 CR, 1 PR (died)	1.5–3.5 y	[33]
SLE ~20			
17	n/a	n/a	[108]
4	3 CR, 1 PR	9 mo–4 y	[110,111]
SSc3	CR	1–5.5 y	[157,158]
JDM 4			
1	PR (died)	n/a	[159] (PV)
2	CR	n/a	(NW)
1	CR	4 y	[160,161]
Vasc 2			
1 PAN	PR	1.5 y	[162]
1 BD	CR	2 y	[163]

Abbreviations: BD, Behçet disease; CR, complete remission; JDM, juvenile dermatomyositis; MA, Mario Abinun, personal communication; n/a, not available; NW, Nico Wulffraat, personal communication; PAN, polyarteritis nodosa; PR, partial remission; PV, Paul Veys, personal communication; SLE, childhood-onset systemic lupus erythematosus (inclusion criteria[18]: in particular evidence for active disease versus progressive chronic change or unresponsiveness to or unacceptable toxicity from standard aggressive therapy); SSc, juvenile systemic sclerosis (inclusion criteria[18]: in particular active, progressive cutaneous disease, pulmonary hypertension and interstitial lung disease); TRM, treatment related mortality; Vasc, childhood systemic vasculitis; y, years.
[a] Patients from the original cohort reported in Ref[23]; Outcome, follow-up, and TRM given for cumulative cohorts (Refs,[23,26–28] and MA).

free with normal HgbA1c for extended periods of time. Nevertheless, it was suggested that the posttransplant insulin independence interval was secondary to a prolonged normal honeymoon period that may occur after T1DM onset.

The authors' subsequent report[117] 2 years later of 23 patients (of whom 14 were younger than 18 years) included follow-up of the first 15 patients, and demonstrated that C-peptide levels increased after autologous HSCT, with peak C-peptide plateau levels occurring 2 to 3 years after transplant. C-peptide is a measure of islet cell mass and its increase after HSCT indicates that posttreatment insulin independence was not secondary to a normal honeymoon effect but rather caused by restoration of islet cell mass. Three patients who either accidentally received corticosteroids or had diabetic ketoacidosis onset, which probably is associated with a severely depleted islet cell mass, did not benefit from HSCT. The other 20 patients all became insulin independent. Eight patients subsequently relapsed (required use of insulin) and 12 patients remained insulin free, with the longest ongoing insulin-free interval being more than 5 years. Two of 8 patients who resumed insulin became insulin independent again after starting sitagliptin, a glucagon-like peptide 1 (GLP-1) sparing agent. The 5-year probability of being insulin free with 95% confidence intervals is presented in **Fig. 1**. Of the 8 patients who returned to using insulin, the C-peptide levels remained significantly higher. Because C-peptide levels correlate inversely with late complications, these patients can be anticipated to benefit from reduced risk of late diabetic complications. A randomized controlled trial comparing autologous HSCT to IIT in adults with new onset T1D has recently received FDA approval.

SUMMARY

A recent review on autologous HSCT for systemic sclerosis has just been published[156] and a summary of reported autologous HSCT for childhood autoimmune diseases is listed in **Table 6**. Early and late toxicity depend on conditioning regimen, extent of graft manipulation (TCD), extent and duration of prior immune suppression, and type and stage of disease at time of transplantation. Phase I/II studies, predominately in adults, demonstrated that heavily pretreated and refractory disease, having tried and exhausted conventional options, responds to autologous HSCT but is at high risk for transplant-related toxicity. Thus, the current focus is to apply safer and less toxic nonmyeloablative autologous HSCT regimens in earlier stage, less advanced, and less chronically immune-suppressed patients.

Although allogeneic HSCT, when compared with autologous HSCT, is generally viewed as a more effective and potentially curative procedure, especially for spontaneously occurring autoimmune diseases (ie, where the autoimmunity is a stem cell disorder), the risks from GVHD and high treatment-related mortality of allogeneic HSCT are currently unacceptable for the pediatric community. Similar to the experience gained from autologous HSCT in adults, performing allogeneic HSCT in adults with safe regimens that demonstrate minimal risk of GVHD will facilitate the application of allogeneic HSCT to children with selected autoimmune diseases.

APPENDIX: SUPPLEMENTARY DATA

Supplementary data associated with this article can be found in the on-line version, at doi:10.1016/j.pcl.2009.12.003.

REFERENCES

1. Burt RK, Marmont A, Oyama Y, et al. Randomized controlled trials of autologous hematopoietic stem cell transplantation for autoimmune diseases: the evolution from myeloablative to lymphoablative transplant regimens. Arthritis Rheum 2006;54(12):3750–60.
2. Loh Y, Oyama Y, Statkute L, et al. Development of a secondary autoimmune disorder after hematopoietic stem cell transplantation for autoimmune diseases: role of conditioning regimen used. Blood 2007;109(6):2643–48.
3. Deeg HJ, Leisenring W, Storb R, et al. Long-term outcome after marrow transplantation for severe aplastic anemia. Blood 1998;91(10):3637–45.
4. Sanders JE, Hawley J, Levy W, et al. Pregnancies following high-dose cyclophosphamide with or without high-dose busulfan or total-body irradiation and bone marrow transplantation. Blood 1996;87(7):3045–52.
5. Frère P, Pereira M, Fillet G, et al. Infections after CD34-selected or unmanipulated autologous hematopoietic stem cell transplantation. Eur J Haematol 2006;76(2):102–8.
6. Ravelli A, Martini A. Juvenile idiopathic arthritis. Lancet 2007;369(9563):767–78.
7. Prahalad S, Glass DN. A comprehensive review of the genetics of juvenile idiopathic arthritis. Pediatr Rheumatol Online J 2008;6:11.
8. Van den Ham HJ, de Jager W, Bijlsma JW, et al. Differential cytokine profiles in juvenile idiopathic arthritis subtypes revealed by cluster analysis. Rheumatology (Oxford) 2009;48(8):899–905.
9. Barnes MG, Grom AA, Thompson SD, et al. Subtype-specific peripheral blood gene expression profiles in recent-onset juvenile idiopathic arthritis. Arthritis Rheum 2009;60(7):2102–12.
10. De Kleer I, Vastert B, Klein M, et al. Autologous stem cell transplantation for autoimmunity induces immunologic self-tolerance by reprogramming autoreactive T cells and restoring the CD4CD25 immune regulatory network. Blood 2006; 107:1696–702.
11. Roord STA, de Jager W, Boon L, et al. Autologous bone marrow transplantation in autoimmune arthritis restores immune homeostasis through CD4CD25Foxp3 regulatory T cells. Blood 2008;111:5233–41.
12. Ilowite NT. Current treatment of juvenile rheumatoid arthritis. Pediatrics 2002; 109(1):109–15.
13. Haskes PJ, Laxer RM. Medical treatment of juvenile idiopathic arthritis. JAMA 2005;294(13):1671–84.
14. Wulffraat N, van Royen A, Bierings M, et al. Autologous haemopoietic stem cell transplantation in four patients with refractory juvenile chronic arthritis. Lancet 1999;353(9152):550–3.
15. Kuis W, Wulffraat NM, Petty RE. Autologous stem cell transplantation: an alternative for refractory juvenile chronic arthritis. Rheumatology (Oxford) 1999;38(8): 737–8.
16. Wulffraat NM, Kuis W, Petty R. Proposed guidelines for autologous stem cell transplantation in juvenile chronic arthritis (Addendum). Pediatric Rheumatology Workshop. Rheumatology (Oxford) 1999;38(8):777–8.
17. Wulffraat NM, Kuis W. Treatment of refractory juvenile idiopathic arthritis. J Rheumatol 2001;28(5):929–31.
18. Barron KS, Wallace C, Woolfrey A, et al. Autologous stem cell transplantation for pediatric rheumatic diseases. NIH Workshop Report. J Rheumatol 2001;28(10): 2337–58.

19. Wulffraat NM, Brinkman D, Ferster A, et al. Long-term follow-up of autologous stem cell transplantation for refractory juvenile idiopathic arthritis. Bone Marrow Transplant 2003;32(Suppl 1):S61–4.
20. Wulffraat NM, Vastert B, Tyndall A. Treatment of refractory autoimmune diseases with autologous stem cell transplantation: focus on juvenile idiopathic arthritis. Bone Marrow Transplant 2005;35(Suppl 1):S27–9.
21. Wedderburn LR, Abinun M, Palmer P, et al. Autologous haematopoietic stem cell transplantation in juvenile idiopathic arthritis. Arch Dis Child 2003;88(3):201–5.
22. Foster HE, Davidson J, Baildam E, et al. Autologous haematopoietic stem cell rescue for severe rheumatic disease in children. Rheumatology 2006;45:1570–1.
23. De Kleer IM, Brinkman DMC, Ferster A, et al. Autologous stem cell transplantation for refractory juvenile idiopathic arthritis: analysis of clinical effects, mortality, and transplant related morbidity. Ann Rheum Dis 2004;63:1318–26.
24. Wedderburn LR, Patel A, King DJ, et al. Long term molecular follow up of immune repertoire after severe immunosuppression and autologous stem cell rescue in children with juvenile idiopathic arthritis [abstract]. Rheumatology 2003;42(Suppl 1):11.
25. Brinkman DMC, van der Zijde CMJ, ten Dam MM, et al. Resetting the adaptive immune system after autologous stem cell transplantation: lessons from responses to vaccines. J clin Immunol 2007;27:647–58.
26. Brinkman DMC, de Kleer IM, ten Cate R, et al. Autologous stem cell transplantation in children with severe progressive systemic or polyarticular juvenile idiopathic arthritis. Long-term follow up of a prospective clinical trial. Arthritis Rheum 2007;56:2410–21.
27. Wulffraat NM, van Rooijen EM, Tewarie R, et al. Current perspectives of autologous stem cell transplantation for severe juvenile idiopathic arthritis. Autoimmunity 2008;41(8):632–8.
28. Abinun M, Flood TJ, Cant AJ, et al. Autologous T cell depleted haematopoietic stem cell transplantation in children with severe juvenile idiopathic arthritis in the UK (2000–2007). Mol Immunol 2009;47(1):46–51.
29. Sykes M, Nikolic B. Treatment of severe autoimmune disease by stem cell transplantation. Nature 2005;435:620–7.
30. Takken T, van den Beuken C, Wullfraat NM, et al. Exercise tolerance in children with juvenile idiopathic arthritis after autologous SCT. Bone Marrow Transplant 2008;42(5):351–6.
31. Quartier P, Prieur AM, Fischer A. Haemopoietic stem cell transplantation for juvenile chronic arthritis. Lancet 1999;353:1885–6.
32. Nakagawa R, Kawano Y, Yoshimura E, et al. Intense immunosuppression followed by purified blood CD34+ cell autografting in a patient with refractory juvenile rheumatoid arthritis. Bone Marrow Transplant 2001;27(3):333–6.
33. Kishimoto T, Hamazaki T, Yasui M, et al. Autologous hematopoietic stem cell transplantation for 3 patients with severe juvenile rheumatoid arthritis. Int J Hematol 2003;78(5):453–6.
34. Vieger AM, Brinkman D, Quartier P, et al. Infection associated MAS in 3 patients receiving ASCT for refractory juvenile chronic arthritis. Bone Marrow Transplant 2000;25(Suppl 1):81.
35. Ten Kate R, Brinkman DM, van Rossum MA, et al. Macrophage activation syndrome after autologous stem cell transplantation for systemic juvenile idiopathic arthritis. Eur J Pediatr 2002;161:685–6.

36. Sreedharan A, Bowyer S, Wallace CA, et al. Macrophage activation syndrome and other systemic inflammatory conditions after BMT. Bone Marrow Transplant 2006;37(7):629–34.

37. Ferreira RA, Vestert SJ, Abinun M, et al. Hemophagocytosis during fludarabine-based SCT for systemic juvenile arthritis. Bone Marrow Transplant 2006;38(3): 249–51.

38. Klein-Gitelman M, Reiff A, Silverman ED. Systemic lupus erythematosus in childhood. Rheum Dis Clin North Am 2002;28:561–77.

39. Miettunen PM, Ortiz-Alvarez O, Petty RE, et al. Gender and ethnic origin have no effect on long-term outcome of childhood onset systemic lupus erythematosus. J Rheumatol 2004;31(8):1650–4.

40. Tucker LB, Menon S, Schaller JG, et al. Adult- and childhood-onset systemic lupus erythematosus: a comparison of onset, clinical features, serology, and outcome. Br J Rheumatol 1995;34(9):866–72.

41. Brunner HI, Silverman ED, To T, et al. Risk factors for damage in childhood-onset systemic lupus erythematosus: cumulative disease activity and medication use predict disease damage. Arthritis Rheum 2002;46(2):436–44.

42. Brunner HI, Gladman DD, Ibañez D, et al. Difference in disease features between childhood-onset and adult-onset systemic lupus erythematosus. Arthritis Rheum 2008;58(2):556–62.

43. Tucker LB, Uribe AG, Fernández M, et al. Adolescent onset of lupus results in more aggressive disease and worse outcomes: results of a nested matched case-control study within LUMINA, a multiethnic US cohort (LUMINA LVII). Lupus 2008;17(4):314–22.

44. Hersh AO, von Scheven E, Yazdany J, et al. Differences in long-term disease activity and treatment of adult patients with childhood- and adult-onset systemic lupus erythematosus. Arthritis Rheum 2009;61(1):13–20.

45. Pluchinotta FR, Schiavo B, Vittadello F, et al. Distinctive clinical features of pediatric systemic lupus erythematosus in three different age classes. Lupus 2007; 16(8):550–5.

46. Ravelli A, Ruperto N, Martini A. Outcome in juvenile onset systemic lupus erythematosus. Curr Opin Rheumatol 2005;17:568–73.

47. Bernatsky S, Boivin JF, Joseph L, et al. Mortality in systemic lupus erythematosus. Arthritis Rheum 2006;54:2550–7.

48. Ruperto N, Buratti S, Duarte-Salazar C, et al. Health-related quality of life in juvenile-onset systemic lupus erythematosus and its relationship to disease activity and damage. Arthritis Rheum 2004;51:458–64.

49. Sullivan KE. Genetics of systemic lupus erythematosus: clinical implications. Rheum Dis Clin North Am 2000;26:229–56.

50. Munoz LE, Gaipl US, Franz S, et al. SLE – a disease of clearance deficiency? Rheumatology 2005;44(9):1101–7.

51. Sturfelt G, Truedsson L. Complement and its breakdown products in SLE. Rheumatology 2005;44(10):1227–32.

52. Mudd PA, Teague BN, Farris AD. Regulatory T cells and systemic lupus erythematosus. Scand J Immunol 2006;64:211–8.

53. Valencia X, Yarboro C, Illei G, et al. Deficient CD4+CD25 (high) T regulatory cell function in patients with active systemic lupus erythematosus. J Immunol 2007; 178:2579–88.

54. Sherer Y, Gorstein A, Fritzler MJ, et al. Autoantibody explosion in systemic lupus erythematosus: more than 100 different antibodies found in SLE patients. Semin Arthritis Rheum 2004;34(2):501–37.

55. Voll RE, Roth EA, Girkontaite I, et al. Histone-specific Th0 and Th1 clones derived from systemic lupus erythematosus patients induce double-stranded DNA antibody production. Arthritis Rheum 1997;40(12):2162–71.
56. Rahman A, Isenberg DA. Systemic lupus erythematosus. N Engl J Med 2008; 358(9):929–39.
57. Avcin T, Silverman ED. Antiphospholipid antibodies in pediatric systemic lupus erythematosus and the antiphospholipid syndrome. Lupus 2007;16(8):627–33.
58. Lehman TJ, Hanson V, Singsen BH, et al. The role of antibodies directed against double-stranded DNA in the manifestations of systemic lupus erythematosus in childhood. J Pediatr 1980;96:657–61.
59. Shergy WJ, Kredich DW, Pisetsky DS. The relationship of anticardiolipin antibodies to disease manifestations in pediatric systemic lupus erythematosus. J Rheumatol 1988;15:1389–94.
60. Oshiro AC, Derbes SJ, Stopa AR, et al. Anti-Ro/SS-A and anti-La/SS-B antibodies associated with cardiac involvement in childhood systemic lupus erythematosus. Ann Rheum Dis 1997;56:272–4.
61. Reichlin M, Broyles TF, Hubscher O, et al. Prevalence of autoantibodies to ribosomal P proteins in juvenile-onset systemic lupus erythematosus compared with the adult disease. Arthritis Rheum 1999;42:69–75.
62. Press J, Palayew K, Laxer RM, et al. Antiribosomal P antibodies in pediatric patients with systemic lupus erythematosus and psychosis. Arthritis Rheum 1996;39:671–6.
63. Male C, Foulon D, Hoogendoorn H, et al. Predictive value of persistent versus transient antiphospholipid antibody subtypes for the risk of thrombotic events in pediatric patients with systemic lupus erythematosus. Blood 2005;106(13):4152–8.
64. Hochberg M. Updating the American College of Rheumatology revised criteria for the classification of systemic lupus erythematosus. Arthritis Rheum 1997; 40(9):1725.
65. Tucker LB. Making the diagnosis of systemic lupus erythematosus in children and adolescents. Lupus 2007;16(8):546–9.
66. Bogdanovic R, Nikolic V, Pasic S, et al. Lupus nephritis in childhood: a review of 53 patients followed at a single center. Pediatr Nephrol 2004;19:36–44.
67. Sibbitt WL Jr, Brandt JR, Johnson CR, et al. The incidence and prevalence of neuropsychiatric syndromes in pediatric onset systemic lupus erythematosus. J Rheumatol 2002;29:1537–42.
68. Levy DM, Ardoin SP, Schanberg LE. Neurocognitive impairment in children and adolescents with systemic lupus erythematosus. Nat Clin Pract Rheumatol 2009;5(2):106–14.
69. Sandborg C, Ardoin SP, Schanberg L. Therapy Insight: cardiovascular disease in pediatric systemic lupus erythematosus. Nat Clin Pract Rheumatol 2008;4(5): 258–65.
70. Lilleby V, Aaløkken TM, Johansen B, et al. Pulmonary involvement in patients with childhood-onset systemic lupus erythematosus. Clin Exp Rheumatol 2006;24(2):203–8.
71. Zonana-Nacach A, Barr SG, Madger LA, et al. Damage in systemic lupus erythematosus and its association with corticosteroids. Arthritis Rheum 2000;43:1801–8.
72. Austin HA III, Klippel JH, Balow JE, et al. Therapy of lupus nephritis. Controlled trial of prednisone and cytotoxic drugs. N Engl J Med 1986;314:614–9.
73. Boumpas DT, Austin HA III, Vaughn EM, et al. Controlled trial of pulse methylprednisolone versus two regimens of pulse cyclophosphamide in severe lupus nephritis. Lancet 1992;340:741–5.

74. Gourley MF, Austin HA III, Scott D, et al. Methylprednisolone and cyclophospha-mide, alone or in combination, in patients with lupus nephritis. A randomized, controlled trial. Ann Intern Med 1996;125:549–57.

75. Flanc RS, Roberts MA, Strippoli GF, et al. Treatment of diffuse proliferative lupus nephritis: a meta-analysis of randomized controlled trials. Am J Kidney Dis 2004;43:197–208.

76. Korbet SM, Lewis EJ, Schwartz MM, et al. Factors predictive of outcome in severe lupus nephritis. Am J Kidney Dis 2000;35:904–14.

77. Ioannidis JPA, Boki KA, Katsorida EM, et al. Remission, relapse, and re-remis-sion of proliferative lupus nephritis treated with cyclophosphamide. Kidney Int 2000;57:258–64.

78. Mok CC, Ying KY, Tang S, et al. Predictors and outcome of renal flares after successful cyclophosphamide treatment for diffuse proliferative lupus glomeru-lonephritis. Arthritis Rheum 2004;50:2559–68.

79. Houssiau FA, Vasconcelos C, D'Cruz D, et al. Immunosuppressive therapy in lupus nephritis, the Euro-Lupus Nephritis Trial, a randomized trial of low-dose versus high-dose intravenous cyclophosphamide. Arthritis Rheum 2002;46: 2121–31.

80. Moore RA, Derry S. Systematic review and meta-analysis of randomized trials and cohort studies of mycophenolate mofetil in lupus nephritis. Arthritis Res Ther 2006;8:R182.

81. Appel GB, Contreras G, Dooley MA, et al. Aspreva Lupus Management Study Group. Mycophenolate mofetil versus cyclophosphamide for induction treat-ment of lupus nephritis. J Am Soc Nephrol 2009;20(5):1103–12.

82. Anolik JH, Barnard J, Cappione A, et al. Rituximab improves peripheral B cell abnormalities in human systemic lupus erythematosus. Arthritis Rheum 2004; 50:3580–90.

83. Looney RJ, Anolik JH, Campbell D, et al. B cell depletion as a novel treatment for systemic lupus erythematosus: a phase I/II dose escalation trial of rituximab. Arthritis Rheum 2004;50:2580–9.

84. Leandro MJ, Edwards JC, Cambridge G, et al. An open study of B lympho-cyte depletion in systemic lupus erythematosus. Arthritis Rheum 2002;46: 2673–7.

85. Cambridge G, Stohl W, Leandro MJ, et al. Circulating levels of B lymphocyte stimulator in patients with rheumatoid arthritis following rituximab treatment: rela-tionships with B cell depletion, circulating antibodies, and clinical relapse. Arthritis Rheum 2006;54:723–32.

86. Available at: http://www.gene.com/gene/news/pressreleases/display.do?method =detail&id=11947. Accessed March 11, 2009.

87. Aringer M, Graninger WB, Steiner G, et al. Safety and efficacy of TNF α- blockade in systemic lupus erythematosus – an open label study. Arthritis Rheum 2004;50:3161–9.

88. A randomized study of the effect of withdrawing hydroxychloroquine sulfate in systemic lupus erythematosus. The Canadian Hydroxychloroquine Study Group. N Engl J Med 1991;324(3):150–4.

89. Tsakonas E, Joseph L, Esdaile JM, et al. A long-term study of hydroxychloro-quine withdrawal on exacerbations in systemic lupus erythematosus. The Cana-dian Hydroxychloroquine Study Group. Lupus 1998;7(2):80–5.

90. Chan TM, Li FK, Tang CS, et al. Efficacy of mycophenolate mofetil in patients with diffuse proliferative lupus nephritis. Hong Kong-Guangzhou Nephrology Study Group. N Engl J Med 2000;343(16):1156–62.

91. Chan TM, Tse KC, Tang CS, et al. Hong Kong Nephrology Study Group. Long-term study of mycophenolate mofetil as continuous induction and maintenance treatment for diffuse proliferative lupus nephritis. J Am Soc Nephrol 2005;16(4): 1076–84.

92. Houssiau FA, Vasconcelos C, D'Cruz D, et al. Early response to immunosuppressive therapy predicts good renal outcome in lupus nephritis: lessons from long-term followup of patients in the Euro-Lupus Nephritis Trial. Arthritis Rheum 2004;50(12):3934–40.

93. Yee CS, Gordon C, Dostal C, et al. EULAR randomised controlled trial of pulse cyclophosphamide and methylprednisolone versus continuous cyclophosphamide and prednisolone followed by azathioprine and prednisolone in lupus nephritis. Ann Rheum Dis 2004;63(5):525–9.

94. Tam LS, Li EK, Wong CK, et al. Double-blind, randomized, placebo-controlled pilot study of leflunomide in systemic lupus erythematosus. Lupus 2004;13(8): 601–4.

95. Contreras G, Pardo V, Leclercq B, et al. Sequential therapies for proliferative lupus nephritis. N Engl J Med 2004;350(10):971–80.

96. Barile-Fabris L, Ariza-Andraca R, Olguín-Ortega L, et al. Controlled clinical trial of IV cyclophosphamide versus IV methylprednisolone in severe neurological manifestations in systemic lupus erythematosus. Ann Rheum Dis 2005;64(4):620–5.

97. Ginzler EM, Dooley MA, Aranow C, et al. Mycophenolate mofetil or intravenous cyclophosphamide for lupus nephritis. N Engl J Med 2005;353(21):2219–28.

98. Ong LM, Hooi LS, Lim TO, et al. Randomized controlled trial of pulse intravenous cyclophosphamide versus mycophenolate mofetil in the induction therapy of proliferative lupus nephritis. Nephrology (Carlton) 2005;10(5):504–10.

99. Bezerra EL, Vilar MJ, da Trindade Neto PB, et al. Double-blind, randomized, controlled clinical trial of clofazimine compared with chloroquine in patients with systemic lupus erythematosus. Arthritis Rheum 2005;52(10):3073–8.

100. Grootscholten C, Ligtenberg G, Hagen EC, et al. Dutch Working Party on Systemic Lupus Erythematosus. Azathioprine/methylprednisolone versus cyclophosphamide in proliferative lupus nephritis. A randomized controlled trial. Kidney Int 2006;70(4):732–42.

101. Grootscholten C, Bajema IM, Florquin S, et al. Dutch Working Party on Systemic Lupus Erythematosus. Treatment with cyclophosphamide delays the progression of chronic lesions more effectively than does treatment with azathioprine plus methylprednisolone in patients with proliferative lupus nephritis. Arthritis Rheum 2007;56(3):924–37.

102. Tseng CE, Buyon JP, Kim M, et al. The effect of moderate-dose corticosteroids in preventing severe flares in patients with serologically active, but clinically stable, systemic lupus erythematosus: findings of a prospective, randomized, double-blind, placebo-controlled trial. Arthritis Rheum 2006;54(11):3623–32.

103. Moroni G, Doria A, Mosca M, et al. A randomized pilot trial comparing cyclosporine and azathioprine for maintenance therapy in diffuse lupus nephritis over four years. Clin J Am Soc Nephrol 2006;1(5):925–32.

104. Wang J, Hu W, Xie H, et al. Induction therapies for class IV lupus nephritis with non-inflammatory necrotizing vasculopathy: mycophenolate mofetil or intravenous cyclophosphamide. Lupus 2007;16(9):707–12.

105. Fortin PR, Abrahamowicz M, Ferland D, et al. Canadian Network For Improved Outcomes in Systemic Lupus. Steroid-sparing effects of methotrexate in systemic lupus erythematosus: a double-blind, randomized, placebo-controlled trial. Arthritis Rheum 2008;59(12):1796–804.

106. Cardiel MH, Tumlin JA, Furie RA, et al. LJP 394-90-09 Investigator Consortium. Abetimus sodium for renal flare in systemic lupus erythematosus: results of a randomized, controlled phase III trial. Arthritis Rheum 2008;58(8):2470–80.

107. Austin HA 3rd, Illei GG, Braun MJ, et al. Randomized, controlled trial of prednisone, cyclophosphamide, and cyclosporine in lupus membranous nephropathy. J Am Soc Nephrol 2009;20(4):901–11.

108. Jayne D, Passweg J, Marmont A, et al. European Group for Blood and Marrow Transplantation; European League Against Rheumatism Registry. Autologous stem cell transplantation for systemic lupus erythematosus. Lupus 2004;13(3): 168–76.

109. Burt RK, Traynor A, Statkute L, et al. Nonmyeloablative hematopoietic stem cell transplantation for systemic lupus erythematosus. JAMA 2006;295(5):527–35.

110. Wulffraat NM, Sanders EAM, Kamphuis SSM, et al. Prolonged remission without treatment after autologous stem cell transplantation for refractory childhood systemic lupus erythematosus. Arthritis Rheum 2001;44(3):728–34.

111. Chen J, Wang Y, Kunkel G, et al. Use of CD34+ autologous stem cell transplantation in the treatment of children with refractory systemic lupus erythematosus. Clin Rheumatol 2005;24:464–8.

112. Muraro PA, Douek DC, Packer A, et al. Thymic output generates a new and diverse TCR repertoire after autologous stem cell transplantation in multiple sclerosis patients. J Exp Med 2005;201(5):805–16.

113. Zhang L, Bertucci AM, Ramsey-Goldman R, et al. Regulatory T cell (TReg) subsets return in patients with refractory lupus following adult stem cell transplantation: TGF-β producing CD8+ Treg (CD8TGF-β Treg) are associated with suppressing lupus into immunologic remission. J immunol 2009;183(10): 6346–58.

114. Alexander T, Thiel A, Rosen O, et al. Depletion of autoreactive immunologic memory followed by autologous hematopoietic stem cell transplantation in patients with refractory SLE induces long-term remission through de novo generation of a juvenile and tolerant immune system. Blood 2009;113(1): 214–23.

115. Burt RK, Loh Y, Cohen B, et al. Autologous non-myeloablative haemopoietic stem cell transplantation in relapsing-remitting multiple sclerosis: a phase I/II study. Lancet Neurol 2009;8(3):244–53.

116. Voltarelli JC, Couri CE, Stracieri AB, et al. Autologous nonmyeloablative hematopoietic stem cell transplantation in newly diagnosed type 1 diabetes mellitus. JAMA 2007;297(14):1568–76.

117. Couri CE, Oliveira MC, Stracieri AB, et al. C-peptide levels and insulin independence following autologous nonmyeloablative hematopoietic stem cell transplantation in newly diagnosed type 1 diabetes mellitus. JAMA 2009;301(15): 1573–9.

118. Gale EAM. The risk of childhood type 1 diabetes in the 20th century. Diabetes 2002;51:3353–61.

119. Knip M, Veijola R, Virtanen SM, et al. Environmental triggers and determinants of β-cell autoimmunity and type 1 diabetes. Diabetes 2005;54(Suppl 2):S125–36.

120. Notkins AL, Lernmark A. Autoimmune type 1 diabetes: resolved and unresolved issues. J Clin Invest 2001;108:1247–52.

121. Nathan DM. Long term complications of diabetes mellitus. N Engl J Med 1993; 328:1676–85.

122. Rubin RR, Peyrot M. Quality of life and diabetes. Diabetes Metab Res Rev 1999; 15:205–18.

123. Todd JA, Walker NM, Cooper JD, et al. Robust associations of four new chromosome regions from genome-wide analyses of type 1 diabetes. Nat Genet 2007; 39:857–64.
124. Tsirogianni A, Pipi E, Soufleros K. Specificity of islet cell autoantibodies and coexistence with other organ specific autoantibodies in type 1 diabetes mellitus. Autoimmun Rev 2009;8(8):687–91.
125. Shehadeh N, Pollack S, Wildbaum G, et al. Selective autoantibody production against CCL3 is associated with human type 1 diabetes mellitus and serves as a novel biomarker for its diagnosis. J Immunol 2009;182(12):8104–9.
126. Bingley PJ, Christie MR, Bonifacio E, et al. Combined analysis of autoantibodies improves prediction of IDDM in islet cell antibody-positive relatives. Diabetes 1994;43:1304–10.
127. Roep BO. The role of T-cells in the pathogenesis of type 1 diabetes: from cause to cure. Diabetologia 2003;46:305–21.
128. Jeitler K, Horvath K, Berghold A, et al. Continuous subcutaneous insulin infusion versus multiple daily insulin injections in patients with diabetes mellitus: systematic review and meta-analysis. Diabetologia 2008;51(6):941–51.
129. Fatourechi MM, Kudva YC, Murad MH, et al. Clinical review: hypoglycemia with intensive insulin therapy: a systematic review and meta-analyses of randomized trials of continuous subcutaneous insulin infusion versus multiple daily injections. J Clin Endocrinol Metab 2009;94(3):729–40.
130. The effect of intensive treatment of diabetes on the development and progression of long term complications in insulin-dependent diabetes mellitus, The Diabetes Control and Complications Trial Research Group. N Engl J Med 1993;329:977–86.
131. Genuth S. Insights from the diabetes control and complications trial/epidemiology of diabetes interventions and complications study on the use of intensive glycemic treatment to reduce the risk of complications of type 1 diabetes. Endocr Pract 2006;12(Suppl 1):34–41.
132. DCCT. The Diabetes Control and Complications Trial Research Group The Effect of Intensive. Treatment of Diabetes on the Development and Progression of Long-Term Complications in Insulin- Dependent Diabetes Mellitus. N Engl J Med 1993;329:977–86.
133. Pavlakis M, Khwaja K. Pancreas and islet transplantation in diabetes. Curr Opin Endocrinol Diabetes Obes 2007;14:146–50.
134. Shapiro AM, Ricordi C, Hering BJ, et al. International trial of the Edmonton protocol for islet transplantation. N Engl J Med 2006;355:1318–30.
135. American Diabetes Association. Pancreas and islet transplantation in type 1 diabetes. Diabetes Care 2006;29(4):935.
136. Steffes MW, Sibley S, Jackson M, et al. Beta-cell function and the development of diabetes-related complications in the Diabetes Control and Complications Trial. Diabetes Care 2003;26(3):832–6.
137. The Diabetes Control and Complications Trial Research Group. Effect of intensive therapy on residual beta-cell function in patients with type 1 diabetes in the Diabetes Control and Complications Trial. Ann Intern Med 1998;128:517–23.
138. Elliott RB, Crossley JR, Berryman CC, et al. Partial preservation of pancreatic beta-cell function in children with diabetes. Lancet 1981;19:631–2.
139. Harrison LC, Colman PG, Dean B, et al. Increase in remission rate in newly diagnosed type 1 diabetic subjects treated with azathioprine. Diabetes 1985;34:1306–8.
140. Cook JJ, Hudson I, Harrison LC, et al. Double-blind controlled trial of azathioprine in children with newly diagnosed type 1 diabetes. Diabetes 1989;38:779–83.

141. Silverstein J, Maclaren N, Riley W, et al. Immunosuppression with azathioprine and prednisone in recent-onset insulin-dependent diabetes mellitus. N Engl J Med 1988;319:599–604.
142. Feutren G, Papoz L, Assan R, et al. Cyclosporin increases the rate and length of remissions in insulin-dependent diabetes of recent onset. Results of a multi-centre double-blind trial. Lancet 1986;2(8499):119–24.
143. Bougneres PF, Carel JC, Castano L, et al. Factors associated with early remission of type I diabetes in children treated with cyclosporine. N Engl J Med 1988; 318(11):663–70.
144. Canadian-European Randomized Control Trial Group. Cyclosporin-induced remission of IDDM after early intervention: association of 1 yr of cyclosporin treatment with enhanced insulin secretion. Diabetes 1988;37:1574–82.
145. Christie MR, Mølvig J, Hawkes CJ, et al. Canadian-European Randomised Control Trial Group. IA-2 antibody-negative status predicts remission and recovery of C-peptide levels in type 1 diabetic patients treated with cyclosporin. Diabetes Care 2002;25(7):1192–7.
146. Martin S, Schernthaner G, Nerup J, et al. Follow-up of cyclosporin A treatment in type 1 (insulin-dependent) diabetes mellitus: lack of long-term effects. Diabetologia 1991;34(6):429–34.
147. Assan R, Feutren G, Sirmai J, et al. Plasma C-peptide levels and clinical remissions in recent-onset type I diabetic patients treated with cyclosporin A and insulin. Diabetes 1990;39(7):768–74.
148. De Filippo G, Carel JC, Boitard C, et al. Long-term results of early cyclosporin therapy in juvenile IDDM. Diabetes 1996;45(1):101–4.
149. Herold KC, Hagopian W, Auger JA, et al. Anti-CD3 monoclonal antibody in new-onset type 1 diabetes mellitus. N Engl J Med 2002;346:1692–8.
150. Keymeulen B, Vandemeulebroucke E, Ziegler AG, et al. Insulin needs after CD3-antibody therapy in new-onset type1 diabetes. N Engl J Med 2005;352: 2598–608.
151. Saudek F, Havrdova T, Boucek P, et al. Polyclonal anti-T-cell therapy for type 1 diabetes mellitus of recent onset. Rev Diabet Stud 2004;1:80–8.
152. Raz I, Elias D, Avron A, et al. Beta-cell function in newly-onset type 1 diabetes and immunomodulation with a heat shock protein peptide (DiaPep277): a randomised, double-blind, phase II trial. Lancet 2001;358:1749–53.
153. Schloot NC, Meierhoff G, Lengyel C, et al. Effect of heat shock protein peptide DiaPep277 on beta-cell function in paediatric and adult patients with recent-onset diabetes mellitus type 1: two prospective, randomized, double-blind phase II trials. Diabetes Metab Res Rev 2007;23(4):276–85.
154. Ludvigsson J, Faresjö M, Hjorth M, et al. GAD treatment and insulin secretion in recent-onset type 1 diabetes. N Engl J Med 2008;359(18):1909–20.
155. Buckingham BA, Sandborg CI. A randomized trial of methotrexate in newly diagnosed patients with type 1 diabetes mellitus. Clin Immunol 2000;96(2):86–90.
156. Milanetti F, Bucha J, Testori A, et al. Autologous hematopoietic stem cell transplantation for systemic sclerosis. Curr Stem Cell Res Ther, in press.
157. Vonk MC, Marjanovic Z, Van Den Hoogen FH, et al. Long-term follow-up results after autologous haematopoietic stem cell transplantation for severe systemic sclerosis. Ann Rheum Dis 2008;67(1):98–104 [Erratum in: Ann Rheum Dis 2008;67(2):280].
158. Rabusin M, Andolina M, Maximova N. Haematopoietic SCT in autoimmune diseases in children: rationale and new perspectives. Bone Marrow Transplant 2008;41(Suppl 2):S96–9.

159. Samarasinghe SR, Cleary G, Veys P, et al. Autologous stem cell transplantation for juvenile dermatomyositis [abstract]. Arch Dis Child 2002;86(Suppl 1):A49.

160. Elhasid R, Rowe JM, Berkowitz D, et al. Disappearance of diffuse calcinosis following autologous stem cell transplantation in a child with autoimmune disease. Bone Marrow Transplant 2004;33:1257–9.

161. Marmont AM, Burt RK. Hematopoietic stem cell transplantation for systemic lupus erythematosus, the antiphospholipid syndrome and bulous skin diseases. Autoimmunity 2008;41(8):639–47.

162. Wedderburn LR, Jeffery R, White H, et al. Autologous stem cell transplantation for paediatric-onset polyarteritis nodosa: changes in autoimmune phenotype in the context of reduced diversity of the T- and B-cell repertoires, and evidence for reversion from the CD45RO(+) to RA(+) phenotype. Rheumatology (Oxford) 2001;40(11):1299–307.

163. Rossi G, Moretta A, Locatelli F. Autologous hematopoietic stem cell transplantation for severe/refractory intestinal Behcet disease. Blood 2004;103(2):748–50.

Management of Acute Graft-Versus-Host Disease in Children

Paul A. Carpenter, MBBS[a,b,]*, Margaret L. MacMillan, MD[c]

KEYWORDS

- Acute GVHD • Graft-versus-host disease
- Children • Management

The most significant immunologic barrier to successful hematopoietic stem cell transplantation (HSCT) is acute graft-versus-host disease (aGVHD), which can result in life-threatening inflammation and tissue destruction. The current model of aGVHD continues to invoke 3 collaborative phases: (1) tissue damage induced by the preparative regimen; (2) priming and activation of donor T cells, with CD8 T cells being stimulated by residual host antigen-presenting cells (APCs) and CD4 T cells being stimulated by donor APCs presenting host-derived antigens; and (3) target tissue damage induced directly by cytotoxic T cells and indirectly by inflammatory cytokines. In addition to $\alpha\beta$ T cells, other cell populations that include natural killer (NK) cells, NK T cells and $\gamma\delta$ T cells, conventional and plasmacytoid dendritic cells, and regulatory T cells (Tregs) seem to have important modulatory functions in aGVHD[1] and further understanding may offer future novel approaches to management. Meanwhile, donor T cells that recognize disparate recipient alloantigens are central mediators of GVHD and remain the focus of current therapies.

The focus of this article is to guide the clinician in the various clinical presentations of aGVHD and initial (primary) therapy. In addition, secondary therapeutic options are reviewed for children who have failed primary therapy and suggestions are offered recognizing that there is no standard approach. Most of what is known about aGVHD therapy has arisen from trials that enrolled on adults with or without children.

This work was supported by Grant No. CA18029 from the National Institutes of Health.

[a] Clinical Research Division, Fred Hutchinson Cancer Research Center, 1100 Fairview Avenue North, Mailstop D5-290, Seattle, WA 98109, USA

[b] Department of Pediatrics, University of Washington, 1959 NE Pacific Street, Health Sciences Building, Seattle, WA 98195, USA

[c] Blood and Marrow Transplant Program, Department of Pediatrics, University of Minnesota Medical School, D-557 Mayo Building, 420 Delaware Street SE, MMC 484, Minneapolis, MN 55455, USA

* Corresponding author. Clinical Research Division, Fred Hutchinson Cancer Research Center, 1100 Fairview Avenue North, Mailstop D5-290, Seattle, WA 98109.

E-mail address: pcarpent@fhcrc.org

Pediatr Clin N Am 57 (2010) 273–295
doi:10.1016/j.pcl.2009.11.007
0031-3955/10/$ – see front matter

Whenever specifics pertain to children, they are highlighted in this paper. The prevention of aGVHD includes the avoidance of known risk factors (predominantly HLA-disparity), immunosuppressive pharmacotherapies, and cellular approaches that are reviewed in the literature.[2–9]

DIAGNOSIS AND CLASSIFICATION OF ACUTE GVHD

Historically, GVHD was categorized as acute or chronic based on time of presentation; GVHD before day 100 was known as acute, and after day 100 it was known as chronic. This classification was based on patients transplanted with HLA-identical sibling bone marrow (BM) after receiving myeloablative conditioning. In the last 20 years, HSCT has become more complex, particularly with the use of different stem cell sources (reviewed by Peters and colleagues elsewhere in this issue), and the development of nonmyeloablative conditioning that is associated with delayed onset aGVHD. These advancements have made the distinction between acute and chronic GVHD based on time of onset no longer accurate. Therefore, it is preferable to recognize aGVHD by the clinicopathologic constellation of combinations of inflammatory dermatitis, enteritis, and hepatitis, which reflects T cell activation with generation of cytotoxic lymphocytes and inflammatory cytokines that cause tissue damage. Chronic GVHD (cGVHD) is now similarly recognized without reference to time after HSCT by the presence of diagnostic or distinct cGVHD manifestations that resemble autoimmune diseases; cGVHD is reviewed by Baird and colleagues in this issue and elsewhere.[10] Thus, for example, secretory diarrhea or erythematous maculopapular dermatitis following a relapsing or indolent course is classified as late persistent aGVHD or cGVHD (with overlap syndrome) if classic manifestations of cGVHD are also present. It remains to be determined whether the type or duration of immunosuppressive therapy should differ based on these clinical distinctions.

GVHD Classification

The severity of aGVHD is determined by the degree (or stage) of involvement in each of the main target organs (skin, liver, and upper and lower gastrointestinal (GI) tract) based on accepted criteria that primarily include the extent of rash, magnitude of hyperbilirubinemia, volume of diarrhea, and presence of nausea (**Table 1**). Various combinations of skin, liver, and GI involvement are then used to assign an overall GVHD severity or grade, as per the modified Glucksberg criteria (Grades I–IV) most commonly or by the International Bone Marrow Transplant Registry (IBMTR) Index (Grades A–D) less commonly (**Table 2**).[11–14]

Mild aGVHD (grade I or A) is essentially cutaneous GVHD (an erythematous maculopapular rash) involving 50% body surface area (BSA) or less, and usually requires no change to systemic GVHD prophylaxis. A rash involving more than 50% BSA requires additional therapy as discussed later. When cellular injury is severe, skin aGVHD may manifest with bulla formation and desquamation. Regardless of surface area involved, this is a severe and often life-threatening form of GVHD (stage 4, overall grade IV).

aGVHD of the GI system may involve the upper GI tract causing anorexia, nausea, and vomiting, and/or the lower GI tract causing profuse watery diarrhea with tenesmus, urgency, and frequency. If severe (stage 4), lower GI GVHD may cause life-threatening bloody diarrhea with cramping abdominal pain. Liver involvement is staged according to the degree of hyperbilirubinemia but is often preceded or accompanied by increased serum transaminase levels (especially alanine aminotransferase [ALT]) and, slightly later, by increased serum alkaline phosphatase level. AGVHD of

Table 1
Acute GVHD staging

	Stage 0	Stage 1	Stage 2	Stage 3	Stage 4
Skin	No rash	Rash <25% BSA	25%–50%	>50% generalized erythroderma	Plus bullae and desquamation
Gut	Adult: <500 mL/d Child: <10 mL/kg/d	Adult: 500–1000 mL/d Child: 10–19.9 mL/kg/d	Adult: 1001–1500 mL/d Child: 20–30 mL/kg/d	Adult: >1500 mL/d Child: >30 mL/kg/d	Severe abdominal pain ± ileus, flank blood, or melena
Upper GI	–	Severe nausea/vomiting	–	–	–
Liver	Bilirubin ≤2 mg/dL	2.1–3 mg/dL	3.1–6 mg/dL	6.1–15 mg/dL	>15 mg/dL

Abbreviation: BSA, body surface area.

the liver rarely occurs without other organ involvement. AGVHD of the gut and/or liver requires systemic therapy in addition to prophylaxis regardless of stage.

Diagnosis of GVHD

The clinical signs of aGVHD are not sufficiently pathognomonic to establish the diagnosis, especially when there is isolated organ involvement and a broad differential diagnosis always needs to be considered (**Table 3**). However, the combination of rash, nausea, and voluminous diarrhea, occurring at the time of, or soon after, neutrophil engraftment makes the diagnosis very likely. Tissue biopsy is recommended to confirm a histologic diagnosis of aGVHD and, most importantly, to exclude opportunistic infection or drug reaction. Skin biopsies and/or upper/lower GI endoscopy and biopsies should be performed depending on the clinical signs and symptoms. Care should be taken performing duodenal biopsies because there is a greater risk

Table 2
Acute GVHD grading systems

Grade[a]	Skin[b]	Liver	GI	Upper GI
Consensus				
I	1–2	0	0	0
II	3	1	1	1
III	–	2–3	2–4	–
IV[c]	4	4	–	–
IBMTR[d]				
A	1	0	0	0
B	2	1–2	1–2	1
C	3	3	3	–
D	4	4	4	–

[a] Each grade is based on maximum stage for each organ involved.
[b] Each column identifies the minimum stage for organ grade.
[c] Grade IV may also include less organ involvement but with extreme decrease in performance status.
[d] Modified as shown to include upper GI GVHD.

Table 3 Differential diagnosis of aGVHD	
aGVHD Manifestation	**Differential Diagnosis**
Rash	Drug reaction Allergic reaction Infection Regimen-related toxicity
Diarrhea	Infection (viral, fungal) Opiate withdrawal
Abdominal pain	Acute pancreatitis Acute cholecystitis (biliary sludge, stones, infection) Narcotic bowel syndrome
Elevated liver enzymes	Sinsusoidal obstruction syndrome Medication toxicities (eg, azoles) Cholangitis lenta (sepsis) Biliary sludge syndrome Viral infections (cytomegalovirus, Epstein-Barr virus, hepatitis B) Hemolysis

for nonhealing ulcerations and intramural hematoma. To avoid bleeding complications, platelet counts should be maintained at more than 50×10^9/L for at least 3 days after GI biopsies. The interpretation of biopsies performed within 3 weeks of myeloablative therapy may be problematic because it is difficult to separate cellular injury induced by chemoradiotherapy from GVHD. The histologic hallmark of GVHD-induced cellular injury is apoptosis, observed in epidermal basal keratinocytes, bile duct, or intestinal crypt epithelial cells, and is often associated with infiltration by lymphocytes.[15,16]

PRIMARY (INITIAL) TREATMENT OF AGVHD

Patients with aGVHD have traditionally continued on GVHD prophylaxis, most commonly a calcineurin inhibitor (CNI), and in some cases the CNI is combined with mycophenolate mofetil (MMF) or sirolimus. Additional therapy depends on the initial grade of aGVHD, the particular organs involved, and is discussed later.

Mild aGVHD (Skin Only)

Grade I aGVHD (see **Table 2**) does not usually require systemic steroid therapy and close observation constitutes acceptable management. A symptomatic rash may be treated with topical therapy using creams or ointments (eg, 0.1% triamcinolone or 0.1% tacrolimus to the body; 1% hydrocortisone cream to the face) applied 3 to 4 times daily. Ultraviolet A and psoralen (PUVA) may also be administered up to 3 times per week.[17] If the rash progresses after 3 to 4 days of topical therapy, or no improvement occurs after 7 days, systemic steroid therapy is needed as outlined for moderate aGVHD (**Fig. 1**).

Moderate to Severe aGVHD

Moderate aGVHD (grade II–III aGVHD) occurs in 30% to 80% of HSCT recipients and is comprised of skin stages 1 to 3 and/or liver stages 1 to 3 and/or lower GI stages 1 to 4, with or without upper GI involvement by the modified Glucksberg criteria.[13]

    Severe aGVHD is grade IV GVHD at onset, or after progression or no response to moderate GVHD therapy. The conventional first-line therapy for grades II to IV aGVHD is systemic glucocorticoids, which are lympholytic and decrease the inflammatory cytokine cascade of aGVHD. The conventional starting dose is 2mg/kg methylprednis-olone (MP) (or prednisone equivalent).[18–20] Patients with skin involvement may also receive topical therapy as discussed earlier.

OPTIONAL APPROACHES FOR AGVHD THERAPY
Modification of the Starting Dose of MP for Patients with Grade II aGVHD

An important goal of therapy is to minimize complications associated with high-dose glucocorticoid therapy. Therefore, some centers have attempted to begin treatment with MP-equivalent doses less than 2 mg/kg for milder GVHD within the spectrum of aGVHD manifestations that warrant systemic therapy as shown by a large retro-spective study of 733 patients.[21] This approach requires further validation, particularly for patients with grades III to IV aGVHD who were not well represented in this study. However, the study findings that overall mortality, relapse mortality, and nonrelapse mortality were similar irrespective of whether patients began therapy with 1 mg/kg or 2 mg/kg MP-equivalent doses, certainly seems generalizable for grade II aGVHD. Mean cumulative MP-equivalent doses at day 100 remained approximately 50% lower for patients who began therapy at 1 mg/kg versus 2 mg/kg. In the multivariate analysis, the risks of invasive fungal infections (hazard ratio [HR] 0.59, 95% confidence interval [CI] 0.3–1.0) and the duration of hospitalization (odds ratio 0.62, 95% CI 0.4–0.9) were also reduced in the low-dose MP group. An important caveat to adopting the approach of intermediate-dose glucocorticoid therapy for mild aGVHD is that MP-equivalent dosing should be escalated to 2 mg/kg/d if aGVHD manifestations are progressing after 3 days of 1 mg/kg.

Nonabsorbable Glucocorticoids for GI Tract GVHD

Another strategy to reduce systemic glucocorticoid exposure has been to incorporate potent topically acting, nonabsorbable glucocorticoids (beclomethasone dipropionate [BDP] or budesonide [BDE]) into the therapy for GI GVHD (see legend to **Fig. 1** for details). Orally administered BDP has been shown to be effective at controlling milder forms of grade II aGVHD[22–24] which these studies defined as rash <50% of the total body surface area (ie, <stage 2), anorexia, nausea, emesis or diarrhea <20 mL/kg/d (ie, <stage 1) and without liver involvement (stage 0). This clinical phenotype has been named grade IIa to delineate it from conventional grade II disease which also includes more extensive rash and allows mild liver involvement. Two of these BDP trials are the first and only randomized clinical trials to suggest a survival advantage for a new treatment of aGVHD (**Table 4**).[23,24] Unfortunately these landmark BDP trials were conducted with a unique BDP formulation that is not currently commercially available. A redesigned phase 3 study in adults with the intent of again seeking FDA approval is ongoing. Further trials in children are also warranted to understand the role of nonabsorbable glucocorticoids in the treatment of GI GVHD and to explore appropriate dose regimens for children.

Upfront Addition of a Second-Line Agent

Recognizing that the overall response of aGVHD to glucocorticoid therapy is roughly 50% (discussed later), and that the durability of those responses is relatively unsatis-factory, several clinical trials have explored ways to improve outcomes; these are summarized in **Table 4**. These studies have included 2 randomized trials that showed no benefit to beginning therapy with MP dosages more than 2 mg/kg/d.[25,26] Other studies have shown the potential benefit of adding several second-line agents to MP as initial therapy for aGVHD but none has been shown definitively to be more

Acute GVHD Treatment Algorithm

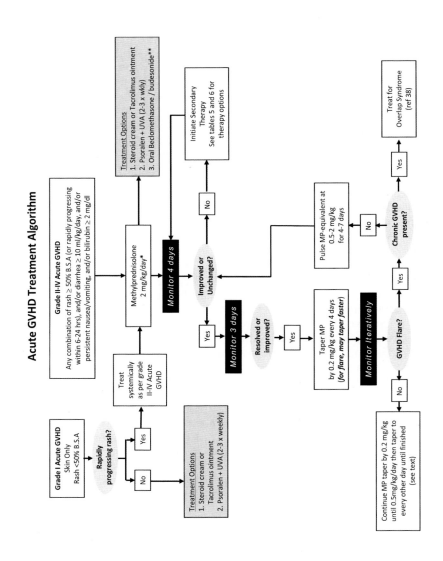

efficacious and safer than MP alone. For example, the results of controlled studies that explored the addition of polyclonal or monoclonal anti-T cell antibodies to MP 2 mg/kg showed either no benefit[12,27] or resulted in inferior survival.[28] In 1 historically controlled phase 2 study, the addition of the anti-tumor necrosis factor (TNF) fusion protein, etanercept, appeared to induce more complete responses.[29] However, among the 4 arms (etanercept, MMF, denileukin diftitox, or pentostatin) of the recently reported prospective BMT Clinical Trials Network (CTN) randomized phase 2 study, it was the combination of MP plus MMF, rather than MP plus etanercept, that showed most promise based on early study endpoints (see **Table 4**).[30] A follow-up phase 3 study by the BMT CTN to more definitively evaluate MMF in this context is imminent.

Fig. 1. Acute GVHD treatment algorithm. *Some centers choose to begin steroid dosing at <2 mg/kg/d for grade II aGVHD (see text). **Seattle uses nonabsorbable gut steroids for children with grade IIa aGVHD defined by anorexia, nausea, emesis or diarrhea less than 20 mL/kg/d, no liver involvement, and rash covering less than 50% of the body surface area (BSA) and not progressing rapidly within the first 6 to 24 hours. Grade IIa aGVHD may be treated with a 10-day induction course of MP 1 mg/kg plus a 50-day course of nonabsorbable glucocorticoids delivered to the GI tract. If GI manifestations are progressing after 3 days of 1 mg/kg and nonabsorbable glucocorticoids, then prednisone should be increased to 2 mg/kg/d. In this latter scenario, the continuation of nonabsorbable glucocorticoids is optional but often invoked as prednisone-sparing therapy. If GI symptoms of anorexia, nausea, and diarrhea less than 10 mL/kg/d without cramping have completely resolved after 10 days, then prednisone is usually successfully tapered rapidly over 1 week to 0.0625 mg/kg/d (or hydrocortisone 7.5 mg/m^2 divided into 2–3 daily doses) and continued until 30 days after nonabsorbable glucocorticoids have stopped. This temporary physiologic replacement therapy is arguably more relevant in small children than adults because adrenal suppression can be clinically relevant as a result of some amount of systemic absorption of the nonabsorbable glucocorticoids. A serum cortisol level less than 19 µg/dL after cosyntropin stimulation, or an early morning baseline cortisol level less than 3.6 µg/dL are often helpful to confirm a diagnosis of suspected adrenal insufficiency. Children with grade IIa GVHD whose diarrheal volumes are between 10 and 20 mL/kg/d, especially with abdominal cramping, may require a slower, more standard taper of prednisone. Landmark trials on beclomethasone dipropionate (BDP) were conducted with a unique BDP formulation, orBec (Soligenix, Princeton, NJ), which is an equipotent mix of plain and enteric-coated tablets designed to deliver 1 mg of BDP to the upper and lower GI tracts, respectively, 4 times daily in adults. Because the US Food and Drug Administration (FDA) Oncology Drugs Advisory Committee voted 7 to 2 that the phase 3 study results were insufficient for orBec to gain approval in 2007 (reviewed in Ref.[31]), this therapy remains commercially unavailable. The group in Seattle currently mimics the approach by prescribing 1 capsule twice daily of EntocortEC (Prometheus, San Diego, CA, USA) which contains 3 mg of micronized, enterically coated BDE, with 1 mg 4 times daily of oral BDP (U.S.P. material, Gallipot, St Paul, MN, www.gallipot.com) emulsion, which is compounded typically in corn or olive oil. Only 11 children (5–17 years of age) received BPD therapy among 231 patients who were treated during the 3 orBec GVHD studies. Therefore, the efficacy of short-course prednisone induction and oral BDP therapy for this indication in children has not been validated. At least 2 other aGVHD studies of BDP[32] or BDE[33] have included children and used adult dosing of BDE and BDP. By analogy, in mild to moderate pediatric Crohn disease, an international survey found that Europeans favored the use of BDE over conventional glucocorticoid therapy.[34] Randomized controlled studies in pediatric Crohn disease have indicated that remission rates were similar in children (mostly teenagers) treated with BDE 3 mg 3 times daily versus prednisone 40 mg daily but side effects were significantly lower in the BDE-treated group (32% vs 71%, P>.05). Induction dosing of BDE 3 mg 4 times daily for 1 month followed by a taper resulted in a trend to higher remission rates without an increase in steroid-associated side effects.[35]

Table 4
Primary therapy trials in aGVHD

Treatment	N	Design	Results and Conclusions	References
Prednisone* 2 mg/kg	443[P]	Retrospective single center. Era: 1990–1999; 40% cohort age <20 y	Day 28 CR/PR 35%/20%. 1-y OS 53% (95% CI 48%–58%). Lower GI ± other organ had worse response. Better OS: age <20 y, T-replete, grade I–II at onset, related or matched unrelated donor	[20]
Prednisone* 1 mg/kg vs 2 mg/kg	733	Retrospective single center. Compared different prednisone starting doses. Era: 2000–2005	For grades II, GVHD control or mortality not compromised at 1 mg/kg vs 2 mg/kg. Lower fungal infection rates and duration of hospitalization for 1 mg/kg. For grades III/IV, small numbers precluded definitive conclusions	[21]
MP 2 mg/kg vs 10 mg/kg	95[P]	Phase 3, multicenter, T-replete MSD BMT. Crossover after 5 days to 10 mg/kg for nonresponders at 2 mg/kg	Compared with 2 mg/kg, 10 mg/kg did not improve response rates (71% vs 68%), TRM, OS, rates of CMV infection, or evolution to grade III–IV aGVHD. TRM 46% among the 55% of nonresponders to 5 days of 2 mg/kg who were rescued with MP 10 mg/kg vs 16% among responders (P = .007)	[25]
MP 2 mg/kg vs 5 mg/kg	211[P]	Phase 3 multicenter. Eligibility: grade I–IV. Day 5 nonresponders (N = 61) randomized to MP 5 mg/kg or 5 mg/kg + rATG	Day 5 CR rate 71% and patients tapered MP from day 6. 5-y TRM cumulative incidence 27% vs 49% (P = .009), and OS 53% vs 35% (P = .007) for responders and nonresponders, respectively. No significant difference in response, TRM, OS between non-ATG and ATG groups	[36]

Prednisone* 1 mg/kg + orBec vs placebo	129[P]	Phase 3 multicenter. Eligibility: grade IIa (anorexia, vomiting, diarrhea <1 L). Randomized (1:1) to 10 days prednisone + 50 days of oral BDP or placebo. Prednisone rapidly tapered from day 11	Among patients eligible for prednisone taper at study day 10, the risk of GVHD treatment failure was lower in the BDP arm at day 80 (HR 0.38). Day 200 posttransplant mortality lower in BDP arm (HR 0.33, P = .03); mostly explained by 91% reduction in day 200 mortality for recipients of unrelated and mismatched grafts (HR 0.09, P = .02). Survival benefit durable to 1 y after randomization	24
Prednisone* + BDE	22[P]	Retrospective single center comparison of patients treated for GI GVHD with MP+BDE 3 mg three times daily to 19 MP-only historical controls	CR 77% in BDE group vs 42% in controls. Two of 8 CRs in controls developed recurrent GI aGVHD during MP taper vs 0 of 17 in BDE group who continued BDE during MP taper. No severe intestinal infections occurred	33
Prednisone* 2 mg/kg + anti-CD5 mAb vs placebo	243[P]	Phase 3, single center, double-blind trial	Higher day 28 CR rate (40% vs 25% P =.019) but similar day 42 CR rate (44% vs 38%), and 1-y survival (49% vs 45%) in anti-CD5 group vs placebo; no long-term benefit of anti-CD5 immunotoxin	12
MP 60 mg/m^2 vs 40 mg/m^2 + ATG	96	Phase 3, single center, open label. Eligibility: REL/URD BMT. Intent-to-treat analysis	Day 42 CR/PR 76% in both arms. More CMV infections and more pneumonitis in MP/ATG arm. EBV PTLD uncommon in either arm. Equivalent OS at day 100, 6 months, and 2 y. ATG should be reserved as second-line therapy	27
MP 2 mg/kg ± infliximab	58	Phase 3, single center, open label	CR + PR rates 63% (MP) vs 66% (infliximab + MP) were similar. Similar death rates in both arms; mainly caused by GVHD and relapse	37

(continued on next page)

Table 4
(continued)

Treatment	N	Design	Results and Conclusions	References
MP 2 mg/kg ± etanercept	61[P]	Retrospective single-center analysis of pilot (N = 20) plus phase 2 (N = 41) prospective studies compared with contemporaneous MP-only controls (N = 99)	Etanercept resulted in more CRs (69% vs 33%; $P < .001$); similar for REL and URD donors. Elevated plasma TNFR1 levels decreased significantly only in patients with CR	29
MP 2 mg/kg ± daclizumab vs placebo	102	Phase 3, multicenter, double blind	Inferior 1-y OS in combination arm (29% vs 60%; $P = .002$) attributed partly to increased relapse/GVHD-related mortality. Study closed early: worse 100-day OS in combination arm (77% vs 94%; $P = .02$). Day 42 CR/PR rates (53% vs 51%)	28
MP 2 mg/kg + human MSCs	32	Phase 2 multicenter. Adults. Randomization: 2×10^6 vs 8.0×10^6 MSC/kg. GVHD grade at onset: II (21), III (8) and IV (3)	Day 28 CR/PR 77%/16%. Both MSC doses similarly effective. No infusional toxicities	38
MP 2 mg/kg + human MSCs vs placebo (1:1 ratio)	192	Phase 3 multicenter, double blind. Third-party commercially prepared MSCs (Prochymal, Osiris)	No difference in proportion of patients surviving at least 90 days who achieved a CR by day 28 (45% vs 46%)	Osiris, press release
MP 2 mg/kg + MMF or etanercept or pentostatin or denileukin diftitox	180[P]	Randomized phase 2 BMT Clinical Trials Network trial. MMF prophylaxis recipients (24%) were randomized to a non-MMF arm. At randomization: aGVHD was grade I–II (68%), III–IV (32%). Visceral organ involvement in 53%	Day 28 CR rates, 9-month OS %, and CI severe infections were: etanercept 26%, 47%, 48%; MMF 60%, 64%, 44%; denileukin 53%, 49%, 62%; pentostatin 38%, 47%, 57%. MMF identified as most promising arm and will be compared with MP alone in phase 3	30

Abbreviations: ATG, antithymocyte globulin; BMT, bone marrow transplant; CMV, cytomegalovirus; CR, complete response; EBV, Epstein-Barr virus; MSC, mesenchymal stem cell; MSD, matched sibling donor; OS, overall survival; P, included children; PR, partial response; PTLD, posttransplant lymphoproliferative disease; REL, related; TNFR1, tumor necrosis factor receptor-1; TRM, treatment-related mortality; URD, unrelated.
* Prednisone or methylprednisolone equivalent.

MONITORING OF RESPONSE AND TAPERING GLUCOCORTICOIDS

All patients with aGVHD should be monitored closely. If aGVHD progresses within 3 to 4 days or no improvement is observed after 5 to 7 days of MP treatment then the GVHD is considered to be steroid refractory (SR-GVHD) and second-line therapy is required as discussed later. Progression is defined as worsening GVHD in 1 or more organ with or without amelioration in any organ.

If on the other hand, GVHD symptoms have resolved after 5 to 7 days of MP therapy, it is reasonable to attempt a taper of prednisone by 10% (of the starting dose) at 4-day intervals (depending on the tempo of the response) beginning 6 to 14 days after starting MP. The goal of glucocorticoid therapy is to treat the acute inflammatory manifestations of GVHD and then to gradually taper the doses of prednisone (or MP) as soon as possible, over the course of 5 to 6 weeks. The literature demonstrates that prolonged use of high-dose glucocorticoids for the treatment of aGVHD is associated with an increased risk of infection, relapse, and death.[25,36,39–44]

The literature has provided little direction on how best to taper glucocorticoids in aGVHD. A European survey indicated that only 36% of 87 centers surveyed used a standard taper schedule.[39] The groups at Minnesota and Seattle use standardized glucocorticoid tapers and although certain details do vary, the principles are similar. If prednisone can be successfully tapered as described earlier then once the total daily dose reaches 0.2 to 0.3 mg/kg (or $\leq$20 mg) a transition is made to alternating day prednisone for the remaining 2 to 3 weeks of the taper to facilitate recovery of the adrenal axis.

After aGVHD manifestations have resolved and the prednisone taper is proceeding, a recurrence (flare) of GVHD activity may emerge. It is important to delineate whether a patient continues to have aGVHD alone, or whether classic cGVHD signs begin to emerge. In the latter scenario of cGVHD with overlap syndrome, it is often preferable to incorporate a less aggressive and more protracted course of immunosuppressive therapy into the plan.[45] If cGVHD is not present then it is reasonable to manage the first flare of aGVHD by boosting the dose of prednisone to 20 mg/m^2 (0.67 mg/kg) for 7 days (Minnesota), or 2 mg/kg for 2 to 4 days (Seattle) and then, once the GVHD is under control, the taper resumes promptly toward the MP-equivalent dose before the flare plus 0.2 to 0.4 mg/kg (see **Fig. 1**). Once steroids have been tapered off for at least a month, consideration can be made to start tapering other immunosuppressive agents, depending on how far out the patient is from HSCT.

TREATMENT OF STEROID-RESISTANT ACUTE GVHD AND OUTCOMES

Approximately half of patients with aGVHD respond to treatment with steroids as initial therapy, with approximately one-third of patients having a durable response.[18–20,46] Factors most commonly associated with a favorable response include HLA matching for the GVHD vector, use of related donor grafts, and early onset of GVHD.[18] Failure of primary therapy (steroid-resistant [SR-aGVHD]) has been defined operationally as the progression of aGVHD symptoms beyond 3 to 4 days after starting MP. Persistence of grade II to IV GVHD after 1 week of initial therapy should also be considered failure of response. The prognosis of aGVHD can be related to its overall severity (grade) and response to glucocorticoids.[18,47] Grades III and IV SR-aGVHD, especially with visceral involvement, generally requires urgent initiation of effective second-line therapy.

Unfortunately, there is no generally accepted therapy for SR-aGVHD but agents that either have been considered or continue to be explored are listed in **Table 5**. Published data for each therapy is summarized in **Table 6** and include key study design points, the era of therapy and whether or not the series included children. Polyclonal

Table 5
Therapy options for steroid-refractory aGVHD

Therapy	Comments
Systemic	
Polyclonal	
Antithymocyte globulin ATGAM,[a] thymoglobulin[b]	Delayed use seems to be very ineffective. Skin responds best
Monoclonal	
Anti-CD2 (OKT3,[c] visilizumab[d])	Currently used infrequently
Anti-IL2 (daclizumab,[d] basilixumab,[e] inolimomab[c])	Also depletes regulatory T cells
Anti-TNFα (infliximab[e])	Consider early for refractory lower GI tract
Anti-CD52 (alemtuzumab[d])	Depletes T and B cells (lower risk EBV PTLD)
Anti-CD2 (alefacept[f])	Selectively depletes memory T cells; needs further study
Fusion proteins	
Anti-IL2 (denileukin diftitox)	Also depletes regulatory T cells
Anti-TNFα (etanercept)	
Macrolides and antimetabolites	
Tacrolimus	Inhibits regulatory T cells
Sirolimus	Does not inhibit regulatory T cells
Mycophenolate mofetil	Enteric-coated formulation may minimize toxicity but liquid formulation not available
Extracorporeal photopheresis	Particularly effective in skin, infrequently associated with opportunistic infections
Mesenchymal stem cells	Recent US multicenter trials did not meet their primary endpoints (see also **Tables 4** and **6**)
Topical	
Glucocorticoids	
BDE	Useful as steroid-sparing agent in GI tract
BDP	Useful as steroid-sparing agent in GI tract but not commercially available
PUVA	Useful for skin only involvement

Abbreviations: ATGAM, equine antithymocyte globulin; EBV, Epstein-Barr virus; PTLD, posttransplant lymphoproliferative disease.
  [a] Equine.
  [b] Rabbit.
  [c] Murine.
  [d] Humanized (and not commercially available).
  [e] Chimeric murine-human.
  [f] Human IgG1-fusion protein.

antithymocyte globulins (ATG), and more recently novel humanized or chimeric monoclonal antibodies, are generally used to treat life-threatening visceral manifestations when urgent control of GVHD is necessary. Unfortunately, longer-term survival has been unusual when visceral manifestations are severe.[48–53] However, early administration of ATG within 14 days of primary therapy was reported in 1 study to be associated with improved survival.[49] It has remained difficult to improve survival after SR-aGVHD because progressive organ dysfunction is often irreversible. Another reason for this observation is that second-line therapies constitute a second hit to an immune system that has already been impaired by cumulative exposure to high-dose prednisone which increases the risk for opportunistic infections. Although more definitive evidence-based practices are needed, the current approach to second-line therapy in Minnesota for SR-aGVHD is equine ATG. In contrast, Seattle has opted for a customized approach based on the severity of involvement in the most involved organ(s). For the skin, PUVA is considered first for mild to moderate SR-aGVHD; MMF or sirolimus are considered next for a rash that is moderately severe and/or PUVA resistant/intolerant. Extracorporeal photopheresis (ECP) is reserved for moderate to severe skin manifestations. For the intestinal tract, topical BDP and BDE are considered first for mild to moderate SR-aGVHD recognizing that topical gut steroids are often incorporated into primary therapy for children in Seattle as detailed earlier. The next consideration for moderate to severe intestinal manifestations is infliximab, with or without weekly ECP. Infliximab 5 mg/kg is used cautiously and generally for no more than 4 doses spaced weekly or every other week depending on the initial response. Since adopting routinely the approach of Ruutu and colleagues[9] using ursodeoxycholic acid prophylaxis in all allogeneic HSCT recipients, liver GVHD has occurred infrequently in Seattle. However, MMF and ECP are considered in resistant cases of liver GVHD that is mild to moderate, or moderate to severe, respectively.

ANTIMICROBIAL PROPHYLAXIS AND SUPPORTIVE CARE

AGVHD is by itself profoundly immunosuppressive as are the therapies used to treat it, leading to an extraordinarily high risk for opportunistic infections and sepsis. Breakdown of skin and intestinal epithelia that occurs in more severe aGVHD forms adds to this risk. High-dose prednisone increases the risk for cytomegalovirus (CMV) reactivation.[41] Similarly, invasive aspergillosis occurs more frequently in patients who develop CMV disease and in patients receiving higher doses of prednisone.[43,44] Therefore, antimicrobial prophylaxis is standard for these patients and always includes an agent to prevent *Pneumocytis jirovecii* pneumonia. Prophylactic and/or preemptive antiviral therapy based on serial monitoring of the blood for early viral reactivation are the main approaches used to avoid life-threatening disease caused by CMV and varicella zoster. In the setting of profound T cell lymphopenia, which is often associated with SR-aGVHD or its treatment, monitoring for Epstein-Barr virus, human herpes virus 6 and adenovirus is prudent to enable preemptive therapy, at least until there is some measure of T cell recovery. Fluconazole is used to prevent yeast (but not mold) infections within the first 75 to 100 days after HSCT but mold-active azoles (eg, voriconazole or posoconazole) or echinocandins are generally substituted when patients have SR-aGVHD or are otherwise receiving high-dose glucocorticoids. Some centers use penicillin or extended spectrum quinolones to provide antibacterial prophylaxis for patients with aGVHD. Immunizations are not indicated for patients with SR-aGVHD as they are unlikely to respond immunologically. The exception is that the injectable form of the influenza vaccination is recommended but not the inhaled live attenuated form (ie, no FluMist) if patients are at least 4 months from HSCT.[54] Patients and their family household contacts should also be vaccinated with the injectable vaccine annually as there is the theoretic risk of shedding live attenuated virus after receipt of the inhaled vaccine.

Adjunctive therapy with ursodeoxycholic acid may improve liver function and a randomized placebo-controlled multicenter study demonstrated that prophylaxis

Table 6
Secondary therapy for AGVHD

Treatment	N	Era	CR/PR (%)	OS (%)	Comments	References
ATGAM	58	1996–1999	30	<10	CR/PR: 79% (S), 40% (GI), 66% (L). Deaths: median 40 days after ATG (mostly infection or PD)	48
ATGAM	54	1989–1998	NA	11	All patients had severe visceral GVHD	Martin (unpublished)
ATGAM	29	1981–1998	NA	12	86% (mostly 3-system) grade III/IV CR/PR: 72% (S), 38% (GI/L). cGVHD in 7/11 survivors	55
ATGAM	79^P	1990–1998	54	32	Cohort: 43% <18 y, 43% grade III/IV. CR/PR 61% (S ± L/GI) vs 27% (GI/L). OS better if ATG within 14 d of starting primary therapy (46% vs 19%, P = .05)	56
ATGAM	69^P	1980–1999	30	5	Cohort: 59% <35 y, 61% grade III/IV; 74% ≥2 organs. ATG initiated at median 25 d after starting primary therapy. CR/PR 59% (S), 15% (L), 32% (GI)	57
Thymoglobulin	36	1996–1999	59	6	89% (mostly 3-system) grade III/IV CR/PR: 96% (S), 46% (GI), 36% (L). Major problem: infections and 25% EBV PTLD rate	49
Daclizumab	43	NA	51	40	Prospective phase 1/2. Day 43 CR 47%. Day 120 OS 53% at OBD. Well tolerated	50
Daclizumab	57^P	1993–2000	54	25	CR/PR 76% if ≤18 y. Best responses: skin only and children. No infusion-related toxicity. Infectious complications in 95%. Careful patient selection and aggressive prophylaxis against viral and fungal infections recommended	58
Daclizumab + infliximab	22^P	2002–2007	86	68	Single center, consecutively treated children. Median response time 15 d from start (second course given to 3/7 with recurrent GVHD). 13 viral reactivations, 4 probable fungal infections but only 2 infection-related deaths (median follow-up 31 mo). 7/22 developed cGHVD	59
Daclizumab	13^P	2002–2006	92	46	At day 30, CR 100% (S), CR/PR 50%/30% (GI), CR/PR 11%/55% (L). 50% developed cGHVD. Most effective in skin or low to moderate GI	60

Denileukin diftitox	32	NA	71	30	Phase 1, single center. OS 58% among 7/12 with CR. Reversible hepatic transaminitis in 22% at maximum tolerated dose	51
Infliximab	21	1999–2001	67	38	Single center, retrospective evaluating 21 of 134 with SR-aGVHD who received single agent infliximab. CR 62%. Well tolerated. Particularly active in GI. Infection rates: fungal (48%), viral (67%), and bacterial (81%)	52
Infliximab	32^P	2000–2004	59	41	Single center, retrospective. Cohort: 22% <14 y, infliximab second/third line: 44%/56%. Median of 3 doses. CR/PR 19%/40%. Best responses: GI, <35 y, longer interval between HSCT and infliximab start. Infection rate 72%. 13/19 responders survived a median 449 d (155–842 d). 13/13 nonresponders died early	61
Infliximab	24^P	1998–2001	82	46*	Retrospective single center (all children). Infliximab 10 mg/kg × median 8 (range 1–162) doses. Evaluable (N=22); CR/PR 55%/27%. Good responses: S, GI. *OS 67% at 6 mo, 46% at 12 mo, 21% at 2 y. Recurrent GVHD common after stopping infliximab. Infection rates: 77% bacterial, 32% viral, 14% molds (invasive probable or proven)	62
Etanercept	13	1995–2005	46	67*	Single center, retrospective (N = 21, 8 had aGVHD). Etanercept 25 mg subcutaneously twice/wk × 4 followed by 25 mg/wk × 4. Organ involvement at start of etanercept: S (14), GI (13), L (5), lung (5), oral (4). GI responses: 64%. In aGVHD: CR/PR = 4/2. Well tolerated. Infection rates: 48% CMV reactivation, 14% bacterial, 19% fungal. *Median follow-up 429 d (range 71–1007 d) for all 21 patients	63
PUVA	103^P	1994–2000	24*	51	Median onset of PUVA was day 46 after HSCT. PUVA second/third line: 83%/17%. Median 16 treatments. Generally well tolerated; 8% discontinued for toxicity. *CR 24% (intent to treat); 37% among those who tolerated PUVA for 6 wk. Mean prednisone dose decreased from 1.6 mg/kg to 0.7 mg/kg by week 6. 57% required no additional therapy for skin GVHD	17
ECP	21	1996–NA	60*	57**	Median age 38 y. Donors: SIB or URD. CRs (*at 3 mo) by grade: 100% (II), 67% (III), 12% (IV) and by organ: 60% (S), 67% (L), 0% (GI). Commonest AEs were cytopenias. **Median follow-up 25 mo after HSCT. 4-y OS 91% among CRs vs 11% non-CR	64

(continued on next page)

Table 6
(continued)

Treatment	N	Era	CR/PR (%)	OS (%)	Comments	References
ECP	59	1996–NA	79.5*	47**	Phase II, single center. Weekly ECP. *CR/PR at a median of 4 cycles (1.3 mo). CR: 82% (S), 61% (L), 61% (GI). **OS at 4 y: 59% among CRs versus 11% non-CRs. Intensified ECP was highly effective in aGVHD	65
ECP	77[P]	1992–2000			Included aGVHD (n = 33) at 4 pediatric hospitals. CR: 76% (S), 60% (L), 75% (GI). 5-y OS 69% among responders vs 12% for nonresponders (P = .001)	66
ECP	31[P]	1999–2005			Unrelated BMT. CR 73%, whereas the good response group had a CR rate of 56% by day 100. 2-y OS/PFS 57%/67% in the good response group vs 85%/87% in the ECP group	67
ECP	23	1996–2006	52	48	SR-aGVHD grade II (10), III (7), IV (6). Median duration of ECP 7 mo (1–33 mo). CR 52% (no responses in grade IV). 12 patients (52%) had complete responses. Average aGVHD grade decreased from 2.8 to 1.4 by day 90 (P = .08). Average MP dose decreased from 2.17 to 0.2 mg/kg/d (P = .004). CR: 66% (S), 27% (L), 40% (GI). Better responses if treated <35 d from onset of aGVHD	68
MMF	36	NA	72	37*	Single center. MMF added to cyclosporine and prednisolone. Overall grade improvement of aGVHD was found in 11 of 17 (65%) patients treated with MMF. Most common AEs: mild to modest cytopenias. *5-y based on 48 patients (12 cGVHD)	69,70
MMF	19	NA	42	16*	Single center. 6 CR and 2 PR. *2-y	71
Sirolimus	21	1996–1999	28*	34*	Single-center pilot trial (all ages). Sirolimus was started 19–78 d (median 37 d) after HSCT for grade III (10) or IV (11) SR-aGVHD. GVHD. High loading dose and/or high maintenance dosing of sirolimus. *Expected toxicities (cytopenias, hyperlipidemia and hemolytic uremic syndrome) were frequent, associated with high serum concentrations, and likely limited efficacy. Among the 18 who received ≥6 doses, 12 responded (5 CR, 7 PR)	72

					Comments	
Pentostatin	23	NA	76	26*	Phase 1, single center. Universal lymphopenia and late infections was the dose-limiting toxicity. Best responses in skin. *Median survival 85 d (5–1258 d). Suggested dose for phase 2 was 1.5 mg/m²/d × 3 d	73
MSCs	1	NA	—	—	Landmark case of haploidentical hMSCs rescuing an adult with resistant grade IV GI and liver aGVHD. Clinical response was striking. The patient was alive and well after 1 year	74
MSCs	8	2001–2005	75	63	Grades III–IV aGVHD and 1 with extensive cGVHD. Median MSC dose 1 × 10⁶ kg from various donors. CR rate 75%. Five patients alive 2 mo to 3 y after HSCT	75
MSCs	55	2001–2007	71	36	Multicenter phase 2 in severe aGVHD using EGBMT ex vivo MSC expansion procedure. Up to 5 doses MSCs; median dose 1.4 × 10⁶/kg. CR + PR = 55% + 16%. No infusion toxicities. 2-y OS among CRs was 53% vs 16% (P = .018)	76
MSCs	12^P	2005–2007	100*	50*	Multicenter, pediatric compassionate use protocol of third-party MSCs (Osiris) for grade III (n = 7), IV (n = 5). MSCs given 2×/wk for 4 wk at 8 × 10⁶/kg/dose in first 2 patients; 2 × 10⁶/kg in next 10 patients. MSC began at median of 119 days post HSCT. No infusion toxicities. Follow-up 102 d (range 36–756 d). CR + PR = 50% + 50%. Six of 12 patients died at median of 68 d (range 36–185 d) from start of therapy: Multiorgan failure (3), infection (3)	77
Human MSCs vs placebo (2:1 ratio)	260^P	2006–2008	—	—	Phase 3 multicenter, double blind. Third-party commercially prepared MSCs (Prochymal, Osiris). *No improvement in durable CR rates (35% vs 30%, primary endpoint) but hMSCs did improve durable liver CRs (29% vs 5%, P = .046, N = 61) and GI responses (88% vs 64%, P = .018, N = 71)	Osiris press release

Abbreviations: AE, adverse event; ATGAM, equine antithymocyte globulin; CMV, cytomegalovirus; CR, complete response; ECP, extracorporeal photopheresis; EGBMT, European Group for Blood and Marrow Transplantation; L, liver; MSC, mesenchymal stem cell; MSD, matched sibling donor; OS, overall survival; ^P, included children; PD, progressive disease; PFS, progression-free survival; PR, partial response; S, skin; SIB, sibling; URD, unrelated.

with ursodeoxycholic acid reduced hepatic problems, severe aGVHD, and improved survival after allogeneic HSCT.[9] In patients with severe GI GVHD, a period of bowel rest and hyperalimentation are usually necessary. The somatostatin analogue, octreotide, may ameliorate large volume diarrhea to some extent.[78] Iatrogenic glucocorticoid-induced myopathy and hyperglycemia need to be kept in mind during the course of aGVHD management as both these complications require appropriate interventions.

SUMMARY

AGVHD remains a major cause of morbidity and mortality after allogeneic HSCT in children. Currently, first-line aGVHD therapy relies on glucocorticoid-induced inhibition of inflammation and donor T cell alloreactivity, usually in combination with 1 or more of the agents chosen for aGVHD prophylaxis. Newer approaches are needed to improve the overall 50% or less durable response rates that have been achieved with systemic glucocorticoids. Because promising agents in small single-center studies alone have not generally led to new standards for primary therapy for aGVHD it is essential to encourage (inter)national participation in well-designed phase 2 and hopefully definitive phase 3 studies so that answers to these important therapy questions can be obtained. Moreover, in the absence of any standard options for the therapy for SR-aGVHD it will be important that the roles of novel cell populations in the pathogenesis of aGVHD be further elucidated, so that follow-on clinical studies can test new approaches with strong rationales in SR-aGVHD. Ideally, the goal of new GVHD therapies should be to minimize the reliance on glucocorticoid-based therapy. Early inclusion of children in GVHD studies is essential so that approaches tested for the most part in adults can have a greater basis when generalized to children.

ACKNOWLEDGMENTS

This work was supported by grant no. CA18029 from the National Institutes of Health.

REFERENCES

1. Morris ES, Hill GR. Advances in the understanding of acute graft-versus-host disease. Br J Haematol 2007;137:3–19.
2. Beatty PG, Hansen JA, Longton GM, et al. Marrow transplantation from HLA-matched unrelated donors for treatment of hematologic malignancies. Transplantation 1991;51:443–7.
3. Lee SJ, Klein J, Haagenson M, et al. High-resolution donor-recipient HLA matching contributes to the success of unrelated donor marrow transplantation. Blood 2007;110:4576–83.
4. Storb R, Deeg HJ, Whitehead J, et al. Methotrexate and cyclosporine compared with cyclosporine alone for prophylaxis of acute graft versus host disease after marrow transplantation for leukemia. N Engl J Med 1986;314:729–35.
5. Beatty PG, Clift RA, Mickelson EM, et al. Marrow transplantation from related donors other than HLA-identical siblings. N Engl J Med 1985;313:765–71.
6. Nash RA, Antin JH, Karanes C, et al. Phase 3 study comparing methotrexate and tacrolimus with methotrexate and cyclosporine for prophylaxis of acute graft-versus-host disease after marrow transplantation from unrelated donors. Blood 2000;96:2062–8.

7. Cutler C, Li S, Ho VT, et al. Extended follow-up of methotrexate-free immunosuppression using sirolimus and tacrolimus in related and unrelated donor peripheral blood stem cell transplantation. Blood 2007;109:3108–14.
8. Kernan NA. T-cell depletion for the prevention of graft-versus-host disease. In: Thomas ED, Blume KG, Forman SJ, editors. Hematopoietic cell transplantation. 2nd edition. Boston: Blackwell Science; 1999. p. 186–96.
9. Ruutu T, Eriksson B, Remes K, et al. Ursodeoxycholic acid for the prevention of hepatic complications in allogeneic stem cell transplantation. Blood 2002;100:1977–83.
10. Filipovich AH, Weisdorf D, Pavletic S, et al. National Institutes of Health consensus development project on criteria for clinical trials in chronic graft-versus-host disease: I. Diagnosis and Staging Working Group report. Biol Blood Marrow Transplant 2005;11:945–56.
11. Glucksberg H, Storb R, Fefer A, et al. Clinical manifestations of graft-versus-host disease in human recipients of marrow from HL-A-matched sibling donors. Transplantation 1974;18:295–304.
12. Martin PJ, Nelson BJ, Appelbaum FR, et al. Evaluation of a CD5-specific immunotoxin for treatment of acute graft-versus-host disease after allogeneic marrow transplantation. Blood 1996;88:824–30.
13. Przepiorka D, Weisdorf D, Martin P, et al. 1994 Consensus conference on acute GVHD grading. Bone Marrow Transplant 1995;15:825–8.
14. Rowlings PA, Przepiorka D, Klein JP, et al. IBMTR severity index for grading acute graft-versus-host disease: retrospective comparison with Glucksberg grade. Br J Haematol 1997;97:855–64.
15. Sale GE. Pathology and recent pathogenetic studies in human graft-versus-host disease. Surv Synth Pathol Res 1984;3:235–53.
16. Sale GE, Shulman HM, Gallucci BB, et al. Young rete ridge keratinocytes are preferred targets in cutaneous graft-versus-host disease. Am J Pathol 1985;118:278–87.
17. Furlong T, Leisenring W, Storb R, et al. Psoralen and ultraviolet A irradiation (PUVA) as therapy for steroid-resistant cutaneous acute graft-versus-host disease. Biol Blood Marrow Transplant 2002;8:206–12.
18. McDonald GB, Bouvier M, Hockenbery DM, et al. Oral beclomethasone dipropionate for treatment of intestinal graft-versus-host disease: a randomized, controlled trial. Gastroenterology 1998;115:28–35.
19. Hockenbery DM, Cruickshank S, Rodell TC, et al. A randomized, placebo-controlled trial of oral beclomethasone dipropionate as a prednisone-sparing therapy for gastrointestinal graft-versus-host disease. Blood 2007;109:4557–63.
20. McDonald GB. Oral beclomethasone dipropionate: a topically active corticosteroid for the treatment of gastrointestinal graft-versus-host disease following allogeneic hematopoietic cell transplantation [review]. Expert Opin Investig Drugs 2007;16:1709–24.
21. Iyer RV, Hahn T, Roy HN, et al. Long-term use of oral beclomethasone dipropionate for the treatment of gastrointestinal graft-versus-host disease. Biol Blood Marrow Transplant 2005;11:587–92.
22. Bertz H, Afting M, Kreisel W, et al. Feasibility and response to budesonide as topical corticosteroid therapy for acute intestinal GVHD. Bone Marrow Transplant 1999;24:1185–9.
23. Levine A, Weizman Z, Broide E, et al. A comparison of budesonide and prednisone for the treatment of active pediatric Crohn disease. J Pediatr Gastroenterol Nutr 2003;36:248–52.

24. Levine A, Kori M, Dinari G, et al. Comparison of two dosing methods for induction of response and remission with oral budesonide in active pediatric Crohn's disease: a randomized placebo-controlled trial. Inflamm Bowel Dis 2009;15:1055–61.
25. van Lint MT, Uderzo C, Locasciulli A, et al. Early treatment of acute graft-versus-host disease with high- or low-dose 6-methylprednisolone: a multicenter randomized trial from the Italian Group for Bone Marrow Transplantation. Blood 1998;92: 2288–93.
26. Vogelsang GB, Hess AD, Santos GW. Acute graft-versus-host disease: clinical characteristics in the cyclosporine era. Medicine 1988;67:163–74.
27. Cragg L, Blazar BR, DeFor T, et al. A randomized trial comparing prednisone with antithymocyte globulin/prednisone as an initial systemic therapy for moderately severe acute graft-versus-host disease. Biol Blood Marrow Transplant 2000;6:441–7.
28. Lee SJ, Zahrieh D, Agura E, et al. Effect of up-front daclizumab when combined with steroids for the treatment of acute graft-versus-host disease: results of a randomized trial. Blood 2004;104:1559–64.
29. Levine JE, Paczesny S, Mineishi S, et al. Etanercept plus methylprednisolone as initial therapy for acute graft-versus-host disease. Blood 2008;111:2470–5.
30. Alousi AM, Weisdorf DJ, Logan BR, et al. Etanercept, mycophenolate, denileukin, or pentostatin plus corticosteroids for acute graft-versus-host disease: a randomized phase 2 trial from the blood and marrow transplant clinical trials network. Blood 2009;114:511–7.
31. Martin PJ, Schoch G, Fisher L, et al. A retrospective analysis of therapy for acute graft-versus-host disease: initial treatment. Blood 1990;76:1464–72.
32. Weisdorf DJ, Snover DC, Haake R, et al. Acute upper gastrointestinal graft-versus-host disease: clinical significance and response to immunosuppressive therapy. Blood 1990;76:624–9.
33. MacMillan ML, Weisdorf DJ, Wagner JE, et al. Response of 443 patients to steroids as primary therapy for acute graft-versus-host disease: comparison of grading systems. Biol Blood Marrow Transplant 2002;8:387–94.
34. Mielcarek M, Storer BE, Boeckh M, et al. Initial therapy of acute graft-versus-host disease with low-dose prednisone does not compromise patient outcomes. Blood 2009;113:2888–94.
35. Baehr PH, Levine DS, Bouvier ME, et al. Oral beclomethasone dipropionate for treatment of human intestinal graft-versus-host disease. Transplantation 1995; 60:1231–8.
36. van Lint MT, Milone G, Leotta S, et al. Treatment of acute graft-versus-host disease with prednisolone: significant survival advantage for day +5 responders and no advantage for nonresponders receiving anti-thymocyte globulin. Blood 2006;107:4177–81.
37. Antin JH, Chen AR, Couriel DR, et al. Novel approaches to the therapy of steroid-resistant acute graft-versus-host disease. Biol Blood Marrow Transplant 2004;10: 655–68.
38. Kebriaei P, Isola L, Bahceci E, et al. Adult human mesenchymal stem cells added to corticosteroid therapy for the treatment of acute graft-versus-host disease. Biol Blood Marrow Transplant 2009;15:804–11.
39. Ruutu T, Niederwieser D, Gratwohl A, et al. A survey of the prophylaxis and treatment of acute GVHD in Europe: a report of the European Group for Blood and Marrow Transplantation (EBMT). Chronic leukaemia working party of the EBMT. Bone Marrow Transplant 1997;19:759–64.
40. Ruutu T, Hermans J, van Biezen A, et al. How should corticosteroids be used in the treatment of acute GVHD? EBMT Chronic Leukemia Working Party. European

Group for Blood and Marrow Transplantation. Bone Marrow Transplant 1998;22: 614–5.

41. Nichols WG, Corey L, Gooley T, et al. Rising pp65 antigenemia during preemptive anticytomegalovirus therapy after allogeneic hematopoietic stem cell transplantation: risk factors, correlation with DNA load, and outcomes. Blood 2001;97: 867–74.

42. Hakki M, Riddell SR, Storek J, et al. Immune reconstitution to cytomegalovirus after allogeneic hematopoietic stem cell transplantation: impact of host factors, drug therapy, and subclinical reactivation. Blood 2003;102: 3060–7.

43. Marr KA, Carter RA, Boeckh M, et al. Invasive aspergillosis in allogeneic stem cell transplant recipients: changes in epidemiology and risk factors. Blood 2002;100: 4358–66.

44. Fukuda T, Boeckh M, Carter RA, et al. Risks and outcomes of invasive fungal infections in recipients of allogeneic hematopoietic stem cell transplants after nonmyeloablative conditioning. Blood 2003;102:827–33.

45. Lee SJ, Vogelsang G, Flowers MED. Chronic graft-versus-host disease. Biol Blood Marrow Transplant 2003;9:215–33.

46. Weisdorf D, Haake R, Blazar B, et al. Treatment of moderate/severe acute graft-versus-host disease after allogeneic bone marrow transplantation: an analysis of clinical risk features and outcome. Blood 1990;75:1024–30.

47. Hings IM, Severson R, Filipovich AH, et al. Treatment of moderate and severe acute GVHD after allogeneic bone marrow transplantation. Transplantation 1994;58:437–42.

48. Khoury H, Kashyap A, Adkins DR, et al. Treatment of steroid-resistant acute graft-versus-host disease with anti-thymocyte globulin. Bone Marrow Transplant 2001; 27:1059–64.

49. McCaul KG, Nevill TJ, Barnett MJ, et al. Treatment of steroid-resistant acute graft-versus-host disease with rabbit antithymocyte globulin. J Hematother Stem Cell Res 2000;9:367–74.

50. Przepiorka D, Kernan NA, Ippoliti C, et al. Daclizumab, a humanized anti-interleukin-2 receptor alpha chain antibody, for treatment of acute graft-versus-host disease. Blood 2000;95:83–9.

51. Ho VT, Zahrieh D, Hochberg E, et al. Safety and efficacy of denileukin diftitox in patients with steroid-refractory acute graft-versus-host disease after allogeneic hematopoietic stem cell transplantation. Blood 2004;104:1224–6.

52. Couriel DR, Saliba RM, Giralt S, et al. Acute and chronic graft-versus-host disease after ablative and nonmyeloablative conditioning for allogeneic hematopoietic transplantation. Biol Blood Marrow Transplant 2004;10:178–85.

53. Carpenter PA, Lowder J, Johnston L, et al. A phase II multicenter study of visilizumab, humanized anti-CD3 antibody, to treat steroid-refractory acute graft-versus-host disease. Biol Blood Marrow Transplant 2005;11:465–71.

54. Tomblyn M, Chiller T, Einsele H, et al. Guidelines for preventing infectious complications among hematopoietic cell transplant recipients: a global perspective. Bone Marrow Transplant 2009;44:453–5.

55. Remberger M, Aschan J, Barkholt L, et al. Treatment of severe acute graft-versus-host disease with anti-thymocyte globulin [review]. Clin Transplant 2001;15: 147–53.

56. MacMillan ML, Weisdorf DJ, Davies SM, et al. Early antithymocyte globulin therapy improves survival in patients with steroid-resistant acute graft-versus-host disease. Biol Blood Marrow Transplant 2002;8:40–6.

57. Arai SM. Poor outcome in steroid-refractory graft-versus-host disease with antithymocyte globulin treatment. Biol Blood Marrow Transplant 2002;8: 155–60.

58. Perales MA, Ishill N, Lomazow WA, et al. Long-term follow-up of patients treated with daclizumab for steroid-refractory acute graft-vs-host disease. Bone Marrow Transplant 2007;40:481–6.

59. Rao K, Rao A, Karlsson H, et al. Improved survival and preserved antiviral responses after combination therapy with daclizumab and infliximab in steroid-refractory graft-versus-host disease. J Pediatr Hematol Oncol 2009; 31:456–61.

60. Miano M, Cuzzubbo D, Terranova P, et al. Daclizumab as useful treatment in refractory acute GVHD: a paediatric experience. Bone Marrow Transplant 2009;43:423–7.

61. Patriarca F, Sperotto A, Damiani D, et al. Infliximab treatment for steroid-refractory acute graft-versus-host disease. Haematologica 2004;89:1352–9.

62. Sleight BS, Chan KW, Braun TM, et al. Infliximab for GVHD therapy in children. Bone Marrow Transplant 2007;40:473–80.

63. Busca A, Locatelli F, Marmont F, et al. Recombinant human soluble tumor necrosis factor receptor fusion protein as treatment for steroid refractory graft-versus-host disease following allogeneic hematopoietic stem cell transplantation. Am J Hematol 2007;82:45–52.

64. Greinix HT, Volc-Platzer B, Kalhs P, et al. Extracorporeal photochemotherapy in the treatment of severe steroid-refractory acute graft-versus-host disease: a pilot study. Blood 2000;96:2426–31.

65. Greinix HT, Knobler RM, Worel N, et al. The effect of intensified extracorporeal photochemotherapy on long-term survival in patients with severe acute graft-versus-host disease. Haematologica 2006;91:405–8.

66. Messina C, Locatelli F, Lanino E, et al. Extracorporeal photochemotherapy for paediatric patients with graft-versus-host disease after haematopoietic stem cell transplantation. Br J Haematol 2003;122:118–27.

67. Calore E, Calo A, Tridello G, et al. Extracorporeal photochemotherapy may improve outcome in children with acute GVHD. Bone Marrow Transplant 2008; 42:421–5.

68. Perfetti P, Carlier P, Strada P, et al. Extracorporeal photopheresis for the treatment of steroid refractory acute GVHD. Bone Marrow Transplant 2008;42: 609–17.

69. Basara N, Blau WI, Kiehl MG, et al. Efficacy and safety of mycophenolate mofetil for the treatment of acute and chronic GVHD in bone marrow transplant recipient. Transplant Proc 1998;30:4087–9.

70. Basara N, Kiehl MG, Blau W, et al. Mycophenolate Mofetil in the treatment of acute and chronic GVHD in hematopoietic stem cell transplant patients: four years of experience. Transplant Proc 2001;33:2121–3.

71. Nash RA, Furlong T, Storb R, et al. Mycophenolate mofetil (MMF) as salvage treatment for graft-versus-host-disease (GVHD) after allogeneic hematopoietic stem cell transplantation (HSCT): safety analysis [abstract]. Blood 1997;90(Suppl 1): 105A, #459.

72. Benito AI, Furlong T, Martin PJ, et al. Sirolimus (Rapamycin) for the treatment of steroid-refractory acute graft-versus-host disease. Transplantation 2001;72: 1924–9.

73. Bolanos-Meade J, Jacobsohn DA, Margolis J, et al. Pentostatin in steroid-refractory acute graft-versus-host disease. J Clin Oncol 2005;23:2661–8.

74. Le Blanc K, Rasmusson I, Sundberg B, et al. Treatment of severe acute graft-versus-host disease with third party haploidentical mesenchymal stem cells. Lancet 2004;363:1439–41.

75. Ringdén O, Uzunel M, Rasmusson I, et al. Mesenchymal stem cells for treatment of therapy-resistant graft-versus-host disease. Transplantation 2006;81:1390–7.

76. Le Blanc K, Frassoni F, Ball L, et al. Mesenchymal stem cells for treatment of steroid-resistant, severe, acute graft-versus-host disease: a phase II study. Lancet 2008;371:1579–86.

77. Prasad VK, Lucas KG, Kleiner GI, et al. Use of mesenchymal stem cells to treat pediatric patients with severe (grade III-IV) acute graft versus host disease refractory to steroid and other agents on a compassionate use basis [abstract]. Blood 2007;118(Part 1):872A–3A, #2971.

78. Ippoliti C, Champlin R, Bugazia N, et al. Use of octreotide in the symptomatic management of diarrhea induced by graft-versus-host disease in patients with hematologic malignancies. J Clin Oncol 1997;15:3350–4.

Chronic Graft-Versus-Host Disease (GVHD) in Children

Kristin Baird, MD[a,*], Kenneth Cooke, MD[b,c,d,e],
Kirk R. Schultz, MD[f,g]

KEYWORDS

- Chronic graft-versus-host disease • GVHD • Children
- Hematopoeitic stem cell transplant

Allogeneic hematopoietic stem cell transplantation (allo-HSCT) is a curative approach for many pediatric diseases. According to the most recent analysis from the Center of International Blood and Marrow Transplant Research (CIBMTR) data, approximately 4500 allo-HSCTs are performed each year in children less than 20 years of age.[1] Most children are transplanted for malignancy, however increasing numbers receive an allo-HSCT for nonmalignant diseases such as bone marrow failure, immunodeficiency, and certain metabolic syndromes/disorders.[2–7] Concurrent with increasing indications for allo-HSCT, there has been a surge of interest in immune modulation to harness the graft-versus-tumor (GVT) effects when this procedure is used for hematologic malignancies. These factors along with improvements in the safety of allo-HSCT have led to an expanding population of long-term survivors, many of whom suffer from long-term toxicities, including chronic graft-versus-host disease (cGVHD).

cGVHD is the most significant nonrelapse cause of morbidity and mortality following allo-HSCT for malignant disease.[8–12] Although the rates of cGVHD tend to be lower in

[a] Pediatric Oncology Branch, Center for Cancer Research, National Cancer Institute, National Institutes of Health, Building 10, Room 1-3750, 9000 Rockville Pike, MSC 1104, Bethesda, MD 20892-1104, USA
[b] Stem Cell and Regenerative Medicine, Case Western Reserve University School of Medicine, Cleveland, OH, USA
[c] Pediatric Blood and Marrow Transplantation Program, Case Western Reserve University School of Medicine, Cleveland, OH, USA
[d] Multidisciplinary Initiative in Graft-vs-Host Disease, Case Western Reserve University School of Medicine, Cleveland, OH, USA
[e] Rainbow Babies and Children's Hospital, Wolstein Research Building, Room 6524, 2103 Cornell Road, Cleveland, OH 44106-7288, USA
[f] Childhood Cancer Research Program of BC Children's Hospital and the Child and Family Research Institute, Vancouver, BC, Canada
[g] Pediatrics, BC Children's Hospital, 4480 Oak Street, A119, Vancouver, BC V6H 3V4, Canada
* Corresponding author.
E-mail address: kbaird@mail.nih.gov

Pediatr Clin N Am 57 (2010) 297–322
doi:10.1016/j.pcl.2009.11.003
0031-3955/10/$ – see front matter. Published by Elsevier Inc.

pediatric.theclinics.com

children (20%–50%) than adults (60%–70%),[13–16] the incidence of cGVHD in the pediatric population is substantial and has increased recently in association with the expanded use of peripheral blood stem cells (PBSCs) and unrelated donors.[17–22] cGVHD has been characterized historically by autoimmune and alloimmune dysregulation occurring after the first 100 days of allo-HSCT.[15,23] A newer set of diagnostic criteria have been developed and the definition of cGVHD has been refined to include the development of diagnostic features of immune dysfunction that may be present before day 100 and almost always occur within 3 years posttransplant.[24] The median onset of cGVHD is approximately 6 months following allo-HSCT.[15] As opposed to acute GVHD (aGVHD), which involves the skin, liver, and gastrointestinal (GI) tract, cGVHD can involve almost any organ of the body. cGVHD leads to significant morbidity, diminished quality of life, and decreased overall survival.

INCIDENCE OF CGVHD IN PEDIATRICS

The rates of cGVHD in the pediatric population depend on several variables and can range from as low as 6% in matched sibling cord blood transplants[25] to as high as 65% in matched unrelated donor (MUD) PBSC transplants.[26] In 2000, Eurocord and the International Bone Marrow Transplant Registry (IBMTR) compared 113 sibling cord blood HSCTs to 2052 HLA-matched sibling bone marrow transplants (BMTs). All of these patients were 15 years of age or younger and received a myeloablative preparative regimen, and most received cyclosporine (CSA)-based GVHD prophylaxis. The cord blood population had a 6% 3-year cumulative incidence of cGVHD versus 15% in the bone marrow recipients.[27] In 2002, Zecca and colleagues[19] published a retrospective analysis of 696 consecutive pediatric patients who underwent transplant in Italy between 1991 and 1999. The indication for transplant was malignancy in two-thirds, almost all patients received bone marrow (BM) as the stem cell source, and two-thirds had HLA-matched sibling donors. The overall incidence of cGVHD in this population was 25%, with a median time to diagnosis of 116 days after transplantation.

PATHOPHYSIOLOGY

The scientific basis for the development of cGVHD is poorly understood and there are limited data specific to pediatrics. Historically, alloreactive donor T cells have been the primary factor implicated in the pathophysiology of cGVHD. However, a recent randomized trial failed to demonstrate that T-cell depletion reduced the incidence of cGVHD.[28] Therefore, the role of direct T-cell–mediated allogeneic immune responses in cGVHD is not clear, and there is no strong correlation between the number of minor histocompatibility antigen–specific T cells and cGVHD.[29,30]

Evidence suggests that B cells also play a role in disease development.[31] B lymphocytes have at least two important functions: production of antibodies and presentation of antigens to T cells, both of which may contribute to cGVHD.[32–35] A coordinated B-T response to minor histocompatibility alloantigens (mHA) is well described,[36,37] as is significant high-titer antibody responses to mHA that correlate with cGVHD in patients.[38] Increased levels of nonspecific auto-(vs allo-) antibodies have repeatedly been described in association with cGVHD and include antinuclear antibody (ANA)[32,33,39]; anti-dsDNA antibody[40]; antimitochondrial antibody[39]; anticardiolipin antibody[39]; antismooth muscle antibody (ASMA); platelet antibodies; and antineutrophil antibodies.[23,33,40–42] In addition, antiplatelet-derived growth factor receptor (PDGFR) antibodies have been associated with sclerotic cGVHD[43] and are implicated in the fibrosis in idiopathic scleroderma, which shares many clinical features with classic cGVHD.[44] Probably the best documented alloantibody association with cGVHD involves the H-Y antigen. Male patients who have received allo-HSCT from female donors are at higher risk for aGVHD and cGVHD.[37,45,46] The Miklos group showed that the H-Y antibodies develop 4 to 12 months after BMT in approximately 50% of male patients receiving allo-HSCT from female donors. The cumulative incidence of cGVHD in the presence of H-Y antibodies was found to be 89% at 5 years post BMT versus 31% in the absence of H-Y antibodies ($P<.0001$). Moreover, responses to the anti-B cell therapy, rituximab (anti-CD20 monoclonal antibody) in steroid-refractory cGVHD strongly suggest that B cells play a significant role in this disease.[31,47]

Soluble factors may also play a role in the pathogenesis of cGVHD. On activation during cGVHD, dendritic cells (DCs) and B lymphocytes secrete inflammatory cytokines after recognition of their cognate antigen. DCs and macrophages produce monocyte chemoattractant protein-1 (MCP-1),[48,49] interleukin (IL)-6,[50,51] transforming growth factor-beta (TGF-β)[52] and interferon-gamma (IFN-γ) which has been implicated in autoimmune disease and GVHD.[53] Soluble IL2 receptor alpha (sIL2Rα), as a marker of activated T cells, correlates with the severity of aGVHD[54–56] and cGVHD[57] and with other autoimmune diseases.[58,59] Specifically, cutaneous cGVHD has been associated with an increase in PDGF,[60,61] cGVHD-associated sclerosis with high levels of TGF-β, fatigue and wasting with high levels of TNF-α, and immunodeficiency with high levels of IL10 and TGF-β.[62] Cytokine polymorphisms of donor and recipient IL1 and IL6 genes, donor TNF receptor type II 169RR-homozygous genotype, recipient IL10 GG-homozygosity, and recipient IL1Rα polymorphisms may also play a role.[31,63–66]

The Children's Oncology Group (COG) recently published an analysis of peripheral blood biomarkers found in 52 children newly diagnosed with extensive cGVHD. Peripheral blood samples were evaluated for 13 known or suspected biomarkers and were compared with 28 time-matched controls with no evidence of cGVHD. Four plasma biomarkers (soluble B-cell–activating factor (sBAFF,) sCD13, anti-dsDNA, and sIL2R α) and 1 cellular biomarker (Toll-like receptor 9 (TLR9) high expressing cytosine-phosphate-guanosine (CpG) responsive B cells) correlated with the diagnosis of cGVHD[67] and in combination, had high specificity (84%) and sensitivity (100%) for the diagnosis of cGVHD. sBAFF, anti-dsDNA antibody, soluble IL2 receptor α, and soluble CD13 were increased in early onset cGVHD compared with controls. Furthermore, sBAFF and anti-dsDNA were increased in late onset cGVHD. Levels of sBAFF and sCD13 were higher in patients with hepatic cGVHD, whereas anti-dsDNA levels were higher in patients with joint, sclerodermatous, and ocular involvement. Increased sBAFF was significantly associated with lichenoid skin rash and joint involvement, increased IL6 and MCP-1 with joint involvement, and increased anticardiolipin antibody with ocular involvement. All of these associations were statistically significant. None of the markers evaluated were associated with gastrointestinal, pulmonary, or musculoskeletal cGVHD.[68] Biomarkers have the potential to predict the risk of developing cGVHD, improving classification, and directing cGVHD research and treatment, but require further investigation and large study validation.

RISK FACTORS

Known risk factors that have been repeatedly associated with higher risks of cGVHD include precedent aGVHD, unrelated donor, mismatched donor, PBSCs as donor source, older recipient or donor age, female donor into a male recipient, the use of total body irradiation (TBI), and malignant disease (**Table 1**).[14,19,27,69,70] By far the

Table 1
cGVHD risk factors

	Patient	Donor/Graft	Transplant
Increased cGVHD risk	Older age Malignancy	Female donor to male patient Mismatched Unrelated Peripheral blood stem cells Donor lymphocyte infusions Older age	Acute GVHD Total irradiation in preparative regimen
Possible increased cGVHD risk	CMV positive CMV reactivation	CD 34+ cell dose	
Decreased cGVHD risk	Younger age	Cord blood	Anti-thyroglobulin in preparative regimen Campath-1H in preparative regimen
Possible decreased cGVHD risk			Methotrexate and cyclosporine prophylaxis

strongest predictor for the development of cGVHD seems to be the severity of aGVHD.[14,19] Conversely, factors that have been found to be associated with lower rates of cGVHD include the use of cord blood stem cells and the use of methotrexate (MTX) with CSA for GVHD prophylaxis.[19,25,27,69] Lower donor or recipient age also reduces the incidence of cGVHD, which has been hypothesized to be due in part to a lower exposure of young donors and recipients to infections.[71,72] The following factors have little or no effect on the risk of developing cGVHD: T-cell depletion of the stem cell graft,[69,73–77] CD34+ cell dose in the graft,[78] or the use of prolonged immunosuppression.[79]

Although ex vivo strategies to deplete donor T cells have not significantly influenced the rates of cGVHD,[69,73–77] the addition of antithymocyte globulin (ATG)[80,81] or Campath-1H to the conditioning regimen[82] does seem to affect the development of cGVHD. ATG is widely used before allo-HSCT, particularly with HLA-matched unrelated donors or mismatched relatives, to prevent graft rejection and GVHD. The addition of ATG has resulted in low rates of GVHD after pediatric mismatched cord blood transplant similar to those found in matched unrelated BM transplants.[80] Many umbilical cord blood (UCB) transplant regimens incorporate ATG suggesting a possible contribution of this agent to the low rates of GVHD. Despite encouraging results, ATG may adversely affect posttransplant immune reconstitution.[83] The reasons why in vivo T cell depletion is more effective in preventing GVHD than ex vivo depletion are incompletely understood. However, agents such as Campath and ATG have a long half-life in the recipient, affecting not only donor T cells but also antigen presenting cells (APCs), natural killer (NK) cells, regulatory T cells, and B cells in the graft and the recipient. The subsequent effects on posttransplant proliferation, cell trafficking and signaling likely promote a more tolerogenic environment.[84,85]

Allo-HSCT using unrelated volunteer donors remains a significant risk factor for the development of cGVHD. Fifty percent of allo-HSCT performed in patients less than 20 years of age are from unrelated donors.[1] Earlier studies of unrelated donor BMT in the pediatric population during the 1980s and early 1990s report high incidences of cGVHD (50%–69%)[86,87] compared with more recent studies showing rates less than 50% (39%–47%).[88–90] Recent improvements and increasing utilization of high-resolution typing of HLA class I and class II loci has further decreased the rates of cGVHD in the unrelated population to 30%, rates comparable to those seen in children transplanted from HLA-identical siblings.[91]

Recently, the impact of hematopoietic stem cell source on the incidence of cGVHD has been investigated. Mobilized PBSCs are now the primary stem cell source in the adult population. However, despite this dramatic increase in adults, BM remains the predominant stem cell source used in pediatric transplantation. CIBMTR data from 2003 to 2006 show that the distribution of stem cell sources for allo-HSCT in children is approximately 42% BM, 37% cord blood, and 21% PBSC.[1] Although still modest, use of PBSCs mobilized by granulocyte colony-stimulating factor (G-CSF) is increasing in pediatrics and is likely to continue to escalate.[17,92] Adult studies have demonstrated higher incidences of cGVHD or refractory cGVHD when using PBSC versus BM.[93,94] Despite increased incidence of cGVHD in adults, the use of PBSC has been associated with decreased treatment-related mortality (TRM) and decreased relapse rates in leukemia patients.[95] The data on children are less clear. One recent study showed no significant differences in TRM, aGVHD, cGVHD, OS, or relapse-free survival in pediatric PBSC recipients (n = 38) compared with marrow (n = 23).[26] This is in contrast to previous studies that consistently show increased rates of cGVHD.[17,96–98] One study of 90 children undergoing PBSC transplants in Spain showed that patients with cGVHD had improved disease-free survival with lower relapse rates and similar TRM.[98] However, a retrospective IBMTR analysis of pediatric PBSC recipients reported poorer survival with PBSC transplants in comparison with BM despite similar rates of relapse. Patients in this study had similar rates of aGVHD, but rates of cGVHD were higher with a relative risk of 1.85 in the PBSC group.[17] Thus, despite the lack of randomized studies in children, it seems that the risk of cGVHD with PBSC is higher than BM, although the overall effects on TRM and relapse-free survival are unclear.[96,97]

Because of the relatively limited stem cell doses in UCB units, this source has been most frequently used in pediatric patients. Most cord blood units are from unrelated donors with only a small fraction coming from a suitably matched sibling. Initially, UCB transplants were associated with poor engraftment and high TRM, however more recent results are promising with high engraftment rates (>80%) and low incidence of acute and chronic GVHD (6%–28%), allowing for a greater degree of HLA mismatch.[19,25,27,99–105] The degree of mismatch does not seem to affect the development of cGVHD in cord blood transplants.[101,105,106] There is also a suggestion that cGVHD in unrelated UCB transplants is more responsive to therapy than in recipients of unrelated BMT.[107]

STAGING AND GRADING

Signs and symptoms of cGVHD typically present 6 to 18 months after allo-HSCT and the onset can be progressive (aGVHD progressing directly to cGVHD), quiescent (precedent aGVHD resolved), or de novo (no history of aGVHD). Grading of cGVHD severity was historically defined as limited or extensive.[23] Although there was prognostic significance to this categorization, investigators have tried to refine prognostic grading scales using survival as the primary endpoint. The two principal grading scales set forth by Akpek (2001) and Lee (2002) show that thrombocytopenia, progressive onset, extensive skin involvement, GI involvement, and low Karnofsky performance status at diagnosis of cGVHD are clearly associated with decreased survival.[108,109] A newly proposed cGVHD diagnosis and scoring system[24] offers an updated definition of cGVHD in which the diagnosis is based on the specificity of signs and histopathology rather than the traditional criterion of time of onset since transplantation (more or <100 days). The National Institutes of Health consensus criteria further refine the grading system based on multiple clinical parameters into mild, moderate, and severe categories.[24] The prognostic and clinical significance of this grading system has yet to be validated.

CLINICAL MANIFESTATIONS

cGVHD most commonly involves the skin, eyes, oral cavity, GI tract, liver, and lungs (**Table 2**). Other organ systems such as the kidneys[110–112] or heart[113,114] can also be affected, although far less frequently. Manifestations of cGVHD can include more inflammatory and acute-type features such as erythematous rash, mucositis, diarrhea, transaminitis, and pulmonary infiltrates, or can be more fibrotic and chronic in nature such as sclerotic or lichen planus-type skin changes, fasciitis, sicca syndrome, esophageal strictures, and bronchiolitis obliterans (BO). Age-based, multidisciplinary, ancillary supportive care is essential to the optimal management of cGVHD in the pediatric patient.[115]

Cutaneous

The skin is the most commonly involved organ of cGVHD. Changes in the skin can be superficial, epidermal (hypo-, hyper-, or depigmentation) or deep into the subcutis and fascial layers. Features commonly seen that may overlap with aGVHD include erythema, maculopapular rash, and pruritis. Diagnostic features of cGVHD include sclerotic, lichen planus-like, morphea-like or lichen sclerosus-like changes and poikiloderma (the combination of atrophy, telangiectasia, and pigmentary changes to the skin). The most severe and difficult-to-treat skin manifestation is sclerotic GVHD. Extensive sclerotic skin changes with superficial or deep subcutaneous or fascial involvement develops in approximately 3% to 4% of patients with cGVHD and can be life threatening.[116] The process is characterized by fibrosis of the skin or subcutaneous tissues and may result in joint contractures, severe wasting, and chest wall restriction. The mean onset of sclerotic skin changes following transplant is late (529 days in 1 study[117]). Other manifestations of disease include ichthyosis, keratosis pilaris, and sweat gland impairment. The skin appendages may also be involved as manifested by nail loss or dystrophia, scalp changes and alopecia, or premature graying. Skin care should include topical moisturizers, antipruritic agents, strict photoprotection, and close surveillance for cutaneous malignancy.

Musculoskeletal

Musculoskeletal involvement of cGVHD in children can result in myositis, fasciitis, muscle weakness, cramping, edema, and pain. Functional limitations from joint contractures, arthralgias and fatigue can be severe, and therefore close monitoring for decreased range of motion and early intervention with physical therapy, occupational therapy, and splinting is essential. Rarely, surgical joint capsular release may be indicated to help preserve range of motion in involved joints although such intervention has been associated with mixed and transient responses.[118] Other commonly seen musculoskeletal complications include osteoporosis and avascular necrosis,[119,120] complications that are the direct result of steroid therapy for cGVHD. Careful follow-up with bone density studies and use of vitamin D and calcium supplementation in conjunction with biphosphonates in select patients are therefore warranted.

Table 2
Manifestations of cGVHD

Organ	Signs	Symptoms
Skin, nails, hair	Sclerosis, lichen sclerosus-like, lichen planus-like features Sweat impairment Ichthyosis Keratosis pilaris Hypo-, hyper -, depigmentation Erythema, poikiloderma Maculopapular rash Nail dystrophy Pterygium unguis Alopecia Scaling, papulosquamous lesions of scalp Hair depigmentation	Pruritus Dryness Longitudinal ridging, splitting of nail Nail loss Thinning of hair Premature graying
Vulvovaginal	Lichen planus-like features Vaginal scarring or stenosis Erosions, fissures, ulcers	Dyspareunia Vaginal dryness
Muscles, fascia, joints	Fasciitis Sclerosis Myositis or polymyositis Edema	Joint stiffness or contractures Muscle cramps or pain Arthralgia or arthritis Weakness
Eyes	Cicatricial conjunctivitis Keratoconjunctivitis sicca Punctate keratopathy Blepharitis	Dry, gritty, or painful eyes Photophobia
Mouth	Erythema Lichen-type features Hyperkeratotic plaques Xerostomia Mucocele Mucosal atrophy Pseudomembrane formation Ulcers Gingivitis, mucositis	Dry mouth Pain Difficulty swallowing Oral sensitivity Change in taste Increased dental caries
GI tract	Esophageal web or strictures Exocrine pancreatic insufficiency Vomiting Diarrhea	Anorexia Nausea Weight loss, failure to thrive Abdominal cramping
Liver	Hyperbilirubinemia Tranaminitis	Jaundice
Lung	Bronchiolitis obliterans BOOP	Dyspnea on exertion
Hematopoeitic/ immune	Anemia, thrombocytopenia, Eosinophilia Hypo- or hyper- gammaglobulinemia Autoantibodies (AIHA, ITP)	
Other	Effusions Peripheral neuropathy Nephrotic syndrome Myasthenia gravis Cardiac conduction abnormality Cardiomyopathy Coronary artery fibrotic changes	Varied

Ocular

GVHD of the eyes affects up to 80% of patients with cGVHD.[121] Patients typically present with dry or gritty eyes (sicca syndrome), photophobia, erythema, or edema. Patients can suffer from lacrimal gland dysfunction and conjunctival inflammation leading to cicatrical conjunctivitis, keratoconjunctivitis, punctate keratopathy, and blepharitis. Topical therapies, such as corticosteroid or cyclosporine drops, can be effective and optimization of these therapies is warranted. Patients may also benefit from local measures such as punctual plugs or scleral lenses, which provide significant symptomatic relief. It is important to follow these patients closely with serial Schirmer tests to assess the degree of wetting and to intervene early at the onset of ocular involvement even before the evolution of symptoms. A Schirmer test without anesthesia may be difficult to perform and is not recommended in younger children; an ophthalmologist's input may be needed for objective scoring in these children.[122] Ocular care consists of photoprotection along with regular evaluation for infection, cataract formation, and increased intraocular pressure. For children who are old enough to tolerate the procedure, routine Schirmer evaluation should be done to monitor tear production. Regional care may include artificial tears, ocular ointments, punctal occlusion, humidified environment, occlusive eye wear, moisture chamber eyeglasses, or gas-permeable scleral contact lens.

Oral

Oral cGVHD can involve the mucosa or the salivary glands. Symptoms include oral pain, dry mouth, taste changes, and food sensitivity. Examination may reveal mucosal erythema, lichen-type changes, xerostomia, mucosal atrophy, mucoceles, and ulcers. The largest single-center series of oral cGVHD in pediatric patients described the findings of 49 patients seen at a multidisciplinary pediatric HSCT clinic at the Dana-Farber Cancer Institute.[123] Oral mucosal involvement was identified in 45% of patients, however only 8% of patients reported mouth pain and all patients reported being able to eat well. The most common manifestation was erythema (42%), followed by reticular (36%) and ulcerative (21%) forms. Forty-five percent of patients required specific therapy for their oral mucosal cGVHD despite being currently treated with at least 1 systemic immunomodulatory agent. Salivary gland and sclerotic diseases were rarely observed.[123] Children with isolated oral cGVHD can often be treated with topical steroid rinses, although responses to topical therapy are varied and many patients require systemic treatment. Other treatment options include topical tacrolimus and agents that stimulate salivary gland function, but no strategy has been shown to have significant benefit over another and some may lead to increased rates of oral squamous cell carcinoma.[124] Secondary infections with viruses (especially herpes simplex) and yeasts are common; therefore using a local antifungal preparation in combination with the steroid rinse is recommended. Patients should adhere to strict oral hygiene and have close regular follow-up with an experienced oral health care specialist.

Gastrointestinal (GI) Tract

Children with cGVHD may have varied GI complaints including nausea, anorexia, abdominal pain, weight loss, cramping, or diarrhea. Although these symptoms may be related to cGVHD, the only finding that is strictly diagnostic of cGVHD of the GI tracts is esophageal sclerosis in the form of an esophageal web or stricture.[24] Many GI symptoms are attributable to other causes including late aGVHD, infection, dysmotility, lactose intolerance, pancreatic insufficiency, or drug-related side effects.[108] As many of these problems can be remedied by other means, full evaluation of symptoms, including upper and lower endoscopy, is important before increasing or continuing immunosuppressive medication, as these may not treat the cause and may actually worsen the child's symptoms.[125]

Weight loss and reduced body mass index (BMI, calculated as weight in kilograms divided by the square of height in meters) remain poorly understood, but they are critical issues in children with multi-organ cGVHD. Maintaining adequate nutrition is essential and careful evaluation of growth and head circumference in infants is required. In adults with cGVHD, low BMI is a predictor for mortality. A retrospective study of 18 children with extensive cGVHD found that patients with multi-organ involvement had a mean maximal decrease in BMI of 20.9% in contrast to patients with 1 organ system involved who had a mean maximal decrease in BMI of 5%. Weight loss often preceded overt signs and symptoms of cGVHD, suggesting an altered metabolic state and/or subclinical malabsorption in these patients. Thus, weight loss and malnutrition (as reflected by a decrease in BMI) are clinically significant issues in children with multisystem cGVHD and are likely systemic manifestations of the disease; they may contribute, to increased mortality in this group.[126] Treatment of GI manifestations may include dietary modification, enzyme supplementation for malabsorption, gastroesophageal reflux management, and esophageal dilatation.

Hepatic

cGVHD of the liver can be one of the most difficult manifestations to diagnose, as many possible causes for liver inflammation and damage exist in this population: infection, drug toxicity, iron overload, focal nodular hyperplasia, and so forth. To confirm the diagnosis evaluation must include viral studies for hepatitis A, B, C, and Epstein-Barr virus, cytomegalovirus (CMV), varicella zoster virus, and adenovirus to exclude infection as a cofactor or cause of hepatic dysfunction. Liver biopsy is often required to confirm the diagnosis; this is particularly important for those patients with no other signs or symptoms of cGVHD. The typical appearance of hepatic cGVHD is that of fibrosis resulting in obstructive jaundice, with increases in alkaline phosphatase, γ-glutamyl transferase (GGT), and serum bilirubin levels. Liver biopsies can show portal fibrosis and bile duct dropout and can ultimately progress to cirrhosis and bridging necrosis.[127] Ursodeoxycholic acid can be used for patients with hyperbilirubinemia. Although cholestasic hepatic cGVHD is the classic manifestation of liver involvement, hepatitic cGVHD is being identified more often, with some patients presenting with isolated increases in serum alanine aminotransferase (ALT) and aspartate aminotransferase (AST) levels.[128,129] First described in adult patients, this hepatitic pattern has also been recognized in pediatric patients. The histologic pattern reveals bile duct epithelial damage, significant portal/periportal inflammation, and lobular necro-inflammation. The clinical and histologic patterns of hepatitic cGVHD described in this pediatric study are similar to that described in adults.[130]

Pulmonary

Two forms of chronic pulmonary dysfunction are common in patients surviving greater than 100 days following allo-HSCT: obstructive lung disease (OLD) and restrictive lung disease (RLD).[131] The incidence of lung toxicity ranges from 30% to 60%.[132] Collagen deposition and the development of fibrosis either in the interstitial (RLD) or peribronchiolar (OLD) space are believed to contribute to lung dysfunction. Although RLD and OLD exist as late onset, noninfectious lung complications following allo-HSCT, they can be distinguished by several clinical parameters as described later (**Table 3**).

Table 3
Clinical factors present in OLD versus RLD

Clinical Factor	OLD	RLD
Diagnostic entity	BO	BOOP
Onset	Late (3–12 months)	Early (within 3 months)
Symptoms	Dyspnea, nonproductive cough	Dyspnea, nonproductive cough
Physical examination	Wheezing	Rales
Pulmonary function tests	Obstructive physiology	Restrictive physiology
FEV_1/FVC	Decreased	Normal
TLC	Normal	Decreased
DL_{CO}	Decreased	Decreased
CT scan findings	Air trapping (expiration) Bronchial wall thickening Ground glass opacities Centrilobular nodules	Fluffy consolidations Ground glass opacities
Laboratory data	Nonspecific	Increased CRP Peripheral neutrophila
Chronic GVHD	Strong association	Variable, positive with BOOP

Abbreviations: CT, computed tomography; DL_{CO}, diffusing capacity of lung for carbon monoxide; FEV,forced expiratory volume; FVC, forced vital capacity; OLD, obstructive lung disease; RLD, restrictive lung disease; TLC, total lung capacity.

The most common and recognizable form of OLD is BO. BO is a serious life-threatening manifestation of cGVHD that is characterized by an inflammatory process resulting in bronchiolar obliteration, fibrosis, and progressive OLD. The presence of BO post transplant is diagnostic for cGVHD.[24] There are no effective therapies for BO, and patients frequently develop progressive and debilitating respiratory failure despite the initiation of enhanced immunosuppression. Mortality approaches 100% in some studies, with a mean fatality rate of 61%[130,133] Patients with BO may be asymptomatic early in the time course of disease, but typically present with a cough, wheezing, or dyspnea on exertion.[24,134] As suggested, pulmonary function tests (PFTs) show obstructive lung mechanics with general preservation of forced vital capacity (FVC), reductions in forced expiratory volume in 1 second (FEV_1) and associated decreases in the FEV_1/FVC ratio with or without significant declines in the diffusing capacity of lung for carbon monoxide (DL_{CO}).

The most recognizable form of RLD after allo-HSCT is BO organizing pneumonia (BOOP). Clinical features include dry cough, shortness of breath, and fever, and radiographic findings show diffuse, peripheral, fluffy infiltrates consistent with airspace consolidation. Although reported in less than 10% of allo-HSCT recipients, the development of BOOP is strongly associated with prior acute and chronic GVHD.[135] The term BOOP should not be used interchangeably with BO to describe a patient with chronic lung dysfunction after allo-HSCT, although such usage is unfortunately widespread.[136] The two disorders differ with respect to histopathology, pulmonary function characteristics, and most importantly, response to therapy; BOOP after HSCT is quite responsive to corticosteroids, whereas BO is not (see **Table 3**).

In addition, other clinical diagnoses (eg, pneumonias, chest wall fibrosis) can be associated with signs and symptoms of lung dysfunction, therefore an extensive workup of the affected individual is recommended. Testing should include a high-resolution, computer-assisted tomography (CT) scan of the chest, which may reveal an infectious process or air trapping, and when clinically possible, serial complete PFTs that include an assessment of lung volumes, spirometry, and DL_{CO}. When evaluating lung function in this context, it is important to keep some key elements in mind. Specifically, pediatric allo-HSCT patients may not continue on the normal growth curves for height and weight. Recipients of total body or chest wall irradiation may not have proportional chest wall growth. Care must therefore be taken to not only follow percent-predicted values but also to evaluate actual lung volumes over time; because PFTs are scored as a percentage of the predicted norms, from healthy age-matched controls, a drop in the percent-predicted value may actually reflect poor lung growth rather than a physiologic drop in lung function. A broncho-alveolar lavage may be necessary to evaluate for possible concurrent infection and aggressive therapy for proven infection is essential. A biopsy may be needed for definitive diagnosis, however this is commonly avoided because of the risks of the procedure. When a definitive tissue diagnosis cannot be made, the term bronchiolitis obliterans syndrome is applied. Pneumothorax, pneumomediastinum, and subcutaneous emphysema are rare and often represent advanced disease. Ancillary support requires infection surveillance, pneumocystis prophylaxis, and treatment of gastroesophageal reflux. Initial therapy for pulmonary cGVHD should include a trial of enhanced systemic immunosuppression. Benefit may also be observed with inhaled corticosteroids, bronchodilators, supplementary oxygen, and pulmonary rehabilitation. As noted earlier, novel targeted therapies may also hold promise. Consideration of lung transplantation is given to the rare appropriate candidate with severe BO.

Hematopoietic System

Cytopenias are common following allo-HSCT. The mechanisms contributing to marrow dysfunction are not clearly defined and are likely to be multifactorial. Cytopenias may result from stromal damage, but antibody-mediated autoimmune neutropenia,[137] anemia,[138] and thrombocytopenia[139] are also common. It is also important to eliminate drug toxicity, infection, graft failure, or disease relapse as the underlying cause. Thrombocytopenia is the most common hematopoeitic manifestation of cGVHD and occurs in approximately 35% of affected patients.[22] Thrombocytopenia alone does not meet the diagnostic criteria for cGVHD, however several studies have shown that thrombocytopenia at the time of cGVHD diagnosis confers a poor prognosis,[108,140] although thrombocytopenia may be a poor prognostic factor independent of GVHD.[141] Eosinophilia is also frequently seen in children and can precede the development of overt cGVHD.[142]

Immune System

Patients with cGVHD have associated immune dysregulation and delayed immune reconstitution as a direct consequence of GVHD and immunosuppressive therapy. In addition, patients with mucosal involvement (skin, oral, or GI) lack intact barriers thus increasing the risk of infections.[143–145] Thus, opportunistic infections are common and remain the leading cause of death in patients with active cGVHD.[23,146,147] Functional asplenia, shown by persistence of Howell-Jolly bodies and a higher incidence of pneumococcal sepsis,[148,149] is also commonly seen and can remain for life despite resolution of cGVHD. Therefore, lifelong prophylaxis against encapsulated organisms is recommended. Patients should also receive prophylaxis against *Pneumocystis jiroveci* until complete resolution of cGVHD and for at least 6 months after discontinuation of immunosuppressive therapy. Supplemental intravenous immunoglobulin (IVIG) replacement is typically used when patients have the combination of severe hypogammaglobulinemia (IgG <400 mg/dL) and recurrent infections. Patients at risk for CMV should be monitored closely with CMV polymerase chain reaction or antigenemia. Patients receiving steroid rinses for oral GVHD are at high risk for local candida infections and topical antifungal prophylaxis (eg, nystatin swishes or clotrimazole troches) should be used. Patients on steroid doses equal to or greater than the equivalent of prednisone 0.8 mg/kg/d should also be given antifungal and antiviral prophylaxis. The decision to discontinue antifungal and antiviral therapy is dependent on each patient and the intensity of the therapy they are receiving. Up-to-date recommendations from the Centers for Disease Control (CDC) and Prevention for infection prophylaxis are available at http://www.cdc.gov/mmwr/preview/mmwrhtml/rr4910a1.htm. Vaccinations are critical to enhance immunity against specific organisms but are typically delayed until 6 to 12 months after HSCT as per institutional guidelines[41] or according to CDC recommendations (http://www.cdc.gov/mmwr/preview/mmwrhtml/rr4910a1.htm). Live vaccines should be avoided in this patient population.

TREATMENT

The treatment of cGVHD in pediatrics is highly variable and mostly extrapolated from the experience in adults. Although there is no proven standard therapy, prednisone and CSA are commonly used as frontline therapy. This combination therapy is based on an alternate day regimen that improved survival in high-risk patients with thrombocytopenia and extensive skin involvement.[140] The general approach to treatment is immediate initiation of therapy, typically high-dose steroids (1–2 mg/kg/d) with calcineurin inhibitor, with steady weaning of steroid until the lowest allowable dose without cGVHD flare is achieved. The mean duration of therapy for patients with cGVHD is 3 years, with approximately half of patients able to discontinue therapy by 5 years post HSCT.[150,151] Patients should be evaluated for response to treatment and monitored for side effects of therapy at a minimum of every 3 months. Therapy is typically continued for at least 3 months after maximal response and weaned off with careful monitoring for a recurrent flare of cGVHD. Investigators at Johns Hopkins observed that 90% of patients who ultimately respond to a therapy show signs of response by 3 months.[152]

SALVAGE REGIMENS
Sirolimus

Sirolimus (rapamycin) is a macrocyclic triene antibiotic with immunosuppressive, antifungal, and antitumor properties; it inhibits signal transduction and cell cycle progression after binding to FKBP12 and inhibiting the mammalian target of rapamycin (mTOR).[153] Sirolimus has been shown to have activity in the prevention and treatment of aGVHD[154–157] and has more recently been evaluated in the chronic setting. Several recent studies show good overall response rates (63%–93%) in cGVHD.[156–158] However, no studies have been performed on a pediatric population so dosing and pharmacokinetics remain incompletely defined and are usually based on data from solid organ transplant populations. Toxicities include hyperlipidemia, cytopenias, and hemolytic uremic syndrome, which may be potentiated by the combination of sirolimus with a calcineurin inhibitor.[156]

Mycophenolate Mofetil (MMF)

MMF is an antimetabolite used as an alternative immunosuppressant that inhibits the proliferation of T and B lymphocytes and is currently in use for aGVHD prophylaxis. MMF is generally well tolerated and when in combination with calcineurin inhibitor, has shown a steroid-sparing effect with response rates ranging from 50% to

79%.[159–163] MMF has been evaluated in several pediatric trials, which show similar response rates and tolerability as seen in the adult trials.[160] Investigators in Seattle reported a promising complete remission rate of 65% in 26 pediatric patients who had previously progressed on therapy with prednisone and CSA. Responses were slow and complete remission was not achieved until up to 3 years following initiation of therapy in several cases. Despite that, the drug was remarkably well tolerated and only 1 patient experienced transient leukopenia.[161] Unfortunately, a large multicenter randomized trial using MMF for the initial treatment of cGVHD was recently closed prematurely secondary to lack of efficacy in the treatment arm.[151]

Pentostatin

Pentostatin is a nucleoside analog that irreversibly inhibits adenosine deaminase resulting in severe immunosuppression. Pentostatin causes decreased T-cell responses to IL2, reduced T-cell number and function, reduced NK cell numbers and lymphocyte counts, thus affecting antibody and nonantibody cytotoxicity.[164,165] In an open-label phase 2 study of pentostatin for patients with steroid-refractory cGVHD, patients were dosed at 4 mg/m^2 intravenously every 2 weeks for 12 doses. Of the 58 patients enrolled, 55% had an objective response, however when stratified for age, younger patients (<33 years) had a better response rate (77%). Twenty percent of patients experienced grade 3 to 4 infection and survival at 2 years was 70%; cGVHD with or without infection accounted for most of the deaths.[166]

Other agents including hydroxychloroquine, a lysosomotropic 4-aminoquinoline anti-malarial drug that has been used to effectively treat autoimmune disorders,[167,168] and thalidomide have been studied in small numbers of pediatric and adult patients. Both agents are reasonably well tolerated and have shown varying degrees of promise (including steroid-sparing effects) in individuals with steroid-refractory cGVHD.[10,169–171]

Extracorporeal Photochemotherapy

Extracorporeal photochemotherapy (ECP) is a therapeutic procedure originally used in clinical medicine for the treatment of cutaneous T-cell lymphoma (CTCL).[172] During ECP, the patient's peripheral blood mononuclear cells are collected by apheresis, incubated with the photoactivatable drug 8-methoxypsoralen (8-MOP), and UV-A irradiation then re-infused into the circulation. Phase 1 and 2 data suggest that ECP is an effective treatment of acute and chronic GVHD, with response rates ranging from 40% to 81%.[173–177] Studies evaluating ECP for GVHD are primarily in adults, but there have been several trials that have either included or exclusively enrolled children. Salvaneschi and colleagues[178] treated 18 children with extensive cGVHD with a 78% response rate and 67% were able to taper steroids. ECP was safe and well tolerated without increase in infections in this study. Messina and colleagues[179] evaluated the use of ECP in 44 pediatric patients with acute and chronic GVHD. They reported an overall response rate of 59%, 44% of patients were able to discontinue all other immunosuppression, and 29% were able to reduce immunosuppression. Currently, a combined phase 2/3, randomized, open-label, multicenter, prospective study comparing the addition of ECP versus calcineurin inhibitor combined with prednisone and sirolimus for the upfront treatment of cGVHD is available through the Blood and Marrow Transplant Clinical Trials Network (BMT-CTN).

Targeted Therapies

Various monoclonal antibodies and anticytokine therapies such as infliximab and etanercept (anti-TNF-α) and daclizumab (anti-IL2R-α), which have been evaluated in the treatment of aGVHD, are being further studied for the treatment of cGVHD.[180] In general, these targeted therapies exhibit more favorable side effect profiles in this patient population. Etanercept (Enbrel) is a recombinant, human, soluble tumor necrosis factor (TNF-α) receptor fusion protein that inhibits TNF-α, a major mediator in the pathogenesis of GVHD. Preliminary data suggest that etanercept may be safe and effective for the treatment of pediatric and adult allo-HSCT recipients with manifestation of cGVHD of the lung.[181] More recently, the safety and efficacy of etanercept was evaluated in 21 patients with steroid-refractory aGVHD (n = 13) and cGVHD (n = 8). Overall, 52% responded to treatment with etanercept, including 5 patients (62%) with cGVHD, with 1 complete remission and 4 partial remissions.[182]

Given the possible contribution of B cells to the pathogenesis of cGVHD, rituximab, an anti-CD20 monoclonal antibody, has been investigated as a novel therapeutic option. Cutler and colleagues[47] evaluated 21 patients who were treated with 38 cycles of rituximab in a phase 1/2 study. Rituximab was well tolerated and toxicity was limited to infectious events. A clinical response rate of 70% was reported, although limited to patients with cutaneous and musculoskeletal manifestations.

A new agent on the horizon of interest to the cGVHD community is imatinib mesylate. After the discovery of stimulatory antibodies to the PDGF receptor and success in the treatment of idiopathic scleroderma patients, investigators looked to identify similar antibodies in patients with cGVHD. Similar antibodies were indeed identified in most patients with cGVHD, higher in patients with skin disease and extensive disease.[42] Several preliminary studies have shown promise in sclerotic skin and nonskin manifestations of cGVHD.[183,184]

Supportive Care

Ancillary and supportive care measures have been reviewed earlier with each organ specific manifestation. In general, topical or local care applied to the skin, eyes, or mouth is strongly encouraged to help minimize the toxicities of systemic therapy. In addition, patients should be monitored closely for neurologic and psychological dysfunction. Individuals may benefit from treatment of depression, pain, or neuropathic syndromes with tricyclic antidepressants, selective serotonin reuptake inhibitors, or anticonvulsants.

TOXICITY AND LATE EFFECTS

The treatment of cGVHD in pediatrics must include consideration of the possible effect that therapy will have on growth, nutrition, organ function, psychosocial functioning, and immune reconstitution. Posttransplant patients are at high risk for many late effects such as osteonecrosis, chronic renal insufficiency, hypothyroidism, growth hormone deficiency, hypogonadism, osteopenia, cataracts, and pulmonary dysfunction.[185] The addition of cGVHD and chronic immunosuppressive agents significantly compounds the risks of these complications. As steroids remain the foundation of cGVHD therapy, the consequences of long-term steroid use in children are well described and long-term deleterious effects on growth and bone density persist even after discontinuation of therapy.[186,187]

Additional concerns for the cGVHD population include impaired functional status and diminished quality of life (QOL). The strongest association between reduced QOL following HSCT is the presence of cGVHD.[188] cGHVD has negative effects on an individual's physical and mental health, and can lead to the development of functional impairments and activity limitations over their lifetime.[109,188,189]

SUMMARY AND FUTURE DIRECTIONS

Five-year survival rates for childhood cancer now exceed 80%[190] and with the significant progress made by the transplant community in developing less toxic conditioning regimens and in the treatment of posttransplant complications, allo-HSCT contributes significantly to that population of long-term survivors. In this context, the acute and long-term toxicities of cGVHD have an ever-increasing effect on organ function, QOL, and survival; patients and families who initially felt great relief to be cured from the primary disease, now face the challenge of a chronic debilitating illness for which preventative and treatment strategies are suboptimal. Hence, the development of novel strategies that reduce and or control cGVHD, preserve GVT effects, facilitate engraftment and immune reconstitution, and enhance survival after allo-HSCT represents one of the most significant challenges facing physician-scientists and patients. Data and research focused on cGVHD in pediatrics are limited; most studies are small and children are often grouped into larger adult series. However, given the impact of cGVHD on nonrelapse mortality, it is critical that clinical trials be designed to include pediatric patients with accrual goals of sufficient numbers to produce statistically significant conclusions. In addition, such trials should integrate biologic studies whenever possible to maximize discovery in pediatric cGVHD.

REFERENCES

1. Pasquini M, Wang Z, Schneider L. Current use and outcome of hematopoietic stem cell transplantation: part I - CIBMTR summary slides, 2007. CIBMTR Newsletter 2007;13:5–9.
2. Notarangelo LD, Forino C, Mazzolari E. Stem cell transplantation in primary immunodeficiencies. Curr Opin Allergy Clin Immunol 2006;6:443–8.
3. Walters MC. Stem cell therapy for sickle cell disease: transplantation and gene therapy. Hematology Am Soc Hematol Educ Program 2005;66–73.
4. Walters MC, Quirolo L, Trachtenberg ET, et al. Sibling donor cord blood transplantation for thalassemia major: experience of the Sibling Donor Cord Blood Program. Ann N Y Acad Sci 2005;1054:206–13.
5. Gaziev J, Lucarelli G. Stem cell transplantation for thalassaemia. Reprod Biomed Online 2005;10:111–5.
6. Kennedy-Nasser AA, Leung KS, Mahajan A, et al. Comparable outcomes of matched-related and alternative donor stem cell transplantation for pediatric severe aplastic anemia. Biol Blood Marrow Transplant 2006;12:1277–84.
7. Peters C, Steward CG. Hematopoietic cell transplantation for inherited metabolic diseases: an overview of outcomes and practice guidelines. Bone Marrow Transplant 2003;31:229–39.
8. Atkinson K. Chronic graft-versus-host disease. Bone Marrow Transplant 1990;5: 69–82.
9. Deeg HJ, Leisenring W, Storb R, et al. Long-term outcome after marrow transplantation for severe aplastic anemia. Blood 1998;91:3637–45.
10. Gilman AL, Chan KW, Mogul A, et al. Hydroxychloroquine for the treatment of chronic graft-versus-host disease. Biol Blood Marrow Transplant 2000;6:327–34.
11. Lee SJ, Klein JP, Barrett AJ, et al. Severity of chronic graft-versus-host disease: association with treatment-related mortality and relapse. Blood 2002;100: 406–14.
12. Goerner M, Gooley T, Flowers ME, et al. Morbidity and mortality of chronic GVHD after hematopoietic stem cell transplantation from HLA-identical siblings

for patients with aplastic or refractory anemias. Biol Blood Marrow Transplant 2002;8:47–56.

13. Storb R, Prentice RL, Sullivan KM, et al. Predictive factors in chronic graft-versus-host disease in patients with aplastic anemia treated by marrow transplantation from HLA-identical siblings. Ann Intern Med 1983;98:461–6.

14. Atkinson K, Horowitz MM, Gale RP, et al. Risk factors for chronic graft-versus-host disease after HLA-identical sibling bone marrow transplantation. Blood 1990;75:2459–64.

15. Sullivan KM, Shulman HM, Storb R, et al. Chronic graft-versus-host disease in 52 patients: adverse natural course and successful treatment with combination immunosuppression. Blood 1981;57:267–76.

16. Ochs LA, Miller WJ, Filipovich AH, et al. Predictive factors for chronic graft-versus-host disease after histocompatible sibling donor bone marrow transplantation. Bone Marrow Transplant 1994;13:455–60.

17. Eapen M, Horowitz MM, Klein JP, et al. Higher mortality after allogeneic peripheral-blood transplantation compared with bone marrow in children and adolescents: the Histocompatibility and Alternate Stem Cell Source Working Committee of the International Bone Marrow Transplant Registry. J Clin Oncol 2004;22:4872–80.

18. Higman MA, Vogelsang GB. Chronic graft versus host disease. Br J Haematol 2004;125:435–54.

19. Zecca M, Prete A, Rondelli R, et al. Chronic graft-versus-host disease in children: incidence, risk factors, and impact on outcome. Blood 2002;100: 1192–200.

20. Busca A, Rendine S, Locatelli F, et al. Chronic graft-versus-host disease after reduced-intensity stem cell transplantation versus conventional hematopoietic stem cell transplantation. Hematology 2005;10:1–10.

21. Lee SJ, Vogelsang G, Flowers ME. Chronic graft-versus-host disease. Biol Blood Marrow Transplant 2003;9:215–33.

22. Akpek G, Lee SJ, Flowers ME, et al. Performance of a new clinical grading system for chronic graft-versus-host disease: a multicenter study. Blood 2003; 102:802–9.

23. Shulman HM, Sullivan KM, Weiden PL, et al. Chronic graft-versus-host syndrome in man. A long-term clinicopathologic study of 20 Seattle patients. Am J Med 1980;69:204–17.

24. Filipovich AH, Weisdorf D, Pavletic S, et al. National Institutes of Health consensus development project on criteria for clinical trials in chronic graft-versus-host disease: I. Diagnosis and staging working group report. Biol Blood Marrow Transplant 2005;11:945–56.

25. Wagner JE, Kernan NA, Steinbuch M, et al. Allogeneic sibling umbilical-cord-blood transplantation in children with malignant and non-malignant disease. Lancet 1995;346:214–9.

26. Meisel R, Laws HJ, Balzer S, et al. Comparable long-term survival after bone marrow versus peripheral blood progenitor cell transplantation from matched unrelated donors in children with hematologic malignancies. Biol Blood Marrow Transplant 2007;13:1338–45.

27. Rocha V, Wagner JE Jr, Sobocinski KA, et al. Graft-versus-host disease in children who have received a cord-blood or bone marrow transplant from an HLA-identical sibling. Eurocord and International Bone Marrow Transplant Registry Working Committee on Alternative Donor and Stem Cell Sources. N Engl J Med 2000;342:1846–54.

28. van Els CA, Bakker A, Zwinderman AH, et al. Effector mechanisms in graft-versus-host disease in response to minor histocompatibility antigens. II. Evidence of a possible involvement of proliferative T cells. Transplantation 1990;50:67–71.

29. de Bueger M, Bakker A, Bontkes H, et al. High frequencies of cytotoxic T cell precursors against minor histocompatibility antigens after HLA-identical BMT: absence of correlation with GVHD. Bone Marrow Transplant 1993;11: 363–8.

30. Mutis T, Gillespie G, Schrama E, et al. Tetrameric HLA class I-minor histocompatibility antigen peptide complexes demonstrate minor histocompatibility antigen-specific cytotoxic T lymphocytes in patients with graft-versus-host disease. Nat Med 1999;5:839–42.

31. Zhang C, Todorov I, Zhang Z, et al. Donor CD4+ T and B cells in transplants induce chronic graft-versus-host disease with autoimmune manifestations. Blood 2006;107:2993–3001.

32. Rouquette-Gally AM, Boyeldieu D, Prost AC, et al. Autoimmunity after allogeneic bone marrow transplantation. A study of 53 long-term-surviving patients. Transplantation 1988;46:238–40.

33. Quaranta S, Shulman H, Ahmed A, et al. Autoantibodies in human chronic graft-versus-host disease after hematopoietic cell transplantation. Clin Immunol 1999; 91:106–16.

34. Allan SE, Crome SQ, Crellin NK, et al. Activation-induced FOXP3 in human T effector cells does not suppress proliferation or cytokine production. Int Immunol 2007;19:345–54.

35. Schultz KR, Paquet J, Bader S, et al. Requirement for B cells in T cell priming to minor histocompatibility antigens and development of graft-versus-host disease. Bone Marrow Transplant 1995;16:289–95.

36. Miklos DB, Kim HT, Zorn E, et al. Antibody response to DBY minor histocompatibility antigen is induced after allogeneic stem cell transplantation and in healthy female donors. Blood 2004;103:353–9.

37. Miklos DB, Kim HT, Miller KH, et al. Antibody responses to H-Y minor histocompatibility antigens correlate with chronic graft-versus-host disease and disease remission. Blood 2005;105:2973–8.

38. Brink R. Regulation of B cell self-tolerance by BAFF. Semin Immunol 2006;18: 276–83.

39. Wechalekar A, Cranfield T, Sinclair D, et al. Occurrence of autoantibodies in chronic graft vs. host disease after allogeneic stem cell transplantation. Clin Lab Haematol 2005;27:247–9.

40. Graze PR, Gale RP. Chronic graft versus host disease: a syndrome of disordered immunity. Am J Med 1979;66:611–20.

41. Vogelsang GB. How I treat chronic graft-versus-host disease. Blood 2001;97: 1196–201.

42. Svegliati S, Olivieri A, Campelli N, et al. Stimulatory autoantibodies to PDGF receptor in patients with extensive chronic graft-versus-host disease. Blood 2007;110:237–41.

43. Baroni SS, Santillo M, Bevilacqua F, et al. Stimulatory autoantibodies to the PDGF receptor in systemic sclerosis. N Engl J Med 2006;354:2667–76.

44. Ferrara JL, Deeg HJ. Graft-versus-host disease. N Engl J Med 1991;324:667–74.

45. Kollman C, Howe CW, Anasetti C, et al. Donor characteristics as risk factors in recipients after transplantation of bone marrow from unrelated donors: the effect of donor age. Blood 2001;98:2043–51.

46. Randolph SS, Gooley TA, Warren EH, et al. Female donors contribute to a selective graft-versus-leukemia effect in male recipients of HLA-matched, related hematopoietic stem cell transplants. Blood 2004;103:347–52.
47. Cutler C, Miklos D, Kim HT, et al. Rituximab for steroid-refractory chronic graft-vs.-host disease. Blood 2006;108(2):756–62.
48. New JY, Li B, Koh WP, et al. T cell infiltration and chemokine expression: relevance to the disease localization in murine graft-versus-host disease. Bone Marrow Transplant 2002;29:979–86.
49. Hildebrandt GC, Duffner UA, Olkiewicz KM, et al. A critical role for CCR2/MCP-1 interactions in the development of idiopathic pneumonia syndrome after allogeneic bone marrow transplantation. Blood 2004;103:2417–26.
50. Imamura M, Hashino S, Kobayashi H, et al. Serum cytokine levels in bone marrow transplantation: synergistic interaction of interleukin-6, interferon-gamma, and tumor necrosis factor-alpha in graft-versus-host disease. Bone Marrow Transplant 1994;13:745–51.
51. Okamoto H, Yamamura M, Morita Y, et al. The synovial expression and serum levels of interleukin-6, interleukin-11, leukemia inhibitory factor, and oncostatin M in rheumatoid arthritis. Arthritis Rheum 1997;40:1096–105.
52. Banovic T, MacDonald KP, Morris ES, et al. TGF-beta in allogeneic stem cell transplantation: friend or foe? Blood 2005;106:2206–14.
53. Theofilopoulos AN, Baccala R, Beutler B, et al. Type I interferons (alpha/beta) in immunity and autoimmunity. Annu Rev Immunol 2005;23:307–36.
54. Foley R, Couban S, Walker I, et al. Monitoring soluble interleukin-2 receptor levels in related and unrelated donor allogenic bone marrow transplantation. Bone Marrow Transplant 1998;21:769–73.
55. Grimm J, Zeller W, Zander AR. Soluble interleukin-2 receptor serum levels after allogeneic bone marrow transplantations as a marker for GVHD. Bone Marrow Transplant 1998;21:29–32.
56. Miyamoto T, Akashi K, Hayashi S, et al. Serum concentration of the soluble interleukin-2 receptor for monitoring acute graft-versus-host disease. Bone Marrow Transplant 1996;17:185–90.
57. Kobayashi S, Imamura M, Hashino S, et al. Clinical relevance of serum soluble interleukin-2 receptor levels in acute and chronic graft-versus-host disease. Leuk Lymphoma 1997;28:159–69.
58. Liu J, Anderson BE, Robert ME, et al. Selective T-cell subset ablation demonstrates a role for T1 and T2 cells in ongoing acute graft-versus-host disease: a model system for the reversal of disease. Blood 2001;98:3367–75.
59. Campen DH, Horwitz DA, Quismorio FP Jr, et al. Serum levels of interleukin-2 receptor and activity of rheumatic diseases characterized by immune system activation. Arthritis Rheum 1988;31:1358–64.
60. Hayashi T, Morishita E, Ontachi Y, et al. Effects of sarpogrelate hydrochloride in a patient with chronic graft-versus-host disease: a case report. Am J Hematol 2006;81:121–3.
61. Chang DM, Wang CJ, Kuo SY, et al. Cell surface markers and circulating cytokines in graft versus host disease. Immunol Invest 1999;28:77–86.
62. Via CS, Rus V, Gately MK, et al. IL-12 stimulates the development of acute graft-versus-host disease in mice that normally would develop chronic, autoimmune graft-versus-host disease. J Immunol 1994;153:4040–7.
63. Cavet J, Dickinson AM, Norden J, et al. Interferon-gamma and interleukin-6 gene polymorphisms associate with graft-versus-host disease in HLA-matched sibling bone marrow transplantation. Blood 2001;98:1594–600.

64. Stark GL, Dickinson AM, Jackson GH, et al. Tumour necrosis factor receptor type II 196M/R genotype correlates with circulating soluble receptor levels in normal subjects and with graft-versus-host disease after sibling allogeneic bone marrow transplantation. Transplantation 2003;76:1742–9.

65. Rocha V, Franco RF, Porcher R, et al. Host defense and inflammatory gene polymorphisms are associated with outcomes after HLA-identical sibling bone marrow transplantation. Blood 2002;100:3908–18.

66. Lin MT, Storer B, Martin PJ, et al. Relation of an interleukin-10 promoter polymorphism to graft-versus-host disease and survival after hematopoietic-cell transplantation. N Engl J Med 2003;349:2201–10.

67. She K, Gilman AL, Aslanian S, et al. Altered Toll-like receptor 9 responses in circulating B cells at the onset of extensive chronic graft-versus-host disease. Biol Blood Marrow Transplant 2007;13:386–97.

68. Fujii H, Cuvelier G, She K, et al. Biomarkers in newly diagnosed pediatric extensive chronic graft-versus-host disease: a report from the Children's Oncology Group. Blood 2008;111(6):3276–85.

69. Saarinen-Pihkala UM, Gustafsson G, Ringden O, et al. No disadvantage in outcome of using matched unrelated donors as compared with matched sibling donors for bone marrow transplantation in children with acute lymphoblastic leukemia in second remission. J Clin Oncol 2001;19:3406–14.

70. Barge RM, Osanto S, Marijt WA, et al. Minimal GVHD following in-vitro T cell-depleted allogeneic stem cell transplantation with reduced-intensity conditioning allowing subsequent infusions of donor lymphocytes in patients with hematological malignancies and solid tumors. Exp Hematol 2003;31:865–72.

71. Langrish CL, Buddle JC, Thrasher AJ, et al. Neonatal dendritic cells are intrinsically biased against Th-1 immune responses. Clin Exp Immunol 2002;128:118–23.

72. Tasker L, Marshall-Clarke S. Functional responses of human neonatal B lymphocytes to antigen receptor cross-linking and CpG DNA. Clin Exp Immunol 2003;134:409–19.

73. Oakhill A, Pamphilon DH, Potter MN, et al. Unrelated donor bone marrow transplantation for children with relapsed acute lymphoblastic leukaemia in second complete remission. Br J Haematol 1996;94:574–8.

74. Fleming DR, Henslee-Downey PJ, Romond EH, et al. Allogeneic bone marrow transplantation with T cell-depleted partially matched related donors for advanced acute lymphoblastic leukemia in children and adults: a comparative matched cohort study. Bone Marrow Transplant 1996;17:917–22.

75. Bunin N, Saunders F, Leahey A, et al. Alternative donor bone marrow transplantation for children with juvenile myelomonocytic leukemia. J Pediatr Hematol Oncol 1999;21:479–85.

76. Green A, Clarke E, Hunt L, et al. Children with acute lymphoblastic leukemia who receive T-cell-depleted HLA mismatched marrow allografts from unrelated donors have an increased incidence of primary graft failure but a similar overall transplant outcome. Blood 1999;94:2236–46.

77. Pavletic SZ, Carter SL, Kernan NA, et al. Influence of T-cell depletion on chronic graft-versus-host disease: results of a multicenter randomized trial in unrelated marrow donor transplantation. Blood 2005;106:3308–13.

78. Baron F, Maris MB, Storer BE, et al. High doses of transplanted CD34+ cells are associated with rapid T-cell engraftment and lessened risk of graft rejection, but not more graft-versus-host disease after nonmyeloablative conditioning and unrelated hematopoietic cell transplantation. Leukemia 2005;19:822–8.

79. Burroughs L, Mielcarek M, Leisenring W, et al. Extending postgrafting cyclo-sporine decreases the risk of severe graft-versus-host disease after nonmyeloa-blative hematopoietic cell transplantation. Transplantation 2006;81:818–25.

80. Wall DA, Carter SL, Kernan NA, et al. Busulfan/melphalan/antithymocyte glob-ulin followed by unrelated donor cord blood transplantation for treatment of infant leukemia and leukemia in young children: the Cord Blood Transplanta-tion study (COBLT) experience. Biol Blood Marrow Transplant 2005;11:637–46.

81. Bacigalupo A, Lamparelli T, Barisione G, et al. Thymoglobulin prevents chronic graft-versus-host disease, chronic lung dysfunction, and late transplant-related mortality: long-term follow-up of a randomized trial in patients undergoing unre-lated donor transplantation. Biol Blood Marrow Transplant 2006;12:560–5.

82. Chakrabarti S, MacDonald D, Hale G, et al. T-cell depletion with Campath-1H "in the bag" for matched related allogeneic peripheral blood stem cell transplanta-tion is associated with reduced graft-versus-host disease, rapid immune consti-tution and improved survival. Br J Haematol 2003;121:109–18.

83. Duval M, Pedron B, Rohrlich P, et al. Immune reconstitution after haematopoietic transplantation with two different doses of pre-graft antithymocyte globulin. Bone Marrow Transplant 2002;30:421–6.

84. Mohty M. Mechanisms of action of antithymocyte globulin: T-cell depletion and beyond. Leukemia 2007;21:1387–94.

85. Giralt S. The role of alemtuzumab in nonmyeloablative hematopoietic transplan-tation. Semin Oncol 2006;33:S36–43.

86. Balduzzi A, Gooley T, Anasetti C, et al. Unrelated donor marrow transplantation in children. Blood 1995;86:3247–56.

87. Davies SM, Wagner JE, Defor T, et al. Unrelated donor bone marrow transplan-tation for children and adolescents with aplastic anaemia or myelodysplasia. Br J Haematol 1997;96:749–56.

88. Bunin N, Carston M, Wall D, et al. Unrelated marrow transplantation for children with acute lymphoblastic leukemia in second remission. Blood 2002;99:3151–7.

89. Talano JA, Margolis DA. Recent molecular and cellular advances in pediatric bone marrow transplantation. Pediatr Clin North Am 2006;53:685–98.

90. Woolfrey AE, Anasetti C, Storer B, et al. Factors associated with outcome after unrelated marrow transplantation for treatment of acute lymphoblastic leukemia in children. Blood 2002;99:2002–8.

91. Giebel S, Giorgiani G, Martinetti M, et al. Low incidence of severe acute graft-versus-host disease in children given haematopoietic stem cell trans-plantation from unrelated donors prospectively matched for HLA class I and II alleles with high-resolution molecular typing. Bone Marrow Transplant 2003;31:987–93.

92. Grupp SA, Frangoul H, Wall D, et al. Use of G-CSF in matched sibling donor pediatric allogeneic transplantation: a consensus statement from the Children's Oncology Group (COG) Transplant Discipline Committee and Pediatric Blood and Marrow Transplant Consortium (PBMTC) Executive Committee. Pediatr Blood Cancer 2006;46:414–21.

93. Cutler C, Antin JH. Peripheral blood stem cells for allogeneic transplantation: a review. Stem Cells 2001;19:108–17.

94. Flowers ME, Parker PM, Johnston LJ, et al. Comparison of chronic graft-versus-host disease after transplantation of peripheral blood stem cells versus bone marrow in allogeneic recipients: long-term follow-up of a randomized trial. Blood 2002;100:415–9.

95. Champlin RE, Schmitz N, Horowitz MM, et al. Blood stem cells compared with bone marrow as a source of hematopoietic cells for allogeneic transplantation. IBMTR Histocompatibility and Stem Cell Sources Working Committee and the European Group for Blood and Marrow Transplantation (EBMT). Blood 2000; 95:3702–9.

96. Watanabe T, Kajiume T, Abe T, et al. Allogeneic peripheral blood stem cell transplantation in children with hematologic malignancies from HLA-matched siblings. Med Pediatr Oncol 2000;34:171–6.

97. Benito AI, Gonzalez-Vicent M, Garcia F, et al. Allogeneic peripheral blood stem cell transplantation (PBSCT) from HLA-identical sibling donors in children with hematological diseases: a single center pilot study. Bone Marrow Transplant 2001;28:537–43.

98. Diaz MA, Gonzalez-Vicent M, Gonzalez ME, et al. Long-term outcome of allogeneic PBSC transplantation in pediatric patients with hematological malignancies: a report of the Spanish Working Party for Blood and Marrow Transplantation in Children (GETMON) and the Spanish Group for Allogeneic Peripheral Blood Transplantation (GETH). Bone Marrow Transplant 2005;36:781–5.

99. Rubinstein P, Carrier C, Scaradavou A, et al. Outcomes among 562 recipients of placental-blood transplants from unrelated donors. N Engl J Med 1998;339: 1565–77.

100. Thomson BG, Robertson KA, Gowan D, et al. Analysis of engraftment, graft-versus-host disease, and immune recovery following unrelated donor cord blood transplantation. Blood 2000;96:2703–11.

101. Yu LC, Wall DA, Sandler E, et al. Unrelated cord blood transplant experience by the pediatric blood and marrow transplant consortium. Pediatr Hematol Oncol 2001;18:235–45.

102. Gluckman E, Rocha V, Chevret S. Results of unrelated umbilical cord blood hematopoietic stem cell transplantation. Rev Clin Exp Hematol 2001;5:87–99.

103. Wagner JE, Barker JN, DeFor TE, et al. Transplantation of unrelated donor umbilical cord blood in 102 patients with malignant and nonmalignant diseases: influence of CD34 cell dose and HLA disparity on treatment-related mortality and survival. Blood 2002;100:1611–8.

104. Barker JN. Who should get cord blood transplants? Biol Blood Marrow Transplant 2007;13(Suppl 1):78–82.

105. Eapen M, Rubinstein P, Zhang MJ, et al. Outcomes of transplantation of unrelated donor umbilical cord blood and bone marrow in children with acute leukaemia: a comparison study. Lancet 2007;369:1947–54.

106. Kamani N, Spellman S, Hurley CK, et al. State of the art review: HLA matching and outcome of unrelated donor umbilical cord blood transplants. Biol Blood Marrow Transplant 2008;14:1–6.

107. Arora M, Nagaraj S, Wagner JE, et al. Chronic graft-versus-host disease (cGVHD) following unrelated donor hematopoietic stem cell transplantation (HSCT): higher response rate in recipients of unrelated donor (URD) umbilical cord blood (UCB). Biol Blood Marrow Transplant 2007;13:1145–52.

108. Akpek G, Zahurak ML, Piantadosi S, et al. Development of a prognostic model for grading chronic graft-versus-host disease. Blood 2001;97:1219–26.

109. Lee S, Cook EF, Soiffer R, et al. Development and validation of a scale to measure symptoms of chronic graft-versus-host disease. Biol Blood Marrow Transplant 2002;8:444–52.

110. Imai H, Oyama Y, Miura AB, et al. Hematopoietic cell transplantation-related nephropathy in Japan. Am J Kidney Dis 2000;36:474–80.

111. Srinivasan R, Balow JE, Sabnis S, et al. Nephrotic syndrome: an under-recog nised immune-mediated complication of non-myeloablative allogeneic haematopoietic cell transplantation. Br J Haematol 2005;131:74–9.

112. Colombo AA, Rusconi C, Esposito C, et al. Nephrotic syndrome after allogeneic hematopoietic stem cell transplantation as a late complication of chronic graft-versus-host disease. Transplantation 2006;81:1087–92.

113. Gilman AL, Kooy NW, Atkins DL, et al. Complete heart block in association with graft-versus-host disease. Bone Marrow Transplant 1998;21:85–8.

114. Rackley C, Schultz KR, Goldman FD, et al. Cardiac manifestations of graft-versus-host disease. Biol Blood Marrow Transplant 2005;11:773–80.

115. Couriel D, Carpenter PA, Cutler C, et al. Ancillary therapy and supportive care of chronic graft-versus-host disease: national institutes of health consensus development project on criteria for clinical trials in chronic graft-versus-host disease: V. Ancillary Therapy and Supportive Care Working Group Report. Biol Blood Marrow Transplant 2006;12:375–96.

116. Chosidow O, Bagot M, Vernant JP, et al. Sclerodermatous chronic graft-versus-host disease. Analysis of seven cases. J Am Acad Dermatol 1992;26:49–55.

117. Penas PF, Jones-Caballero M, Aragues M, et al. Sclerodermatous graft-vs-host disease: clinical and pathological study of 17 patients. Arch Dermatol 2002;138:924–34.

118. Beredjiklian PK, Drummond DS, Dormans JP, et al. Orthopaedic manifestations of chronic graft-versus-host disease. J Pediatr Orthop 1998;18:572–5.

119. Stern JM, Chesnut CH 3rd, Bruemmer B, et al. Bone density loss during treatment of chronic GVHD. Bone Marrow Transplant 1996;17:395–400.

120. Tauchmanova L, De Rosa G, Serio B, et al. Avascular necrosis in long-term survivors after allogeneic or autologous stem cell transplantation: a single center experience and a review. Cancer 2003;97:2453–61.

121. Franklin RM, Kenyon KR, Tutschka PJ, et al. Ocular manifestations of graft-vs-host disease. Ophthalmology 1983;90:4–13.

122. Pavletic SZ, Martin P, Lee SJ, et al. Measuring therapeutic response in chronic graft-versus-host disease: National Institutes of Health Consensus Development Project on Criteria for Clinical Trials in Chronic Graft-versus-Host Disease: IV. Response Criteria Working Group Report. Biol Blood Marrow Transplant 2006;12:252–66.

123. Treister NS, Woo SB, O'Holleran EW, et al. Oral chronic graft-versus-host disease in pediatric patients after hematopoietic stem cell transplantation. Biol Blood Marrow Transplant 2005;11:721–31.

124. Imanguli MM, Pavletic SZ, Guadagnini JP, et al. Chronic graft versus host disease of oral mucosa: review of available therapies. Oral Surg Oral Med Oral Pathol Oral Radiol Endod 2006;101:175–83.

125. Jacobsohn DA, Montross S, Anders V, et al. Clinical importance of confirming or excluding the diagnosis of chronic graft-versus-host disease. Bone Marrow Transplant 2001;28:1047–51.

126. Browning B, Thormann K, Seshadri R, et al. Weight loss and reduced body mass index: a critical issue in children with multiorgan chronic graft-versus-host disease. Bone Marrow Transplant 2006;37:527–33.

127. Shulman HM, Sharma P, Amos D, et al. A coded histologic study of hepatic graft-versus-host disease after human bone marrow transplantation. Hepatology 1988;8:463–70.

128. Strasser SI, Shulman HM, Flowers ME, et al. Chronic graft-versus-host disease of the liver: presentation as an acute hepatitis. Hepatology 2000;32:1265–71.

129. Akpek G, Boitnott JK, Lee LA, et al. Hepatitic variant of graft-versus-host disease after donor lymphocyte infusion. Blood 2002;100:3903–7.
130. Melin-Aldana H, Thormann K, Duerst R, et al. Hepatitic pattern of graft versus host disease in children. Pediatr Blood Cancer 2007;49:727–30.
131. Cooke KR, Yanik G. Lung injury following hematopoietic cell transplantation. In: Appelbaum FR, Forman SJ, Negrin RS, et al, editors. Thomas' hematopoietic cell transplantation. 4th edition. Wiley-Blackwell; 2009.
132. Afessa B, Litzow MR, Tefferi A. Bronchiolitis obliterans and other late onset non-infectious pulmonary complications in hematopoietic stem cell transplantation. Bone Marrow Transplant 2001;28:425–34.
133. Dudek AZ, Mahaseth H, DeFor TE, et al. Bronchiolitis obliterans in chronic graft-versus-host disease: analysis of risk factors and treatment outcomes. Biol Blood Marrow Transplant 2003;9:657–66.
134. Ratanatharathorn V, Ayash L, Lazarus HM, et al. Chronic graft-versus-host disease: clinical manifestation and therapy. Bone Marrow Transplant 2001;28: 121–9.
135. Freudenberger TD, Madtes DK, Curtis JR, et al. Association between acute and chronic graft-versus-host disease and bronchiolitis obliterans organizing pneumonia in recipients of hematopoietic stem cell transplants. Blood 2003;102: 3822–8.
136. Yoshihara S, Yanik G, Cooke KR, et al. Bronchiolitis obliterans syndrome (BOS), bronchiolitis obliterans organizing pneumonia (BOOP), and other late-onset noninfectious pulmonary complications following allogeneic hematopoietic stem cell transplantation. Biol Blood Marrow Transplant 2007;13: 749–59.
137. Khouri IF, Ippoliti C, Gajewski J, et al. Neutropenias following allogeneic bone marrow transplantation: response to therapy with high-dose intravenous immunoglobulin. Am J Hematol 1996;52:313–5.
138. Au WY, Lo CM, Hawkins BR, et al. Evans' syndrome complicating chronic graft versus host disease after cadaveric liver transplantation. Transplantation 2001; 72:527–8.
139. Tomonari A, Tojo A, Lseki T, et al. Severe autoimmune thrombocytopenia after allogeneic bone marrow transplantation for aplastic anemia. Int J Hematol 2001;74:228–32.
140. Sullivan KM, Witherspoon RP, Storb R, et al. Prednisone and azathioprine compared with prednisone and placebo for treatment of chronic graft-v-host disease: prognostic influence of prolonged thrombocytopenia after allogeneic marrow transplantation. Blood 1988;72:546–54.
141. Nevo S, Enger C, Hartley E, et al. Acute bleeding and thrombocytopenia after bone marrow transplantation. Bone Marrow Transplant 2001;27:65–72.
142. Jacobsohn DA, Schechter T, Seshadri R, et al. Eosinophilia correlates with the presence or development of chronic graft-versus-host disease in children. Transplantation 2004;77:1096–100.
143. Siadak M, Sullivan KM. The management of chronic graft-versus-host disease. Blood Rev 1994;8:154–60.
144. Storek J, Witherspoon RP, Webb D, et al. Lack of B cells precursors in marrow transplant recipients with chronic graft-versus-host disease. Am J Hematol 1996;52:82–9.
145. Maury S, Mary JY, Rabian C, et al. Prolonged immune deficiency following allogeneic stem cell transplantation: risk factors and complications in adult patients. Br J Haematol 2001;115:630–41.

146. Atkinson K. Reconstruction of the haemopoietic and immune systems after marrow transplantation. Bone Marrow Transplant 1990;5:209–26.
147. Storek J, Witherspoon RP, Maloney DG, et al. Improved reconstitution of CD4 T cells and B cells but worsened reconstitution of serum IgG levels after allogeneic transplantation of blood stem cells instead of marrow. Blood 1997;89: 3891–3.
148. Rege K, Mehta J, Treleaven J, et al. Fatal pneumococcal infections following allogeneic bone marrow transplant. Bone Marrow Transplant 1994;14:903–6.
149. Kulkarni S, Powles R, Treleaven J, et al. Chronic graft versus host disease is associated with long-term risk for pneumococcal infections in recipients of bone marrow transplants. Blood 2000;95:3683–6.
150. Stewart BL, Storer B, Storek J, et al. Duration of immunosuppressive treatment for chronic graft-versus-host disease. Blood 2004;104:3501–6.
151. Martin PJ, Storer BE, Rowley SD, et al. Evaluation of mycophenolate mofetil for initial treatment of chronic graft-versus-host disease. Blood 2009;113: 5074–82.
152. Wingard JR, Piantadosi S, Vogelsang GB, et al. Predictors of death from chronic graft-versus-host disease after bone marrow transplantation. Blood 1989;74: 1428–35.
153. Sehgal SN. Rapamune (Sirolimus, rapamycin): an overview and mechanism of action. Ther Drug Monit 1995;17:660–5.
154. Benito AI, Furlong T, Martin PJ, et al. Sirolimus (rapamycin) for the treatment of steroid-refractory acute graft-versus-host disease. Transplantation 2001;72: 1924–9.
155. Cutler C, Antin JH. Sirolimus for GVHD prophylaxis in allogeneic stem cell transplantation. Bone Marrow Transplant 2004;34:471–6.
156. Couriel DR, Saliba R, Escalon MP, et al. Sirolimus in combination with tacrolimus and corticosteroids for the treatment of resistant chronic graft-versus-host disease. Br J Haematol 2005;130:409–17.
157. Johnston LJ, Brown J, Shizuru JA, et al. Rapamycin (sirolimus) for treatment of chronic graft-versus-host disease. Biol Blood Marrow Transplant 2005;11:47–55.
158. Jurado M, Vallejo C, Perez-Simon JA, et al. Sirolimus as part of immunosuppressive therapy for refractory chronic graft-versus-host disease. Biol Blood Marrow Transplant 2007;13:701–6.
159. Mookerjee B, Altomonte V, Vogelsang G. Salvage therapy for refractory chronic graft-versus-host disease with mycophenolate mofetil and tacrolimus. Bone Marrow Transplant 1999;24:517–20.
160. Busca A, Saroglia EM, Lanino E, et al. Mycophenolate mofetil (MMF) as therapy for refractory chronic GVHD (cGVHD) in children receiving bone marrow transplantation. Bone Marrow Transplant 2000;25:1067–71.
161. Yusuf USJ, Stephan V. Mycophenolate mofetil (MMF) as salvage treatment for steroid-refractory chronic graft-versus-host-disease (GVHD) in children [abstract]. Blood 2001;98:398a.
162. Lopez F, Parker P, Nademanee A, et al. Efficacy of mycophenolate mofetil in the treatment of chronic graft-versus-host disease. Biol Blood Marrow Transplant 2005;11:307–13.
163. Krejci M, Doubek M, Buchler T, et al. Mycophenolate mofetil for the treatment of acute and chronic steroid-refractory graft-versus-host disease. Ann Hematol 2005;84:681–5.
164. Giblett ER, Anderson JE, Cohen F, et al. Adenosine-deaminase deficiency in two patients with severely impaired cellular immunity. Lancet 1972;2:1067–9.

165. Saven A, Piro L. Newer purine analogues for the treatment of hairy-cell leukemia. N Engl J Med 1994;330:691–7.
166. Jacobsohn DA, Chen AR, Zahurak M, et al. Phase II study of pentostatin in patients with corticosteroid-refractory chronic graft-versus-host disease. J Clin Oncol 2007;25:4255–61.
167. Mackenzie AH. Antimalarial drugs for rheumatoid arthritis. Am J Med 1983;75: 48–58.
168. Olson NY, Lindsley CB. Adjunctive use of hydroxychloroquine in childhood dermatomyositis. J Rheumatol 1989;16:1545–7.
169. Vogelsang GB, Farmer ER, Hess AD, et al. Thalidomide for the treatment of chronic graft-versus-host disease. N Engl J Med 1992;326:1055–8.
170. Cole CH, Rogers PC, Pritchard S, et al. Thalidomide in the management of chronic graft-versus-host disease in children following bone marrow transplantation. Bone Marrow Transplant 1994;14:937–42.
171. Rovelli A, Arrigo C, Nesi F, et al. The role of thalidomide in the treatment of refractory chronic graft-versus-host disease following bone marrow transplantation in children. Bone Marrow Transplant 1998;21:577–81.
172. Edelson R, Berger C, Gasparro F, et al. Treatment of cutaneous T-cell lymphoma by extracorporeal photochemotherapy. Preliminary results. N Engl J Med 1987; 316:297–303.
173. Greinix HT, Volc-Platzer B, Kalhs P, et al. Extracorporeal photochemotherapy in the treatment of severe steroid-refractory acute graft-versus-host disease: a pilot study. Blood 2000;96:2426–31.
174. Couriel D, Hosing C, Saliba R, et al. Extracorporeal photopheresis for acute and chronic graft-versus-host disease: does it work? Biol Blood Marrow Transplant 2006;12:37–40.
175. Couriel DR, Hosing C, Saliba R, et al. Extracorporeal photochemotherapy for the treatment of steroid-resistant chronic GVHD. Blood 2006;107:3074–80.
176. Foss FM, DiVenuti GM, Chin K, et al. Prospective study of extracorporeal photopheresis in steroid-refractory or steroid-resistant extensive chronic graft-versus-host disease: analysis of response and survival incorporating prognostic factors. Bone Marrow Transplant 2005;35:1187–93.
177. Rubegni P, Cuccia A, Sbano P, et al. Role of extracorporeal photochemotherapy in patients with refractory chronic graft-versus-host disease. Br J Haematol 2005;130:271–5.
178. Salvaneschi L, Perotti C, Zecca M, et al. Extracorporeal photochemotherapy for treatment of acute and chronic GVHD in childhood. Transfusion 2001;41: 1299–305.
179. Messina C, Locatelli F, Lanino E, et al. Extracorporeal photochemotherapy for paediatric patients with graft-versus-host disease after haematopoietic stem cell transplantation. Br J Haematol 2003;122:118–27.
180. Srinivasan R, Chakrabarti S, Walsh T, et al. Improved survival in steroid-refractory acute graft versus host disease after non-myeloablative allogeneic transplantation using a daclizumab-based strategy with comprehensive infection prophylaxis. Br J Haematol 2004;124:777–86.
181. Yanik GA, Uberti JP, Ferrara JLM, et al. Etanercept for sub-acute lung injury following allogeneic stem cell transplantation. Blood 2003;102:471a.
182. Busca A, Locatelli F, Marmont F, et al. Recombinant human soluble tumor necrosis factor receptor fusion protein as treatment for steroid refractory graft-versus-host disease following allogeneic hematopoietic stem cell transplantation. Am J Hematol 2007;82:45–52.

183. Magro L, Mohty M, Catteau B, et al. Imatinib mesylate as salvage therapy for refractory sclerotic chronic graft-versus-host disease. Blood 2009;114:719–22.
184. Olivieri A, Locatelli F, Zecca M, et al. Imatinib for refractory chronic graft-versus-host disease with fibrotic features. Blood 2009;114:709–18.
185. Leung W, Ahn H, Rose SR, et al. A prospective cohort study of late sequelae of pediatric allogeneic hematopoietic stem cell transplantation. Medicine (Baltimore) 2007;86:215–24.
186. Falcini F, Taccetti G, Trapani S, et al. Growth retardation in juvenile chronic arthritis patients treated with steroids. Clin Exp Rheumatol 1991;9(Suppl 6): 37–40.
187. Lai HC, FitzSimmons SC, Allen DB, et al. Risk of persistent growth impairment after alternate-day prednisone treatment in children with cystic fibrosis. N Engl J Med 2000;342:851–9.
188. Baker KS, Fraser CJ. Quality of life and recovery after graft-versus-host disease. Best Pract Res Clin Haematol 2008;21:333–41.
189. Lee SJ, Kim HT, Ho VT, et al. Quality of life associated with acute and chronic graft-versus-host disease. Bone Marrow Transplant 2006;38:305–10.
190. Oeffinger KC, Mertens AC, Sklar CA, et al. Chronic health conditions in adult survivors of childhood cancer. N Engl J Med 2006;355:1572–82.

The Burden of Cure: Long-term Side Effects Following Hematopoietic Stem Cell Transplantation (HSCT) in Children

K. Scott Baker, MD, MS[a], Dorine Bresters, MD, PhD[b],
Jane E. Sande, MD[c],*

KEYWORDS

- Late effects • Pediatric bone marrow transplantation
- Long-term follow-up

In the last several decades, hematopoietic stem cell transplantation (HSCT) has become accepted as a standard-of-care treatment modality for an increasing number of malignant and nonmalignant diseases of children. Advances in patient and donor selection, preparative regimen design and delivery, and supportive care have led to improved patient survival. As more children survive HSCT, however, the price of survival has become increasingly apparent in the protean manifestations of the late effects of treatment.

Late effects following treatment of childhood cancer are increasingly well studied; less is known about late effects specifically attributable to HSCT, although several studies document more complications in transplant survivors than in those treated with chemotherapy alone for similar diseases. Very little is known about late complications following reduced-intensity conditioning regimens, or HSCT for nonmalignant disorders.

[a] Survivorship Program, Fred Hutchinson Cancer Research Center, University of Washington, 1100 Fairview Avenue N, Mailstop D5-280, PO Box 19024, Seattle, WA 98109-1024, USA
[b] Department of Pediatric Immunology, Hemato-Oncology, and Bone Marrow Transplantation, Leiden University Medical Center, Postbus 9600, 2300 RC Leiden, The Netherlands
[c] Blood and Marrow Transplant Program, Division of BMT and Immunology, Center for Cancer and Blood Disorders, Children's National Medical Center, The George Washington University, 111 Michigan Avenue NE, Washington, DC 20010, USA
* Corresponding author.
E-mail address: jsande@cnmc.org

Pediatr Clin N Am 57 (2010) 323–342
doi:10.1016/j.pcl.2009.11.008   **pediatric.theclinics.com**
0031-3955/10/$ – see front matter © 2010 Elsevier Inc. All rights reserved.

This article reviews recent literature on the study of childhood HSCT survivors through a systems-based approach and provides current references for topics of interest.

SYSTEMS-BASED REVIEW
Cardiovascular

The risks for late cardiovascular (CV) disease or events in survivors after HSCT have not yet been studied in detail. For the HSCT patient, the risk is cumulative, and in addition to pretransplant conditioning therapy, pre-HSCT treatment exposures including cumulative doses of anthracyclines and exposure to radiation therapy that may have included the heart or mediastinum, have to be accounted for. For anthracyclines the risk is dose and age dependent, with the highest risk for cardiomyopathy seen at doses of 550 mg/m^2 or higher in patients older than 18 years, and at doses of 300 mg/m^2 or higher in patients less than 18 years at the time of treatment.[1,2] However, higher risks are associated with the combined exposure to radiation therapy. In HSCT patients there is frequently the additional exposure to high-dose cyclophosphamide (CY), which has been described as a cause of acute cardiotoxicity, and to total body irradiation (TBI). In practice the CY/TBI regimen is a commonly used transplant regimen, and there does not seem to be a great deal of clinical evidence on the long-term risk of cardiomyopathy in HSCT patients who do not have significant pre-HSCT exposure to cardiotoxic therapies.

A higher risk of CV mortality has been described in childhood cancer survivors; the standardized mortality ratio for cardiac-related deaths was 8.2 (95% confidence interval [CI] 6.4–10.4) among 5-year or longer survivors of childhood cancer, and 3.8 (95% CI 1.5–7.6) for leukemia survivors.[3] Although CV mortality has not been specifically evaluated in a population of pediatric survivors after HSCT, large studies of late mortality after HSCT that have included children have shown a higher risk of mortality from CV events compared with the general population. The Bone Marrow Transplant Survivor Study has evaluated selected CV risk factors, and survivors of allogeneic HSCT were found to be 3.65 times (95% CI 1.82–7.32) more likely to report diabetes mellitus than siblings and 2.06 times (95% CI 1.39–3.04) more likely to report hypertension compared with siblings.[4] Allogeneic HSCT survivors were also more likely to develop hypertension (OR = 2.31, 95% CI1.45–3.67) than autologous recipients and TBI exposure was associated with an increased risk of diabetes mellitus (OR = 3.42, 95% CI 1.55–7.52). The patients in this cohort were relatively young (mean age at survey completion was 39.3 years); thus, the concern is that the higher risk of these outcomes at a relatively young age will lead to a higher than expected risk of CV events as these individuals grow older. Long-term screening for the development of hypertension and diabetes mellitus and screening for other CV risk factors such as lipid abnormalities and obesity are certainly indicated in HSCT survivors.

Metabolic Syndrome

The metabolic syndrome (central obesity, insulin resistance, glucose intolerance, dyslipidemia, and hypertension) is associated with a substantially increased risk for type 2 diabetes mellitus and atherosclerotic cardiovascular disease (CVD).[5–7] Although limited, there is evidence to suggest that long-term childhood cancer survivors may be at high risk for premature development of characteristics associated with the metabolic syndrome.[8–10] In 1 study, 23 long-term survivors (median age 20 years), who were 3–18 years post HSCT for leukemia, 13 patients in remission from leukemia without HSCT, and 23 healthy age- and sex-matched controls were evaluated for metabolic syndrome parameters. Hyperinsulinemia, impaired glucose tolerance, hypertriglyceridemia, low high-density lipoprotein (HDL)-cholesterol, and abdominal obesity were more common among the HSCT survivors than among the non-HSCT group of leukemia patients or the healthy controls.[11] Core signs of the metabolic syndrome were found in 39% of HSCT survivors versus 8% of leukemia controls and 0% of healthy controls. Fifty-two percent of HSCT patients were found to have hyperinsulinemia and 43% had abnormal glucose metabolism, compared with none of the healthy controls ($P = .0002$ and 0.001 respectively). Variables associated with hyperinsulinemia in the HSCT patients were time from transplantation ($P = .01$), presence of chronic graft-versus-host disease (GVHD) ($P = .01$), and hypogonadism ($P = .04$). Another study in 34 children and adolescents after either autologous or allogeneic HSCT compared with 21 age- and sex-matched controls found that the 18 patients who received TBI had a significantly higher first phase insulin response and insulinemia/glycemia ratio on glucose tolerance testing compared with patients who received only lymphoid radiation, no radiation, or controls.[12] These results suggest that TBI may play a role in the development of insulin resistance.

In ongoing studies of CV risk in survivors of HSCT for hematologic malignancy, measures of insulin resistance, fasting glucose, insulin, lipids, anthropometry, blood pressure, and carotid artery compliance and distensibility were determined in 106 children and young adults (current age 26.6 years) who had received HSCT for hematologic malignancy during childhood (mean age at HSCT 9.9 years) and 72 healthy sibling controls. Sixty-two patients received TBI, 20 received cranial radiation before TBI (TBI + cranial radiation), and 24 received no TBI or cranial radiation (noXRT) before or during HSCT. Metabolic syndrome was present in 15/106 (14.2%) HSCT survivors and 4/72 (5.6%) controls (odds ratio [OR] 2.3, 95% CI 0.7–7.7, $P = .16$). However, 2 or more components of metabolic syndrome were present in 39/106 (37%) survivors and only 10/72 (13.9%) controls (OR, 2.7, 95% CI 1.2–5.9, $P = .015$). Compared with siblings, there were no differences between groups for glucose, body mass index (BMI, calculated as weight in kilograms divided by the square of height in meters), waist circumference, percent body fat, or blood pressure. However, HSCT survivors who had TBI or TBI + cranial radiation all had significantly higher total cholesterol, low-density lipoprotein (LDL)-cholesterol, triglycerides, and insulin. Those who received TBI + cranial radiation had significantly lower HDL-cholesterol and were also more insulin resistant. However, for the patients who did not receive any radiation before or during HSCT, there were no differences in any of the CV risk factors compared with controls. These findings are of concern and suggest that even at a relatively young age, and independent of obesity, survivors of HSCT for childhood hematologic malignancies have increased CV risk factors that are associated with exposure to TBI and/or cranial radiation. These abnormalities may ultimately contribute to a higher risk of early CV morbidity and mortality; thus early screening and management of modifiable CV and metabolic risk factors should be considered in HSCT survivors.[13]

Pulmonary Late Effects

Pulmonary toxicity of HSCT is a major cause of morbidity and mortality in the first year after transplant and impaired pulmonary function (PF) after transplant is a common late effect. Obstructive pattern PF is present in bronchiolitis obliterans within the context of chronic GVHD, typically in the first year after transplant. Obstructive PF is only found in up to 10% of childhood HSCT survivors, but has a high morbidity and mortality.[14–19] Restrictive and impaired diffusion pattern PF have been shown to be much more common long-term after HSCT. Restrictive PF and/or impaired diffusion capacity have been found in 20% to 40% and 35% to 80% of childhood HSCT survivors, respectively.[14,17,19,20] It has been shown that PF may be abnormal even before HSCT, likely as a result of previous treatment, such as chemotherapy or radiation for malignant disease.[15,16,19,21] After HSCT, PF may deteriorate in the first 1 to 2 years, with some improvement in the years thereafter.[15,16,19,22] However, PF does not normalize or return to pretransplant values and 5 to 10 years after HSCT, restrictive PF abnormality and impaired diffusion persist.[14,16,17] Currently, the course of the PF abnormalities more than 10 years after HSCT in childhood is unknown. Only 1 cross-sectional study analyzed PF in pediatric HSCT survivors more than 10 years after HSCT.[20] Fortunately, most children have only mild to moderate impairment of PF and are asymptomatic, with impaired function detected by PF tests only.[14,16,17,19] Analysis of risk factors for impaired PF after HSCT has been hampered by small patient numbers in most studies; some patients received pulmotoxic treatment of their underlying malignant disease pre-HSCT and most conditioning regimens include at least 1 pulmotoxic modality. Busulfan and TBI in the conditioning regimen have been determined to be risk factors for impaired PF.[16,22]

Although childhood cancer survivors are noted to have an increased risk of recurrent infection and chronic cough,[23] no such data exist for children who have undergone HSCT. Additional information is required with regard to long-term PF in children who have undergone transplantation.

Endocrine

There is a high prevalence of endocrine dysfunction in children who survive HSCT. This is attributed to the conditioning regimens used, whether or not they contain radiation or high-dose chemotherapy only. Disturbances in thyroid function, onset of puberty, fertility, bone health, and growth and development, all are commonly reported.

Thyroid dysfunction

Thyroid dysfunction is common post HSCT and is reported in up to 50% of survivors.[24–27] The wide variation in incidence may be attributed to time post transplant, with those surviving longest at highest risk.[24,28,29]

Abnormalities described include sick euthyroid syndrome, especially occurring early post HSCT,[28] overt hypothyroidism, compensated hypothyroidism, thyrotoxicosis (rarely), and secondary thyroid carcinomas. The use of radiation was initially felt to be the primary cause of thyroid dysfunction. However, recent data have also implicated chemotherapy-only regimens, particularly those using busulfan.[24,29,30]

Puberty and fertility

Normal pubertal development is a result of complex interactions between the hypothalamus (gonadotropin-releasing hormone), the pituitary (luteinizing hormone (LH) and follicle-stimulating hormone (FSH) production), sex steroid hormone production and secretion, and target organ responsiveness. For most individuals studied post HSCT, the hypothalamic-pituitary axis appears intact, with increased production of LH and FSH in the setting of delayed puberty, amenorrhea, and/or azoospermia. In general, for women, hormonal function correlates with fertility. Prepubertal females can tolerate higher doses of alkylating agents than pubertal females due to decreasing ovarian follicle reserves with age, but high doses of radiation and busulfan can lead to premature ovarian failure. For males, endocrine function is retained at higher doses of radiation or alkylating agents than females, but spermatogenesis is much more vulnerable. High-dose chemotherapy and radiation result in damage to the germinal epithelium, with increased LH levels but usually normal testosterone levels, reflecting the

Leydig cells' resistance to cytotoxic agents relative to Sertoli cells.[25,31–36] Puberty is often delayed for these boys. Girls receiving chemotherapy and fractionated radiation before puberty may enter and progress through puberty normally; postpubertal girls often experience amenorrhea, with few experiencing ovarian function recovery over time. Preparative regimens that include busulfan and radiation are strongly associated with ovarian failure and azoospermia.[36–38] In contrast, children receiving cyclophosphamide alone usually enter and progress through puberty normally, although ovarian failure has been observed in these patients.

There have been several reports of successful pregnancies in women who have undergone HSCT or are married to men who underwent HSCT. Congenital anomalies are not increased more than that of the general population; however, there is a higher incidence of cesarean section, preterm delivery, and low birthweight in babies born to transplant survivors compared with the general population.[32,39,40]

Growth
Like puberty, growth is dependent on the complex interplay of several factors. Several studies have demonstrated significant growth delay in children undergoing HSCT. Radiation, especially craniospinal radiation, is implicated as the primary cause of growth failure post HSCT. The hypothalamic-pituitary axis can be damaged by cranial radiation, resulting in decreased growth hormone (GH) production. Radiation can also damage the epiphyseal growth plates of bone, leading to premature fusion. In addition, the pubertal growth spurt, which is dependent on the interaction between sex steroids and GH, will not occur in the setting of poor gonadal function. Growth deficiency has been documented in children receiving TBI,[31,33,41] TBI plus craniospinal irradiation,[31,41,42] and in children who received TBI who also were treated for chronic GVHD.[31] Fractionated TBI seems to have less effect than single-dose radiation, but still produces overall reduced final height (although still within population norms). In documented GH deficiency, GH replacement has been helpful in minimizing the growth loss associated with HSCT-related therapies, but it does not seem to result in catch-up growth.[43–46]

Bone health
There are several retrospective and cross-sectional studies of bone mineral density (BMD) in pediatric HSCT survivors, and 1 prospective study.[47–52] Whether decreased BMD is related to transplant or caused by pretransplant conditions is unclear. Childhood cancer survivors, for example, are known to be at high risk for osteopenia and osteoporosis, conditions that predispose to or are associated with decreased BMD. Recently, however, studies have shown that children with nonmalignant diseases may also have decreased BMD before undergoing transplantation.[47,50] BMD loss for children undergoing HSCT has been shown to be more profound than that of adults. This is highly significant, as BMD loss in childhood may result in relatively decreased peak bone mass and increased risk or early onset osteoporosis and fractures later in life.[51] A prospective study from the University of Minnesota showed the most profound loss of BMD within the first 6 months following HSCT, similar to what is reported in adults. Some children recovered; however, 33% remained osteopenic and 19% osteoporotic at 1 year following HSCT.[52]

Risk factors for BMD loss during HSCT include chemo- and radiotherapy, glucocorticoid use, prolonged physical inactivity, transient estrogen insufficiency in females, and use of total parenteral nutrition.[53] A retrospective study from Seattle suggests that the use of bisphosphonates in addition to supplemental vitamin D and calcium may reverse osteopenia and osteoporosis post HSCT.[54] This intervention requires further study.

Renal

Acute and chronic renal dysfunction have long been associated with HSCT. Multiple factors contribute to acute renal insufficiency in the immediate posttransplant setting, including chemotherapy and radiation, medications used during HSCT (particularly calcineurin inhibitors), extreme fluid shifts, venoocclusive disease of the liver, hepatorenal syndrome, sepsis, and the antimicrobial agents used to treat infections. Chronic renal insufficiency following HSCT has often been attributed to radiation-induced renal injury but has also been associated with chronic GVHD.[55–59] There are 3 prospective studies reporting on renal function in children post HSCT.[57–59] Kist-van Holthe and colleagues[57] found acute renal insufficiency post HSCT to be associated with venoocclusive disease of the liver, high serum cyclosporine levels, and foscarnet therapy, but not with radiation. In addition, they found that acute renal insufficiency was the only risk factor for development of chronic renal disease. Patzer and colleagues[59] found glomerular filtration rates to be normal post HSCT, but significantly lower than pre-HSCT testing. Unlike Kist-van Holthe and colleagues these investigators found no correlation between renal insufficiency early after transplant and chronic renal insufficiency. Frisk and colleagues[58] was the only study to find a correlation between renal insufficiency and radiation. These investigators found that TBI was associated with chronic renal insufficiency.

Gastrointestinal/Hepatic Late Effects

Most HSCT procedures are complicated by gastrointestinal mucosal injury. The gastrointestinal tract is also commonly involved in acute GVHD. However, late luminal gastrointestinal problems after HSCT have not been reported to date and acute gastrointestinal problems seem to be reversible in most children.

By contrast, elevated liver enzymes are a common occurrence in the acute phase after HSCT and long-term, with studies in children and adults showing a prevalence of recurrent or persistently abnormal liver enzymes 1 to 10 years after transplant that varies from 10% to 57%.[60–64] Only 3 studies have focused on late (1–6 years post HSCT) hepatic effects after transplant in childhood.[60,61,64] These studies showed a prevalence of abnormal liver enzymes in childhood allogeneic HSCT survivors of 25%[60,64] and 53%,[61] respectively. In the study by Locasciulli and colleagues[61] this was explained in more than half of the patients by hepatitis C virus (HCV) and/or hepatitis B virus (HBV) infection in children who had received blood transfusion before HCV screening was implemented. Abnormal liver enzymes late after HSCT have been found to be caused by chronic viral hepatitis B or C, iron overload, chronic GVHD, and autoimmune hepatitis.[61–67] As a result of the implementation of screening of blood products for HBV and HCV, transfusion-acquired viral hepatitis is less common in survivors of HSCT transplanted more recently.[60,64] Chronic GVHD as a cause of abnormal liver enzymes is more prevalent in adults compared with children after HSCT.[60,62,64] In a proportion of HSCT survivors with elevated liver enzymes, no apparent cause is found.[61,62,64]

In most HSCT survivors with elevated liver enzymes, synthetic and metabolic liver function is normal and no signs or symptoms of liver disease are found.[61,62,64] Pediatricians are obviously reluctant to perform liver biopsies in these children, and histopathologic correlates are thus unknown. It is uncertain, especially in cases of unknown cause, how liver function may evolve in these patients over time and if survivors are at risk for cirrhosis.

Another reported late hepatic effect of chemotherapy and/or HSCT is the development of focal nodular hyperplasia (FNH).[68,69] FNH is the second most common benign tumor of the liver and may mimic metastases and secondary malignant tumors. Magnetic resonance images are diagnostic and no further investigations are needed, but long-term imaging surveys are recommended.[68,69] Neither complications nor malignant transformation of FNH have been reported to date.

Oral/Dental Late Effects

Reported oral and dental problems after cancer treatment and/or HSCT include xerostomia, gingivitis, abnormal development of teeth (tooth agenesis, hypodontia, microdontia, enamel hypoplasia, malformed roots, taurodontia), delayed eruption, over-retention of primary teeth, and increased caries index.[70–77] Disturbances in craniofacial growth may be seen[78] and a higher risk of developing secondary oral tumors exists.[79] Adverse effects on mineralized dental tissues are typically irreversible and may affect the quality of life (QoL) of survivors permanently. Some studies have indicated that xerostomia is a significant problem in childhood HSCT survivors, even in those who did not receive TBI.[70,71] Fibrosis of the salivary gland ducts may occur in the context of chronic GVHD.

Chemotherapy and radiotherapy have been described as risk factors for dental late effects.[71–77] Children less than 5 years old at the time of HSCT have been shown to have the highest risk for dental late effects, especially involving developmental problems but also including caries and gingival problems.[72,73] Dental late effects are less common in children aged 12 years or older at the time of transplant. The development of permanent teeth and their roots starts at about 3 years of age and may last up to the age of 7.5 years. Chemotherapy and radiotherapy given at this time will therefore likely interfere with dental development.

Regular dental care by a dentist familiar with HSCT-related oral and dental late effects is important in children and adults after HSCT in childhood.

Ocular Late Effects

Cataracts are the most commonly reported ocular late effect of pediatric HSCT, with cumulative incidence rates ranging from 28% to 78% in various studies.[80–85] The development of cataracts is strongly associated with the use of TBI in conditioning regimens, but in some studies is also influenced by steroid administration and the presence of chronic GVHD. Ocular sicca syndrome (associated with chronic GVHD) and microvascular retinopathy have also been reported.

Neurocognitive Late Effects

As more and more children survive HSCT, progress through school, and enter adulthood, more attention is being focused on neurocognitive and psychosocial outcomes. Several recent prospective studies have evaluated neurocognitive function before and after HSCT, with patients evaluated from 1 to 5 years post transplant. All studies suffer from high attrition rates. In addition, measurement scales are not consistent across ages and developmental stages, which makes longitudinal comparison of outcomes problematic.

Kupst and colleagues[86] found virtually no decline in neurocognitive function in 74 survivors followed up to 2 years post HSCT. Socioeconomic status and pre-HSCT full scale intelligence quotient (IQ) measures correlated strongly with post-HSCT outcomes. Phipps and colleagues,[87] who followed children prospectively for 5 years post HSCT, found a very slight global decline in IQ (2 IQ points, within the margin of error for the testing performed). There were small but significant declines in IQ in children transplanted for malignant disorders, those who received TBI or craniospinal radiation, and those who developed acute GVHD. Again, socioeconomic status was the most important determinant of cognitive and academic function. Kramer and colleagues[88] found a modest but significant decline in mean IQ 1 year post HSCT, with no significant further decline at 3-year follow-up. However, more than 40% of children in this study experienced declines in IQ of greater than 2 standard deviations from baseline measures. Again, pre-HSCT IQ was the most significant predictor of post-BMT functioning; there was no association with age at HSCT, the use of TBI and/or busulfan-containing regimens, or any other factors related to treatment or diagnosis. Most of these patients were less than 6 years of age when transplanted, so may have been more susceptible to deleterious effects. Barrera and colleagues[89] found normal to higher than average verbal, performance, and full IQ scores 2 years post transplant; however, these children had mean arithmetical scores significantly less than normal. This is consistent with data from survivors of childhood leukemia and central nervous system tumors, and requires further investigation.

In the studies referred to earlier, patients with multiple pretransplant diagnoses were pooled. In a recent study including only children with hematologic malignancies, the Stanford group found significant declines in verbal skills 3 years post HSCT. When evaluated 5 years following transplantation, this group showed continued declines in verbal skills, performance skills, and long-term and overall memory. All declines were significant compared with sibling controls.[90] When children who underwent HSCT that included a conditioning regimen with craniospinal radiation were compared with those who had not received craniospinal radiation, the former group was found to have significantly worse scores in cognitive function, performance skills, and short- and long-term memory.

Immune Reconstitution

Immune reconstitution following HSCT is extremely complex and dependent on various factors. Recipient factors include age, the underlying disease for which the transplant is being performed, prior treatment, and general physical condition. Stem cell source (autologous, allogeneic matched related or unrelated, umbilical cord blood, bone marrow or peripheral stem cells, manipulated (ie, T-cell depleted) or unmanipulated) also affects immune reconstitution,[91–94] as do the conditioning and GVHD prophylaxis regimens used. The occurrence of GVHD has a profound effect on immune reconstitution. A thorough review of immune reconstitution is beyond the scope of this article, but several excellent review articles are available.[95–98]

Children commonly require revaccination following recovery from HSCT. The United States Centers for Disease Control (CDC) and the European Blood and Marrow Transplant Group (EBMT) have established somewhat arbitrary timetables for the initiation of revaccination following HSCT; the CDC recommends beginning killed vaccines at 1 year post HSCT and live viral vaccines at 2 years, whereas the EBMT recommends initiation of vaccination as early as 6 months post HSCT.[99] It is by no means clear that all children will be sufficiently immune-replete to mount a protective response to vaccines at these time points. Many individual centers, therefore, have developed their own approaches for revaccination, including the evaluation of surrogate markers (ie, CD4+ counts, IgG levels, and so forth.) of immune reconstitution before initiating vaccines. This is an area requiring further study and careful standardization of practice.

Chronic GCHD (cGVHD) and Multisystem Effects

cGVHD in children can result in significant long-term morbidity and mortality. cGVHD, reviewed elsewhere in this issue, can certainly lead to multiple long-term

complications for patients after HSCT.[100] The manifestations from skin and joint involvement, with sclerodermatous features and joint contractures, can lead to impairment in mobility and function with subsequent difficulties with activities of daily living, school, and work. Liver involvement can result in abnormalities of liver function, persistent jaundice, and in severe cases, liver failure. Pulmonary involvement with significant obstructive pulmonary disease is one of the most devastating consequences of cGVHD. Pulmonary involvement can be very difficult to treat and can lead to significant disability. cGVHD and the ongoing immunosuppressive therapies required for its treatment can result in significant suppression of immune function and the risk for secondary bacterial, viral, or fungal infections.

Other common features of cGVHD that can result in long-term problems include xerostomia and keratoconjunctivitis sicca. Both can be medically managed, but these conditions do have an adverse effect on a patient's QoL. When prolonged therapy for cGVHD is required, steroids are a necessary part of the management. Thus, children with cGVHD receiving months to years of steroid therapy are also at high risk for the long-term complications of steroid therapy such as avascular necrosis, growth failure, glucose intolerance, hypertension, and others.

SPECIAL SITUATIONS
Sequelae for Infants

Infants requiring HSCT are one of the most significant challenges for pediatric transplant centers. The long-term complications that can occur after HSCT in infants result from exposures to pretransplant chemotherapy (and possibly central nervous system (CNS)-directed radiation therapy [CRT]), and the high-dose chemotherapy with or without TBI associated with the transplant preparative regimen. There are only a handful of studies on the long-term complications after HSCT for infants. One from the University of Minnesota examined the long-term follow-up of 17 children who underwent HSCT for acute myeloblastic leukemia or acute lymphoblastic leukemia (ALL) at less than 3 years of age.[101] Eleven patients (65%) received TBI (none received CRT) and 7 received preparative regimens with busulfan and cyclophosphamide. Median follow-up was 11.5 years after HSCT. Medical outcomes and complications of HSCT that occurred in survivors included GH deficiency (58.8%), hypothyroidism (35.3%), abnormal pubertal development (11.8%), osteopenia/osteoporosis (23.5%), short stature (47.1%), dental abnormalities (47.1%), and cataracts (47.1%). Dyslipidemias were present in 58.8% of patients, hyperinsulinemia in 17.6%, and hypertension in 11.8%, all characteristics associated with the metabolic syndrome. All patients underwent neuropsychological testing. Survivors were found to perform more poorly on measures of sustained attention, inhibition, response speed, and consistency of attentional effort ($P<.001$). They also performed more poorly on measures of fine motor speed/dexterity ($P<.001$) and visual-motor integration skills ($P<.006$). However, performance on measures of general intellectual ability and academic achievement were within expectations based on population norms. In addition, measures of QoL in survivors were not different compared with population norms. Although two-thirds of patients in this study received TBI and showed a range of neuropsychological deficits, most were actually functioning at an average academic level or higher. This study was unable to make any definitive comparisons between preparative regimens with and without TBI.

A similar study from St Jude Children's Research Hospital reported on the late sequelae of 34 children diagnosed with acute leukemia at age 12 months or younger.[102] These patients were divided into 3 groups based on treatment exposures: group A, chemotherapy alone (n = 10); group B, chemotherapy and CRT (n = 17); and group C, chemotherapy, HSCT, and CRT (n = 7, [cranial only n = 2, craniospinal n = 1, TBI n = 4]). From a growth standpoint, compared with patients in group A, patients in group B had a greater decrease in height Z scores, and patients in group C had the greatest decrease in height Z scores with 71% of them decreasing by more than 2 standard deviations. Other endocrine abnormalities included hypothyroidism (21%, from groups B and C only). Three patients had precocious puberty (from groups B and C) and 1 patient from group B had delayed puberty after testicular radiation. Two patients developed mild cardiac dysfunction and 2 exposed to TBI developed cataracts. Neuropsychological evaluations found that 50% did not have any academic difficulties that required special tutoring or special education classes, whereas the other 50% did require these services. Patients in groups B and C had higher incidences of academic difficulties (59% and 86%, respectively) compared with 10% in group A. The odds of academic difficulties were inversely related to age, and increased by 18% for each month of age younger at the time of CRT.

More data are needed to better define the impact of non-TBI conditioning regimens in infants undergoing HSCT and to account for the additive effect of pretransplant treatment exposures on the ultimate development of chronic medical conditions. In addition, the factors associated with HSCT that influence the success rate of the HSCT itself, such as TBI for children with ALL, and whether the same holds true for infants, must be taken into account.

Transplant for Nonmalignant Disease

There are a wide variety of nonmalignant disorders for which HSCT is a common therapeutic option, including immune deficiency disorders, metabolic storage disorders, nonmalignant hematologic diseases such as thalassemia and sickle cell disease, congenital bone marrow failure syndromes, and others. Late complications in these patients can be associated with the transplant conditioning regimen but also to issues specific to the underlying disease, including iron overload with cardiac, growth, hepatic, and endocrine consequences for thalassemia, sickle cell disease, and other bone marrow failure diseases for which large numbers of transfusions have been administered. Patients with mucopolysaccharide storage diseases may have cardiac, musculoskeletal,[103] and neurologic[104] complications that become more problematic as they age, because their life expectancy is prolonged after successful HSCT. Patients with Fanconi anemia and other diseases with underlying genetic instability have an inherent risk of certain types of malignancies and these risks may be further amplified by the exposure to certain chemotherapeutic agents or to TBI. Thus, children transplanted for these types of disorders require not only standard posttransplant long-term follow-up but also surveillance for additional complications that may be related to their underlying disease.

SECONDARY MALIGNANT NEOPLASMS

Although the risk of secondary malignancy for those undergoing HSCT during childhood is certainly increased compared with age-matched controls, the risk may also be increased compared with individuals undergoing transplantation at older ages. In a study of more than 19,000 HSCT patients, 3200 of whom had survived more than 5 years, Curtis and colleagues[79] documented a cumulative incidence rate of secondary malignancy of 2.2% 5 years after HSCT, increasing to 6.7% in those who survived 15 years or longer. Survivors undergoing HSCT at less than 10 years of age had a risk of new malignant neoplasms 36.6 times the general population;

this risk decreased to 4.6-fold for those transplanted between the ages of 10 and 29 years and reached parity for those transplanted after the age of 29 years. The most common secondary cancers were brain tumors (9/13 patients), significantly associated with craniospinal irradiation, and thyroid carcinoma; when these 2 tumors were excluded, there was no difference in incidence of secondary malignancy between younger and older patients in this study. Cohen and colleagues[105] also identified an increased risk of secondary thyroid carcinoma following HSCT, the strongest relative risk in children undergoing HSCT at less than 10 years of age, with additional risk factors including female gender, chronic GVHD, and the use of ionizing radiation. An additional study evaluating children transplanted for leukemia showed a cumulative risk of secondary solid tumors of 11% 15 years following HSCT.[106] The risk was highest among the youngest children and those who had received high-dose TBI; in this study, cGVHD was associated with a decreased risk of a second malignancy (relative risk 3.1), although others have reported an increased risk with cGVHD.

The risk of secondary malignancy may increase with prolonged survival post HSCT. Although no pediatric-specific data were included, Kolb and colleagues[107] reported a 3.5% actuarial incidence of secondary malignancy at 10 years post HSCT, increasing to 12.8% at 15 years. Of 3182 children receiving allogeneic HSCTs for leukemia reported to the International Bone Marrow Transplant Registry, 45 developed secondary malignancies, 25 with invasive solid tumors, and 20 with posttransplant lymphoproliferative disorders (PTLD). The most common solid tumors reported were thyroid carcinoma, malignant melanoma, osteosarcoma, carcinomas of the tongue and salivary gland, and malignant fibrous histiocytoma. Younger age at time of transplant and use of high-dose TBI conferred a higher relative risk of invasive solid tumors. Patients at increased risk of PTLD had significantly higher incidence of cGVHD, unrelated donor stem cell source, or related donor mismatched at greater than 2 HLA antigens, T-cell depleted grafts, and use of antithymocyte globulin as prophylaxis or treatment of acute GVHD.[108]

BURDEN OF LATE EFFECTS AND LATE MORTALITY

Two important studies on the burden of late effects in childhood cancer survivors, with a median follow-up of 25 and 17 years, have been published.[109,110] The cumulative incidence of late effects in childhood cancer survivors was shown to be 73% and 75%, respectively. Forty-two percent and 40% of survivors, respectively, had severe, disabling and/or life-threatening late effects or died as a result of an adverse effect of cancer treatment.[109,110]

Only a few studies have been published on the cumulative incidence and severity, or burden, of late effects in survivors of childhood HSCT. Most of these studies have focused on survivors with a particular disease, age, and/or conditioning regimen (eg, including TBI) and have described the cumulative incidence of each late effect separately, but not the total burden of late effects.[81,101,111,112] In 1 single-center study, the burden of late effects was established according to the Common Terminology Criteria for Adverse Events (CTCAE vs 3.0), as has been done in the childhood cancer survivor studies mentioned earlier.[109,110,113] Compared with childhood cancer survivors, pediatric HSCT survivors have a higher cumulative incidence of late effects, with 93% of survivors having at least 1 late effect after a median follow-up of only 7 years. In 25% of pediatric HSCT survivors late effects were severe, disabling, or life-threatening.[113] Although the cumulative incidence of severe late effects is less than described in childhood cancer survivors, follow-up was only 7 years compared with 17 and 25 years in the childhood cancer survivor studies; late effects are known to increase with time after treatment.[109,110,113]

The most frequent late effects in childhood HSCT survivors are discussed in this article, including pulmonary dysfunction, endocrine problems, cataracts, bone complications, and dental problems.[81,101,111–113] Because follow-up in most studies has been only 5 to 10 years, the incidence of secondary malignancies is expected to increase with time after transplant and will likely impose an even higher burden of late effects on childhood HSCT survivors. TBI-containing regimens, older age at transplant, and chronic GvHD also contribute to this burden, as described earlier.[81,109,110,113]

Late Mortality

Only 1 study has been published on late mortality in HSCT survivors, including adults and children. This study showed a standardized mortality ratio at 15 years after HSCT of 2.2, with relapse of primary disease and cGVHD as the leading causes of premature death in 29% and 22%, respectively.[114] In childhood cancer survivors the standardized mortality ratio was shown to increase with time after treatment up to a ratio of 8.2 at 30 years after diagnosis, with secondary malignancy as the main late cause of death, followed by pulmonary and cardiac late effects[115]; such data has not matured for childhood HSCT survivors.

QOL

Despite the high burden of late effects in childhood HSCT survivors, their QoL has been shown to be good. A systematic review of the limited literature on QoL of survivors of HSCT for pediatric malignancy found that health-related quality of life (HRQL) was already compromised pretransplant, further impaired following conditioning, but improved 4 to 12 months post HSCT.[116] Six months to 8 years post transplant HRQL was comparable with or better than population norms.[116] However, a recent study by Löf and colleagues[117] showed that adult survivors of pediatric HSCT experience a HRQL that is poorer than age-matched norms. Yet most patients in this study rated their own health as good in the subjective symptom inventory. A higher burden of late effects has been shown to have no or limited effect on the HRQL.[117–119]

Most studies of QoL in survivors of HSCT in childhood are limited by retrospective or cross-sectional design; older studies were also hampered by lack of standardized pediatric QoL measures. Several studies report that, although most survivors report good QoL, a minority report functional limitations that prevent them from working or going to school.[120–122] A recent comparison study showed survivors have significantly lower HRQL than their siblings,[123] but a longitudinal study comparing QoL before transplant to QoL 2 years following transplant reported that the QoL of survivors was better 2 years following transplantation than it had been before.[124]

In conclusion, although pediatric HSCT survivors seem to have a higher burden of late effects compared with childhood cancer survivors who did not undergo transplant, they experience a good QoL. Unfortunately, because follow-up in most studies on childhood HSCT survivors is relatively short, more morbidity and mortality from late effects may be seen in the near future.

RECOMMENDATIONS FOR FOLLOW-UP

Given the nature and complexity of long-term side effects following HSCT in children, it is necessary for them to receive frequent and thorough evaluations to detect problems as early as possible. Early diagnosis can lead to early intervention and may at least partially ameliorate the manifestations of many late effects, such as delayed growth and pubertal development, restrictive lung disease, the metabolic syndrome, and many others. Some survivors have access to comprehensive HSCT late effects clinics, but many do not. It often falls to the primary care provider to detect and initiate treatment of 1 or more of the myriad potential side effects following HSCT.

The European Group for Blood and Marrow Transplantation, the Center for International Blood and Marrow Transplant Research, and the American Society of Blood and Marrow Transplantation have published joint recommendations for long-term follow-up of HSCT.[125] Additional information, especially useful for those transplanted for childhood malignancies, can be found online in the Children's Oncology Group Survivorship Guidelines.[126]

REFERENCES

1. Kremer LC, van Dalen EC, Offringa M, et al. Frequency and risk factors of anthracycline-induced clinical heart failure in children: a systematic review. Ann Oncol 2002;13:503–12.
2. Kremer LC, van der Pal HJ, Offringa M, et al. Frequency and risk factors of subclinical cardiotoxicity after anthracycline therapy in children: a systematic review. Ann Oncol 2002;13:819–29.
3. Mertens AC, Yasui Y, Neglia JP, et al. Late mortality experience in five-year survivors of childhood and adolescent cancer: the Childhood Cancer Survivor Study. J Clin Oncol 2001;19:3163–72.
4. Baker KS, Ness KK, Steinberger J, et al. Diabetes, hypertension, and cardiovascular events in survivors of hematopoietic cell transplantation: a report from the Bone Marrow Transplant Survivor Study. Blood 2007;109:1765–72.
5. Reusch JE. Current concepts in insulin resistance, type 2 diabetes mellitus, and the metabolic syndrome. Am J Cardiol 2002;90:19G–26G.
6. Trevisan M, Liu J, Bahsaa FB, et al. Syndrome X and mortality: a population-based study. Risk Factor and Life Expectancy Research Group. Am J Epidemiol 1998;148:958–66.
7. Lakka HM, Laaksonen DE, Lakka TA, et al. The metabolic syndrome and total and cardiovascular disease mortality in middle-aged men. JAMA 2002;288:2709–16.
8. Nuver J, Smit AJ, Postma A, et al. The metabolic syndrome in long-term cancer survivors, an important target for secondary preventive measures. Cancer Treat Rev 2002;28:195–214.
9. Talvensaari KK, Knip M. Childhood cancer and later development of the metabolic syndrome. Ann Med 1997;29:353–5.
10. Talvensaari KK, Lanning M, Tapanainen P, et al. Long-term survivors of childhood cancer have an increased risk of manifesting the metabolic syndrome. J Clin Endocrinol Metab 1996;81:3051–5.
11. Taskinen M, Saarinen-Pihkala UM, Hovi L, et al. Impaired glucose tolerance and dyslipidaemia as late effects after bone marrow transplantation in childhood. Lancet 2000;356:993–7.
12. Lorini R, Cortona L, Scaramuzza A, et al. Hyperinsulinemia in children and adolescents after bone marrow transplantation. Bone Marrow Transplant 1995;15:873–7.
13. Majhail NS, Challa TR, Mulrooney DA, et al. Hypertension and diabetes mellitus in adult and pediatric survivors of allogeneic hemtopoietic cell transplantation. Biol Blood Marrow Transplant 2009;15(9):1100–7.

14. Cerveri I, Zoia MC, Flugoni P, et al. Late pulmonary sequelae after childhood bone marrow transplantation. Thorax 1999;54(2):131–5.
15. Fanfulla F, Locatelli F, Zoia MC, et al. Pulmonary complications and respiratory function changes after bone marrow transplantation in children. Eur Respir J 1997;10(10):2301–6.
16. Frisk P, Arvidson J, Bratteby LE, et al. Pulmonary function after autologous bone marrow transplantation in children: a long-term prospective study. Bone Marrow Transplant 2004;33(6):645–50.
17. Nysom K, Holm K, Hesse B, et al. Lung function after allogeneic bone marrow transplantation for leukaemia or lymphoma. Arch Dis Child 1996; 74(5):432–6.
18. Savani BN, Montero A, Srinivasan R, et al. Chronic GVHD and pretransplantation abnormalities in pulmonary function are the main determinants predicting worsening pulmonary function in long-term survivors after stem cell transplantation. Biol Blood Marrow Transplant 2006;12(12):1261–9.
19. Wieringa J, van Kralingen KW, Sont JK, et al. Pulmonary function impairment in children following hematopoietic stem cell transplantation. Pediatr Blood Cancer 2005;45(3):318–23.
20. Hoffmeister PA, Madtes DK, Storer BE, et al. Pulmonary function in long-term survivors of pediatric hematopoietic cell transplantation. Pediatr Blood Cancer 2006;47(5):594–606.
21. Leneveu H, Bremont F, Rubie H, et al. Respiratory function in children undergoing bone marrow transplantation. Pediatr Pulmonol 1999;28(1):31–8.
22. Bruno B, Souillet G, Bertrand Y, et al. Effects of allogeneic bone marrow transplantation on pulmonary function in 80 children in a single paediatric centre. Bone Marrow Transplant 2004;34(2):143–7.
23. Mertens AC, Yasui Y, Liu Y, et al. Pulmonary complications in survivors of childhood and adolescent cancer. A report from the Childhood Cancer Survivor Study. Cancer 2002;95(11):2431–41.
24. Berger C, Le-Gallop B, Donadieu J, et al. Late thyroid toxicity in 153 long-term survivors of allogeneic bone marrow transplantation for acute lymphoblastic leukemia. Biol Blood Marrow Transplant 2005;35:991–5.
25. Cohen A, Bekassy AN, Gaiero A, et al. Endocrinological late complications after hematopoietic SCT in children. Bone Marrow Transplant 2008;41:S43–8.
26. Dahllof G, Hingorani SR, Sanders JE. Late effects following hematopoietic cell transplantation for children. Biol Blood Marrow Transplant 2008;14:88–93.
27. Legault L, Bonny Y. Endocrine complications of bone marrow transplantation in children. Pediatr Transplant 1999;3:60–6.
28. Matsumoto M, Ishiguro H, Tomita Y, et al. Changes in thyroid function after bone marrow transplant in young patients. Pediatr Int 2004;46:291–5.
29. Sanders JE, Hoffmeister PA, Woolfrey AE, et al. Thyroid function following hematopoietic cell transplantation in children: 30 years' experience. Blood 2009;113: 306–8.
30. Slatter MA, Gennery AR, Cheetham TD, et al. Thyroid dysfunction after bone marrow transplantation for primary immunodeficiency without the use of total body irradiation in conditioning. Bone Marrow Transplant 2004;33:949–53.
31. Sanders JE, Pritchard S, Mahoney P, et al. Growth and development following marrow transplantation for leukemia. Blood 1986;68(5):1129–35.
32. Sanders JE, Hawley J, Levy W, et al. Pregnancies following high-dose cyclophosphamide with or without high-dose busulfan or total-body irradiation and bone marrow transplantation. Blood 1996;87:3045–52.

33. Clement-De Boers A, Oostdijk W, Van Weel-Sipman MH, et al. Final height and hormonal function after bone marrow transplantation in children. J Pediatr 1996; 129:544–50.

34. Sarafoglou K, Boulad F, Gillio A, et al. Gonadal function after bone marrow transplantation for acute leukemia during childhood. J Pediatr 1997;130:210–6.

35. Hovi L, Saarinen-Pihkala UM, Taskinen M, et al. Subnormal androgen levels in young female bone marrow transplant recipients with ovarian dysfunction, chronic GvHD and receiving glucocorticoid therapy. Bone Marrow Transplant 2004;33:503–8.

36. Thibaud E, Rodriguez-Macias K, Trivin C, et al. Ovarian function after bone marrow transplantation during childhood. Bone Marrow Transplant 1998;21:287–90.

37. Hovi L, Tapanainen P, Saarinen-Pihkala UM, et al. Impaired androgen production in female adolescents and young adults after total body irradiation prior to BMT in childhood. Bone Marrow Transplant 1997;20:561–5.

38. Teinturier C, Hartmann O, Valteau-Couanet D, et al. Ovarian function after autologous bone marrow transplantation in childhood: high-dose busulfan is a major cause of ovarian failure. Bone Marrow Transplant 1998;22:989–94.

39. Anserini P, Chiodi S, Spinelli S, et al. Semen analysis following allogeneic bone marrow transplantation. Additional data for evidence-based counseling. Bone Marrow Transplant 2002;30:447–51.

40. Salooja N, Szydlo RM, Socie G, et al. Pregnancy outcomes after peripheral blood or bone marrow transplantation: a retrospective survey. Lancet 2001; 358:271–6.

41. Sanders JE. Growth and development after hematopoietic cell transplant in children. Bone Marrow Transplant 2008;41:223–7.

42. Cohen A, Duell T, Socie G, et al. Nutritional status and growth after bone marrow transplantation (BMT) during childhood: EBMT late-effects working party retrospective data. Bone Marrow Transplant 1999;23:1043–7.

43. Giorgiani G, Bozzola M, Locatelli F, et al. Role of busulfan and total body irradiation on growth of prepubertal children receiving bone marrow transplantation and results of treatment with recombinant growth hormone. Blood 1995;86(2):825–31.

44. Cohen A, Rovelli A, Bakker B, et al. Final height of patients who underwent bone marrow transplantation for hematological disorders during childhood: a study by the Working Party for Late Effects-EBMT. Blood 1999;93(12):4109–15.

45. Sanders JE, Guthrie KA, Hoffmeister PA, et al. Final adult height of patients who received hematopoietic cell transplantation in childhood. Blood 2005;105: 1348–54.

46. Chemaitilly W, Boulad F, Heller G, et al. Final height in pediatric patients after hyperfractionated total body irradiation and stem cell transplantation. Bone Marrow Transplant 2007;40:29–35.

47. Nandagopal R, Laverdiere C, Mulrooney D, et al. Endocrine late effects of childhood cancer therapy: a report from the Children's Oncology Group. Horm Res 2008;69:65–74.

48. Nysom K, Holm K, Michaaelsen KF, et al. Bone mass after allogeneic BMT for childhood leukemia or lymphoma. Bone Marrow Transplant 2000;25:191–6.

49. Kaste SC, Shidler TJ, Tong X, et al. Bone mineral density and osteonecrosis in survivors of childhood allogeneic bone marrow transplantation. Bone Marrow Transplant 2004;22:435–41.

50. Klopfenstein KJ, Clayton J, Rosselet R, et al. Prevalence of abnormal bone density of pediatric patients prior to blood or marrow transplant. Pediatr Blood Cancer 2009;53:675–7.

51. Bhatia S, Ramsay NKC, Weisdorf D, et al. Bone mineral density in patients undergoing bone marrow transplantation for myeloid malignancies. Bone Marrow Transplant 1998;22:87–90.
52. Petryk A, Bergemann TL, Polga KM, et al. Prospective study of changes in bone mineral density and turnover in children after hematopoietic cell transplantation. J Clin Endocrinol Metab 2006;91:899–905.
53. Ferrone M, Geraci M. A review of the relationship between parenteral nutrition and metabolic bone disease. Nutr Clin Pract 2007;22:329–39.
54. Carpenter PA, Hoffmeister P, Chesnut CH III, et al. Bisphosphonate therapy for reduced bone mineral density in children with chronic graft-versus-host disease. Biol Blood Marrow Transplant 2007;13:683–90.
55. Gronroos MG, Bolme P, Winiarski J, et al. Long-term renal function following bone marrow transplantation. Bone Marrow Transplant 2007;39:717–23.
56. Kist-van Holthe JE, Bresters D, Ahmed-Ousenkova YM, et al. Long-term renal function after hemopoietic stem cell transplantation. Bone Marrow Transplant 2005;36:605–10.
57. Kist-van Holthe JE, Goedvolk CA, Brand R, et al. Prospective study of renal insufficiency after bone marrow transplantation. Pediatr Nephrol 2002;17:1032–7.
58. Frisk P, Bratteby LE, Carlson K, et al. Renal function after autologous bone marrow transplantation in children: a long-term prospective study. Bone Marrow Transplant 2002;29:129–36.
59. Patzer L, Ringelmann F, Kentouche K, et al. Renal function in long-term survivors of stem cell transplantation in childhood. A prospective trial. Bone Marrow Transplant 2001;27:319–27.
60. Frisk P, Lonnerholm G, Oberg G. Disease of the liver following bone marrow transplantation in children: incidence, clinical course and outcome in a long-term perspective. Acta Paediatr 1998;87(5):579–83.
61. Locasciulli A, Testa M, Valsecchi MG, et al. Morbidity and mortality due to liver disease in children undergoing allogeneic bone marrow transplantation: a 10-year prospective study. Blood 1997;90(9):3799–805.
62. Tomas JF, Pinilla I, Garcia-Buey ML, et al. Long-term liver dysfunction after allogeneic bone marrow transplantation: clinical features and course in 61 patients. Bone Marrow Transplant 2000;26(6):649–55.
63. Strasser SI, Sullivan KM, Myerson D, et al. Cirrhosis of the liver in long-term marrow transplant survivors. Blood 1999;93(10):3259–66.
64. Bresters D, van Gils ICM, Dekker FW, et al. Abnormal liver enzymes two years after haematopoietic stem cell transplantation in children: prevalence and risk factors. Bone Marrow Transplant 2008;41(1):27–31.
65. Ivantes CA, Amarante H, Ioshii SO, et al. Hepatitis C virus in long-term bone marrow transplant survivors. Bone Marrow Transplant 2004;33(12):1181–5.
66. McKay PJ, Murphy JA, Cameron S, et al. Iron overload and liver dysfunction after allogeneic or autologous bone marrow transplantation. Bone Marrow Transplant 1996;17(1):63–6.
67. Strasser SI, Kowdley KV, Sale GE, et al. Iron overload in bone marrow transplant recipients. Bone Marrow Transplant 1998;22(2):167–73.
68. Bouyn CI, Leclere J, Raimondo G, et al. Hepatic focal nodular hyperplasia in children previously treated for a solid tumor. Incidence, risk factors, and outcome. Cancer 2003;97(12):3107–13.
69. Sudour H, Mainard L, Baumann C, et al. Focal nodular hyperplasia of the liver following hematopoietic SCT. Bone Marrow Transplant 2009;43(2):127–32.

70. Bagesund M, Viniarski J, Dahllof G. Subjective xerostomia in long-term surviving children and adolescents after pediatric bone marrow transplantation. Transplantation 2000;69(5):822–6.
71. Dahllof G, Bagesund M, Ringden O. Impact of conditioning regimens on salivary function, caries-associated microorganisms and dental caries in children after bone marrow transplantation. A 4-year longitudinal study. Bone Marrow Transplant 1997;20(6):479–83.
72. Holtta P, Hovi L, Saarinen-Pihkala UM, et al. Disturbed root development of permanent teeth after pediatric stem cell transplantation. Dental root development after SCT. Cancer 2005;103(7):1484–93.
73. Holtta P, Alaluusua S, Saarinen-Pihkala UM, et al. Agenesis and microdontia of permanent teeth as late adverse effects after stem cell transplantation in young children. Cancer 2005;103(1):181–90.
74. Pajari U, Lanning M. Developmental defects of teeth in survivors of childhood ALL are related to the therapy and age at diagnosis. Med Pediatr Oncol 1995;24(5):310–4.
75. Uderzo C, Fraschini D, Balduzzi A, et al. Long-term effects of bone marrow transplantation on dental status in children with leukaemia. Bone Marrow Transplant 1997;20(10):865–9.
76. Vaughan MD, Rowland CC, Tong X, et al. Dental abnormalities after pediatric bone marrow transplantation. Bone Marrow Transplant 2005;36(8):725–9.
77. Wogelius P, Dahllof G, Gorst-Rasmussen A, et al. A population-based observational study of dental caries among survivors of childhood cancer. Pediatr Blood Cancer 2008;50(6):1221–6.
78. Dahllof G. Craniofacial growth in children treated for malignant diseases. Acta Odontol Scand 1998;56(6):378–82.
79. Curtis RE, Rowlings PA, Deeg HJ, et al. Solid cancers after bone marrow transplantation. N Engl J Med 1997;336(13):897–904.
80. Faraci M, Bekassy AN, De Fazio V, et al. Non-endocrine late complications in children after allogeneic haematopoietic SCT. Bone Marrow Transplant 2008; 41:S49–57.
81. Ferry C, Gemayel G, Rocha V, et al. Long-term outcomes after allogeneic stem cell transplantation for children with hematological malignancies. Bone Marrow Transplant 2007;40:219–24.
82. Gurney JG, Ness KK, Rosenthal J, et al. Visual, auditory, sensory, and motor impairments in long-term survivors of hematopoietic stem cell transplantation performed in childhood: results from the Bone Marrow Transplant Survivor Study. Cancer 2006;106(6):1402–8.
83. Leung W, Ahn H, Rose SR, et al. A prospective cohort study of late sequelae of pediatric allogeneic hemtopoietic stem cell transplantation. Medicine 2007; 86(4):215–24.
84. Van Kempen-Harteveld ML, Belkacemi Y, Kal HB, et al. Dose-effect relationship for cataract induction after single-dose total body irradiation and bone marrow transplantation for acute leukemia. Int J Radiat Oncol Biol Phys 2002;52(5): 1367–74.
85. Van Kempen-Harteveld ML, Struikmans H, Kal HB, et al. Cataract after total body irradiation and bone marrow transplantation: degree of visual impairment. Int J Radiat Oncol Biol Phys 2002;52(5):1375–80.
86. Kupst MJ, Penati B, Debban B, et al. Cognitive and psychosocial functioning of pediatric hematopoietic stem cell transplant patients: a prospective longitudinal study. Bone Marrow Transplant 2002;30:609–17.

87. Phipps S, Rai SN, Leung W-H, et al. Cognitive and academic consequences of stem cell transplantation in children. J Clin Oncol 2008;26:2027–33.
88. Kramer JH, Crittenden MR, DeSantes K, et al. Cognitive and adaptive behavior 1 and 3 years following bone marrow transplantation. Bone Marrow Transplant 1997;19:607–13.
89. Barrera M, Atenafu E, Andrews GS, et al. Factors related to changes in cognitive, educational and visual motor integration in children who undergo hematopoietic stem cell transplant. J Pediatr Psychol 2008;33(5):536–46.
90. Shah AJ, Epport K, Azen C, et al. Progressive decline in neurocognitive function among survivors of hematopoietic stem cell transplantation for pediatric hematologic malignancies. J Pediatr Hematol Oncol 2008;30:411–8.
91. Szabolcs P, Niedzwiecki D. Immune reconstitution in children after unrelated transplantation. Cytotherapy 2007;9(2):111–22.
92. Brown J, Boussiotis VA. Umbilical cord blood transplantation: basic biology and clinical challenges to immune reconstitution. Clin Immunol 2008;127(3):286–97.
93. Szabolcs P, Niedzwiecki D. Immune reconstitution in children after unrelated cord blood transplantation. Biol Blood Marrow Transplant 2008;14(9):66–72.
94. Handgretinger R, Chen X, Pfeiffer M, et al. Cellular immune reconstitution after haploidentical transplantation in children. Biol Blood Marrow Transplant 2008; 14(1S1):59–65.
95. Eyrich M, Wollny G, Tzaribaschev N, et al. Onset of thymic recovery and plateau of thymic output are differentially regulated after stem cell transplantation in children. Biol Blood Marrow Transplant 2005;11(3):194–205.
96. Fry TJ, Mackall CL. Immune reconstitution following hematopoietic progenitor cell transplantation: challenges for the future. Bone Marrow Transplant 2005; 35:S53–7.
97. Lum LG. The kinetics of immune reconstitution after human marrow transplantation. Blood 1987;69:369–80.
98. Peggs KS. Reconstitution of adaptive and innate immunity following allogeneic hematopoietic stem cell transplantation in humans. Cytotherapy 2006;8:427–36.
99. Small T. Vaccination of children following allogeneic stem cell transplantation. Biol Blood Marrow Transplant 2008;14(1 Suppl 1):54–8.
100. Carpenter PA. Late effects of chronic graft-versus-host-disease. Best Pract Res Clin Haematol 2008;21:309–31.
101. Perkins JL, Kunin-Batson AS, Youngren NM, et al. Long-term follow-up of children who underwent hematopoietic cell transplant (HCT) for AML or ALL at less than 3 years of age. Pediatr Blood Cancer 2007;49:958–63.
102. Leung W, Hudson M, Zhu Y, et al. Late effects in survivors of infant leukemia. Leukemia 2000;14:1185–90.
103. Odunusi E, Peters C, Krivit W, et al. Genu valgum deformity in Hurler syndrome after hematopoietic stem cell transplantation: correction by surgical intervention. J Pediatr Orthop 1999;19(2):270–4.
104. Peters C, Shapiro EG, Krivit W. Neuropsychological development in children with Hurler Syndrome following hematopoietic stem cell transplantation. Pediatr Transplant 1998;2:250–3.
105. Cohen A, Rovelli A, Merlo DF, et al. Risk for secondary thyroid carcinoma after hematopoietic stem cell transplantation: an EBMT Late Effects Working Party Study. J Clin Oncol 2007;25(17):2449–54.
106. Socie G, Curtis RE, Deeg HJ, et al. New malignant diseases after allogeneic marrow transplantation for childhood acute leukemia. J Clin Oncol 2000;18: 348–57.

107. Kolb HJ, Socie G, Duell T, et al. Malignant neoplasms in long-term survivors of bone marrow transplantation. Ann Intern Med 1999;131:738–44.
108. Baker KS, DeFor TE, Burns LJ, et al. New malignancies after blood or marrow stem cell transplantation in children and adults: incidence and risk factors. J Clin Oncol 2003;21(7):1352–8.
109. Geenen MM, Cardous-Ubbink MC, Kremer LC, et al. Medical assessment of adverse health outcomes in long-term survivors of childhood cancer. JAMA 2007;297(24):2705–15.
110. Oeffinger KC, Mertens AC, Sklar CA, et al. Chronic health conditions in adult survivors of childhood cancer. N Engl J Med 2006;355(15):1572–82.
111. Faraci M, Barra S, Cohen A, et al. Very late nonfatal consequences of fractionated TBI in children undergoing bone marrow transplant. Int J Radiat Oncol Biol Phys 2005;63(5):1568–75.
112. Leahey AM, Teunissen H, Friedman DL, et al. Late effects of chemotherapy compared to bone marrow transplantation in the treatment of pediatric acute myeloid leukemia and myelodysplasia. Med Pediatr Oncol 1999;32(3):162–9.
113. Bresters D, van Gils I, Kollen WJ, et al. High burden of late effects after haematopoietic stem cell transplantation in childhood: a single-centre study. Bone Marrow Transplant 2009;5:4. DOI: 10.1038/bmt.2009.92.
114. Bhatia S, Francisco L, Carter A, et al. Late mortality after allogeneic hematopoietic cell transplantation and functional status of long-term survivors: report from the Bone Marrow Transplant Survivor Study. Blood 2007; 110(10):3784–92.
115. Mertens AC, Liu Q, Neglia JP, et al. Cause-specific late mortality among 5-year survivors of childhood cancer: the Childhood Cancer Survivor Study. J Natl Cancer Inst 2008;100(19):1368–79.
116. Clarke SA, Eiser C, Skinner R. Health-related quality of life in survivors of BMT for paediatric malignancy: a systematic review of the literature. Bone Marrow Transplant 2008;42(2):73–82.
117. Löf CM, Winiarski J, Giesecke A, et al. Health-related quality of life in adult survivors after paediatric allo-SCT. Bone Marrow Transplant 2009;43(6):461–8.
118. Forinder U, Löf C, Winiarski J. Quality of life and health in children following allogeneic SCT. Bone Marrow Transplant 2005;36(2):171–6.
119. Michel G, Bordigoni P, Simeoni MC, et al. Health status and quality of life in long-term survivors of childhood leukaemia: the impact of haematopoietic stem cell transplantation. Bone Marrow Transplant 2007;40(9):897–904.
120. Ortega JJ, Olive T, de Heredia CD, et al. Secondary malignancies and quality of life after stem cell transplantation. Bone Marrow Transplant 2005;35:S83–7.
121. Helder DI, Bakker B, de Heer P, et al. Quality of life in adults following bone marrow transplantation during childhood. Bone Marrow Transplant 2004;33: 329–36.
122. Ness KK, Bhatia S, Baker KS, et al. Performance limitations and participation restrictions among childhood cancer survivors treated with hematopoietic stem cell transplantation: the Bone Marrow Transplant Survivor Study. Arch Pediatr Adolesc Med 2005;159:706–13.
123. Barrera M, Atenafu E. Cognitive, educational, psychosocial adjustment and quality of life of children who survive hematopoietic SCT and their siblings. Bone Marrow Transplant 2008;42:15–21.
124. Barrera M, Atenafu E, Hancock K. Longitudinal health-related quality of life outcomes and related factors after pediatric SCT. Bone Marrow Transplant 2009;44:249–56.

125. Rizzo JD, Wingard JR, Tichelli A, et al. Recommended screening and preventive practices for long-term survivors after hematopoietic cell transplantation: joint recommendations of the European Group for Blood and Marrow Transplantation, the Center for International Blood and Marrow Transplant Research, and the American Society of Blood and Marrow Transplantation. Biol Blood Marrow Transplant 2006;12(2):138–51.

126. Children's Oncology Group Survivorship Guidelines. Available at: http://www.survivorshipguidelines.org. Accessed September 15, 2009.

Index

Note: Page numbers of article titles are in **boldface** type.

A

Acid lipase deficiency (Wolman disease), 127, 136
Acid-sphingomyelinase deficiency, 136
Adenovirus infections, adoptive T-cell therapy for, 85–88
Adoptive immunotherapy, T-cell, 85–90
Adrenoleukodystrophy, 126, 130–133
Anemia
    Diamond-Blackfan, 149, 158–160
    Fanconi, 147–154, 332
    in thalassemia. *See* Thalassemia.
    sickle cell. *See* Sickle cell disease.
Antibiotics, for graft-versus-host disease, 285, 290
Antithymocyte globulins, for graft-versus-host disease, 284, 286
Arthritis, juvenile idiopathic, 241–245
Arylsulfatase A deficiency, mesenchymal stromal cells for, 111
Aspartylglucosaminuria, 127
Aspergillosis, adoptive T-cell therapy for, 85–88
Autoimmune diseases, HSCT for, 245–251
    diabetes mellitus type 1, 255–261
    juvenile idiopathic arthritis, 241–245
    rationale for, 240–241
    systemic lupus erythematosus, 245–255
Autoimmune lymphoproliferative syndrome, 219

B

B cells
    in graft-versus-host disease, 298–299
    in graft-versus-tumor effect, 71
    mesenchymal stromal cell interactions with, 107, 109
Bare lymphocyte syndrome, 214
Beclomethasone, for graft-versus-host disease, 277
Beta cells, antibodies to, in diabetes mellitus, 255–258
Bone disorders, in long-term survivors, 327–328
Bone marrow
    failure of, **147–170**
        congenital amegakaryocytic thrombocytopenia, 157–158
        Diamond-Blackfan anemia, 158–160
        dyskeratosis congenita, 149, 156–157
        Fanconi anemia, 147–154, 332
        Shwachman-Diamond syndrome, 154–156, 332
    for HSCT, for leukemia, 30–31, 33–35

Pediatr Clin N Am 57 (2010) 343–352
doi:10.1016/S0031-3955(10)00037-4
0031-3955/10/$ – see front matter © 2010 Elsevier Inc. All rights reserved.

pediatric.theclinics.com

Bronchiolitis obliterans and bronchiolitis obliterans organizing pneumonia
   in graft-versus-host disease, 306
   in long-term survivors, 325–326
Budesonide, for graft-versus-host disease, 277
Burkitt lymphoma, HSCT for, 50
Busulfan, for reduced intensity conditioning, 223–224

C

Calcitriol, for osteopetrosis, 174
Cancer
   natural killer cell surveillance for, 99
   secondary, 332–333
   vaccines for, 83–85
Carbonic anhydrase deficiency, in osteopetrosis, 173
Cardiomyopathy, in long-term survivors, 324
Cardiovascular disorders, in long-term survivors, 324
Cartilage hair hypoplasia, 214–215
Cataract, in long-term survivors, 329
Cathepsin defects, in osteopetrosis, 173
Chediak-Higashi syndrome, 219
Chemotherapy
   for Hodgkin's disease, 48–49
   for juvenile myelomonocytic leukemia, 11
   for leukemia
      acute lymphoblastic, 2
      acute myeloid, 7
      chronic myelogenous, 10
   for lymphoma, 50
   for myelodysplastic syndromes, 11
Chimeric immunoreceptors, for neuroblastoma, 58
Chronic granulomatous disease, 217, 227–228
Conditioning regimens, for primary immunodeficiency disease treatment, 219–228
Congenital amegakaryocytic thrombocytopenia, 149, 157–158
Conjunctivitis, in graft-versus-host disease, 304
Corticosteroids
   for Diamond-Blackfan anemia, 159
   for graft-versus-host disease, 277–283
   for osteopetrosis, 174
Cyclophosphamide, for reduced intensity conditioning, 225
Cytomegalovirus infections, adoptive T-cell therapy for, 87–88
Cytopenia, in graft-versus-host disease, 307

D

Daclizumab, for graft-versus-host disease, 282, 286, 309–310
Dendritic cells, mesenchymal stromal cell interactions with, 107, 109
Dental disorders, in long-term survivors, 329
Diabetes mellitus
   type 1, HSCT for, 255–261
   type 2, in long-term survivors, 324

Diamond-Blackfan anemia, 149, 158–160
Dry mouth, in graft-versus-host disease, 304
Dyskeratosis congenita, 149, 156–157
Dyslipidemia, in long-term survivors, 324–325

E

Edema, in graft-versus-host disease, 302
Endocrine disorders, in long-term survivors, 326–328
Epstein-Barr virus infections, adoptive T-cell therapy for, 85–88
Esophageal sclerosis, in graft-versus-host disease, 304–305
Etanercept, for graft-versus-host disease, 282, 287, 309–310
Ewing sarcoma
    HSCT for, 50–51
    natural killer cells and, 104
Eye disorders
    in graft-versus-host disease, 303–304
    in long-term survivors, 329

F

Fanconi anemia, HSCT for, 147–154
    from matched unrelated donors, 152–153
    from umbilical cord blood, 153–154
    long-term outcome of, 332
    with leukemia, 154
    with myelodysplasia, 154
Farber disease, 127
Fasciitis, in graft-versus-host disease, 302
Fertility, in long-term survivors, 326–327
Fibrosis, hepatic, in graft-versus-host disease, 305
Fludarabine, for reduced intensity conditioning, 220–226
Focal nodular hyperplasia, in long-term survivors, 329
Fucosidosis, 126

G

Galactocerebrosidase deficiency (Krabbe disease), 126, 133–134
Gangliosidosis, 136
Gastrointestinal disorders
    in graft-versus-host disease, 303–305
    in long-term survivors, 328–329
Gaucher disease, 127, 136
Gene therapy
    for inherited metabolic disorders, 137–138
    for osteopetrosis, 175
Globoid-cell leukodystrophy (Krabbe disease), 126, 133–134
Glucksburg criteria, for graft-versus-host disease, 274
Glucocerebrosidase deficiency, 136
Glucose intolerance, in long-term survivors, 324–325
Graft failure, after thalassemia treatment, 186

Graft-versus-host disease
   acute, **273–295**
      antimicrobial prophylaxis for, 285
      classification of, 274–275
      diagnosis of, 275–276
      mild, 276
      moderate to severe, 276–277
      primary treatment of, 276–290
      steroid-resistant, 283–289
   after leukemia treatment, 13
   after severe combined immunodeficiency disease treatment, 212–213
   after thalassemia treatment, 186
   chronic, **297–322**
      clinical manifestations of, 302–308
      in long-term survivors, 330–331
      incidence of, 298
      pathophysiology of, 298–299
      risk factors for, 299–301
      staging of, 301–302
      treatment of, 308–310
   graft-versus-tumor effect and, 67–81
   mesenchymal stromal cells for, 111–112
Graft-versus-leukemia effect, 13
Graft-versus-tumor effect, **67–81**
   biology of, 69–71
   enhancement of, 71–75
   evidence for, 68
   versus type of malignancy, 68–69
Growth retardation
   in graft-versus-host disease, 305
   in long-term survivors, 327
   in thalassemia, 187

H

Hematopoietic stem cell transplantation
   allogeneic, for solid tumors, 56
   autologous, principles of, 48
   failure of, 111, 186
   for autoimmune diseases, **239–271**
   for bone marrow failure syndromes, **147–170**
   for hemoglobinopathies, **181–205**
   for leukemia, **1–25, 27–46**
      clinical outcomes of, 33–38
      graft procurement in, 29–33
   for metabolic disorders, **123–145**
   for osteopetrosis, **171–180**
   for primary immunodeficiency diseases, **207–237**
   for solid tumors, **47–66**
   graft-versus-host disease in. See Graft-versus-host disease.
   graft-versus-tumor effect in, **67–81**

history of, 27–29
immunotherapy and, **97–121**
long-term effects of, **323–342**
   burden of, 333–334
   cardiovascular, 324
   chronic graft-versus-host disease, 330–331
   dental, 329
   endocrine, 326–328
   follow-up recommendations for, 334–335
   gastrointestinal, 328–329
   immunologic, 330
   in infants, 331–332
   in nonmalignant disease, 332
   metabolic syndrome, 324–325
   mortality, 333–334
   neurocognitive, 329–330
   ocular, 329
   oral, 329
   pulmonary, 325–326
   quality of life and, 334
   renal, 328
   secondary malignancy, 332–333
T-cell–based, **83–96**
Hematopoietic system, graft-versus-host disease of, 303
Hemoglobinopathies. *See* Sickle cell disease; Thalassemia.
Hemophagocytic lymphohistiocytosis, 218–219, 226–227
Hepatitis B, in long-term survivors, 328–329
Hepatitis C
   in long-term survivors, 328–329
   in thalassemia, 186–187
Hodgkin disease
   adoptive T-cell therapy for, 88–90
   HSCT for, 48–50
HSCT. *See* Hematopoietic stem cell transplantation.
Hunter syndrome, 124, 126
Hurler syndrome, 124–126, 128–129
Hydrocortisone, for graft-versus-host disease, 276
Hyper Ig-M syndrome, 216–217
Hypertension, in long-term survivors, 324–325
Hyperthyroidism, in long-term survivors, 326
Hypothyroidism, in long-term survivors, 326

I

Imatinib, for graft-versus-host disease, 310
Immune dysregulation, polyendocrinopathy, enteropathy, X-linked syndrome, 219
Immune reconstitution, in long-term survivors, 330
Immunodeficiency
   in graft-versus-host disease, 307–308
   primary. *See* Primary immunodeficiency diseases.
Immunoreceptors, chimeric, for neuroblastoma, 58

Immunotherapy
    for leukemia, 71–74
    for neuroblastoma, 57–59
    mesenchymal stromal cells in, 104–112
    natural killer cells in, 97–104
    T-cell–based, **83–96**
Inborn errors of metabolism. *See* Metabolic disorders, inherited; *specific disorders.*
Infections
    adoptive T-cell therapy for, 85–88
    in graft-versus-host disease, 285, 290, 307–308
Infliximab, for graft-versus-host disease, 281, 285–287, 309–310
Insulin resistance, in long-term survivors, 324–325
Intelligence quotient, in long-term survivors, 329–330
Interferon(s), for osteopetrosis, 174
Iron overload, in thalassemia, 186–187

J

Jaundice, in graft-versus-host disease, 305
Juvenile idiopathic arthritis, HSCT for, 241–245

K

Keratitis, in graft-versus-host disease, 304
Keratopathy, in graft-versus-host disease, 304
Kidney disorders, in long-term survivors, 328
Krabbe disease, 126, 133–134

L

Leukemia, **1–25**
    acute lymphoblastic, 1–7
    acute lymphoid, 33–34
    acute myeloid, 7–10, 34, 154
    chronic myelogenous, 10–11
    graft-versus-tumor effect in, 67–81
    juvenile myelomonocytic, 11–13
    myelodysplastic syndromes, 11–13
    natural killer cells and, 99–103
Leukocyte adhesion deficiency, 217, 228
Leukodystrophy
    globoid-cell, 126, 133–134
    metachromic, 134–136
Liver
    graft-versus-host disease of, 303, 305
    long-term effects on, 328–329
Lung
    graft-versus-host disease of, 303, 305–307
    long-term effects on, 325–326
Lymphohistiocytosis, hemophagocytic, 218–219, 226–227
Lymphoma
    adoptive T-cell therapy for, 88–90
    HSCT for, 50

M

Mannosidosis, 126, 136
Maroteaux-Lamy syndrome, 124, 126, 130
Melphalan, for reduced intensity conditioning, 220–223
Mendelian susceptibility to mycobacterial disease, 217–218
Mesenchymal stromal cells, 104–112
    animal studies of, 108, 110
    biology of, 104–105
    characterization of, 105
    clinical results of, 110–112
    expansion methods for, 105–106
    for graft-versus-host disease, 282, 289
    for inherited metabolic disorders, 137
    immune modulatory properties of, 106–107
    immunosuppressive mechanisms of, 108
    sources of, 105
Metabolic disorders, inherited. *See also specific disorders.*
    HSCT for, **123–145,** 332
Metabolic syndrome, in long-term survivors, 324–325
Metachromic leukodystrophy, 111, 126, 134–136
Metaiodobenzylguanidine, for neuroblastoma, 55–56
Methylprednisolone, for graft-versus-host disease, 277–282
Minimal residual disease, in leukemia, 74–75
Mixed chimerism, after thalassemia treatment, 185–186
Monoclonal antibodies
    for graft-versus-host disease, 284, 309–310
    for reduced intensity conditioning, 225
Morquio syndrome, 136
Mortality, late, 333–334
Mouth, disorders of
    in graft-versus-host disease, 303–304
    in long-term survivors, 329
Mucolipidosis, 127
Mucopolysaccharidoses, 124–130, 136, 332
Musculoskeletal disorders, in graft-versus-host disease, 302–303
Mycobacterial disease, Mendelian susceptibility to, 217–218
Mycophenolate mofetil, for graft-versus-host disease, 285, 288, 308–309
Myeloablation, for HSCT, for hemoglobinopathies, 191–192
Myelodysplasia, Fanconi anemia with, 154
Myositis, in graft-versus-host disease, 302

N

Natural killer cells
    in graft-versus-tumor effect, 71
    in immunotherapy
        biology of, 97–99
        cancer and, 99
        for hematologic malignancies, 102–103
        for solid tumors, 104
        HSCT and, 99–102

Natural (*continued*)
  mesenchymal stromal cell interactions with, 107, 109
Neuroblastoma
  HSCT for, 51–59
  natural killer cells and, 104
Neurocognitive disorders, in long-term survivors, 329–330
Neutropenia
  in graft-versus-host disease, 307
  severe congenital, 218
Niemann-Pick disease, 127, 136

O

Obesity, in long-term survivors, 324–325
Obstructive lung disease, in graft-versus-host disease, 305–307
Omenn syndrome, 213–214
Oral disorders
  in graft-versus-host disease, 303–304
  in long-term survivors, 329
Osteoclast dysfunction, in osteopetrosis, 172–174
Osteogenesis imperfecta, mesenchymal stromal cells for, 111
Osteopenia, in long-term survivors, 327–328
Osteopetrosis, **171–180**
  classification of, 172
  clinical features of, 171–172
  osteoclast function in, 172–174
  treatment of
    gene therapy, 175
    HSCT for, 175–178
    medical, 174–175

P

Pentostatin, for graft-versus-host disease, 282, 289, 309
Peripheral blood progenitor cells, for HSCT, for leukemia, 31–32, 37–38
Phagocyte dysfunction, immunodeficiency diseases in, 217–218
Photophoresis, 287–288, 309
Pompe disease, 127
Posttransplant lymphoproliferative disease, adoptive T-cell therapy for, 85–88
Prednisone, for graft-versus-host disease, 280, 283
Primary immunodeficiency diseases, HSCT for, **207–237**
  causes related to, 209–210
  combined nonclassical, 213–215
  in immune dysregulation, 218–219
  modified conditioning for, 219–228
  non-severe combined, 215–217
  severe combined, 208–213
Psychosocial outcomes, in long-term survivors, 329–330
Puberty, in long-term survivors, 326–327
Purine nucleoside phosphorylase deficiency, 214
PUVA therapy, for graft-versus-host disease, 287

Q

Quality of life, in long-term survivors, 334

R

Radiation therapy, for reduced intensity conditioning, 224–225
Rash, in graft-versus-host disease, 302
Receptor activator nuclear factor-κB and ligand (RANK and RANKL), in osteopetrosis, 172–174
Restrictive lung disease
    in graft-versus-host disease, 305–307
    in long-term survivors, 325–326
Rhabdomyosarcoma
    HSCT for, 51
    natural killer cells and, 104
Rituximab, for graft-versus-host disease, 310

S

Sandhoff disease, 127, 136
Sanfilippo syndrome, 126, 130
Scheie syndrome, 126
Severe combined immunodeficiency syndromes, 208–213
Severe congenital neutropenia, 218
Shwachman-Diamond syndrome, 149, 154–156, 218
Sicca syndrome
    in graft-versus-host disease, 304
    in long-term survivors, 329, 331
Sick euthyroid syndrome, in long-term survivors, 326
Sickle cell disease
    HSCT for, 187–191
        family attitudes toward, 188–189
        from umbilical cord blood, 192, 194
        indications for, 187–188
        organ recovery after, 189, 191
        reduced-intensity conditioning for, 191–193
        results of, 189–190
        with unrelated donors, 194–195
    overview of, 183–184
Sirolimus, for graft-versus-host disease, 285, 288, 308
Skin disorders, in graft-versus-host disease, 302
Sly syndrome, 126, 136
Systemic lupus erythematosus, 245–255

T

T cells
    in graft-versus-tumor effect, 71
    in immunotherapy, **83–96**
        adoptive, 85–90
        effectiveness of, 90–92
        vaccines, 83–85

T cells (*continued*)
    mesenchymal stromal cell interactions with, 106–107, 109
Tacrolimus, for graft-versus-host disease, 276
Tay-Sachs disease, 127, 136
T-cells, augmentation with, for neuroblastoma, 57–58
Teeth, problems with, in long-term survivors, 329
Thalassemia
    HSCT for
        current experience of, 185–186
        from umbilical cord blood, 192, 194
        historical experience of, 184–185
        management after, 186–187
        reduced-intensity conditioning for, 191–193
        with unrelated donors, 194
    overview of, 182–183
Thrombocytopenia
    congenital amegakaryocytic, 149, 157–158
    in graft-versus-host disease, 307
Thymoglobulin, for graft-versus-host disease, 286
Thyroid dysfunction, in long-term survivors, 326
Tolerance, in tumors, 69
Transplantation, stem cell. *See* Hematopoietic stem cell transplantation.
Treosulfan, for reduced intensity conditioning, 224
Triamcinolone, for graft-versus-host disease, 276
Tumors, vaccines for, 83–85

U

Umbilical cord blood, for HSCT
    for Fanconi anemia, 153–154
    for hemoglobinopathies, 192, 194
    for leukemia, 32–33, 35–37
    for severe combined immunodeficiency diseases, 211–212
    history of, 28–29
Ursodeoxycholic acid, for graft-versus-host disease, 285, 290

V

Vaccines
    after HSCT, 330
    T-cell–based, for tumors, 83–85

W

Weight loss, in graft-versus-host disease, 305
Wiskott-Aldrich syndrome, 215–216, 227
Wolman syndrome, 127, 136

X

Xerostomia, in long-term survivors, 331

Z

Zap-70 deficiency, 214

Moving?

Make sure your subscription moves with you!

To notify us of your new address, find your **Clinics Account Number** (located on your mailing label above your name), and contact customer service at:

Email: journalscustomerservice-usa@elsevier.com

800-654-2452 (subscribers in the U.S. & Canada)
314-447-8871 (subscribers outside of the U.S. & Canada)

Fax number: 314-447-8029

Elsevier Health Sciences Division
Subscription Customer Service
3251 Riverport Lane
Maryland Heights, MO 63043

*To ensure uninterrupted delivery of your subscription, please notify us at least 4 weeks in advance of move.